Crohn's Disease

Alessandro Fichera • Mukta K. Krane
Editors

Crohn's Disease

Basic Principles

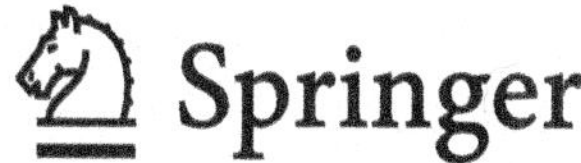

Editors
Alessandro Fichera
Department of Surgery
University of Washington Medical Center
Seattle, WA, USA

Mukta K. Krane
Department of Surgery
University of Washington Medical Center
Seattle, WA, USA

ISBN 978-3-319-35627-3 ISBN 978-3-319-14181-7 (eBook)
DOI 10.1007/978-3-319-14181-7

Springer Cham Heidelberg New York Dordrecht London

Softcover reprint of the hardcover 1st edition 2015

Printed on acid-free paper

Springer International Publishing AG Switzerland is part of Springer Science+Business Media (www.springer.com)

Foreword

Crohn's disease remains a very elusive clinical entity for more than 80 years since the original description. The scientific community has clearly come a long way, but there are still many unknowns.

While new and more effective drugs are developed and tested, we still do not clearly know the basic etiology and pathogenesis of the disease as we are targeting several different steps of the uncontrolled and self-destructive inflammatory cascade. This is clearly not the whole story as remission rates, while better than ever before, are not overwhelming and recurrences are not the exception as proven by the steady rates of surgical interventions in these patients.

Racial, geographic, and genetic predispositions, considered a landmark of the disease in the past, do not apply any longer as the incidence of Crohn's disease is increasing dramatically in Asia, and in the USA the disease is not sparing minorities any longer. Several reasons for such a change have been hypothesized, but no theory has been proven correct.

The medical and surgical approach to the disease has changed significantly as well. Effective maintenance therapy, after remission is achieved, is now part of the therapeutic options with acceptable long-term side effects. The same applies to surgically induced remission now routinely surveyed to direct further therapy. Multiple surgeries in the lifetime of these patients, previously an expected outcome, are now the exception and potentially avoidable. This trend will continue to improve as new therapeutic agents are developed.

Surgery for Crohn's disease has evolved dramatically. The radical extended resections via a full laparotomy are things of the past and belong to the history museum. Laparoscopy, in experienced hands, is the standard of care. Medical preoperative optimization together with bowel sparing approaches, such as very advanced strictureplasty techniques, has allowed us to limit the amount of intestine resected, thus avoiding the devastating sequelae of short bowel syndrome. New anastomotic techniques have shown promising results in terms of reduction of postoperative recurrences.

Eighty years in medicine nowadays is a very long time; the advances that have taken place in the field of inflammatory bowel disease in general and Crohn's disease in particular have revolutionized the management of this disease. The level of complexity is now such that dedicated specialists (IBD gastroenterologists and surgeons) are needed to properly treat these patients. This is now a true multidisciplinary disease that should only be managed in the context of a multispecialty group that includes gastroenterologists, surgeons, radiologists, pathologists, enterostomal therapists, psychologists, nutritionists, and pediatricians all working together based on the needs of the individual patient. The concept of personalized medicine totally applies to this patient population.

With these concepts in mind we have invited to contribute a premier group of specialists, each with decades of experience in the field of Crohn's disease, to offer a comprehensive overview of the current standards and future directions. The title of this book is somewhat deceiving, since there is nothing basic about Crohn's disease any longer; our knowledge is only scratching the surface.

Seattle, WA, USA Alessandro Fichera

Acknowledgements

To the patients affected by this lifelong disease. The nature of Crohn's disease is such that a very close relationship with the treating team naturally develops. By going through the highs and lows of their journey, I have learnt a great deal and I continue to learn every day. Mentors and colleagues have played a major role in my personal growth as a Crohn's disease surgeon and many of them have contributed to this book. This is a totally inadequate way to thank them for their support. Lastly without the love and understanding of my wife Lia and my twins Paolo and Patrizio, this book would not have been possible. The countless hours taken away from you all cannot be repaid in any way.

Alessandro Fichera

To my mentors, many of whom have contributed to this book, who have not only taught me everything I know about Crohn's disease but also set an incredible example of how to be an expert and compassionate IBD surgeon. To the patients with Crohn's disease who entrust us to care for them and are always willing to participate in research. I continue to grow and be a better doctor through our interactions. Lastly to my husband Jerry and my two children Nathaniel and Maya—your limitless love and support allow me to "have it all."

Mukta K. Krane

Contents

Contributors

Cheguevara Afaneh, MD Department of Surgery, New York-Presbyterian Hospital/Weill Cornell Medical Center, New York, NY, USA

Felipe Bellolio-Roth, MD Department of Digestive Surgery, Pontificia Universidad Catolica de Chile, Santiago, Chile

Julia Berian, MD Department of Surgery, University of Chicago, Chicago, IL, USA

Joseph E. Bornstein, MD Division of Colon and Rectal Surgery, Department of Surgery, Icahn School of Medicine at Mount Sinai, New York, NY, USA

Emma Calabrese, MD, PhD Gastroenterology Unit, Department of Systems Medicine, University of Rome Tor Vergata, Rome, Italy

Britt Christensen, BSc, MBBS, MPH Section of Gastroenterology, Hepatology and Nutrition, The University of Chicago Medicine, Chicago, IL, USA

Kindra Clark-Snustad, DNP, ARNP Inflammatory Bowel Disease Research Program, University of Washington, Seattle, WA, USA

Russell D. Cohen, MD Department of Medicine, Inflammatory Bowel Disease Center, The University of Chicago Medicine, Chicago, IL, USA

Janice C. Colwell, RN, MS, CWOCN, FAAN Advanced Practice Nurse: Wound Ostomy and Skin Care, Department of General Surgery, The University of Chicago Medicine, Chicago, IL, USA

Tara M. Connelly Division of Colon and Rectal Surgery, Milton S. Hershey Medical Center, Penn State College of Medicine, Hershey, PA, USA

Kara De Felice, MD Mayo Clinic Hospital-Rochester Methodist Campus, Rochester, MN, USA

Manjiri K. Dighe, MD Department of Radiology, University of Washington, Seattle, WA, USA

Rebecca A. Fausel, MD Division of Gastroenterology, University of Washington Medical Center, Seattle, WA, USA

Alessandro Fichera, MD, FACS, FASCRS Division of General Surgery, Department of Surgery, University of Washington Medical Center, Seattle, WA, USA

Jessica Fisher Division of Gastroenterology, University of Washington, Seattle, WA, USA

Larry J. Gottlieb, MD, FACS Department of Surgery, Section of Plastic and Reconstructive Surgery, University of Chicago, Chicago, IL, USA

Amy L. Halverson, MD, FACS, FASCRS Department of Surgery, Section of Colon and Rectal Surgery, Northwestern University Feinberg School of Medicine, Chicago, IL, USA

Roger D. Hurst, MD, FRCS(Ed), FACS University of Chicago Pritzker School of Medicine, Chicago, IL, USA

Amila Husic, MD Division of Colorectal Surgery, Mayo Clinic College of Medicine, Phoenix, AZ, USA

Malak Itani, MD Department of Radiology, University of Washington Hospitals, Seattle, WA, USA

Diane R. Javelli, RDCD Department of Outpatient Nutrition, University of Washington Medical Center, Seattle, WA, USA

Walter A. Koltun Division of Colon and Rectal Surgery, Milton S. Hershey Medical Center, Penn State College of Medicine, Hershey, PA, USA

Toru Kono, MD, PhD, FACS Advanced Surgery Center, Department of Surgery, Sapporo Higashi Tokushukai Hospital, Sapporo, Hokkaido, Japan

Mukta K. Krane, MD Department of Surgery, University of Washington School of Medicine, Seattle, WA, USA

Essie Kueberuwa, MD Section of Plastic and Reconstructive Surgery, Department of Surgery, University of Chicago, Chicago, IL, USA

Sachin S. Kumbhar, MD Department of Radiology, University of Washington, Seattle, WA, USA

Neeraj Lalwani, MD Department of Radiology, University of Washington, Seattle, WA, USA

Scott David Lee, MD Division of Gastroenterology, Clinical Inflammatory Bowel Disease Program, University of Washington, Seattle, WA, USA

Robin S. McLeod, MD Department of Surgery, University of Toronto, Toronto, ON, Canada

Michael F. McNeeley, MD Department of Radiology, University of Washington Hospitals, Seattle, WA, USA

Fabrizio Michelassi, MD Department of Surgery, New York-Presbyterian Hospital/Weill Cornell Medical Center, New York, NY, USA

J.W. Milsom, MD Minimally Invasive New Technologies, Section of Colon and Rectal Surgery, Center for Advanced Digestive Care, Weill Cornell Medical College, New York Presbyterian Hospital, New York, NY, USA

Ryan B. O'Malley, MD Department of Radiology, University of Washington, Seattle, WA, USA

Aytekin Oto, MD Department of Radiology, University of Chicago, Chicago, IL, USA

Joel Pekow, MD Department of Gastroenterology, Hepatology, and Nutrition, University of Chicago, Chicago, IL, USA

Laura E. Raffals, MD Department of Gastroenterology and Hepatology, May Clinic, Rochester, MN, USA

Patricia L. Roberts, MD Department of Colon and Rectal Surgery, Division of Surgery, Lahey Hospital and Medical Center, Burlington, MA, USA

Tufts University School of Medicine, Boston, MA, USA

Charles A. Rohrmann Jr., MD Department of Radiology, University of Washington Hospitals, Seattle, WA, USA

David T. Rubin, MD Section of Gastroenterology, Hepatology and Nutrition, The University of Chicago Medicine, Chicago, IL, USA

S.K. Sharma, MD Minimally Invasive New Technologies, Section of Colon and Rectal Surgery, Center for Advanced Digestive Care, Weill Cornell Medical College, New York Presbyterian Hospital, New York, NY, USA

Randolph M. Steinhagen, MD Division of Colon and Rectal Surgery, Mount Sinai Medical Center, New York, NY, USA

Joseph H. Yacoub, MD, MS, FACS, FASCRS Department of Radiology, Loyola University Chicago, Stritch School of Medicine, Maywood, IL, USA

Tonia M. Young-Fadok, MD, MS, FACS, FASCRS Division of Colorectal Surgery, Mayo Clinic College of Medicine, Phoenix, AZ, USA

Timothy L. Zisman, MD, MPH Division of Gastroenterology, University of Washington Medical Center, Seattle, WA, USA

Francesca Zorzi, MD, PhD Gastroenterology Unit, Department of Systems Medicine, University of Rome Tor Vergata, Rome, Italy

History of Crohn's Disease

1

Joseph E. Bornstein and Randolph M. Steinhagen

Introduction

There is no doubt that the existence of Crohn's disease has pre-dated our ability to understand and define it. In fact, a precise definition continues to elude us to this day, relying mostly on phenotype to describe the diverse presentations of the disease. This lack of precision, compounded by rudimentary and perfunctory specimen evaluation techniques of the past, left Crohn's disease an undiscovered entity until the 1932 seminal paper by Crohn and Ginzburg and Oppenheimer (CGO) [1]. We now recognize the incidence rate to be as high as 16 per 100,000 worldwide [2–4]. The history of Crohn's disease is a tale of discovery that is far from complete and has utilized many of the advances of medical science to improve the precision of both diagnosis and treatment. Surgical therapy has evolved from primary treatment to being reserved for medically refractory or complicated cases. Medical therapy, once predominated by therapeutic nihilism between surgical episodes, has evolved with more sophisticated trials and therapies now including narrowly targeted drugs. Herein, we review the early descriptions of Crohn's disease prior to its initial description, its origins at The Mount Sinai Hospital and the medical revolution that has occurred subsequent to the landmark 1932 article.

J.E. Bornstein, MD
Division of Colon and Rectal Surgery, Department of Surgery, Icahn School of Medicine at Mount Sinai, New York, NY 10029, USA

R.M. Steinhagen, MD (✉)
Division of Colon and Rectal Surgery, Mount Sinai Medical Center, One Gustave L. Levy Place, Box 1259, New York, NY 10029, USA
e-mail: Randolph.steinhagen@mountsinai.org; randolph.steinhagen@mssm.edu

Crohn's Disease Pre-1932

Reports consistent with Crohn's disease abound in past literature, although definitive diagnosis in these prior case reports is conjectural at best. The clinical and anatomic descriptions of Crohn's disease were often confused with complicated appendicitis, intussusception, intestinal tumor, or infection (e.g., tuberculosis). Prior medical historians have reviewed old literature to find numerous cases suspected of Crohn's disease including the King of France, Louis the XIII (1601–1643) [5, 6]. Louis the XIII's medical record unveils a history of multiple chronic gastrointestinal complaints including perianal abscesses, bowel obstructions, and chronic diarrhea [7]. Autopsy showed ulcerations of the small and large bowel with fistulas [6]. The famous Italian pathologist G.B. Morgagni (1682–1771), in his 80th year, published the "De Sedibus et Causis Morborum per Anatomen Indagatis," a collection of cases and autopsies which also describes likely instances of inflammatory bowel disease [8]. One of the first well-described cases of Crohn's disease is

A. Fichera and M.K. Krane (eds.), *Crohn's Disease: Basic Principles*,
DOI 10.1007/978-3-319-14181-7_1, © Springer International Publishing Switzerland 2015

attributed to Combe and Saunders in 1806 in which they published an account of stricture and thickening of the terminal ileum [9]. Additional reports in the early 1800s are found within a series of case reports published by Abercrombie in 1828 entitled "Pathological and Practical Researches on Diseases of the Stomach, the Intestinal Canal, the Liver and other Viscera of the Abdomen" [10]. Abercrombie described cases suggestive of ileitis with associated bowel obstruction including that of a 63-year-old who died of a bowel obstruction with "great thickening and induration of the ileum" and a 20-year-old with "extensive inflammation of the ileum; the inflamed parts were extensively glued together, and pressed down into the cavity of the pelvis" [10]. Lack of routine pathologic evaluation and rudimentary techniques available to study specimens limited the ability to differentiate cases of Crohn's disease from other entities. At that time, many patients were diagnosed on the basis of gross anatomic findings rather than strict histologic or culture based evidence.

In the late 1800s and early 1900s, increased rigor in the examination of anatomic and microscopic pathology of surgical specimens led to identification and study of non-malignant inflammatory abdominal masses of the ileocecal region [11–23]. Many of the great names of surgery such as Billroth, Bassini, and Hartmann have been referenced describing cases of chronic fibrotic or ulcerative ileocecal disease which were often believed to be due to tuberculosis [19, 24, 25]. A notable report in 1900 came from Lartigau, a pathologist from Columbia College of Physicians and Surgeons, in which he presented an abstract before the New York Pathological Society describing an ileocecal lesion of "such a character that the inflammatory hyperplasia or 'pseudo-neoplasm' may easily be mistaken clinically for tumor-formation of the locality resembling carcinoma" [16]. In his review, he commented upon many case reports in the literature which he believed to be tuberculous lesions of the ileum and cecum, which may instead have represented Crohn's disease in a number of instances. Dieluafoy's textbook of medicine published in 1911 extensively reviewed surgical cases of stenosis of the terminal ileum and cecum with non-caseating necrosis and bowel obstruction believed to be either tuberculosis or lymphosarcoma (i.e., lymphoma) [24]. Despite the likelihood of Crohn's disease present in these reports, its differentiation from intestinal tuberculosis is not trivial, even now, in the endemic population, so definitive conclusions should be withheld [26, 27]. Notable case reports and series were published by Moynihan [12] and Braun [15]. Glasgow surgeon T. Kennedy Dalziel in 1913 published a series of cases with similarity to tuberculosis pathology of intestinal specimens; however, he was unable to prove bacterial pathogenesis [18]. In 1923, A.O. Wilensky and Eli Moschowitz from the Mount Sinai Hospital in New York published a review of four cases of chronic and nonspecific granuloma of the intestine which had been assumed to be tuberculosis or neoplastic but these were histologically ruled out [20]. Further reports soon followed recognizing cases of nonspecific intestinal granuloma [21]. Certainly many additional examples of patients likely afflicted with Crohn's disease exist beyond what was published or widely known pre-1932, as the true disease prevalence was not affected by our defining it. These were the important events leading up to the identification of Crohn's disease as a separate clinical entity in the 1932 CGO paper.

The Story Behind CGO Collaboration

Crohn, Ginzburg, and Oppenheimer all graduated from Columbia University's College of Physicians and Surgeons and subsequently succeeded in becoming house staff at the Mount Sinai Hospital. Their careers were certainly lifted by their publications on Crohn's disease. Crohn became a private practice gastroenterologist. Ginzburg continued at The Mount Sinai Hospital and later became Chief of Surgery at the Beth Israel Hospital in New York. Oppenheimer specialized in Urology and served as Chief of Urology at Mount Sinai.

Despite the appearance of shared collaboration in the authorship on the title page of the CGO paper, controversy exists over the significance of each of the individual's contribution to the publication. The significance of the paper itself is all that is truly important to medical progress; however, there exists a degree of drama that underlies the work and is of historical interest. The Mount Sinai Hospital Levy Library Archives holds copies of many correspondence, letters and speeches given by Crohn and Ginzburg regarding the origins of Crohn's disease at Mount Sinai. Within these letters and autobiographical articles, the original authors reflected on their lives some 50 years later to tell of the controversy beneath their discovery. Amongst these, Ginzburg and Crohn report a disparate sequence of events.

According to Ginzburg's account, the story begins with his interest in inflammatory granulomatous diseases in 1925 when he was on the surgical service of Dr. A.A. Berg (attending surgeon) and continued thereafter when he was an attending in his private practice [28, 29]. Dr. Berg had an extremely busy clinical practice and had operated on many cases of inflammatory masses of the intestines dating back to 1920. Ginzburg recruited Oppenheimer who was working in surgical pathology as an assistant, at that time, to help him begin his research. They collaborated to retrospectively review all the cases that involved surgical excision for an inflammatory mass of the large or small intestine. Using pathological analysis, they attempted to classify these cases, which amounted to 52 in total. Twelve of these patients disease had disease limited to the terminal ileum and did not fit any well-described pathological process. Dr. Ginzburg recalls that he and Dr. Oppenheimer referred to this group as "segmental, hypertrophic ulcerative stenosis of the terminal ileum." They attempted to study these cases more intensively, and owing to their limitations with more advanced pathologic evaluation, sought assistance from the Department of Pathology. It was this group of patients that, in collaboration with gastroenterology colleague Burrill B. Crohn, ultimately culminated in the Crohn, Ginzburg, Oppenheimer 1932 publication entitled "Regional ileitis: a pathologic and clinical entity" which included 14 cases (two added by Dr. Crohn). The larger group of 52 patients, put together by Ginzburg and Oppenheimer alone was published soon after in the Annals of Surgery 1933 [29].

The story of their collaboration is where the controversy begins. As recounted by Dr. Ginzburg, this began when Crohn approached Ginzburg during lunch, about two cases of Dr. Berg's he was involved with, who had inflammatory tumor of the terminal ileum [30]. Dr. Crohn inquired in the pathology lab and was referred to speak to Ginzburg who was actively researching the topic. Dr. Berg requested that Dr. Crohn be given a copy of the draft publication. Unbeknownst to Ginzburg, Crohn reviewed the research and presented it at the A.M.A. meeting in New Orleans in 1932. Crohn further prepared the document originally written by Ginzburg and Oppenheimer, added to it and submitted it for publication without further discussion with them. Ginzburg, notably, had disdain for Crohn. He believed that Crohn intentionally omitted their names from the program of the 1932 meeting to claim the science as his own (see Fig. 1.1). Ginzburg emphatically reported that Dr. Crohn played "no role <u>whatsoever</u> in the development of either the concept, the research, the interpretation or the writing of the original draft of 'regional enteritis'" [30]. A committee was created within Mount Sinai to review possible academic misconduct of Crohn, chaired by Dr. Berg after the presentation in New Orleans. No minutes or records were kept and per Ginzburg's account, the matter was swept aside with the promise of shared authorship on the final paper.

Crohn's recollection of the history of the collaboration was quite different. In 1983, Kovalecik recounted Crohn' version of event as described by Crohn in Gastroenterology in 1967 [31].

> ...we were enabled to see and to examine for the first time a specimen of typical granulomatous terminal ileitis. Within two years Dr. Berg and I were able to gather 13 more cases of identical nature which constituted the basis for the first publication. Dr. Berg, with unnecessary modesty, declined or preferred not to act as co-author, but suggested that the two younger men, Ginzburg and Oppenheimer, who were then engaged in the study of intestinal granulomas, act as co-authors. [32]

Ginzburg regarded this description of events as "sheer fantasy" [30] and further outlined his view of events in a letter to the editor of Gastroenterology dated September 20, 1985 [33]. Much of Ginzburg's consternation of the events likely has to do with the recognition Crohn received in the years following the initial report (Fig. 1.2).

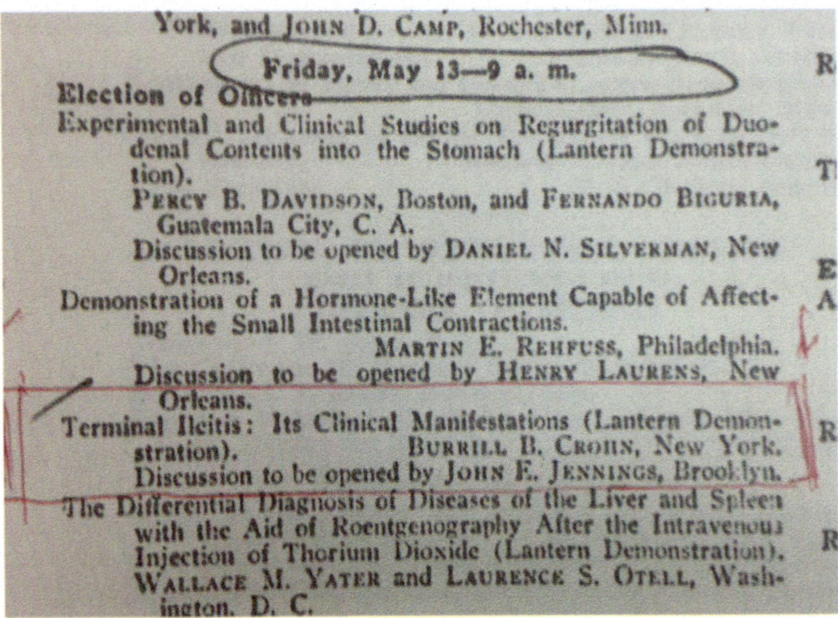

York, and JOHN D. CAMP, Rochester, Minn.

Friday, May 13—9 a. m.

Election of Officers

Experimental and Clinical Studies on Regurgitation of Duodenal Contents into the Stomach (Lantern Demonstration).
PERCY B. DAVIDSON, Boston, and FERNANDO BIGURIA, Guatemala City, C. A.
Discussion to be opened by DANIEL N. SILVERMAN, New Orleans.

Demonstration of a Hormone-Like Element Capable of Affecting the Small Intestinal Contractions.
MARTIN E. REHFUSS, Philadelphia.
Discussion to be opened by HENRY LAURENS, New Orleans.

Terminal Ileitis: Its Clinical Manifestations (Lantern Demonstration). BURRILL B. CROHN, New York.
Discussion to be opened by JOHN E. JENNINGS, Brooklyn.

The Differential Diagnosis of Diseases of the Liver and Spleen with the Aid of Roentgenography After the Intravenous Injection of Thorium Dioxide (Lantern Demonstration).
WALLACE M. YATER and LAURENCE S. OTELL, Washington, D. C.

Fig. 1.1 Photocopy of the 1932 meeting program as reproduced by Ginzburg (provided by The Levy Library, Mount Sinai Hospital)

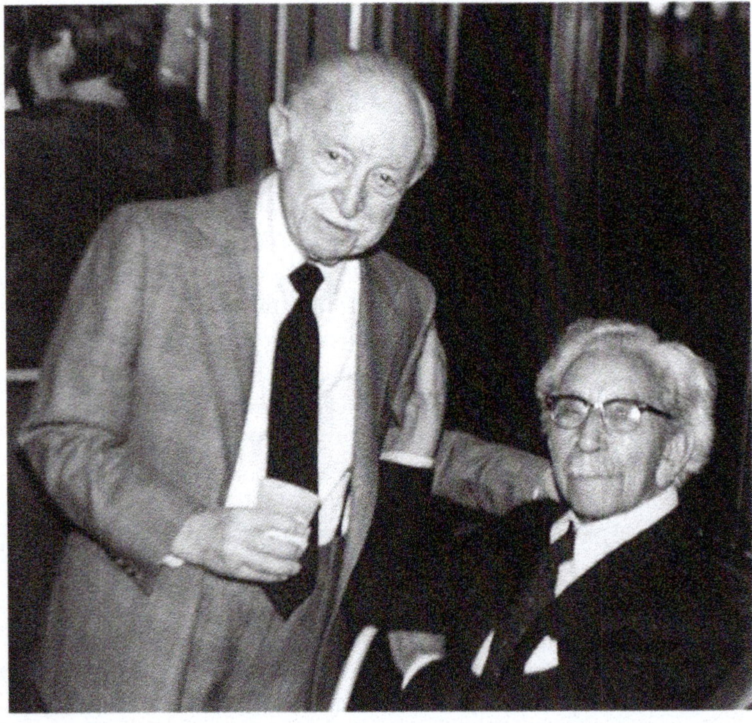

Fig. 1.2 Ginzburg (*left*) and Crohn at the 50th Anniversary IBD symposium at Mount Sinai in New York, May, 1982. (Courtesy of Arthur H. Aufuses Jr. M.D.)

Following publication of the landmark 1932 article, the eponym "Crohn" appeared in the literature almost immediately. Crohn was the first author on the publication purely as a function of alphabetical order. It is interesting to speculate that had A.A. Berg not declined to have his name included on the paper, we would today be discussing "Berg's disease." This, in addition to Crohn's advocacy and charisma, likely led to his name becoming the identifier of the disease. The first article known to use Crohn's name as a synonym for the disease was published in 1933 by Harris et al. entitled "Chronic cicatrizing enteritis: Regional ileitis (Crohn)" and later in 1937 it appeared as the disease name in the British Encyclopedia of Medical Practice [34, 35]. The authors of both of those articles were known personally to Crohn, and any personal involvement, on Crohn's part, promoting the use of his name is purely speculative [33]. One exception to the universal acceptance of "Crohn's disease" exists in Poland where the disease is referred to as Lésniowski-Crohn's disease to commemorate the Polish surgeon Lésniowski who published case reports of likely Crohn's disease cases in 1903 [36]. Despite the appellation of the disease with his own name, Crohn maintained that it was not specific enough a designation and preferred the name "Regional ileitis"; however, as the spectrum of the disease widened, a title more suitable to the syndrome was necessary and the eponym became widely used.

CGO and Beyond

To understand the historical evolution of the disease, a review of its initial definition is critical. In 1932, Crohn, Ginzburg, and Oppenheimer identified 14 cases of inflammatory disease of the terminal ileum which they believed to be a newly defined entity called "regional ileitis." The key diagnostic findings outlined by the authors included "1) a mass in the right iliac region, 2) evidence of fistula formation, 3) emaciation and anemia, 4) the scar of previous appendectomy, and 5) evidence of intestinal obstruction" [1]. The mass in the right iliac region was inflamed, thickened ileum. Fistula was near universal finding and was noted to form readily to adjacent bowel, often sigmoid, or ascending colon. In at least half of the cases, the appendix had been removed at a prior operation indicating likely previous diagnostic confusion, but not definitively ruled out as a potential causative factor in pathogenesis. Lastly, the ultimate presentation was that of intestinal obstruction noted to be occasionally "visible through the emaciated abdominal wall." In his comments, Crohn noted the great lengths to which Dr. Paul Klemperer, the pathologist, had gone to painstakingly exhaust alternative diagnoses such as tuberculosis, symphilis, actinomycosis, Hodgkin's disease, and lymphosarcoma.

An important contribution to the definition of the disease was published in JAMA by Kantor in 1934, which created a more formal roentgenographic description of disease [37]. Dr. Kantor endowed the term "string sign" to the stricture often seen roentgenographically in the terminal ileum of advanced cases. Additional "chief changes" as described by Kantor included (1) filling defect just proximal to the cecum, (2) abnormality in contour of the last filled loop of ileum, and (3) dilation of ileum proximal to the lesion (Fig. 1.3).

Throughout the remainder of the 1930s into the early 1940s, numerous case reports and small case series began to emerge, confirming and expanding upon the findings of Crohn et al. [37–49]. The early experience was clouded by uncertainty as to the correct operation and high mortality associated with the stage of presentation (see Fig. 1.4). In 1935, Mixter published 11 operative cases from the Beth Israel Hospital in Boston [41]. Six patients were treated with a single stage ileocecal resection, while five required staged resection all of which were complicated by fistula or abscesses postoperatively. In 1937, Pemberton et al. published the Mayo Clinic series of 39 cases (36 operative) with 47 major surgical procedures and an associated mortality rate of 4.2 % [39]. Amongst these early reports, operations commonly performed included bypass procedures (ileo-ileostomy, ileocolostomy, ileosigmoidostomy), resection and ileo-colonic anastomosis, or drainage alone without resection (Fig. 1.4). These early series included patients with proximal small

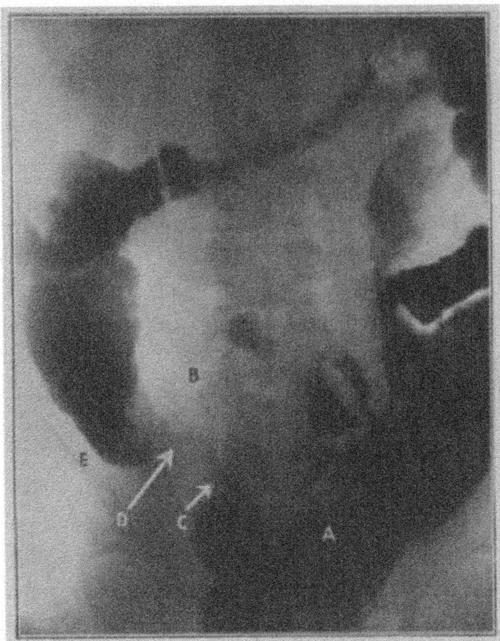

Fig. 1.3 Roentgenographic findings of regional (terminal) ileitis as shown by Kantor, 1934 JAMA [37]. Although not recognized at the time, note the obvious disease in the distal transverse colon

bowel lesions in addition to the terminal ileum, beginning the expansion of the clinical definition [50]. With additional cases being brought to the literature, the clinical spectrum and epidemiology became elucidated. These early case reports were encouraging for the success of surgical management as gross recurrence was rarely encountered in the early experience and surgery was believed to be curative.

Despite the initial description that the pathology was limited to the distal ileum, early series of Crohn's disease soon revealed more widespread gastrointestinal tract disease [51]. Dr. Ralph Colp at The Mount Sinai Hospital is credited with the first description implicating Crohn's colitis as an associated entity in 1934 [43]. Two years later Crohn reported being "loath to accept the fact that ileitis of any type could involve the colon in an analogous inflammatory process" however did ultimately accept this association later in his career [44]. In a 1954 publication, Crohn described the finding of both ileitis and colitis as a "bewildering combination of two disease processes" [52]. Associated colonic inflammation was believed to be either an innocent bystander from disease "spread," or a separate synchronous illness such as ulcerative colitis [53–55]. It was not until the late 1950s and early 1960s that there was acceptance of Crohn's (granulomatous) colitis as a distinct entity [55–57]. In 1952, Wells was the first to definitively use the description "Crohn's disease of the colon" [55]. Differentiation between alternative forms of colitis was challenging. In 1960, Lockhart-Mummery described 25 cases of regional enteritis of the large intestine with criteria to differentiate it from ulcerative colitis [57]. By the 1970s, Crohn's colitis was a well-established entity [58, 59]. Descriptions of involvement of other portions of the intestinal tract followed in parallel, including that of perianal disease, and gastroduodenal disease [60, 61]. Bissell, in 1934, reported an association between regional ileitis and perianal disease [62]. Penner and Crohn in 1938 expanded upon this significantly with a series of patients with regional ileitis who also had perianal and rectovaginal fistula [45]. While no etiology was suggested, they astutely recognized that in a series of 56 patients, 14 % were diagnosed with fistula in ano. This was a rate which far exceeded any known association with routine diarrheal illnesses. In 1950, Comfort et al. reported the first accounts of gastroduodenal granulomatous inflammation and its relationship with regional ileitis [60]. In the early 1950s, extraintestinal manifestations of the disease were noted, specifically the association with arthritis which was later expanded upon in larger retrospective reviews in the 1970s [63–68].

Likely impeding a wider recognition of the disease process earlier was the inability to precisely define the pathophysiology or epidemiology. Leading opinions of the 1930s were a yet undetermined microbiologic pathogen (bacterial, toxin-mediated, viral, protozoa), fecal stagnation due to the ileocecal valve, foreign body reaction, lymphangitis, vascular insult, or hereditary [49, 51]. Early case series speculated that there was a link to Jewish ancestry as hospitals with large

Author, Year	Institution	Number of Operative Cases	Operations Performed (number performed)	Overall Mortality
Mixter 1935[41]	Beth Israel, Boston, MA	11	Single Stage Ileocecal Resection (6), Multi-Stage resection (5)	36%
Ravdin 1937[38]	Hospital of the University of Pennsylvania, Philadephia, PA	4	Ileocolostomy (2), Single Stage Ileocecal Resection (2)	0%
Pemberton 1937[39]	Mayo Clinic, Rochester, Minn.	36	Ileocolostomy w/ delayed resection (10), Single Stage Ileocecal Resection (5), Small Bowel Resection (2), Ileoileostomy (1), Ileocolostomy (5), Other (3)	4% (in-hospital), 16% at 8 months
Ginzburg 1942[48]	Mt. Sinai Hospital, New York, NY	77	Ileocolostomy (54), Ileocecal resection (23)	5% (all from ileocecal resection)
Holloway 1943[49]	Cleveland Clinic, Cleveland, OH	13	Exploration alone +/- Appendectomy (6), Multi - Stage resection (1), Single Stage Ileocecal Resection (6)	0%
Marshall 1940 [46]	Lahey Clinic, Boston, MA	29	Single Stage Ileocecal Resection (5), Diversion followed by resection (4), Ileocolostomy (4), Mikulicz-type multi-stage resection 13	7%

Fig. 1.4 Results of early case series of regional ileitis

Jewish populations were amongst the first to report cases. Genetic associations were first suggested by noting familial clustering as early as the 1930s [69, 70] and were confirmed decades later by identifying common polymorphisms (i.e., NOD2, ATG16L1) that affect host–microbe interactions in the intestinal tract and autophagy, respectively [71–73]. Many more genetic associations have been since described [72].

The early surgical treatment of Crohn's disease was surrounded by controversy given the difficulty in diagnosis and the unknown prognosis. Initial case series reported that patients frequently underwent appendectomy when in retrospect the clinical picture and gross operative findings were more consistent with acute ileitis. With improved recognition of the disease, controversy existed as to the best operative strategy. Resection was mandated by some groups, while others advocated for surgical bypass of the affected bowel [46–49, 74]. In groups advocating resection, further debate existed as to the merits of a single or multi-stage operations which included a first stage bypass followed by delayed resection of abnormal bowel [74]. At the Mount Sinai Hospital, Dr. Berg initially advocated for right colectomy as performed for cancer but later changed his preference to bypass owing to lower surgical mortality rates [48]. The bypass procedure was adopted as the procedure of choice at The Mount Sinai Hospital and was initially planned as a part of a staged operation and not definitive therapy [48]. However, clinical improvement following bypass alone resulted in its being adopted as sole surgical therapy. Principles touted by Ginzburg, in a 1942 review of cases at The Mount Sinai Hospital, included the need to evaluate the entire small bowel for skip lesions and that ileotransverse colostomy with exclusion should be the definitive surgical procedure, as he found a 0 % mortality rate when this procedure was performed [48]. Diffuse involvement of the small bowel was widely considered to be a contraindication to surgery because of the significant risk of short bowel syndrome [52]. Improvement in surgical mortality in successive decades likely had more to do with improvements in anesthesia and perioperative care rather than choice of procedure.

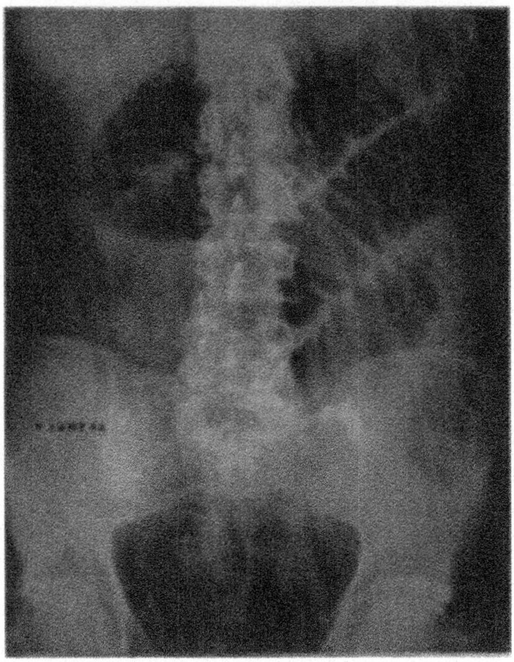

Fig. 1.5 President Dwight D. Eisenhower's Abdominal Roentgenogram performed on June 9th, 1956 [75]

One particularly historic case of Crohn's disease involved the 34th President of the United States, Dwight David Eisenhower. His illness and treatment were subsequently reported in detail by Lt. Gen. Leonard Heaton et al. [75]. In 1956, at 65 years of age, President Eisenhower presented with vague lower abdominal discomfort. Symptoms progressed to include obstipation, abdominal distention, and bilious emesis. After initial fluid resuscitation, he was brought to Walter Reed Army Hospital. He had a history of prior appendectomy and was known to have suffered from bouts of recurrent abdominal pain (Fig. 1.5).

On June 9th, he underwent laparotomy via a right paramedian incision. Gross description of the findings depicted a long strictured segment of terminal ileum with "claw-like" projections of mesenteric fat towards the antimesenteric border and no identifiable skip lesions. Ileotransverse colostomy was performed. His post-operative course was notable for passage of flatus on POD#5 and full resumption of administrative duties. He was ultimately discharged on post-operative day 21. There was significant criticism of the choice of operation at the time, since it did

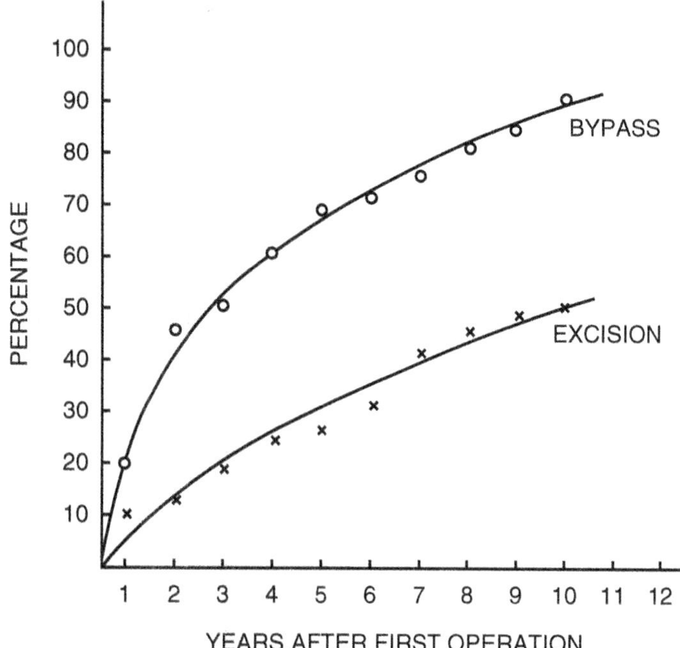

Fig. 1.6 Cumulative risk of recurrence requiring a second operation after primary surgery for ileitis [81]

not involve resection. The surgeons concluded that a bypass was the most expeditious conservative operation given the President's preoperative state and his recent myocardial infarction.

During the 1950s, increasing experience lead clinicians to recognize that despite surgery, the disease process resulted in high recurrence rates [76, 77]. Large retrospective series from the major teaching institutions in the 1950s became available, and further scrutiny of the optimal operative strategy developed [78–80]. These series allowed direct comparisons of patients who underwent the two predominating operations of the time: resection versus bypass. Endpoints such as disease persistence and clinical recurrence were compared directly and were shown to favor resection with primary anastomosis [76, 81–83] (Fig. 1.6). Soon, additional concerns about the bypass procedure developed. Greenstein et al. from The Mount Sinai Hospital in the 1970s, published reports of carcinoma in the excluded bowel segment [84, 85].

With high rates of surgical recurrence prevalent, even when all macroscopic disease was resected, there was significant controversy over the necessity of disease free margins. The effect of residual microscopic disease at the resection margins was evaluated for both recurrence risk and its potential for post-operative complication (e.g., anastomotic dehiscence). Retrospective reviews showed positive microscopic margins in up to 50 % of resections; however, no statistically significant effect was found on the rate of anastomotic complications [86]. Early retrospective reviews suggested that the risk of recurrence was unaffected by presence of microscopic disease at the surgical margin [87]. A randomized trial by Fazio et al., at the Cleveland Clinic, in 1996 concluded that recurrence rates did not differ when extended resection was performed even when microscopic disease was present at the margin [88]. This provided further support to the practice of limiting extent of bowel resection in order to preserve as much intestinal length and absorptive surface as possible.

The presence of proximal small bowel lesions was considerably troublesome, and was widely considered a contraindication to surgery, as reiterated by Crohn in the 1950s [52]. Common practice, when small bowel strictures were symptomatic, was either to avoid surgery with supportive care alone, perform limited resections or to bypass involved proximal segments of bowel. Surgical conservatism led to the principles of management still held today which involve treating specific complications (i.e., refractory obstruction, perforation) of the disease, and conserving as much bowel as possible. Stricturoplasty as a technique to relieve stricture was reportedly first employed in 1961 by Bryan Brooke and has subsequently been shown to be a useful adjunct to surgical management [89, 90]. The first case of Crohn's disease treated with stricturoplasty was published by Lee and Papaioannou in 1982 [91]. They noted that many others were already describing this technique at meetings, but were reticent to publish their results due to fears that this technique would not provide long-term benefit, and would result in high morbidity due to the risks of leak and fistula. Their data, however, confirmed its safety.

The reduction of surgical morbidity has continued with the advent and dissemination of minimally invasive techniques. Contained perforation resulting in abscess formation is now readily managed with image-guided drainage. More recent advances in surgery have brought about the era of laparoscopic surgery for Crohn's disease. Laparoscopic ileocecal resection is now a well-validated option without any significant disease specific outcome disadvantages [92–97].

Major advances in the medical treatment of Crohn's disease have paralleled improved understanding of its pathophysiology. The initial treatment was believed to be surgical with therapeutic nihilism being the standard of care between relapses and supportive care for chronic symptoms. High rates of recurrence, need for reoperation, and medical consequences of wide resection (i.e., B12 deficiency, bile salt deficiency, chronic malnutrition, anemia) were frequently reported [76, 77, 81, 98–100]. Furthermore, because of the morbidity associated with extensive small bowel resections, patients with "jejunoileitis" were largely considered non-operative cases [50]. In the 1950s and 1960s, groups reported the first cases of remission with use of ACTH and corticosteroids [101–105]. The side effects of chronic steroid use, however, provided the impetus for study of non-steroid agents to induce and maintain remission, and also led to the development of steroid medication with low systemic absorption such as budesonide, which was evaluated with a double-blind randomized trial in the early 1990s [106]. Immunomodulatory agents including methotrexate, cyclosporine, azathioprine, and 6-mercaptopurine were tested throughout the 1980s and 1990s [107–111]. With design and scaled production of monoclonal antibodies, development of anti-TNF-α antibodies has had significant success at inducing remission in steroid resistant patients with severe active disease [112–114].

Despite over 80 years of familiarity with the many facets of Crohn's disease, medical and surgical decision making remains challenging. Our current ability to provide a precise treatment to those afflicted with this disease mirrors our ability to define the precise mechanisms of disease.

Acknowledgments The authors wish to acknowledge the invaluable contributions made by Arthur H. Aufses, Jr., M.D., who was kind enough to critically review the manuscript, and who provided us with access to his personal photographs, and by Barbara J. Niss, Archivist of the Mount Sinai Medical Center, who provided us with access to the Mount Sinai Levy Library Archives.

References

1. Crohn BB, Ginzburg L, Oppenheimer GD. Regional ileitis: a pathologic and clinical entity. JAMA. 1932;99(16):1323–9.
2. Lakatos PL. Recent trends in the epidemiology of inflammatory bowel diseases: up or down? World J Gastroenterol. 2006;12(38):6102–8.
3. Russel MG. Changes in the incidence of inflammatory bowel disease: what does it mean? Eur J Intern Med. 2000;11(4):191–6.
4. Sedlack RE, et al. Incidence of Crohn's disease in Olmsted County, Minnesota, 1935–1975. Am J Epidemiol. 1980;112(6):759–63.
5. Kirsner J. Crohn's disease. In: Origins and directions of inflammatory bowel disease. Netherlands: Springer; 2001. p. 55–101.
6. Bernier JJ, et al. Louis XIII's disease. Intestinal tuberculosis or Crohn's disease? Nouv Presse Med. 1981;10(27):2243. 2247–50.
7. Goldfischer S, Janis M. A 42-year-old king with a cavitary pulmonary lesion and intestinal perforation. Bull N Y Acad Med. 1981;57(2):139–43.
8. Morgagni G. The seats and causes of diseases investigated by anatomy; in five books, containing a great variety of dissections, with remarks. To which are added copious indexes. Translated from Latin of John Baptist Morgagni by Benjamin Alexander. London: A. Millar; and T. Cadell, his successor; 1769.

9. Combe C, Saunders W. A singular case of stricture and thickening of the ileum. Med Trans R Soc Med. 1806:16–8.
10. Abercrombie J. Pathological and practical researches on diseases of the stomach, the intestinal tract and other viscera of the abdomen. Edinburgh: Waugh and Innes; 1830.
11. Wilmanns R. Ein fall von darmstenose infolge cronisch etzundlicher vrdickung der ieocacal kappe. Beit z Klin Chir. 1905;46:221–32.
12. Moynihan B. The mimicry of malignant disease in the large bowel. Edinburgh Med J. 1907;21:203–28.
13. Robson AW. An address ON SOME ABDOMINAL TUMOURS SIMULATING MALIGNANT DISEASE, AND THEIR TREATMENT: delivered before the Torquay Medical Society. Br Med J. 1908;1(2460):425–8.
14. Nixon PI. Inflammatory tumors of the abdomen. Ann Surg. 1918;67(3):306–11.
15. Braun H. Ueber Enzandlichesgeschwfilste am Darm. Deutsch Ztschr f Chir. 1909;100:1–12.
16. Lartigau AJ. A study of chronic hyperplastic tuberculosis of the small intestine, with report of a case. J Exp Med. 1901;6(1):23–51.
17. von Bergmann A. Tumorbildung bei appendicitis und ihre radikale behandlung. St Petersburger Med Wochschr. 1911;36:512–23.
18. Dalziel TK. Chronic interstitial enteritis. Br Med J. 1913;2:1068–70.
19. Homer Gage EH. Hypertrophic ileo-caecal tuberculosis. New Engl J Med. 1917;176:259–66.
20. Moschowitz EW, Wilensky AO. Non-specific granulomata of the intestine. Am J Med Sci. 1923;166: 48–66.
21. Coffen TH. Nonspecific granuloma of the intestine causing intestinal obstruction. JAMA. 1925;85: 2303–4.
22. Moore N. Stricture of intestine at the ileocecal valve. Trans Pathol Soc Lond. 1882;34:112.
23. Jones N, Eisenberg AA. Inflammatory neoplasms of the intestine simulating malignancy. Surg Gynecol Obstet. 1918;27:420–423.
24. Dieulafoy G, Collins VE, Liebmann JA. A text-book of medicine. D. Appleton: New York; 1911.
25. The Medical and Surgical Reporter. Crissy & Markley, Printers; 1893.
26. Almadi MA, Ghosh S, Aljebreen AM. Differentiating intestinal tuberculosis from Crohn's disease: a diagnostic challenge. Am J Gastroenterol. 2009;104(4): 1003–12.
27. Kim BJ, et al. Prospective evaluation of the clinical utility of interferon-gamma assay in the differential diagnosis of intestinal tuberculosis and Crohn's disease. Inflamm Bowel Dis. 2011;17(6):1308–13.
28. Ginzburg L. The road to regional enteritis. Mt Sinai J Med. 1974;41(2):272–5.
29. Ginzburg L, Oppenheimer GD. Non-specific granulomata of the intestines: inflammatory tumors and strictures of the bowel. Ann Surg. 1933;98(6): 1046–62.
30. Ginzburg L. Letter April 30, 1984 to Dr. Kirsner. Levy Library Archives at the Mount Sinai Hospital; 1984. p. 3.
31. Kovalicik PJ. Early history of regional enteritis. Curr Surg. 1982;39(6):395–400.
32. Crohn BB. Granulomatous diseases of the small and large bowel. A historical survey. Gastroenterology. 1967;52(5):767–72.
33. Ginzburg L. Letter to the editor of gastroenterology. Mount Sinai Levy Library Archives; 1985.
34. Harris FI. Chronic cicatrizing enteritis of the ileum; regional ileitis (Crohn). Surg Gynecol Obstet. 1933;57.
35. Hurst AF. Crohn's disease. In: British encyclopedia of medical practice [as referenced by Ginzburg's 1984 letter]; 1937. p. 503–5.
36. Lichtarowicz AM, Mayberry JF. Antoni Lesniowski and his contribution to regional enteritis (Crohn's disease). J R Soc Med. 1988;81(8):468–70.
37. Kantor JL. Regional (terminal) ileitis: its Roentgen diagnosis. JAMA. 1934;103(26):2016–21.
38. Ravdin IS, Rhoads JE. Regional ileitis and fibroplastic appendicitis. Ann Surg. 1937;106(3):394–406.
39. Pemberton JD, Brown PW. Regional ileitis. Ann Surg. 1937;105(5):855–70.
40. Probstein JG, Gruenfeld GE. Acute regional ileitis. Ann Surg. 1936;103(2):273–8.
41. Mixter CG. Regional ileitis. Ann Surg. 1935; 102(4):674–94.
42. Bockus HL, Lee WE. Regional (terminal) ileitis. Ann Surg. 1935;102(3):412–21.
43. Colp R. A case of nonspecific granuloma of the terminal ileum and cecum. Surg Clin North Am. 1934;14:443–9.
44. Crohn BB, Rosenak BD. A combined form of ileitis and colitis. JAMA. 1936;106(1):1–7.
45. Penner A, Crohn BB. Perianal fistulae as a complication of regional ileitis. Ann Surg. 1938;108(5): 867–73.
46. Marshall SF. Regional ileitis. New Engl J Med. 1940;222(10):375–82.
47. Graham WL. Regional ileitis. Can Med Assoc J. 1941;44(2):168–71.
48. Ginzburg L, Garlock JH. Regional ileitis. Ann Surg. 1942;116(6):906–12.
49. Holloway JW. Regional ileitis. Ann Surg. 1943;118(3):329–42.
50. Brown P, Bargen JA, Weber H. Chronic inflammatory lesions of the small intestine (regional enteritis). Am J Dig Dis. 1934;1(6):426–31.
51. Radin IS, Johnston CJ. Regional ileitis. A summary of the literature. Am J Med Sci. 1939;198(2):269–91.
52. Crohn BB. Indications for surgical intervention in regional ileitis. AMA Arch Surg. 1957;74(3):305–11.
53. Bargen JA. The present status of ulcerative colitis and regional enteritis. Bull N Y Acad Med. 1944; 20(1):34–45.
54. McCready FJ, et al. Involvement of the ileum in chronic ulcerative colitis. New Engl J Med. 1949;240(4):119–27.

55. Wells C. Ulcerative colitis and Crohn's disease. Ann R Coll Surg Engl. 1952;11(2):105–20.
56. Cornes JS, Stecher M. Primary Crohn's disease of the colon and rectum. Gut. 1961;2:189–201.
57. Lockhart-Mummery HE, Morson BC. Crohn's disease (regional enteritis) of the large intestine and its distinction from ulcerative colitis. Gut. 1960;1: 87–105.
58. Glotzer DJ, et al. Comparative features and course of ulcerative and granulomatous colitis. New Engl J Med. 1970;282(11):582–7.
59. Zetzel L. Granulomatous (ileo) colitis. New Engl J Med. 1970;282(11):600–5.
60. Comfort MW, et al. Nonspecific granulomatous inflammation of the stomach and duodenum; its relation to regional enteritis. Am J Med Sci. 1950;220(6):616–32.
61. Fielding JF, et al. Crohn's disease of the stomach and duodenum. Gut. 1970;11(12):1001–6.
62. Bissell AD. Localized chronic ulcerative ileitis. Ann Surg. 1934;99(6):957–66.
63. Lindstrom C, Wramsby H, Ostberg G. Granulomatous arthritis in Crohn's disease. Gut. 1972;13(4):257–9.
64. Frayha R, Stevens MB, Bayless TM. Destructive monarthritis and granulomatous synovitis as the presenting manifestations of Crohn's disease. Johns Hopkins Med J. 1975;137(4):151–5.
65. Bayless TM, Stevens MB. Granulomatous synovitis and Crohn's disease. New Engl J Med. 1976; 294(16):903.
66. Greenstein AJ, Janowitz HD, Sachar DB. The extra-intestinal complications of Crohn's disease and ulcerative colitis: a study of 700 patients. Medicine (Baltimore). 1976;55(5):401–12.
67. Cornell A. The extra-intestinal manifestations of regional ileitis: some comparisons with chronic ulcerative colitis. J Mt Sinai Hosp N Y. 1955; 22(3):170–4.
68. Soren A. Joint affections in regional ileitis. Arch Intern Med. 1966;117(1):78–83.
69. Kirsner JB, Spencer JA. Family occurrences of ulcerative colitis, regional enteritis, and ileocolitis. Ann Intern Med. 1963;59(2):133–44.
70. John GEHEL. Regional ileitis in mother and son. Br Med J. 1956;2(4984):85.
71. Abraham C, Cho JH. Inflammatory bowel disease. New Engl J Med. 2009;361(21):2066–78.
72. Barrett JC, et al. Genome-wide association defines more than 30 distinct susceptibility loci for Crohn's disease. Nat Genet. 2008;40(8):955–62.
73. Orholm M, et al. Familial occurrence of inflammatory bowel disease. New Engl J Med. 1991;324(2): 84–8.
74. Pratt FW, Simpson SL. Regional ileitis. Br Med J. 1942;1(4246):634–7.
75. Heaton LD, et al. President Eisenhower's operation for regional enteritis: a footnote to history. Ann Surg. 1964;159:661–6.
76. De Dombal FT, Burton I, Goligher JC. Recurrence of Crohn's disease after primary excisional surgery. Gut. 1971;12(7):519–27.
77. Garlock JH, et al. An appraisal of the long-term results of surgical treatment of regional ileitis. Gastroenterology. 1951;19(3):414–23.
78. Crohn BB, Janowitz HD. Reflections on regional ileitis, twenty years later. J Am Med Assoc. 1954;156(13):1221–5.
79. Van Patter WN, et al. Regional enteritis. Gastroenterology. 1954;26(3):347–450.
80. Jackson BB. Chronic regional enteritis; a survey of one hundred twenty-six cases treated at the Massachusetts General Hospital from 1937 to 1954. Ann Surg. 1958;148(1):81–7.
81. Alexander-Williams J, Fielding JF, Cooke WT. A comparison of results of excision and bypass for ileal Crohn's disease. Gut. 1972;13(12):973–5.
82. Lock MR, et al. Recurrence and reoperation for Crohn's disease. New Engl J Med. 1981;304(26): 1586–8.
83. Homan WP, Dineen P. Comparison of the results of resection, bypass, and bypass with exclusion for ileocecal Crohn's disease. Ann Surg. 1978; 187(5):530.
84. Greenstein AJ, et al. Cancer in Crohn's disease after diversionary surgery. A report of seven carcinomas occurring in excluded bowel. Am J Surg. 1978; 135(1):86–90.
85. Greenstein AJ, Janowitz HD. Cancer in Crohn's disease. The danger of a by-passed loop. Am J Gastroenterol. 1975;64(2):122–4.
86. Pennington L, et al. Surgical management of Crohn's disease. Influence of disease at margin of resection. Ann Surg. 1980;192(3):311.
87. Heuman R, et al. The influence of disease at the margin of resection on the outcome of Crohn's disease. Br J Surg. 1983;70(9):519–21.
88. Fazio VW, et al. Effect of resection margins on the recurrence of Crohn's disease in the small bowel. A randomized controlled trial. Ann Surg. 1996; 224(4):563.
89. Alexander-Williams J, Haynes IG. Conservative operations for Crohn's disease of the small bowel. World J Surg. 1985;9(6):945–51.
90. Fazio VW, et al. Strictureplasty in Crohn's disease. Ann Surg. 1989;210(5):621–5.
91. Lee E, Papaioannou N. Minimal surgery for chronic obstruction in patients with extensive or universal Crohn's disease. Ann R Coll Surg Engl. 1982;64(4): 229–33.
92. Dasari BV, McKay D, Gardiner K. Laparoscopic versus open surgery for small bowel Crohn's disease. Cochrane Database Syst Rev. 2011(1): Cd006956.
93. Polle SW, et al. Short-term outcomes after laparoscopic ileocolic resection for Crohn's disease. A systematic review. Dig Surg. 2006;23(5–6): 346–57.
94. Lowney JK, et al. Is there any difference in recurrence rates in laparoscopic ileocolic resection for Crohn's disease compared with conventional surgery? A long-term, follow-up study. Dis Colon Rectum. 2006;49(1):58–63.

95. Bergamaschi R, Pessaux P, Arnaud JP. Comparison of conventional and laparoscopic ileocolic resection for Crohn's disease. Dis Colon Rectum. 2003;46(8):1129–33.
96. Wu JS, et al. Laparoscopic-assisted ileocolic resections in patients with Crohn's disease: are abscesses, phlegmons, or recurrent disease contraindications? Surgery. 1997;122(4):682–8. discussion 688-9.
97. Kim NK, et al. Long-term outcome after ileocecal resection for Crohn's disease. Am Surg. 1997;63(7):627–33.
98. Truelove SC, Pena AS. Course and prognosis of Crohn's disease. Gut. 1976;17(3):192–201.
99. Greenstein AJ, et al. Reoperation and recurrence in Crohn's colitis and ileocolitis. Crude and cumulative rates. N Engl J Med. 1975;293(14):685–90.
100. Hardison WGM, Rosenberg IH. Bile-salt deficiency in the steatorrhea following resection of the ileum and proximal colon. New Engl J Med. 1967;277(7):337–42.
101. Kirsner JB, Palmer WL, Klotz AP. ACTH in severe chronic regional enteritis: observations in four patients. Gastroenterology. 1952;20(2):229–33.
102. Cooke WT, Fielding JF. Corticosteroid or corticotrophin therapy in Crohn's disease (regional enteritis). Gut. 1970;11(11):921–7.
103. Fielding JF, Cooke WT. Corticosteroids (including ACTH) in Crohn's disease. Gut. 1969;10(12):1054.
104. Gray SJ, Reifenstein RW, Benson JA. ACTH therapy in ulcerative colitis and regional enteritis. New Engl J Med. 1951;245(13):481–7.
105. Jones JH, Lennard-Jones JE. Corticosteroids and corticotrophin in the treatment of Crohn's disease. Gut. 1966;7(2):181–7.
106. Greenberg GR, et al. Oral budesonide for active Crohn's disease. New Engl J Med. 1994;331(13):836–41.
107. Brynskov J, et al. A placebo-controlled, double-blind, randomized trial of cyclosporine therapy in active chronic Crohn's disease. New Engl J Med. 1989;321(13):845–50.
108. Present DH, et al. Infliximab for the treatment of fistulas in patients with Crohn's disease. New Engl J Med. 1999;340(18):1398–405.
109. Present DH, et al. Treatment of Crohn's disease with 6-mercaptopurine. New Engl J Med. 1980;302(18):981–7.
110. Malchow H, et al. European Cooperative Crohn's Disease Study (ECCDS): results of drug treatment. Gastroenterology. 1984;86(2):249–66.
111. Summers RW, et al. National Cooperative Crohn's Disease Study: results of drug treatment. Gastroenterology. 1979;77(4 Pt 2):847–69.
112. Targan SR, et al. A short-term study of chimeric monoclonal antibody cA2 to tumor necrosis factor alpha for Crohn's disease. Crohn's Disease cA2 Study Group. N Engl J Med. 1997;337(15):1029–35.
113. van Dullemen HM, et al. Treatment of Crohn's disease with anti-tumor necrosis factor chimeric monoclonal antibody (cA2). Gastroenterology. 1995;109(1):129–35.
114. Behm BW, Bickston SJ. Tumor necrosis factor-alpha antibody for maintenance of remission in Crohn's disease. Cochrane Database Syst Rev. 2008(1):Cd006893.

Molecular and Genetic Factors in Crohn's Disease

2

Tara M. Connelly and Walter A. Koltun

Introduction

The precise etiology of Crohn's disease (CD) is not yet known. However, research in the fields of immunology, microbiology, and genetics suggests an interplay between host and environmental factors. Environmental factors may be external agents that a patient has been exposed to such as NSAIDs or cigarette smoking or present within the host, such as the microbes and pathogens that comprise the microbiome. Host factors relate to the individual's immunologic response to these external factors, which increasingly appear to be genetically defined or programmed early in life. This interplay between host physiology and external agents ultimately leads to an alteration in the host's inflammatory homeostasis and maintenance of the gut mucosal integrity (Fig. 2.1) resulting in unchecked inflammation, enteric bacterial invasion, and worsening tissue destruction. Additionally, the variation in the multitude of factors that interact within the individual patient presumably results in the dozens of different phenotypes of CD (stricturing, fistulizing, inflammatory, ileal, colonic, etc.).

Although over 40 microbes including bacteria, viruses, and yeasts, and over 100 genes have been implicated in the pathophysiology of the disease, no one factor alone causes CD [1, 2]. Thus, the current working hypothesis is that this is a disease caused by a widely variable set of environmental insults presented to a genetically predisposed and uniquely immune compromised host [3–5].

The Immune System in Crohn's Disease

The development of a healthy immune system requires exposure to a variety of pathogens, particularly early in life. The lack of such environmental exposure has been suggested to play a role in the development of CD. This concept, known as the "hygiene hypothesis," suggests that lack of such exposure causes an impairment in tolerance to both self and foreign pathogens and a subsequent exaggerated immune response when the individual is exposed to pathogens later in life [6]. Supporting this hypothesis is the inability to induce IBD-like colitis in genetically predisposed mice as long as these mice are kept in germ free environments. When removed from the germ free environment, these mice rapidly develop severe colitis [7].

Additionally, patients with CD tend to cluster geographically with higher incidences found in urban areas where more sanitary conditions and decreased exposure to pathogens is the norm.

T.M. Connelly • W.A. Koltun (✉)
Division of Colon and Rectal Surgery, Milton S. Hershey Medical Center, Penn State College of Medicine, Hershey, PA, USA
e-mail: wkoltun@hmc.psu.edu

A. Fichera and M.K. Krane (eds.), *Crohn's Disease: Basic Principles*,
DOI 10.1007/978-3-319-14181-7_2, © Springer International Publishing Switzerland 2015

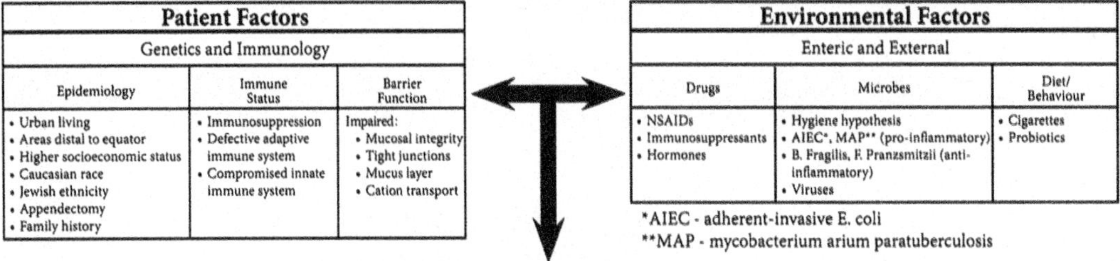

Fig. 2.1 The etiology of Crohn's disease. The current hypothesis on the etiology of Crohn's disease suggests an interplay between patient and environmental factors. Patient factors involve epidemiological and demographic variables, immune status, and intestinal epithelial barrier function. Environmental factors are enteric and external. These factors include drugs, enteric pathogens (bacteria, viruses, and fungi), and drugs

Exposure to helminthes, which are less commonly found in western countries, is a newer studied topic in the pathogenesis and potential treatment of CD. Interestingly, the administration of helminthes such as Trichuris suis, a porcine whipworm has been shown to improve the symptoms of CD in early trials [33]. However, the hygiene hypothesis does not entirely account for the development of CD as migration from a low risk geographic area (with a high amount of childhood exposure to a variety of pathogens) to a higher risk area increases one's risk of developing CD to that of the new, local population within the same generation [34–36].

The most studied and implicated areas of immunology in CD are innate immunity including epithelial barrier function, bacterial recognition, and autophagy and adaptive immunity, mainly focusing on the T cell response.

The History of CD Genetic Research

Early CD genetic research was based on the observation of multiple affected family members which led to the theory that the disease was due to a pathogen that was passed between family members. One such pathogen, Mycobacterium avium subspecies paratuberculosis (MAP) which has been implicated in Johne's disease, a CD-like disease in hoofed livestock was the focus of many early studies [37]. However, this theory and MAP have now been disproven as causes of CD. Research now focuses on genetic alterations that may be causative of the disease and/or modify its course. Much of this research is the result of several landmark IBD-twin studies originating from Scandinavia's carefully maintained national twin registries. These and other familial studies have demonstrated that:

1. No single gene is causative
2. Inheritance is not simple, Mendelian inheritance
3. The presence of a family member with IBD is the number one risk factor for developing the disease [38].

In fact, up to 35 % of IBD patients have an affected family member [38]. The risk to an individual increases to 50 % if his or her monozygotic twin has CD. If a non-twin sibling is affected, the risk is still elevated above the normal population risk but is much less than the identical twin rate [39]. Additionally, "IBD families" are generally concordant for CD location, behavior, and age of onset [40–43].

Using available technology at the time, early CD genetic research was slow moving and tedious. Methods included genetic investigation of sibling pairs, searching for high rates of shared alleles [44], linkage studies, and candidate gene studies investigating the few known IBD associated loci at that time. These techniques led to the discovery of the first IBD-associated genes including nucleotide-binding oligomerization domain protein 2/ caspase recruitment domain-containing peptide 15 (NOD2/CARD15) [45].

Since that early work, the subsequent development of whole genome sequencing and the completion of the HapMap project has led to several genome wide association studies (GWAS) studying thousands of genes in thousands of diseased and control patients that defined the most common allelic variations in these genes associated with IBD. This led to a rapid advance in the field of IBD genetics. To date, over 300 single nucleotide polymorphisms (SNPs, single base pair substitutions in the genetic code, for example a guanine is found where the majority of the population have a adenine) corresponding to over 100 genes have been associated with IBD with approximately 30 loci being exclusively associated with CD [46, 47]. Whole exome sequencing, covering the 1 % of the genome that actually codes for proteins, and whole genome sequencing, covering the entire genome, will soon become affordable for use in translational clinical studies and, eventually, for use in a personalized medicine approach. This personalized approach will use the genetic information obtained from sequencing to predict disease behavior including response to medication and surgical therapy in the individual patient with CD.

The majority of the genes associated with CD discovered to date have roles in the main categories of innate immunity including intestinal barrier function and autophagy as well as adaptive immunity [4]. In CD, in response to antigenic insult, the innate immune system triggers proinflammatory cascades and activates the adaptive immune system. As a result, inflammation occurs. When this process is dysregulated, cell damage with subsequent further inflammation and innate and adaptive immunoactivation occurs (Fig. 2.2).

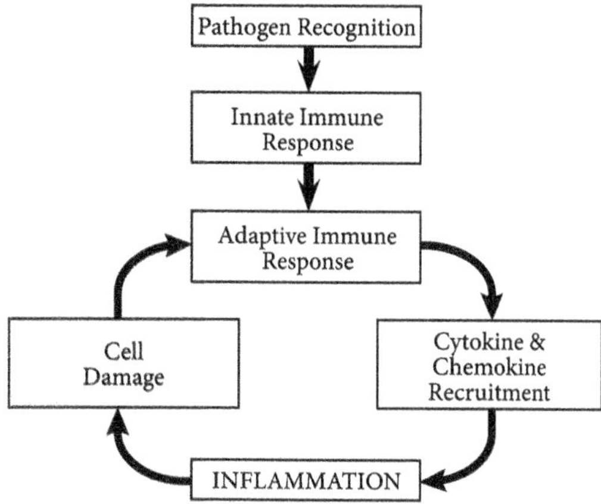

Fig. 2.2 In CD, in response to antigenic insult, the innate immune system triggers proinflammatory cascades and activates the adaptive immune system. As a result, inflammation occurs. When this process is dysregulated, cell damage with subsequent further inflammation and innate and adaptive immunoactivation occurs

Innate Immunity

As the first line of immune mediated defense, the innate immune system rapidly senses and responds to the presence of cell injury or the infiltration of microbes using several molecular processes including the secretion of IgA, Toll-like receptor (TLRs) mediated recognition, and autophagy. The key cellular players are epithelial Paneth cells, macrophages, and dendritic cells [48] (Fig. 2.3). Over 92 SNPs associated with IBD have been correlated with regions of the genome that actively regulate immune cells and the intestinal epithelium in a 2014 functional genetics study [49].

The innate immune response is triggered by the recognition of a molecular signature from a luminal pathogen in the form of a pathogen-associated molecular pattern (PAMP) or intracellularly in the form of a damage associated molecular pattern (DAMP) resulting from cell stress or injury (Fig. 2.4). After recognition by pattern recognizing receptors (PRRs) located on effector cells, a series of inflammation inducing pathways is activated. Conversely, when these pathogens are removed, inflammation resolves. This is demonstrated in CD as in when the fecal stream is diverted via an upstream stoma, the inflammation and symptoms of downstream CD often improve [50, 51]. These receptor mediated responses are involved in the sampling of the individual's intestinal microflora and, in health, prevent dysbiosis or "bacterial imbalance." Dysbiosis and reduced diversity of intestinal

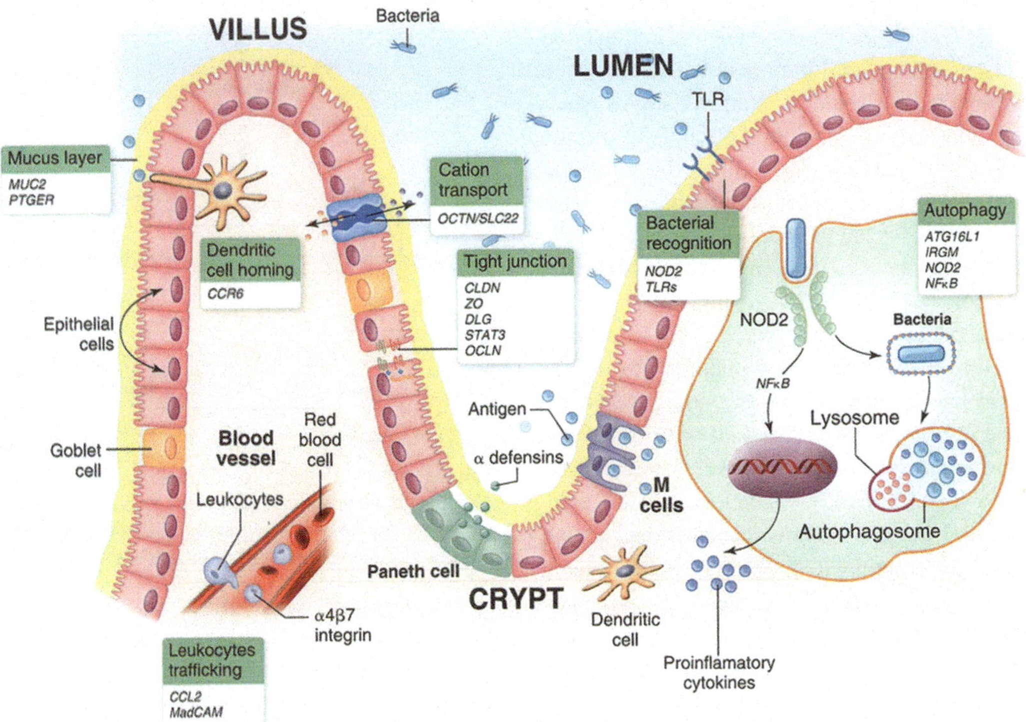

Fig. 2.3 The innate immune system in Crohn's disease. The functions of the innate immune system most recognized as affected in Crohn's include (1) epithelial barrier function, (2) bacterial recognition, and (3) autophagy. The mucus layer is key to the integrity and protection of the epithelial barrier. Tight junctions protect the intestine from an unregulated influx of bacteria from the lumen. Other mechanisms including the secretion of proinflammatory cytokines, dendritic cell homing, and leukocyte trafficking address bacteria at the surface or that have entered the intestine from the lumen. These bacteria are then broken down and digested through autophagy or travel on antigen presenting cells to activate the adaptive immune system. Key genes associated with dysregulation in these individual processes are listed under each process

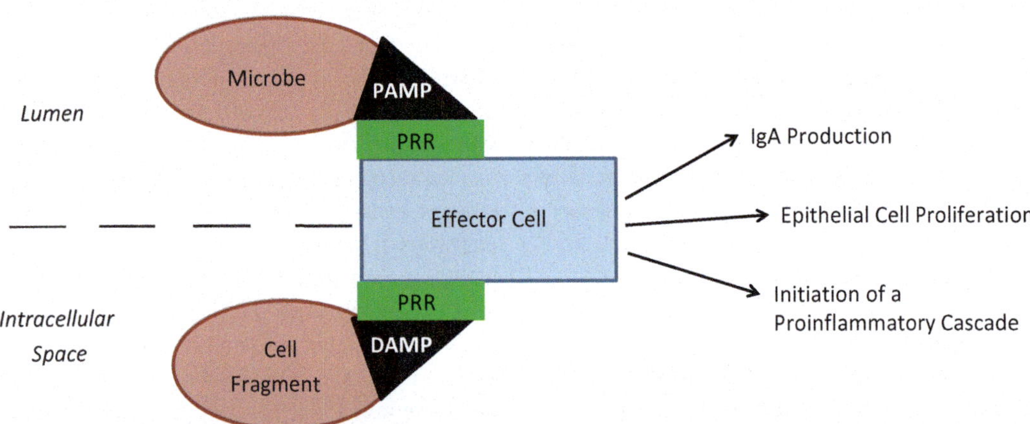

Fig. 2.4 Pattern recognition receptors (PRRs). In the lumen, PRRs recognize pathogen associated molecular pattern (PAMPs) on the surface of bacteria, viruses, and fugi. In the intracellular space, PRRs recognize pathogen damage associated molecular patterns (DAMPs) derived from cell fragments or waste products. Such PAMP and DAMP mediated recognition leads to an immune response inclusive of IgA and proinflammatory cytokine production and epithelial proliferation

microbiota have been demonstrated in CD patients when compared to healthy controls. However, CD patients are frequently treated with antibiotics and other microbiome altering medications, complicating interpretation of this phenomenon [51–57].

The Epithelium

At the interface between the gut tissue and luminal contents with its multitude of bacteria, the epithelial barrier is key in the pathogenesis of CD. In the small bowel, four main cell types are found, goblet cells, enteroendocrine cells, Paneth cells, and enterocytes. After differentiation, goblet cells, enteroendocrine cells, and enterocytes migrate to the villi and Paneth cells migrate to the base of the intestinal crypts. In the colon, Paneth cells are not found and, as villi are not present, enteroendocrine, goblet cells, and enterocytes migrate to the surface of the colon.

Toll-Like Receptors

TLRs are the subset of PRRs most commonly studied in CD. These are located on epithelial cell surfaces or within endosomes and span the cell membrane. Although several subtypes of TLR are involved in the pathogenesis of IBD, TLR2 and 4 are the most studied. TLR2 detects bacterial proteins. TLR4 detects lipopolysaccharide (LPS), an outer membrane component of gram negative bacteria. Once presented with a PAMP or DAMP, TLRs activate inflammatory pathways including the adapter protein myeloid differentiation factor 88 (MyD88) dependent pathway. The activation of this pathway results in the production of several proinflammatory cytokines. TLR4 can also more directly activate inflammatory mediators such as interferons (IFNs) and tumor necrosis factor alpha (TNFα) through a MyD88 independent pathway. CD patients have significantly higher intestinal TLR4 expression than healthy controls which may lead to an increased inflammatory response [58].

NOD2/CARD15

NOD2 also known as CARD15, another type of PRR, an NLR (nucleotide-binding domain leucine rich repeat (LRR)-containing receptor), is highly expressed in Paneth cells and monocytes. NOD2 is a regulator of autophagy and recruits the autophagy associated protein, ATG16L1 to the cell membrane. Discovered in 2001, the NOD2 gene was the first discovered IBD gene and still has the most commonly and strongest replicated association with IBD [45, 59].

Located on chromosome 16, the NOD2/ gene's protein product, CARD15, is involved in the recognition of the bacterial cell wall component, muramyl dipeptide (MDP) [59]. MDP recognition activates NOD2 leading to the dimerization of its subunits and translocation into the cell nucleus for the activation of the MAPK (mitogen activated protein kinase) and NFκB (nuclear factor kappa B) pathways [60]. These pathways play a key role in the immune and inflammatory responses and are involved in the regulation of several genes involved in the production of proinflammatory cytokines such as interleukins (IL) 1β, IL6, IL8, IL12, and TNF-α.

Three NOD2 SNPs, R702W, G908R and 1007fs located within or near the MDP sensing area of the gene (the LRR sequence) have been most frequently associated with IBD. Up to half of all European and North American CD patients tested for these mutations had at least one mutation, compared with 10–15 % of the healthy population [61]. Downstream effects of these mutations include impaired activation of NFκB with subsequent decreased production of inflammatory cytokines [62].

Neutrophils and Macrophages

Macrophages secrete proinflammatory cytokines which activate natural killer (NK) cells. INFγ secretion by NK cells in turn activates dendritic cells. Dendritic cells then secrete TNFα, recruiting more inflammatory cells to the area [63]. In the peritoneum the Macrophage stimulating 1 (MST1) gene has been shown to induce phagocytosis. SNPs in this gene have been shown to be associated with CD in multiple GWAS studies [64, 65].

MadCAM-1

Bacterial recognition also leads to neutrophil recruitment for phagocytosis and subsequent recruitment of macrophages. In the setting of increased cytokine expression such as IL-1, TNFα, leukotrienes, and a multitude of chemokines, leukocytes travel through the blood vessels and traverse the endothelial surface using mediators such as surface integrins which bind to homing molecules such a mucosal addressin cell adhesion molecule-1 (MAdCAM-1) on the endothelium [63, 66]. The integrins that bind to these adhesion molecules are the targets of some of the newest CD drugs [66]. MadCAM-1 has been shown to be overexpressed in the epithelium of the gut during active CD [67].

The Mucus Layer and Goblet Cells

Goblet cells store and secrete mucus into the intestinal lumen forming a protective physical barrier over the intestinal mucosa. Intestinal mucus also contains immunoglobulins such as IgA and plays a role in the regulation of inflammation and epithelial repair. The main component of intestinal mucus is the Muc glycoprotein family, particularly MUC2. Murine models with mutations in MUC2 develop CD-like colitis [1]. Similarly, polymorphisms that affect the MUC19 gene, a mucin component, have been associated with the development of CD in humans [60]. Anti-inflammatory prostaglandins such as prostaglandin E2 are involved in epithelial mucosal repair. Polymorphisms associated with the gene encoding its receptor, prostaglandin E receptor 4 (PTGER4) have been associated with the development of CD [60].

Paneth Cells

Paneth cells are the main source of antimicrobial peptides in the small intestine. These cells increase in number distally with the maximum concentration found in the ileum [48]. Their main role is the secretion of antimicrobial peptides that form a chemical barrier aiding in the epithelial defense of pathogens. The most abundant antimicrobial peptide produced is α defensin, however; other antimicrobial peptides including lysozyme a phospholipase A2, are also produced. Alpha defensins are hydrophobic peptides that form pores in bacterial membranes causing bacterial lysis and death [63]. Murine models of colitis with dysfunctional Paneth cells have dysfunctional secretion of antimicrobial peptides [1, 68].

Cation Transport

Epithelial cells contain cation transporters that move charged ions in and out of the cell to maintain homeostasis. It is not fully understood how these cells are involved in the pathogenesis of CD. However, mutations within genes encoding these proteins have been repeatedly associated with CD by GWAS. The organic cation transporter genes (OCT) genes OCTN1 and 2, also known as the solute carrier family 22, member 4 (SLC22A4) and SLC22A5, respectively, are located in the IBD5 locus on chromosome 5 [69]. Although associated with CD overall and with colonic involvement and anal disease in particular in multiple GWAS, the exact mechanism of these genes in the disease process is not yet known [69].

Intraepithelial Junctions

Tight junctions are connections between adjacent epithelial cells. Intact tight junctions maintain intestinal homeostasis by controlling permeability and are necessary to avoid the passage of microbes from the lumen into the underlying lamina propria and the systemic circulation. Increased space between these junctions [60] and a more permeable intestinal barrier have been demonstrated in CD patients before the onset of disease and in unaffected family members of CD patients, compared to controls [70, 71]. Occludin and claudin are transmembrane bridging proteins found between epithelial cells that are key to tight junction formation and maintenance. They interact with scaffolding proteins including the Zo family linking them to the actin cytoskeleton [72, 73]. An absence of Zo-1 in experimental colitis models and aberrant claudin and occludin have been demonstrated in murine models of colitis and in mucosal samples from CD patients [74, 75]. Claudin family protein expression levels have been demonstrated to correspond to severity of inflammation in Crohn's colitis [76].

Miscellaneous Epithelial Integrity Genes

Intelectin-1 (ITLN1), STAT3 and DLG

The protein product of ITLN1 is expressed in the brush border of enterocytes and plays an important role in membrane stabilization. It is also involved in protecting the glycolipid barrier from pathogens [77]. Part of the Janus kinase signal transducer and activator of transcription (JAK–STAT) signal transmission pathway, STAT3 has a paradoxical effect in CD with its activation in innate immune cells enhancing mucosal barrier function but its activation in T cells exacerbating colitis [77]. STATs are located in the cytoplasm and are latent until, in response to cytokines and growth factors, such as IL2, IL3, IL5 IL7, erythropoietin, GM-CSF, and thrombopoietin, they become activated by receptor-associated tyrosine kinases from the JAK family. They then dimerize, translocate to the cell nucleus, and act as transcription activators [78–80]. The DLG5 (Drosophila Discs large) protein, a member of the guanylate kinase family, is located at the cell–cell junction and SNPs associated with the gene have been associated with CD [81].

Autophagy

Originally believed to be an energy conserving mechanism for the recycling of nutrients to the cell, an immunological role for autophagy has since been discovered [82]. Autophagy or the process of degrading and re-using cellular components is now known to also be involved in suppressing inflammatory responses and to participate in T and B cell differentiation. However, the mechanism of these T and B cell associated phenomena is poorly understood [1].

The cellular material for degradation is engulfed by the autophagosome which then fuses with a lysosome for degradation within the cell's cytoplasm. The degraded peptides can then be presented to HLA Class II molecules for further processing. Intracellular pathogens including bacteria such as Mycobacterium and listeria may also be degraded directly by autophagy or by the inflammatory pathways activated by the process [1]. In macrophages genetically programmed to be unable to perform autophagy, high levels of proinflammatory cytokines including IL1B and IL18 are produced [1]. IL8 and IFNγ production leads to macrophage maturation and the formation of multinucleate giant cells [70]. These cells together with Th1 cells and bacteria, form granulomas, hallmarks of CD. The granulomas themselves then act as APCs and release proinflammatory cytokines potentiating T cell activation and further inflammation [63].

ATG16L1

The ATG16L1 gene is found on chromosome 2q37. ATG16L1 is expressed by APCs, T cells and intestinal epithelial cells and, along with NOD2, this gene must be functional in dendritic cells for autophagy to occur. Paneth cell abnormalities, increased levels of inflammatory cytokines, and an impaired ability to breakdown intracellular bacteria have been demonstrated in both CD patients with mutations in ATG16L1 and ATG16L1 murine knockdown models [1, 70].

IRGM

Located on chromosome 5, a chromosome containing several IBD related genes, the IRGM (immunity-related GTPase family M protein) codes for proteins necessary for the IFNγ mediated clearance of intracellular pathogens. Similar to ATG16L1 knockdown mice, IRGM knockdown mice demonstrate defective autophagy with increased survival of pathogens including *Mycobacterium tuberculosis, Toxoplasma gondii,* and *Listeria monocytogenes* [83, 84]. A 2013 meta-analysis of 25 studies inclusive of 20,590

IBD cases and 27,670 controls demonstrated 3 IRGM SNPs to be associated with IBD. Stratification by ethnicity revealed that a significantly increased CD risk was demonstrated in Europeans but not in Asians [85].

Antigen Presenting Cells

Antigen presenting cells (APCs) bridge the innate and adaptive immune systems and recognize both "self" and "outside" peptides. The "boomerangs of immunity," these cells travel to the site of a pathogen that has either breached the epithelial barrier or that is in the lumen but within easy reach through the junction between two epithelial cells. APCs bind these antigens and return to lymphoid tissue for presentation to T cells in a process guided by homing molecules [66]. Dendritic cells are the most prevalent APCs in CD. One theory on lack of tolerance to normal flora and/or hyper responsiveness seen in CD is that a faulty or "leaky" epithelial barrier may lead to increased DC-antigen contact and an overstimulation of the immune system [82].

DCs reach bacteria in the lumen by extending armlike dendrites through the tight junctions or by interacting with M (microfold) cells, which are unique, specialized cells located in the small intestine that take up antigen directly from the lumen via endocytosis and transport it to dendritic and T cells in a basolaterally located pocket [1]. DCs have several subsets with some involved in tolerance and others in pro-inflammatory responses. One such subset produces the proinflammatory cytokine IL23 in the intestine (see IL23 section). The secretion of IL12 by dendritic cells drives the differentiation of naïve T cells to the Th1 subset which secretes IL2, a key cytokine involved in T cell activation and survival.

CCR6 (Chemokine Receptor 6)

This gene encodes a homing receptor that is expressed by immature dendritic and memory T cells. It is key in CD and T cell migration in response to epithelial inflammation and pathogen exposure. Mutations in this gene have been associated with CD on GWAS [77].

Adaptive Immunity

T cells are the main adaptive immunity cells in CD. The role of the B cells, other than the secretion of the key immunological defense molecule IgA, is less understood in CD [86]. T cells are predominately located in the lamina propria and subdivided into two main categories: CD4 (memory T cells) and CD8 (cytotoxic T cells). CD4 cells have the predominant role in CD. The main role for CD8 cells is the production of IFNγ [66].

T Cell Activation and Differentiation

After APCs bind with antigen and travel back through the lymphatic vessels to the gut associated lymphoid tissue (GALT), such as mesenteric lymph nodes and the [87] lymphoid patches known as Peyers' patches, the antigen is presented to the naïve T cell and T cell activation occurs. After activation, under the influence of cytokines in the cellular milieu (Fig. 2.5), naïve T cells differentiate into subsets. A bias towards the Th1 (T helper one) subset with subsequent IL12, IFNγ, and TNF production has been documented as the main pattern of differentiation in CD [46, 88]. Although some T cells differentiate into Th2 cells (with subsequent production of IL4, 5 and 13), a far less substantial role for this subset is seen in CD. Th2 cell bias is more commonly associated with ulcerative colitis. The IL17 secreting Th17 subset is associated with both UC and CD but has a slightly stronger association with CD. Several known IBD associated genes including IL12B, STAT3, JAK2, TNFSF15, and CCR6 are involved in Th17 differentiation.

The more newly discovered T regulatory (Treg) subset has been found to have a strong role in CD pathogenesis. These cells promote tolerance to dietary antigens and gut microbiota and suppress immune responses [89].

Human Leucocyte Antigen

Human leucocyte antigen (HLA) also known as major histocompatibility complex (MHC) class I and II molecules are coded for by genes on a

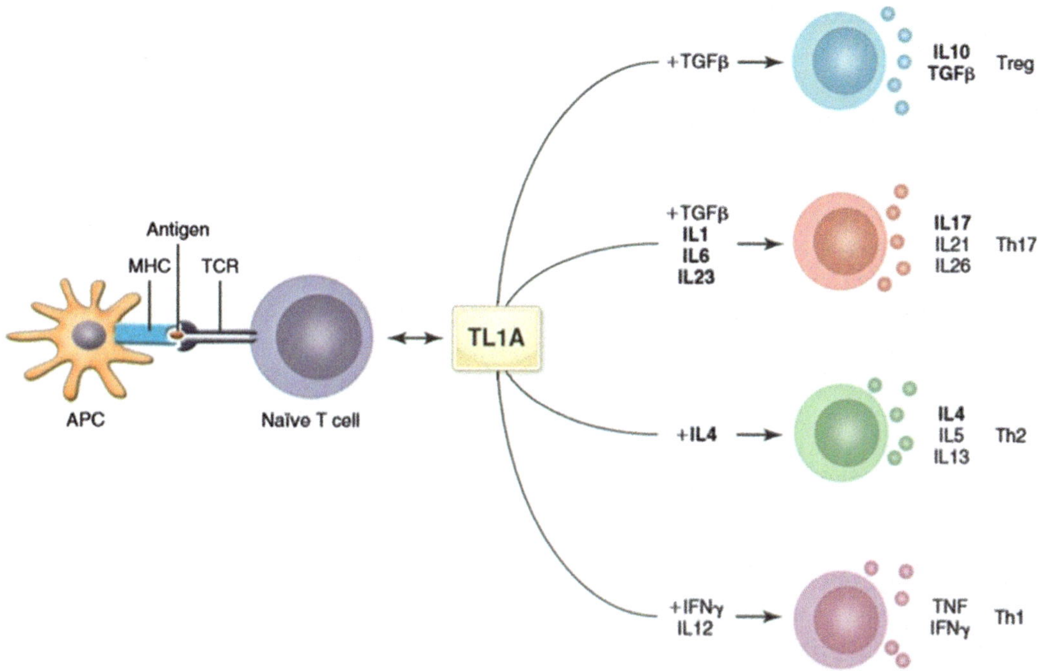

Fig. 2.5 T cell differentiation. After T cell activation resulting from contact with an antigen on the major histocompatibility complex (MHC) on an antigen presenting cell (APC), in response to cytokines in the cellular milieu, the T cell differentiates into one of four subsets; T helper 17 (Th17), T regulatory (Treg), Th1 and Th2. These cells then secrete characteristic cytokines. Th1, Th17, and Tregs are most commonly associated with CD

locus on chromosome 6 [90]. The HLA protein complex on the APC cell surface binds antigen. Expressed in fibroblasts, dendritic cells and endothelial cells, Class I HLA gene expression increases in response to viral and bacterial exposure. Class II HLA genes, which are more commonly studied in IBD, are expressed in macrophages, activated T cells, endothelial, dendritic, and epithelial cells. IBD studies focus particularly on HLA-DRB1 due to the role of this subgroup in antigen presentation to T cells. Although conventionally thought of as UC associated, subtypes of HLA genes such as DR7, DRB3, and DQ4 have also been associated with CD [8, 91–93]. Notably this gene has been associated with the extra intestinal manifestations of IBD [91].

MHC molecules expressed on the surface of intestinal epithelial cells are capable of antigen sampling. However, these molecules do not have the necessary costimulatory molecules needed for activation of the adaptive immune system [66]. Thus, their main role in the epithelium is the secretion of cytokines including TGFβ [1].

TNFSF15

The tumor necrosis factor superfamily member 15 (TNFSF15) gene which is also known as the vascular endothelial growth inhibitor (VEGI) gene and the TNF superfamily ligand A (TL1A) gene is found on chromosome 9. The TNFSF15 gene has both angiostatic and immunological functions [94]. Its protein product, TL1A is produced by DCs, monocytes, T lymphocytes, and endothelial cells and binds to death domain receptor 3 (DR3) which is expressed predominately on T lymphocytes [89, 95]. When stimulated through the NFκB pathway, TNFSF15 is involved in the differentiation of naïve T cells into the main T helper subsets, particularly Th1 and 17 [89, 96, 97]. It also enhances IL2 and IFNγ production by T cells in IBD patients with marked increases found in CD patients vs controls [96, 98]. Additionally, TL1A is involved in apoptosis and the induction of metalloproteinases involved in intestinal barrier function [99–101]. IBD patients with certain allelic variations in TNFSF15 have been shown to have a more aggressive course to their disease [102]. Interestingly, this gene has also been associated with diverticulitis requiring surgery suggesting a more broad based role in intestinal inflammatory disease [103].

Cytokine Signaling

Several cytokines play a role in the induction, maintenance or interruption of pathways involved in CD. Several are mentioned in the above sections.

IL10

Unlike the majority of known CD-related cytokines, IL10 is an anti-inflammatory cytokine. Thus mutations affecting the gene or its receptor result in increased inflammation, often leading to a severe clinical phenotype. IL10 is perhaps the best known cytokine in CD due to the 2009 UK pediatric study of a small cohort of patients with extremely severe, early onset, medically refractory CD with dramatic anal disease who were found to have IL10 receptor mutations. Subsequently, these patients were successfully treated by bone marrow transplantation [17]. An association with severe, very early onset disease has since been replicated [30].

IL23

Similar to several other IBD associated genes, the IL23R gene is also associated with other immune mediated diseases such as ankylosing spondylitis and rheumatoid arthritis [86]. IL23 is secreted by activated macrophages, monocytes, and dendritic cells. As part of the IL23/IL17 axis, its secretion leads to Th17 differentiation from the naïve T cell and causes macrophages and monocytes to release TNFα and IL's 1 and 6 [104]. IL23R (interleukin23 receptor) is a key connector of the innate and adaptive immune systems and functions to promote naïve T cell differentiation into the Th17 class.

Several cell lines express IL23R including NK and memory and effector T cells with particularly high levels seen in Th17 cells [86]. After production by activated macrophages and dendritic cells, IL23 binds to the IL23R, activating the Janus kinase 2 gene (JAK2). Downstream recruitment and dimerization of the two subunits of the signal transducer and activator of transcription 3 (STAT3) transcription activator occurs making STAT3 able to translocate into the cell nucleus to promote the transcription of proinflammatory mediators [104]. The IL23 signaling pathway also activates another pathway which plays an important role in $CD4^+$ T helper cell differentiation, the retinoic acid-binding orphan receptor-γt (ROR-γt) pathway. The production of IL17, IL6 and TNFα cytokines resulting from activation of this pathway also leads to inflammation and differentiation of Th17 cells [104].

Using Genetics to Improve Patient Care

The course of CD is unpredictable. As the disease evolves, phenotype can change. Additionally, disease phenotype varies between patients resulting in difficulty in determining the manner in which the disease will progress in severity and in anatomic location and if a patient will respond to medical and/or surgical treatment. Thus several aspects of CD lend themselves to characterization using genetic markers. These include (1) classification of disease phenotype, (2) determining prognosis or the natural history of the disease, (3) predicting response to therapy, and (4) genetic counselling. With several CD–gene associations established to date, a move towards utilizing these correlations between genetic variants and clinical phenotype has begun.

Classification of Disease Phenotype

When all possible combinations of disease location, behavior, and extraintestinal manifestations are considered, several dozen phenotypes of CD are possible. Systems such as the Montreal classification have attempted to provide a general phenotypic categorization system. However, such classification systems are imperfect due to the evolving nature of the disease [105]. By correlating the over 160 SNPs associated with CD with different aspects of the disease in carefully clinically defined patients, it is hoped that a more exact, gene-based classification system may be created in the near future. Possible clinical implications of the development of such a system may include curative colectomy in CD patients whose disease is known to be definitively limited to the colon and favoring intestinal sparing stricturoplasties instead of resection in patients predicted to have recurrent small bowel disease [106]. Identifying such genetic–clinical correlates is difficult however, and confounded by numerous factors, which need to be carefully kept in mind with such studies (Tables 2.1 and 2.2). Known genotype–phenotype associations are shown in Fig. 2.6.

Small Bowel Disease

In an early 2002 genotype–phenotype study of the few CD-associated genes known at that time NOD2 was the first gene to be identified with a disease phenotype, namely ileal disease [9]. This association has been replicated in several subsequent studies [8, 10–12]. As a greater number of CD-associated genes have been discovered, the TNFSF15 gene has also been associated with ileal disease and stricturing behavior with levels of gene expression correlating with severity of inflammation and fibrostenosis [13, 14, 107].

The autophagy gene ATG16L1 and its associated SNP rs2241880 have also been linked with ileal disease in multiple studies including a large Scottish study on familial and sporadic IBD [22]. A separate UK study demonstrated a twofold risk of disease involving the ileum in patients GG homozygous for the same SNP [23]. Similarly, mutations within the IRGM, the neutrophil cytosolic factor 4 (NCF4), TNFSF1a and HLADRB1*07 genes, and the IBD5 locus have also been associated with ileal disease [8, 11, 12, 29]. NCF4 is involved in phagocytosis of pathogens.

These SNP associations can be combined into "risk haplotypes" as seen in a 2012 study by Duraes et al. The authors demonstrated an increasing risk for ileal or ileocolic disease as the number of risk alleles in the ATG16L1, IRGM, and ITLN1 genes present within the individual patient increased in a cohort of 511 CD patients versus 626 controls. A model for the correlation of the number of risk alleles present with the likelihood of ileal or ileocolonic disease was then constructed with an OR of 7.10 for ileal disease in those with all risk alleles seen [24]. A Canadian group similarly found CARD15 and HLA-DRB1 to be associated with ileal disease in their cohort and suggested a similar risk model based on number of combined "risk SNPs" [32].

Non-small Bowel Disease

The STAT5 gene has been associated with small bowel sparing CD [16]. STAT5 has been shown to inhibit Th17 cell differentiation [108] and apoptosis and enhance IL4 secretion by mast cells [109]. Several genes associated with colonic CD such as HLA DRB1*0103 and OCTN1 and OCTN2 are also associated with ulcerative colitis highlighting the overlap between the two diseases [8, 11, 12, 32, 110, 111]. Anal disease is a common and often distressing disease manifestation in CD [112, 113]. SNPs associated with at least four genes have been implicated in severe, fistulizing anal CD, IL10, TAGAP (an adaptive immunity regulating gene) the cation transporter, OCTN1/2 (also known as SLC22A4) [17, 18, 26, 30] and

Table 2.1 Phenotype–genotype correlations

Disease location			Disease behavior			Response to therapy		
Small bowel	Ileocolic	Colonic	Stricturing	Fistulizing	Anal disease	IFX requirement	IFX response	Requirement for surgery
NOD2 [8–14]	IRGM [15]	STAT5A [16]	TNFSF15 [13]	IL10 (pediatrics study) [17]	TAGAP [18]	HLADRB1*0103 [8]	ATG16L1 (pediatric study) [19]	MDR [20, 21]
TNFSF15 [22–24]	ITLN1	OCTN1/2 [8]	NOD2 [25]	OCTN1/2 [26]	OCTN1/2 [26]	MDR1 [27]	5q31 (pediatric study) [19]	TNF (pediatric study) [28]
ATG16L1 [24, 29]	TNFSF15 [13]	TNFSF15 [8]			IL10 [17, 30]		IL1B [31]	IL12B [25]
IRGM [11, 29]		HLADRB1*0103 [8]			NOD2 [25]			IL23R [25]
NCF4 [12, 32]								C11orf30 [25]
TNFSF1a [24]								NOD2 [25]
HLADRB1*07 [24, 32]								
ITLN1 [24]								
IRGM [24]								
NOD2 [32]								

Table 2.2 Key points in critically evaluating a genotype–phenotype study in CD

Gene–phenotype associations may be specific to a certain ethnicity or ethnicities
Studies on disease location are often not limited to a single anatomic location, i.e., studies on ileal disease often include ileocolic disease as well
Due to the variability in disease course, genetic studies on disease location and severity should have a long follow-up with disease carefully categorized clinically
Studies should utilize a statistical correction (such as a Bonferroni correction) of raw p values in light of multiple comparisons inherent to large SNP and gene association studies
Multiple family members should not typically be included in the same study as their similar genetics may affect results

NOD2 [25] offering insight into the pathogenesis of this aspect of the disease [106].

Prediction of Response to Treatment

Predicting Disease Recurrence

Recurrence of ileocolic disease after surgery is common and typically occurs as the result of a stricturing phenotype [114–116]. Recurrence is more common in those who require surgery shortly after diagnosis and in smokers [117]. Medication use, anastomosis type, and family history have been studied as potential predictors of recurrence but results are inconsistent leading

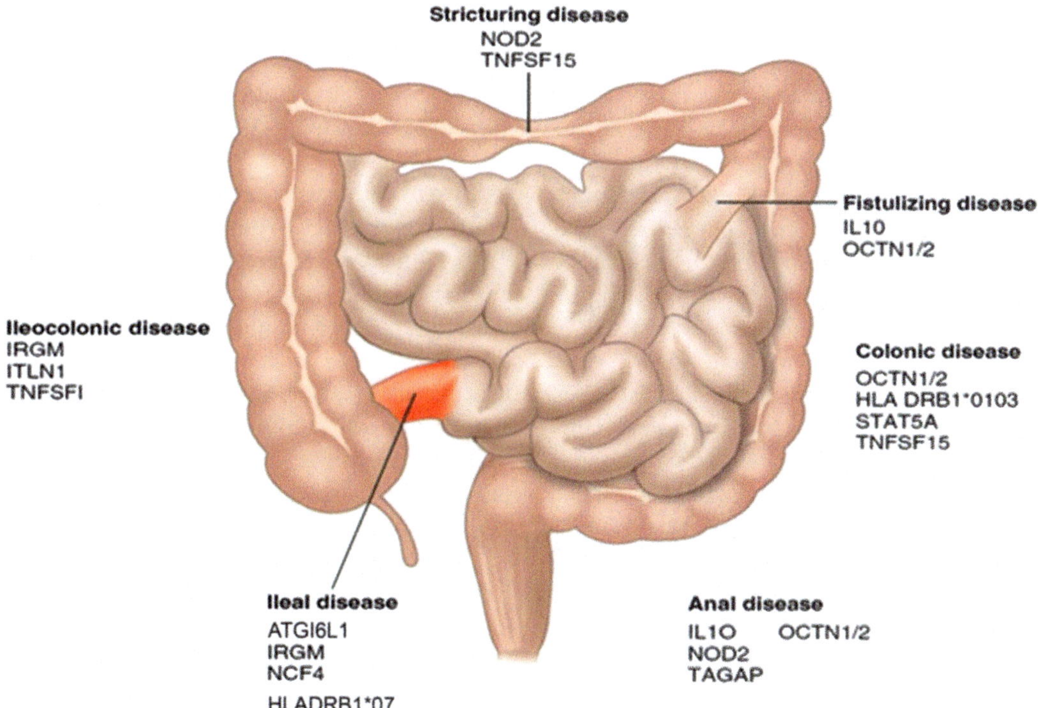

Fig. 2.6 Clinical Correlates of Genetic Suseptibility. Several genotype–phenotype associations in CD have been determined. Behavioral phenotypes such as fistulizing and stricturing disease have genetic correlates. Disease location (small bowel, ileocolic, and colonic) has also been correlated with different genes as demonstrated in the figure

to the search for a genetic marker. The IRGM gene has been associated with early recurrence. In Seghal et al.'s study of over 70 IBD associated SNPs, patients with the IRGM SNP rs4958847 required more frequent ileocolectomies and had an earlier time to reoperation. One surgery was required every 6.8 years in patients with the at risk genotype vs. every 11.4 years in patients with the wildtype allele [15]. In a study by Seiderer et al., 80 patients with small bowel CD were genotyped for the three most common NOD2/CARD15 variants. The presence of at least one variant was seen in over 60 % of patients with stenotic disease. Over 60 % of patients with the 1007fs variant required surgical intervention for stenosis [15].

Medical Therapy Requirement and Response

Due to the side effects, expense and/or propensity of CD drugs to lose their effect with time, a genetic predictor of response to these drugs is being sought. Gene associations with severe disease requiring medical treatment such as HLA DRB1*0103 and MDR1 and the requirement for infliximab [8, 27] and recent studies focusing on the anti-TNF drug class have suggested a genetic component to drug responses. In a GWAS of pediatric IBD and anti-TNF drug response, a small group of CD patients demonstrated that the presence of risk alleles in several CD associated genes including ATG16L1 and the IBD locus 5q31 correlated with a lack of response to infliximab, a member of the anti-TNF drug family [19]. A subsequent adult IBD study inclusive of 29 CD patients failed to show a correlation between polymorphisms in the TNF gene promoter region and response to anti-TNFs. However, the C allele of the IL1B SNP rs1143634 was associated with poorer clinical remission after 14 weeks of infliximab treatment [31].

Due to effects of glucocorticoid use on growth and the delay in widespread use of anti-TNF treatment in the pediatric population, genetic associations with glucocorticoid effectiveness have undergone greater study in the pediatric population. In a study of only four genes in 154 pediatric IBD patients treated with steroids for 30 days, 82 of whom had CD, on multivariate analysis, BclI mutations were significantly associated with response while NACHT leucine-rich-repeat protein 1 (NALP1) mutations were associated with lack of response [118]. However, one study on adult CD patients demonstrated that the presence of a polymorphism in the macrophage migration inhibitory factor (MIF) gene involved in the innate immune response was associated with the need for increased dosages of corticosteroids [119]. A recent study has correlated NOD2/CARD15 mutations with poor response to antibiotics in septic anal disease in 55 CD patients [120].

Although multiple genetic associations with medication response have been suggested, none are currently in use except for the clinical testing of the thiopurine methyl transferase (TPMT) gene and the metabolism of azathioprine and 6 mercaptopurine (6-MP). This commonly administered genetic test determines the presence or absence of a genetic variation that is associated with increased cytotoxicity or lack of drug effectiveness due to altered enzyme activity [59].

Failure of Medical Treatment/The Requirement for Surgery

The new field of "Surgical Genetics" correlates genotype with operative outcomes [3, 106]. Predicting the need for surgery and the likelihood of postoperative recurrence, particularly in ileocolic disease, have been the two foci of surgical genetics in CD to date. In an early genetic study by Farrell et al., multidrug resistance (MDR) gene expression levels in peripheral blood lymphocytes was studied to predict failure of steroid treatment and the need for surgery. Higher expression was demonstrated in these patients. The MDR gene codes for a drug efflux pump [20]. In a pediatric study, patients with a TNF polymorphism (308A allele), demonstrated an OR of 2.1 for requiring surgery compared to patients with the wildtype allele [21]. A more recent study by Dubinsky et al. correlated genotyping results at over 70 known IBD loci in over 1,000 CD patients to discover three CD associated loci that were independently associated with the requirement for surgery within 5 years of diagnosis; IL12B, IL23R, and the transcription regulator, Chromosome 11 open reading frame 30 (C11orf30). They also demonstrated two CD susceptibility loci, 9q34 and 7q21 to be associated with early surgery [28]. The immunoregulatory TNFSF15 gene discussed above has also been associated with medically refractory IBD requiring surgery in UC. It has not yet been studied as a predictor of the requirement for surgery in CD [107].

Genetic Counselling

Due to the increased likelihood of IBD developing in a family member of Crohn's patient, genetic correlations may in the future be used to (1) identify family members who are predetermined to develop IBD, (2) predict the disease phenotype in newly diagnosed patients, (3) select appropriate medical treatment, and (4) select appropriate surgical treatment. No single gene or combination of IBD associated genes has been identified to date for these potential future aims. However, with more focused study, the hope will be that patients identified as high risk by genetic criteria could then be treated either prophylactically to avoid development of the disease or alter the environmental half of the host/environment etiology of the disease pathophysiology to then avoid the development of CD later in life.

References

1. Stappenbeck TS, Rioux JD, Mizoguchi A, Saitoh T, Huett A, Darfeuille-Michaud A, et al. Crohn disease: a current perspective on genetics, autophagy and immunity. Autophagy. 2011;7(4):355–74.
2. Wagner J, Sim WH, Lee KJ, Kirkwood CD. Current knowledge and systematic review of viruses associated with Crohn's disease. Rev Med Virol. 2013;23(3):145–71.
3. Koltun WA. Diagnosis and evaluation. In: Beck DE, Roberts PL, Saclarides TJ, editors. The ASCRS textbook of colon and rectal surgery. 2nd ed. New York: Springer; 2011. p. 449–62.
4. Cho JH, Brant SR. Recent insights into the genetics of inflammatory bowel disease. Gastroenterology. 2011;140(6):1704–12.
5. Ponder A, Long MD. A clinical review of recent findings in the epidemiology of inflammatory bowel disease. Clin Epidemiol. 2013;5:237–47.
6. Bernstein CN, Shanahan F. Disorders of a modern lifestyle: reconciling the epidemiology of inflammatory bowel diseases. Gut. 2008;57(9):1185–91.
7. Nell S, Suerbaum S, Josenhans C. The impact of the microbiota on the pathogenesis of IBD: lessons from mouse infection models. Nat Rev Microbiol. 2010;8(8):564–77.
8. Hancock L, Beckly J, Geremia A, Cooney R, Cummings F, Pathan S, et al. Clinical and molecular characteristics of isolated colonic Crohn's disease. Inflamm Bowel Dis. 2008;14(12):1667–77.
9. Cuthbert AP, Fisher SA, Mirza MM, King K, Hampe J, Croucher PJ, et al. The contribution of NOD2 gene mutations to the risk and site of disease in inflammatory bowel disease. Gastroenterology. 2002;122(4): 867–74.
10. Bhat M, Nguyen GC, Pare P, Lahaie R, Deslandres C, Bernard EJ, et al. Phenotypic and genotypic characteristics of inflammatory bowel disease in French Canadians: comparison with a large North American repository. Am J Gastroenterol. 2009;104(9):2233–40.
11. Fernandez L, Mendoza JL, Martinez A, Urcelay E, Fernandez-Arquero M, Garcia-Paredes J, et al. IBD1 and IBD3 determine location of Crohn's disease in the Spanish population. Inflamm Bowel Dis. 2004;10(6):715–22.
12. Ahmad T, Armuzzi A, Bunce M, Mulcahy-Hawes K, Marshall SE, Orchard TR, et al. The molecular classification of the clinical manifestations of Crohn's disease. Gastroenterology. 2002;122(4):854–66.
13. Barrett R, Zhang X, Koon HW, Vu M, Chang JY, Yeager N, et al. Constitutive TL1A expression under colitogenic conditions modulates the severity and location of gut mucosal inflammation and induces fibrostenosis. Am J Pathol. 2012;180(2):636–49.
14. Shih DQ, Barrett R, Zhang X, Yeager N, Koon HW, Phaosawasdi P, et al. Constitutive TL1A (TNFSF15) expression on lymphoid or myeloid cells leads to mild intestinal inflammation and fibrosis. PLoS One. 2011;6(1):e16090.
15. Sehgal R, Berg A, Polinski JI, Hegarty JP, Lin Z, McKenna KJ, et al. Mutations in IRGM are associated with more frequent need for surgery in patients with ileocolonic Crohn's disease. Dis Colon Rectum. 2012;55(2):115–21.
16. Connelly TM, Koltun WA, Berg AS, Hegarty JP, Brinton D, Deiling S, et al. A single nucleotide polymorphism in the STAT5 gene favors colonic as opposed to small-bowel inflammation in Crohn's disease. Dis Colon Rectum. 2013;56(9):1068–74.
17. Glocker EO, Kotlarz D, Boztug K, Gertz EM, Schaffer AA, Noyan F, et al. Inflammatory bowel disease and mutations affecting the interleukin-10 receptor. N Engl J Med. 2009;361(21):2033–45.
18. Connelly TM, Sehgal R, Berg AS, Hegarty JP, Deiling S, Stewart DB, et al. Mutation in TAGAP is

protective of anal sepsis in ileocolic Crohn's disease. Dis Colon Rectum. 2012;55(11):1145–52.
19. Dubinsky MC, Mei L, Friedman M, Dhere T, Haritunians T, Hakonarson H, et al. Genome wide association (GWA) predictors of anti-TNFalpha therapeutic responsiveness in pediatric inflammatory bowel disease. Inflamm Bowel Dis. 2010;16(8):1357–66.
20. Farrell RJ, Murphy A, Long A, Donnelly S, Cherikuri A, O'Toole D, et al. High multidrug resistance (P-glycoprotein 170) expression in inflammatory bowel disease patients who fail medical therapy. Gastroenterology. 2000;118(2):279–88.
21. Cucchiara S, Latiano A, Palmieri O, Canani RB, D'Inca R, Guariso G, et al. Polymorphisms of tumor necrosis factor-alpha but not MDR1 influence response to medical therapy in pediatric-onset inflammatory bowel disease. J Pediatr Gastroenterol Nutr. 2007;44(2):171–9. PMID: 17255827.
22. Van Limbergen J, Russell RK, Nimmo ER, Drummond HE, Smith L, Anderson NH, et al. Autophagy gene ATG16L1 influences susceptibility and disease location but not childhood-onset in Crohn's disease in Northern Europe. Inflamm Bowel Dis. 2008;14(3):338–46.
23. Prescott NJ, Fisher SA, Franke A, Hampe J, Onnie CM, Soars D, et al. A nonsynonymous SNP in ATG16L1 predisposes to ileal Crohn's disease and is independent of CARD15 and IBD5. Gastroenterology. 2007;132(5):1665–71.
24. Duraes C, Machado JC, Portela F, Rodrigues S, Lago P, Cravo M, et al. Phenotype–genotype profiles in Crohn's disease predicted by genetic markers in autophagy-related genes (GOIA study II). Inflamm Bowel Dis. 2013;19(2):230–9.
25. Seiderer J, Brand S, Herrmann KA, Schnitzler F, Hatz R, Crispin A, et al. Predictive value of the CARD15 variant 1007fs for the diagnosis of intestinal stenoses and the need for surgery in Crohn's disease in clinical practice: results of a prospective study. Inflamm Bowel Dis. 2006;12(12):1114–21.
26. Vermeire S, Pierik M, Hlavaty T, Claessens G, van Schuerbeeck N, Joossens S, et al. Association of organic cation transporter risk haplotype with perianal penetrating Crohn's disease but not with susceptibility to IBD. Gastroenterology. 2005;129(6):1845–53.
27. Potocnik U, Ferkolj I, Glavac D, Dean M. Polymorphisms in multidrug resistance 1 (MDR1) gene are associated with refractory Crohn disease and ulcerative colitis. Genes Immun. 2004;5(7):530–9.
28. Dubinsky MC, Kugathasan S, Kwon S, Haritunians T, Wrobel I, Wahbeh G, et al. Multidimensional prognostic risk assessment identifies association between IL12B variation and surgery in Crohn's disease. Inflamm Bowel Dis. 2013;19(8):1662–70.
29. Roberts RL, Hollis-Moffatt JE, Gearry RB, Kennedy MA, Barclay ML, Merriman TR. Confirmation of association of IRGM and NCF4 with ileal Crohn's disease in a population-based cohort. Genes Immun. 2008;9(6):561–5.
30. Begue B, Verdier J, Rieux-Laucat F, Goulet O, Morali A, Canioni D, et al. Defective IL10 signaling defining a subgroup of patients with inflammatory bowel disease. Am J Gastroenterol. 2011;106(8):1544–55.
31. Lacruz-Guzman D, Torres-Moreno D, Pedrero F, Romero-Cara P, Garcia-Tercero I, Trujillo-Santos J, et al. Influence of polymorphisms and TNF and IL1beta serum concentration on the infliximab response in Crohn's disease and ulcerative colitis. Eur J Clin Pharmacol. 2013;69(3):431–8.
32. Newman B, Silverberg MS, Gu X, Zhang Q, Lazaro A, Steinhart AH, et al. CARD15 and HLA DRB1 alleles influence susceptibility and disease localization in Crohn's disease. Am J Gastroenterol. 2004;99(2):306–15.
33. Summers RW, Elliott DE, Urban Jr JF, Thompson R, Weinstock JV. Trichuris suis therapy in Crohn's disease. Gut. 2005;54(1):87–90.
34. Binder V. Genetic epidemiology in inflammatory bowel disease. Dig Dis. 1998;16(6):351–5.
35. Probert CS, Jayanthi V, Pinder D, Wicks AC, Mayberry JF. Epidemiological study of ulcerative proctocolitis in Indian migrants and the indigenous population of Leicestershire. Gut. 1992;33(5):687–93.
36. Montgomery SM, Morris DL, Pounder RE, Wakefield AJ. Asian ethnic origin and the risk of inflammatory bowel disease. Eur J Gastroenterol Hepatol. 1999;11(5):543–6.
37. Greenstein RJ. Is Crohn's disease caused by a mycobacterium? Comparisons with leprosy, tuberculosis, and Johne's disease. Lancet Infect Dis. 2003;3(8):507–14.
38. Farmer RG, Michener WM, Mortimer EA. Studies of family history among patients with inflammatory bowel disease. Clin Gastroenterol. 1980;9(2):271–7.
39. Halme L, Paavola-Sakki P, Turunen U, Lappalainen M, Farkkila M, Kontula K. Family and twin studies in inflammatory bowel disease. World J Gastroenterol. 2006;12(23):3668–72.
40. Peeters M, Nevens H, Baert F, Hiele M, de Meyer AM, Vlietinck R, et al. Familial aggregation in Crohn's disease: increased age-adjusted risk and concordance in clinical characteristics. Gastroenterology. 1996;111(3):597–603.
41. Colombel JF, Grandbastien B, Gower-Rousseau C, Plegat S, Evrard JP, Dupas JL, et al. Clinical characteristics of Crohn's disease in 72 families. Gastroenterology. 1996;111(3):604–7.
42. Satsangi J, Grootscholten C, Holt H, Jewell DP. Clinical patterns of familial inflammatory bowel disease. Gut. 1996;38(5):738–41.
43. Bayless TM, Tokayer AZ, Polito 2nd JM, Quaskey SA, Mellits ED, Harris ML. Crohn's disease: concordance for site and clinical type in affected family members – potential hereditary influences. Gastroenterology. 1996;111(3):573–9.

44. Parkes M, Jewell D. Ulcerative colitis and Crohns disease: molecular genetics and clinical implications. Expert Rev Mol Med. 2001;2001:1–18.
45. Hugot JP, Chamaillard M, Zouali H, Lesage S, Cezard JP, Belaiche J, et al. Association of NOD2 leucine-rich repeat variants with susceptibility to Crohn's disease. Nature. 2001;411(6837):599–603.
46. Jostins L, Ripke S, Weersma RK, Duerr RH, McGovern DP, Hui KY, et al. Host-microbe interactions have shaped the genetic architecture of inflammatory bowel disease. Nature. 2012;491(7422):119–24.
47. Budarf ML, Labbe C, David G, Rioux JD. GWA studies: rewriting the story of IBD. Trends Genet. 2009;25(3):137–46. PMID: 19217684.
48. Santaolalla R, Abreu MT. Innate immunity in the small intestine. Curr Opin Gastroenterol. 2012;28(2):124–9.
49. Mokry M, Middendorp S, Wiegerinck CL, Witte M, Teunissen H, Meddens CA, et al. Many inflammatory bowel disease risk loci include regions that regulate gene expression in immune cells and the intestinal epithelium. Gastroenterology. 2014;146(4):1040–7.
50. Rutgeerts P, Goboes K, Peeters M, Hiele M, Penninckx F, Aerts R, et al. Effect of faecal stream diversion on recurrence of Crohn's disease in the neoterminal ileum. Lancet. 1991;338(8770):771–4.
51. Man SM, Kaakoush NO, Mitchell HM. The role of bacteria and pattern-recognition receptors in Crohn's disease. Nat Rev Gastroenterol Hepatol. 2011;8(3):152–68.
52. Frank DN, St Amand AL, Feldman RA, Boedeker EC, Harpaz N, Pace NR. Molecular-phylogenetic characterization of microbial community imbalances in human inflammatory bowel diseases. Proc Natl Acad Sci U S A. 2007;104(34):13780–5.
53. Sokol H, Seksik P, Furet JP, Firmesse O, Nion-Larmurier I, Beaugerie L, et al. Low counts of Faecalibacterium prausnitzii in colitis microbiota. Inflamm Bowel Dis. 2009;15(8):1183–9.
54. Hviid A, Svanstrom H, Frisch M. Antibiotic use and inflammatory bowel diseases in childhood. Gut. 2011;60(1):49–54.
55. Kronman MP, Zaoutis TE, Haynes K, Feng R, Coffin SE. Antibiotic exposure and IBD development among children: a population-based cohort study. Pediatrics. 2012;130(4):e794–803.
56. Shaw SY, Blanchard JF, Bernstein CN. Association between the use of antibiotics in the first year of life and pediatric inflammatory bowel disease. Am J Gastroenterol. 2010;105(12):2687–92.
57. Virta L, Auvinen A, Helenius H, Huovinen P, Kolho KL. Association of repeated exposure to antibiotics with the development of pediatric Crohn's disease – a nationwide, register-based Finnish case-control study. Am J Epidemiol. 2012;175(8):775–84.
58. Cario E, Podolsky DK. Differential alteration in intestinal epithelial cell expression of toll-like receptor 3 (TLR3) and TLR4 in inflammatory bowel disease. Infect Immun. 2000;68(12):7010–7.
59. McCauley JL, Abreu MT. Genetics in diagnosing and managing inflammatory bowel disease. Gastroenterol Clin North Am. 2012;41(2):513–22.
60. Abraham C, Cho JH. Inflammatory bowel disease. N Engl J Med. 2009;361(21):2066–78.
61. Kosovac K, Brenmoehl J, Holler E, Falk W, Schoelmerich J, Hausmann M, et al. Association of the NOD2 genotype with bacterial translocation via altered cell–cell contacts in Crohn's disease patients. Inflamm Bowel Dis. 2010;16(8):1311–21.
62. Bonen DK, Ogura Y, Nicolae DL, Inohara N, Saab L, Tanabe T, et al. Crohn's disease-associated NOD2 variants share a signaling defect in response to lipopolysaccharide and peptidoglycan. Gastroenterology. 2003;124(1):140–6.
63. Petersen HJ, Smith AM. The role of the innate immune system in granulomatous disorders. Front Immunol. 2013;4:120.
64. Fisher SA, Tremelling M, Anderson CA, Gwilliam R, Bumpstead S, Prescott NJ, et al. Genetic determinants of ulcerative colitis include the ECM1 locus and five loci implicated in Crohn's disease. Nat Genet. 2008;40(6):710–2.
65. Wellcome Trust Case Control Consortium. Genome-wide association study of 14,000 cases of seven common diseases and 3,000 shared controls. Nature. 2007;447(7145):661–78.
66. Eksteen B, Liaskou E, Adams DH. Lymphocyte homing and its role in the pathogenesis of IBD. Inflamm Bowel Dis. 2008;14(9):1298–312.
67. Biancheri P, Di Sabatino A, Rovedatti L, Giuffrida P, Calarota SA, Vetrano S, et al. Effect of tumor necrosis factor-alpha blockade on mucosal address in cell-adhesion molecule-1 in Crohn's disease. Inflamm Bowel Dis. 2013;19(2):259–64.
68. Adolph TE, Tomczak MF, Niederreiter L, Ko HJ, Bock J, Martinez-Naves E, et al. Paneth cells as a site of origin for intestinal inflammation. Nature. 2013;503(7475):272–6.
69. Van Limbergen J, Wilson DC, Satsangi J. The genetics of Crohn's disease. Annu Rev Genomics Hum Genet. 2009;10:89–116.
70. Marks DJ, Rahman FZ, Sewell GW, Segal AW. Crohn's disease: an immune deficiency state. Clin Rev Allergy Immunol. 2010;38(1):20–31.
71. Schreiber S, Rosenstiel P, Albrecht M, Hampe J, Krawczak M. Genetics of Crohn disease, an archetypal inflammatory barrier disease. Nat Rev Genet. 2005;6(5):376–88.
72. Fanning AS, Jameson BJ, Jesaitis LA, Anderson JM. The tight junction protein ZO-1 establishes a link between the transmembrane protein occludin and the actin cytoskeleton. J Biol Chem. 1998;273(45):29745–53.
73. Poritz LS, Garver KI, Green C, Fitzpatrick L, Ruggiero F, Koltun WA. Loss of the tight junction protein ZO-1 in dextran sulfate sodium induced colitis. J Surg Res. 2007;140(1):12–9.
74. Reuter BK, Pizarro TT. Mechanisms of tight junction dysregulation in the SAMP1/YitFc model of Crohn's disease-like ileitis. Ann N Y Acad Sci. 2009;1165:301–7.
75. Kucharzik T, Walsh SV, Chen J, Parkos CA, Nusrat A. Neutrophil transmigration in inflammatory bowel disease is associated with differential expression of

epithelial intercellular junction proteins. Am J Pathol. 2001;159(6):2001–9.
76. Weber CR, Nalle SC, Tretiakova M, Rubin DT, Turner JR. Claudin-1 and claudin-2 expression is elevated in inflammatory bowel disease and may contribute to early neoplastic transformation. Lab Invest. 2008;88(10):1110–20.
77. Barrett JC, Hansoul S, Nicolae DL, Cho JH, Duerr RH, Rioux JD, et al. Genome-wide association defines more than 30 distinct susceptibility loci for Crohn's disease. Nat Genet. 2008;40(8):955–62.
78. Piazza F, Valens J, Lagasse E, Schindler C. Myeloid differentiation of FdCP1 cells is dependent on Stat5 processing. Blood. 2000;96(4):1358–65.
79. Snow JW, Abraham N, Ma MC, Herndier BG, Pastuszak AW, Goldsmith MA. Loss of tolerance and autoimmunity affecting multiple organs in STAT5A/5B-deficient mice. J Immunol. 2003; 171(10):5042–50.
80. Shuai K, Liu B. Regulation of JAK–STAT signalling in the immune system. Nat Rev Immunol. 2003;3(11):900–11.
81. Stoll M, Corneliussen B, Costello CM, Waetzig GH, Mellgard B, Koch WA, et al. Genetic variation in DLG5 is associated with inflammatory bowel disease. Nat Genet. 2004;36(5):476–80.
82. Nys K, Agostinis P, Vermeire S. Autophagy: a new target or an old strategy for the treatment of Crohn's disease? Nat Rev Gastroenterol Hepatol. 2013;10(7):395–401.
83. Massey DC, Parkes M. Genome-wide association scanning highlights two autophagy genes, ATG16L1 and IRGM, as being significantly associated with Crohn's disease. Autophagy. 2007;3(6):649–51.
84. Singh SB, Davis AS, Taylor GA, Deretic V. Human IRGM induces autophagy to eliminate intracellular mycobacteria. Science. 2006;313(5792):1438–41.
85. Lu XC, Tao Y, Wu C, Zhao PL, Li K, Zheng JY, et al. Association between variants of the autophagy related gene – IRGM and susceptibility to Crohn's disease and ulcerative colitis: a meta-analysis. PLoS One. 2013;8(11):e80602.
86. Cho JH. The genetics and immunopathogenesis of inflammatory bowel disease. Nat Rev Immunol. 2008;8(6):458–66.
87. Brand S. Crohn's disease: Th1, Th17 or both? The change of a paradigm: new immunological and genetic insights implicate Th17 cells in the pathogenesis of Crohn's disease. Gut. 2009;58(8):1152–67.
88. Bouma G, Strober W. The immunological and genetic basis of inflammatory bowel disease. Nat Rev Immunol. 2003;3(7):521–33.
89. Plevy SE, Targan SR. Future therapeutic approaches for inflammatory bowel diseases. Gastroenterology. 2011;140(6):1838–46.
90. Rodriguez-Bores L, Fonseca GC, Villeda MA, Yamamoto-Furusho JK. Novel genetic markers in inflammatory bowel disease. World J Gastroenterol. 2007;13(42):5560–70.
91. Ahmad T, Marshall SE, Jewell D. Genetics of inflammatory bowel disease: the role of the HLA complex. World J Gastroenterol. 2006;12(23):3628–35.
92. Stokkers PC, Reitsma PH, Tytgat GN, van Deventer SJ. HLA-DR and -DQ phenotypes in inflammatory bowel disease: a meta-analysis. Gut. 1999;45(3): 395–401.
93. Silverberg MS, Mirea L, Bull SB, Murphy JE, Steinhart AH, Greenberg GR, et al. A population- and family-based study of Canadian families reveals association of HLA DRB1*0103 with colonic involvement in inflammatory bowel disease. Inflamm Bowel Dis. 2003;9(1):1–9.
94. Yang CR, Hsieh SL, Teng CM, Ho FM, Su WL, Lin WW. Soluble decoy receptor 3 induces angiogenesis by neutralization of TL1A, a cytokine belonging to tumor necrosis factor superfamily and exhibiting angiostatic action. Cancer Res. 2004;64(3):1122–9.
95. Bamias G, Martin 3rd C, Marini M, Hoang S, Mishina M, Ross WG, et al. Expression, localization, and functional activity of TL1A, a novel Th1-polarizing cytokine in inflammatory bowel disease. J Immunol. 2003;171(9):4868–74.
96. Michelsen KS, Thomas LS, Taylor KD, Yu QT, Mei L, Landers CJ, et al. IBD-associated TL1A gene (TNFSF15) haplotypes determine increased expression of TL1A protein. PLoS One. 2009;4(3):e4719.
97. Cavallini C, Lovato O, Bertolaso A, Pacelli L, Zoratti E, Zanolin E, et al. The TNF-family cytokine TL1A inhibits proliferation of human activated B cells. PLoS One. 2013;8(4):e60136.
98. Jones GW, Stumhofer JS, Foster T, Twohig JP, Hertzog P, Topley N, et al. Naive and activated T cells display differential responsiveness to TL1A that affects Th17 generation, maintenance, and proliferation. FASEB J. 2011;25(1):409–19.
99. Meylan F, Song YJ, Fuss I, Villarreal S, Kahle E, Malm IJ, et al. The TNF-family cytokine TL1A drives IL-13-dependent small intestinal inflammation. Mucosal Immunol. 2011;4(2):172–85.
100. Young HA, Tovey MG. TL1A: a mediator of gut inflammation. Proc Natl Acad Sci U S A. 2006;103(22):8303–4.
101. Kang YJ, Kim WJ, Bae HU, Kim DI, Park YB, Park JE, et al. Involvement of TL1A and DR3 in induction of pro-inflammatory cytokines and matrix metalloproteinase-9 in atherogenesis. Cytokine. 2005;29(5):229–35.
102. Targan SR. Crohn's disease: therapeutic implications of disease subtypes. In: Bayless TM, Hanauer S, Hanauer SB, editors. Advanced therapy in inflammatory Bowel disease, vol. 2. 2nd ed. Shelton: PMPH-USA; 2011. p. 633.
103. Connelly T, Koltun W. The TNFSF15 gene single nucleotide polymorphism rs7848647 is associated with surgical diverticulitis. Ann Surg. 2014;259(6):1132–7.
104. Shih DQ, Targan SR, McGovern D. Recent advances in IBD pathogenesis: genetics and immunobiology. Curr Gastroenterol Rep. 2008;10(6):568–75.
105. Satsangi J, Silverberg MS, Vermeire S, Colombel JF. The Montreal classification of inflammatory

bowel disease: controversies, consensus, and implications. Gut. 2006;55(6):749–53.
106. Connelly TM, Koltun WA. The role of genetics in the surgical management of inflammatory bowel disease. Semin Colon Rectal Surg. 2012;23(2): 44–50.
107. Haritunians T, Taylor KD, Targan SR, Dubinsky M, Ippoliti A, Kwon S, et al. Genetic predictors of medically refractory ulcerative colitis. Inflamm Bowel Dis. 2010;16(11):1830–40.
108. O'Shea JJ, Lahesmaa R, Vahedi G, Laurence A, Kanno Y. Genomic views of STAT function in CD4+ T helper cell differentiation. Nat Rev Immunol. 2011;11(4):239–50. PMID: 21436836.
109. Budagian V, Bulanova E, Paus R, Bulfone-Paus S. IL-15/IL-15 receptor biology: a guided tour through an expanding universe. Cytokine Growth Factor Rev. 2006;17(4):259–80.
110. Trachtenberg EA, Yang H, Hayes E, Vinson M, Lin C, Targan SR, et al. HLA class II haplotype associations with inflammatory bowel disease in Jewish (Ashkenazi) and non-Jewish Caucasian populations. Hum Immunol. 2000;61(3):326–33.
111. Gazouli M, Mantzaris G, Archimandritis AJ, Nasioulas G, Anagnou NP. Single nucleotide polymorphisms of OCTN1, OCTN2, and DLG5 genes in Greek patients with Crohn's disease. World J Gastroenterol. 2005;11(47):7525–30.
112. Koltun WA. A paradigm for the management of complex perineal Crohn's disease in the anti-TNF era. Semin Colon Rectal Surg. 2006;17:61–7.
113. Tozer PJ, Burling D, Gupta A, Phillips RK, Hart AL. Review article: medical, surgical and radiological management of perianal Crohn's fistulas. Aliment Pharmacol Ther. 2011;33(1):5–22.
114. Greenstein AJ, Lachman P, Sachar DB, Springhorn J, Heimann T, Janowitz HD, et al. Perforating and non-perforating indications for repeated operations in Crohn's disease: evidence for two clinical forms. Gut. 1988;29(5):588–92.
115. Fichera A, Lovadina S, Rubin M, Cimino F, Hurst RD, Michelassi F. Patterns and operative treatment of recurrent Crohn's disease: a prospective longitudinal study. Surgery. 2006;140(4):649–54.
116. Maconi G, Colombo E, Sampietro GM, Lamboglia F, D'Inca R, Daperno M, et al. CARD15 gene variants and risk of reoperation in Crohn's disease patients. Am J Gastroenterol. 2009;104(10): 2483–91.
117. Cristaldi M, Sampietro GM, Danelli PG, Bollani S, Bianchi Porro G, Taschieri AM. Long-term results and multivariate analysis of prognostic factors in 138 consecutive patients operated on for Crohn's disease using "bowel-sparing" techniques. Am J Surg. 2000;179(4):266–70.
118. De Iudicibus S, Stocco G, Martelossi S, Londero M, Ebner E, Pontillo A, et al. Genetic predictors of glucocorticoid response in pediatric patients with inflammatory bowel diseases. J Clin Gastroenterol. 2011;45(1):e1–7.
119. Griga T, Wilkens C, Wirkus N, Epplen J, Schmiegel W, Klein W. A polymorphism in the macrophage migration inhibitory factor gene is involved in the genetic predisposition of Crohn's disease and associated with cumulative steroid doses. Hepatogastroenterology. 2007;54(75):784–6.
120. Freire P, Portela F, Donato MM, Ferreira M, Andrade P, Sofia C. CARD15 mutations and perianal fistulating Crohn's disease: correlation and predictive value of antibiotic response. Dig Dis Sci. 2011;56(3):853–9.

Medical Therapy for Crohn's Disease: The Present

3

Rebecca A. Fausel and Timothy L. Zisman

Introduction

Treatment options for Crohn's disease have been developing and expanding rapidly over the past 10 years. Multiple classes of medications are currently available to treat Crohn's disease, including 5-aminosalicylates (5-ASA), antibiotics, glucocorticoids, thiopurine immunosuppressives, methotrexate, tumor necrosis factor (TNF) alpha antagonists, and anti-integrin therapies. Goals of treatment have expanded beyond relief of symptoms to include maintenance of long-term remission, avoidance of corticosteroids and their associated side effects, and prevention of disease complications such as fistulas, strictures, and abscesses. Additional aims of therapy are to avoid the need for surgical intervention, minimize the risk of colorectal cancer, and to maintain adequate nutrition and improve quality of life. The benefits of medications in achieving these outcomes must be balanced with the potential drawbacks, including the increased risks of serious infections, malignancies, and substantial financial burden for both individual patients and society.

R.A. Fausel, MD • T.L. Zisman, MD, MPH (✉)
Division of Gastroenterology, University of Washington Medical Center, 1959 NE Pacific Street, Box 356424, Seattle, WA 98195, USA
e-mail: rfausel@medicine.washington.edu; tzisman@medicine.washington.edu; tzisman@uw.edu

Aminosalicylates

Sulfasalazine is composed of 5-aminosalicylic acid (5-ASA) linked to sulfapyridine by an azo-bond that is cleaved in the presence of colonic bacteria to release the active 5-ASA (mesalamine) component. Other 5-ASA formulations have various delayed- and sustained-release formulations to promote absorption in targeted segments of the GI tract, typically aimed at the distal small bowel and/or colon. The mechanism of action of 5-ASA is incompletely understood, but thought to include topical anti-inflammatory properties, including inhibition of cytokine synthesis, free radical scavenging, and impairment of white blood cell adhesion and function [1].

Aminosalicylates have been widely used with success for ulcerative colitis, but evidence of benefit in Crohn's disease is less compelling with studies demonstrating mixed results. Early studies of sulfasalazine demonstrated a modest benefit in inducing remission (but not maintaining remission) in patients with Crohn's colitis, using a dose of approximately 1 gram per 15 kg of body weight [2]. However, subsequent studies of mesalamine, including a 2004 meta-analysis showed only a modest and clinically insignificant treatment effect [3, 4].

Subsequent to this, a Cochrane meta-analysis in 2010 showed a small benefit with sulfasalazine: it was more likely to induce remission than

A. Fichera and M.K. Krane (eds.), *Crohn's Disease: Basic Principles*,
DOI 10.1007/978-3-319-14181-7_3, © Springer International Publishing Switzerland 2015

placebo (RR 1.38), with a benefit seen mostly in patients with disease confined to the colon [5]. Mesalamine was not more effective than placebo for inducing remission or response. Similarly, a 2011 meta-analysis of 22 randomized controlled trials showed a trend toward benefit of sulfasalazine over placebo for active Crohn's disease (RR 0.83 of failure to achieve remission), but no clear benefit of mesalamine over placebo for the same purpose [6]. Neither sulfasalazine nor mesalamine was effective for preventing relapse of quiescent Crohn's disease, and neither has demonstrated a steroid-sparing effect. Without clear evidence supporting its efficacy in Crohn's disease, aminosalicylate therapy is not widely used or recommended at this time. However, sulfasalazine may have a role in treating mild-moderate Crohn's colitis.

Adverse effects of sulfasalazine lead to discontinuation of the medication in about 20–25 % of patients and are generally related to the sulfapyridine component [7]. Idiosyncratic reactions include rash, hepatitis, pancreatitis, pneumonitis, agranulocytosis, aplastic anemia, lupus-like reactions, Stevens–Johnson syndrome, and allergic reactions to the sulfa moiety. Agranulocytosis typically occurs within the first 3 months of treatment and can rarely be fatal. Compete blood cell counts and liver function tests should be monitored frequently during the first 6 months of therapy. Dose related effects can include nausea, anorexia, dyspepsia, leukopenia, hemolytic anemia, and headache. Sulfasalazine is also associated with oligospermia in men, which is reversible after discontinuation. Folic acid supplementation is recommended during sulfasalazine treatment to prevent the effects of medication-induced folic acid deficiency [7]. Adverse effects of mesalamine are less common, but can include nausea, headache, diarrhea, pancreatitis, and pneumonitis. Rarely, patients can develop worsening of their colitis symptoms, sometimes associated with fever and rash [8]. Nephrotoxicity is also a rare side effect, most often caused by acute or chronic interstitial nephritis with a risk of approximately 1 per 4,000 patients per year, and so renal function should be monitored periodically during therapy [9].

Antibiotics

Antibiotics have a role in treating infectious complications of Crohn's disease, including perianal and intra-abdominal abscesses, and in the longer term management of perianal fistulizing disease, and prevention of recurrence after ileocecal resection. Antibiotics may also play a role to a lesser extent in reducing mucosal inflammation in luminal Crohn's disease. It is hypothesized that the effect of antibiotics on intestinal inflammation may be mediated through alterations of the intestinal microbiota, resulting in a decreased antigenic stimulus in patients with a genetic predisposition to immune dysregulation.

Antibiotics that have historically been used for Crohn's disease include metronidazole and ciprofloxacin, although more recent studies have evaluated a potential role for rifaximin. Studies of metronidazole in active Crohn's disease have not consistently signaled a clear benefit over placebo, although there has been a suggestion of symptom reduction in patients with colonic disease [10]. A small randomized controlled trial of combination ciprofloxacin and metronidazole versus methylprednisolone in active Crohn's disease showed similar rates of clinical remission at 12 weeks [11]. Unfortunately, long-term use of metronidazole is associated with many side effects, including peripheral neuropathy, dysgeusia, and nausea, causing a significant percentage of patients to discontinue the therapy [12].

In the treatment of perianal fistulizing disease, an open-label study of metronidazole showed complete or advanced healing in 15 of 18 patients treated with metronidazole [13]. However, only 28 % of patients were able to stop the medication without fistula recurrence. In patients with recurrent fistulizing disease after cessation of metronidazole, healing was again observed when metronidazole was re-introduced [14]. A small pilot study of ciprofloxacin for perianal disease showed a numerical improvement in patients with complete fistula closure (40 % versus 12.5 %), but this was not statistically significant given the small sample size [15]. Two other studies have shown that antibiotics can enhance the effect of TNF inhibitors for healing of perianal fistulas. A recent study of adalimumab in combination with ciprofloxacin showed that patients treated with the antibiotic and anti-TNF agent together had a significantly greater rate of clinical response (defined as 50 % closure of fistulas) and remission (defined as complete closure of fistulas) at week 12, compared with those patients treated with adalimumab alone [16]. However, this effect was not sustained at week 24 after the antibiotic was stopped. In a similar study of infliximab plus ciprofloxacin, there was a trend toward improved efficacy using the combination of medications compared with infliximab monotherapy (73 % versus 39 %), but this was not statistically significant given the small sample size [17].

Rifaximin is a non-absorbable antibiotic with a broad-spectrum of activity against intestinal microbes. The lack of absorption results in fewer systemic side effects and improved long-term tolerability, making rifaximin an appealing candidate for treatment of Crohn's disease. Several studies have demonstrated a modest clinical benefit for rifaximin in maintaining steroid-induced remission, and inducing response or remission in active luminal disease [18–20].

In a meta-analysis of antimicrobial therapy for Crohn's disease, antibiotics as a general category were superior to placebo for induction of remission (RR 0.85 for lack of remission), and rifamycin derivatives including rifaximin appeared to be most effective for this purpose. Antibiotics also reduced fistula drainage (RR 0.8) and relapse of quiescent disease (RR 0.62) [21]. Overall, antibiotics may be more effective for colonic disease, due to the higher burden of bacteria in this area, and they have a particular role as adjunctive therapy for healing of perianal fistulas. However, traditional antibiotics including metronidazole and ciprofloxacin require continued therapy to maintain effectiveness and have frequent side effects, thus limiting their use. Studies of rifaximin suggest a benefit for treating mucosal inflammation without major identified side effects, although the benefits appear to be relatively small at this point.

Glucocorticoids

Glucocorticoids are highly effective for the short-term control of Crohn's disease-related symptoms, but they are less effective for maintenance of remission, and have significant adverse effects that preclude safe long-term administration [22]. They work by interacting with glucocorticoid receptors in the cell nucleus to alter expression of inflammatory genes, inhibit the expression of adhesion molecules, and inhibit the migration of inflammatory cells into tissues [23].

In a 23-year population-based study of the natural history of Crohn's disease, the short-term benefit of steroids was substantial with 84 % of patients demonstrating complete or partial response at 30 days [24]. However, only 32 % of these patients were able to maintain remission at the end of a year without ongoing steroid use. Another 28 % were steroid dependent and 39 % required surgery by 1 year. This study highlights the excellent short-term efficacy of steroids but also underscores the need for steroid-sparing therapy to maintain the initial response to steroids. Several other studies have confirmed the efficacy of systemic glucocorticoids for induction of remission in active Crohn's disease [25, 26].

Despite their benefit for induction of remission, systemic glucocorticoids have numerous adverse effects that prohibit sustained administration. Short-term side effects can include psychiatric disturbances such as anxiety, emotional lability, psychosis, and insomnia. Other potential effects can include hypertension, hyperglycemia, acne, fungal, viral, and bacterial infections, and weight gain. Long-term effects can include cataracts, glaucoma, osteoporosis, avascular necrosis, diabetes mellitus, steroid induced myopathy, and adrenal insufficiency. In a safety registry of Crohn's disease patients, corticosteroid use was independently associated with higher risk of mortality (HR 2.14) and serious infection (HR 1.57) [27].

Because of the multiple side effects associated with these medications, budesonide has been studied as an alternative glucocorticoid treatment.

Budesonide is a topical glucocorticoid with high affinity for the glucocorticoid receptors (200 times that of prednisolone) that delivers steroid locally to the distal ileum and proximal colon [28]. Because of extensive first pass metabolism in the liver, only 10–15 % of the oral dose is systemically active, leading to fewer side effects compared with traditional glucocorticoids. Abnormal responses to ACTH tests were less common in budesonide-treated patients compared to those receiving systemic glucocorticoids, but still more common than in patients receiving placebo, confirming there is a small degree of systemic activity with budesonide [29]. Budesonide is more effective than placebo but less effective than prednisone in inducing remission in patients with active luminal Crohn's disease, and the greatest benefit appears to be in patients with ileal or proximal colonic disease. Budesonide is not effective for the prevention of relapse in patients with quiescent Crohn's disease [26].

With regard to maintenance therapy, a 2003 meta-analysis of corticosteroids showed no benefit as maintenance therapy at 6, 12, and 24 months when compared with placebo [30]. Meta-analyses of budesonide have similarly demonstrated a lack of improvement over placebo in maintenance of remission at 3, 6, and 12 months [31]. Because of their potential side effects and lack of maintenance efficacy data, corticosteroids are typically only used for short-term treatment of an acute disease exacerbation, or as a bridge to maintenance therapy with a steroid-sparing agent.

Thiopurine Immunosuppressives

Azathioprine is a pro-drug that is converted into 6-mercaptopurine (6-MP) and is subsequently metabolized by one of three different enzymes to form either active or inactive metabolites [32]. There is substantial inter-individual variation in azathioprine metabolism so an understanding of these mechanisms is essential to safe and effective administration of thiopurine therapy. Metabolism of 6-MP by xanthine oxidase produces 6-thiouric acid, which is inactive. Metabolism by hypoxanthine phosphoribosyltransferase produces the active 6-thioguanine (6-TG) nucleotides which are associated with improved efficacy in Crohn's disease, but also an increased risk of leukopenia. Lastly, metabolism by thiopurine methyltransferase (TPMT) produces an inactive metabolite, 6-methylmercaptopurine (6-MMP), which can be hepatotoxic at higher concentrations. The active metabolite, 6-TG, is a purine analogue that incorporates into cellular DNA, inhibits proliferation of lymphocytes, and stimulates apoptosis of T cells in the lamina propria. There are genetic polymorphisms in TPMT enzyme activity that profoundly impact the metabolism of azathioprine. It is advised to check TPMT activity prior to initiating thiopurines in order to select optimal dosing and avoid toxicity. One in 300 patients has very low or absent TPMT activity, which can lead to severe leukopenia even with small doses of azathioprine and another 11 % have intermediate enzyme activity and may require dose reduction [32]. For patients with a high 6-MMP to 6-TG ratio, a xanthine oxidase inhibitor, allopurinol, can be added in conjunction with thiopurine dose reduction in order to favorably alter the 6-TG and 6-MMP metabolite profile. The addition of allopurinol in these patients has been shown to improve disease activity scores, reduce daily prednisone dosage, and decrease aminotransferase levels [33]. However, this strategy carries a significant risk of leukopenia and requires close follow-up and careful monitoring [34].

The initial report of successful azathioprine use for IBD was in 1969 in a case series of six patients with severe Crohn's disease [35]. Subsequently a 2-year randomized controlled trial in Crohn's disease showed patients who received 6-MP were more likely to experience clinical improvement (67 % versus 8 %), closure of fistulas, and reduction in steroid dosing than those who received placebo. The response to azathioprine took between 3 and 6 months to see full effect [36]. A second randomized controlled trial in 1995 evaluated patients concurrently treated with a 12-week tapering course of prednisolone in addition to azathioprine 2.5 mg/kg versus placebo [37]. This landmark trial showed a significant difference in steroid-free remission at 15 months, but no difference at 12 weeks, again suggesting that thiopurines are effective in maintaining remission in Crohn's disease, but may not be effective for short-term induction therapy.

Despite these early studies showing significant benefit for thiopurines, enthusiasm for this class of medication has been tempered by recent prospective studies with larger patient enrollment demonstrating a more modest treatment benefit. A 2013 open-label trial of adults recently diagnosed with Crohn's disease (within 6 months) evaluated the early use of azathioprine compared with conventional management (defined as azathioprine only in case of steroid dependency, frequent flares, severe perianal disease, or poor steroid response) [38]. There was no difference in time spent in steroid and anti-TNF free remission during the first 3 years when comparing the two groups, although there was a lower rate of perianal surgery in the early azathioprine group. By then end of the study 61 % of the patients in the conventional therapy group had been started on azathioprine. A similar double blind prospective study of azathioprine versus placebo within 8 weeks of disease diagnosis (only other medication allowed was corticosteroids) showed no difference in corticosteroid free remission at 76 weeks, although azathioprine did reduce the rate of moderate-severe relapse [39]. These studies suggest there is limited benefit to monotherapy with thiopurines early in the course of disease, for the endpoint of steroid-free remission [40]. Long-term cohort studies have shown that early azathioprine use within 3 years of initial diagnosis was associated with a reduced risk of initial abdominal surgery (HR 0.45), recurrent abdominal surgery (HR 0.44), and perianal surgery (HR 0.30) [41]. Overall, the risk of first major abdominal surgery in this cohort was 17.5 % at 1 year, 28.4 % at 5 years, and 39.5 % at 10 years. Similarly, a recently published large meta-analysis of 17 observational studies and 21,632 patients showed a 40 % reduced risk of surgical resection in patients who received thiopurines [42]. These studies suggest that thiopurine therapy may have important long-term protective effects, perhaps unseen in shorter efficacy studies.

Side effects with thiopurines are common and are an important consideration when treating patients with Crohn's disease. In a long-term prospectively maintained database of Spanish IBD patients on thiopurines over a median follow-up of 44 months, 17 % of patients discontinued treatment due to adverse events [43]. The most frequent side effects were nausea (8 %), hepatotoxicity (4 %), myelotoxicity (4 %), and pancreatitis (4 %). Other potential adverse events associated with azathioprine include allergic reactions, rash, fever, headache, fatigue, anorexia, cholestatic hepatitis, and arthralgias. Approximately 50 % of patients who discontinue azathioprine due to adverse events can subsequently tolerate 6-MP, but this should not be prescribed to patients who experienced bone marrow suppression or pancreatitis [44].

As many as 1.8 % of patients experience a serious infection with long-term azathioprine use [45]. Interestingly, in a 5-year follow-up analysis of the TREAT registry (a large prospective observational research program to evaluate the long-term safety of medications for Crohn's), thiopurine immunosuppressives were not independently associated with a significantly increased risk of serious infection or mortality [27].

Studies have demonstrated an approximately three to sevenfold increased risk of non-Hodgkin's lymphoma in patients treated with thiopurines, although the absolute risk is still very low [46]. This risk increases with age, and also increases significantly after 1–2 years of thiopurine exposure, but returns to baseline after thiopurines are stopped [46–48]. Cases of hepatosplenic T cell lymphoma have been reported in IBD patients taking thiopurines. This is a rare, aggressive, almost universally fatal extranodal lymphoma that primarily affects males younger than 35 [49]. Among reported cases, the vast majority had at least 2 years of thiopurine exposure, with a median duration of 5 years [49]. Thiopurines are also associated with an increased risk of non-melanoma skin cancer with a pooled adjusted hazard ratio of 2.28 [50]. Interestingly, the statistical significance was lost when studies with shorter follow-up (less than 6 years) were excluded, suggesting a possible surveillance bias.

Regardless, patients receiving thiopurines should be counseled on the importance of sun protection and regular skin exams.

Methotrexate

Methotrexate is a structural analogue of folic acid that competitively inhibits its binding to its receptors and has demonstrated effectiveness for treating several autoimmune diseases, including rheumatoid arthritis and psoriasis. Possible mechanisms of its anti-inflammatory action include increased concentrations of adenosine, inhibition of methylation functions necessary for cell replication, and apoptosis of T cells [51]. A randomized placebo-controlled trial evaluating the use of intramuscular methotrexate for induction therapy in patients with active Crohn's disease showed a significant benefit in inducing clinical remission at 16 weeks (39 % versus 19 %), as well as a reduction in prednisone dosing [52]. Adverse events leading to discontinuation occurred in 17 % of the methotrexate group, primarily due to serum aminotransferase elevations or nausea. Patients who achieved clinical remission in this study were then re-randomized to a maintenance trial of continued methotrexate 15 mg weekly versus placebo for 40 more weeks. Those who received maintenance methotrexate were more likely to remain in remission and less likely to require steroids, compared with those who received placebo (65 % versus 39 %) [53]. In a few small, randomized controlled trials, oral methotrexate monotherapy has not shown any benefit for treatment of Crohn's [54, 55].

In addition to nausea and liver function test abnormalities, side effects of methotrexate can include stomatitis, diarrhea, headache, hair loss, infections, bone marrow depression, and interstitial pneumonitis. Hepatic fibrosis has been seen with long-term methotrexate use and requires vigilant monitoring of liver enzymes with dose reduction or discontinuation of methotrexate if hepatotoxicity occurs [56]. Methotrexate is highly teratogenic, so women of childbearing capacity should be counseled about this risk and are advised to use highly effective contraception while on methotrexate. Additionally, methotrexate can induce a reversible oligospermia and the safety of male partner methotrexate use during conception is unknown. Consequently, men are counseled to discontinue methotrexate at least 3 months in advance of trying to conceive a pregnancy. Folic acid supplementation is recommended uniformly to prevent folate deficiency and reduce side effects [1]. In recognition of the lack of high quality data and the slow onset of action, methotrexate is not currently endorsed as a first line option for induction of remission in Crohn's disease, but may have a role in treating patients who have failed other options [57]. In current practice, methotrexate is more commonly used in combination with anti-TNF agents, and its use in this capacity will be discussed later in this review.

Tumor Necrosis Factor-Alpha (TNF-α) Inhibitors

TNF-α is a pro-inflammatory cytokine that plays a pivotal role in the pathogenesis of IBD and has been found in increased concentrations in the mucosa and stool of patients with Crohn's disease. There are currently three available anti-TNF monoclonal antibodies approved for use in Crohn's disease. Infliximab is a chimeric mouse-human IgG1 monoclonal antibody, whereas adalimumab is a humanized IgG1 antibody and certolizumab pegol is a pegylated Fab' fragment. All three TNF inhibitors bind with high specificity and affinity to soluble and membrane-bound TNF-α, leading to neutralization of its biological activity. Infliximab and adalimumab, but not certolizumab pegol, also induce apoptosis of TNF expressing cells.

The first randomized controlled trial of infliximab in 1997 evaluated a single infusion in 108 patients with active Crohn's disease and demonstrated clinical response at week 2 in 81 % of the infliximab-treated patients versus 17 % of the placebo-treated patients [58]. Subsequently, the ACCENT 1 trial evaluated the use of repeated infliximab infusions for maintenance therapy in moderate-severe Crohn's disease [59]. In total,

58 % of patients responded within 2 weeks to the initial infusion of infliximab, and those randomized to receive ongoing infusions achieved a 39 % remission rate at week 30, compared with 21 % of placebo-treated patients. When all patients treated with infliximab were pooled, the odds ratio of sustained clinical remission with infliximab compared to placebo was 2.7 and three times as many patients in the infliximab group were able to discontinue steroids. Interestingly, the real life experience with infliximab seems to be even better than the clinical trials. In a Canadian cohort of 130 patients, most on concurrent immunomodulators, 83 % maintained clinical response at 30 weeks and 64 % at 54 weeks [60]. Another study detailing a large single center experience with infliximab showed an 82 % response to infliximab induction, and a 66 % sustained clinical benefit [61].

Infliximab has also proven effective for treatment of fistulas in Crohn's disease. The initial study of its use for this indication included 94 patients with draining abdominal or perianal fistulas [62]. Of the patients who received 5 mg/kg infliximab induction dosing, 68 % had a reduction of at least 50 % in the number of draining fistulas, compared to 26 % of the placebo group, and 55 % of the patients in the infliximab group had complete closure of their fistulas. Subsequently, the landmark ACCENT II trial demonstrated that continued infusions of infliximab every 8 weeks was more effective than placebo in maintaining fistula closure [63]. In this study 36 % of patients in the infliximab arm had a complete absence of draining fistulas at week 54, a statistically significant increase from the placebo group. In this same trial, infliximab was effective for inducing and maintaining closure of rectovaginal fistulas, and reducing the number of hospital days, surgeries, and procedures [64, 65].

Adalimumab has shown similar efficacy for induction of moderately to severely active Crohn's disease, with 59 % of patients demonstrating response and 36 % achieving remission at 4 weeks [66]. Among initial responders to induction therapy, more than one third were still in remission at 1 year with maintenance doses of adalimumab [67]. Rates of response and remission were inversely correlated with duration of disease [68]. A secondary analysis of patients with fistulizing disease showed a significant improvement in mean number of draining fistulas per day in the adalimumab group compared with placebo [69]. At the end of 56 weeks, 33 % of patients on adalimumab had complete fistula healing versus (13 % placebo) and among these patients 90 % maintained fistula healing after an additional year of adalimumab. Adalimumab is also effective for patients with prior exposure to infliximab who developed a secondary loss of response or intolerance. However, the response and remission rates are lower than in TNF-naïve patients [67, 70].

The most recently approved TNF-α inhibitor used in the treatment of Crohn's disease is certolizumab pegol, a pegylated humanized Fab' fragment. Unlike infliximab and adalimumab, certolizumab has not been shown to induce apoptosis of inflammatory cells. The initial study evaluating certolizumab showed, among patients with an elevated CRP, 37 % of patients had a clinical response at week 6, compared with 26 % in the placebo group [71]. At week 26, there was no significant difference in rates of remission. In the PRECISE II study of certolizumab maintenance, 64 % of patients responded to induction therapy by 6 weeks [72]. Among these initial responders, those who continued to receive certolizumab had a 48 % remission rate at week 26 versus 29 % of the placebo group. A sub-analysis showed that patients with a shorter disease duration (<1 year) at study entry had a significantly greater rate of clinical response and remission than those with longer disease duration [73]. Certolizumab therapy was also associated with a significantly increased chance of perianal fistula closure in an open-label study and has been shown to be effective in patients who have experienced secondary failure of infliximab [74, 75].

Unfortunately, many patients who initially respond to anti-TNF therapy will eventually experience loss of response [76, 77]. One of the common and well-recognized mechanisms for attenuation of response is mediated by the development of anti-drug antibodies [78]. These antibodies directed against the TNF antagonist molecule can result in drug-neutralization or accelerated clearance, leading to loss of clinical effectiveness. Strategies to prevent anti-drug antibody development include an induction dosing regimen, scheduled rather than episodic maintenance therapy, and co-administration of a thiopurine immunosuppressive or methotrexate [78, 79]. If loss of response does occur, this can often be overcome by dose escalation or switch to another TNF antagonist and this management decision can be guided by monitoring of drug levels and anti-drug antibodies. Severe disease activity (as indicated by high CRP, high TNF levels, and low albumin) is also associated with accelerated clearance of TNF antagonists [78]. This observation suggests that TNF antagonists should not be reserved for use only as a rescue therapy in the setting of severe disease, and when they are used in this setting higher doses may be required.

Potential adverse events associated with anti-TNF therapies include injection site or infusion reactions, neutropenia, demyelinating disease, hepatotoxicity, serious infections, congestive heart failure, rash and induction of autoimmunity. Worsening of demyelinating disorders has been described with anti-TNF agents and consequently it is recommended to avoid these medications in patients with a history of demyelinating neurologic disease [80]. In general, TNF inhibitors should also be avoided in patients with advanced heart failure, as they have been associated with increased mortality in these patients [81]. Approximately 50 % of patients receiving infliximab develop antinuclear antibodies after 2 years, but drug-induced lupus is rare [82]. Paradoxical development of a psoriasiform rash has been described with TNF antagonists and often resolves with cessation of the anti-TNF agent. The risk of recurrence of psoriasis with a second TNF antagonist is about 50 % [83]. Serious infections occur in 2–4 % of patients treated with anti-TNF therapy annually [84]. Patients and their providers should be aware of this risk and vigilant monitoring and early workup of infectious symptoms is advised. Tuberculosis and Hepatitis B testing should be performed prior to initiating therapy, with initiation of treatment or vaccination for these infections as appropriate.

Lymphomas have been described in patients on TNF antagonists at rates higher than the general population [85]. It is difficult to definitively attribute the lymphoma risk to TNF inhibitors alone, since most patients in whom this risk was studied were on concurrent or previous thiopurine therapy [86, 87]. Regardless, the absolute risk of lymphoma with a TNF antagonist and thiopurine in combination is low [86]. Hepatosplenic T cell lymphoma is a rare and particularly aggressive form of lymphoma that is seen primarily in young male patients with IBD on combination therapy with TNF antagonists and thiopurines [49]. Consequently combination therapy should be carefully considered in this high risk group. Patients on TNF inhibitors may also have a two to threefold increased risk of non-melanoma skin cancer, although studies have been mixed [88]. Additionally, there is likely a small increased risk of melanoma [89]. Patients taking TNF inhibitor therapy should be advised on the importance of sun protection and regular skin exams. Despite the small increased risk of lymphomas and skin cancers, overall malignancy risk is not elevated in patients on TNF antagonist therapy [90].

Anti-Integrin Therapies

Integrins are glycoproteins expressed on the surface of circulating leukocytes and mediate their adhesion to the vascular endothelium and their subsequent migration into adjacent tissue. Anti-integrin therapies have been developed to selectively block this critical step in the recruitment of leukocytes to the gut in patients with inflammatory bowel disease. Natalizumab, the first anti-integrin therapy studied in Crohn's disease is a humanized IgG4 monoclonal antibody that leads to inhibition of both $\alpha 4\beta 7$ integrin (responsible for leukocyte trafficking to the GI tract) and $\alpha 4\beta 1$ (responsible for leukocyte trafficking to the central nervous system). As a result, natalizumab induces a selective immunosuppression of both the GI tract and the brain and has demonstrated benefit in treating both Crohn's disease and multiple sclerosis. Results of the pivotal ENCORE and ENACT studies showed that natalizumab was superior to placebo for induction and maintenance of response and remission in patients with moderately to severely active Crohn's disease [91–93]. The benefit of natalizumab was most pronounced for patients with an elevated CRP at baseline and in those previously treated with anti-TNF therapy.

Unfortunately, use of natalizumab has been associated with an increased risk of progressive multifocal leukoencephalopathy (PML), a rare but devastating demyelinating disease of the CNS caused by reactivation of the JC polyomavirus [94, 95]. PML usually presents with sub-acute neurologic deficits, including cognitive deficits (48 %), motor deficits (37 %), language disturbances (31 %), and visual difficulties (26 %) [95]. Although JC virus infection is quite common (affecting up to 86 % of the general population) PML is only seen in immunosuppressed individuals, suggesting that depletion of CNS lymphocytes is responsible for the increased risk in natalizumab-treated patients. Among patients receiving natalizumab, concomitant immunosuppression, longer duration of natalizumab therapy, and a positive JC virus antibody test at baseline or during treatment are all associated with a higher risk of PML [96]. In recognition of the risk of PML, patients receiving natalizumab must be enrolled in a safety monitoring program that involves periodic testing for JC virus antibody, avoidance of adjunctive immunosuppression, and consideration of drug holidays for patients on long-term therapy.

Vedolizumab is a humanized monoclonal IgG1 antibody specific for the $\alpha4\beta7$ integrin that does not cross-react with $\alpha4\beta1$, and does not interfere with leukocyte migration to the CNS. This is supported by studies showing no alteration of the lymphocyte composition in the cerebrospinal fluid of patients treated with vedolizumab [97]. Additionally, no cases of PML have been observed among the 3,000 patients who received vedolizumab in clinical trials, including nearly 1,000 patients with 2 years or more of continuous exposure [98, 99]. The efficacy of vedolizumab for inducing remission in active Crohn's disease was modest with 14.5 % of patients achieving remission at week 6, compared to 6.8 % of patients receiving placebo [98]. However, the maintenance data were better with 39 % of vedolizumab patients and 21 % of placebo patients in remission at week 52. Among patients with previous anti-TNF treatment, there was no statistically significant difference in clinical remission at 6 weeks, but there was a statistical benefit at 10 weeks, suggesting that vedolizumab has a slower onset of effect than anti-TNF agents, but is effective in patients with prior anti-TNF failure [99]. The only adverse effect that occurred more frequently in the vedolizumab group was nasopharyngitis, but the long-term safety of this novel therapy is not yet established. Additionally, the benefit of vedolizumab for treatment of fistulizing disease, extra-intestinal manifestations or prevention of post-operative recurrence remain to be determined.

Treatment Strategy

The natural history of Crohn's disease involves fluctuating periods of disease quiescence punctuated by episodes of exacerbation. Cumulative bowel injury occurs over time with chronic smoldering inflammation and is accelerated by disease flares such that there is a progression from inflammatory to fibrostenotic or penetrating disease behavior [100]. This understanding of Crohn's disease implies that there is a window of opportunity to treat with medical therapy before permanent structural intestinal damage has occurred, and that effective treatment early in the disease course is essential to mitigate the risks of strictures, abscesses, and fistulas. This conceptual model of Crohn's disease is supported by empiric evidence demonstrating that patients with shorter disease duration have a greater likelihood of responding to medical therapy [68, 73].

Currently the most effective treatment available for induction of remission in moderate to severe Crohn's disease is the combination of a TNF antagonist and a thiopurine immunosuppressant. In the SONIC trial, a landmark study of induction therapy for active Crohn's disease, the combination of infliximab and azathioprine was more effective than either infliximab alone or azathioprine alone in achieving remission [101].

There were no significant differences in serious infections among the 3 treatment groups. A study looking at methotrexate in combination with infliximab did not show any benefit over infliximab alone for maintenance of steroid-induced remission [102]. This may be in part because both the combination therapy group and the infliximab monotherapy group received steroids, so the additional benefit of methotrexate may have been masked. Patients who received methotrexate did have higher infliximab levels and were less likely to have anti-infliximab antibodies, indicating methotrexate may have had some beneficial effect in reducing the immunogenicity of infliximab [103]. Taken together these studies support a role for early introduction of effective therapy for moderate to severe Crohn's disease, and highlight a role for combination therapy with a TNF antagonist partnered with a thiopurine or methotrexate. Whether to continue combination therapy indefinitely or to discontinue one agent or the other in select patients remains a subject of ongoing investigation.

Unfortunately, many patients who initially respond to TNF antagonist therapy will eventually lose response. In this setting, dose intensification of the TNF antagonist can often recapture clinical response. Measuring drug levels and anti-drug antibodies can inform decisions about switching to a second TNF antagonist or changing to another drug class. Vedolizumab should be considered for patients with moderate to severe disease who have a primary nonresponse to dual therapy with a TNF antagonist, or those with contraindications to anti-TNF therapy.

Treatment of penetrating Crohn's disease first requires control of infection with antibiotics, and possibly bowel rest and percutaneous drainage of any accessible fluid collections. Once source control of infection is achieved, immunosuppression can be initiated [104]. TNF antagonists are the preferred option for treatment of fistulizing Crohn's disease because of their superior efficacy and faster onset of action than other Crohn's disease therapies in this setting [63].

The optimal management of mild Crohn's disease remains uncertain. For patients with disease isolated to the colon, 5-aminosalicylates may be a reasonable treatment option. Other available options include monotherapy with a thiopurine or methotrexate. Steroids are useful for rapid disease control in the setting of exacerbation, but long-term use is limited by lack of sustained effect and by an unfavorable side effect profile. Consequently, steroids are primarily used as a bridge while waiting for slower acting therapies to take effect. Vedolizumab offers the promise of a targeted-intestinal immune suppression with a better safety profile. However, clinical experience with both safety and efficacy of vedolizumab are limited at this time, so the optimal positioning of vedolizumab in the treatment algorithm remains undefined.

Conclusion

Medical therapy for Crohn's disease has seen substantial advancements over the past few decades. Aminosalicylates and corticosteroids which were once the mainstay of treatment are now used only in unique situations. Thiopurines, methotrexate, and TNF antagonists have become the preferred treatment because of their improved efficacy and safety over prior therapies. The success of these therapies in regulating disease activity has allowed gastroenterologists to expand our goals of care beyond simply short-term symptom control. We now aim to induce and maintain durable steroid-free remission and to prevent long-term disease complications such as strictures, fistulas, and colorectal cancer. Anti-integrin therapies represent a novel therapeutic approach with selective blockade of intestinal lymphocytes and offer the promise of disease control without the adverse consequences of systemic immunosuppression.

References

1. Sands BE, Siegel CA. Chapter 111: Crohn's disease. In: Sleisenger MH, Feldman M, Friedman LS, Brandt LJ, editors. Sleisenger and Fordtran's gastrointestinal and liver disease pathophysiology, diagnosis, management. 9th ed. Philadelphia: Saunders/Elsevier; 2010. p. 1 online resource (2 volumes (xxv, 2299, xc pages)).

2. Summers RW, Switz DM, Sessions Jr JT, Becktel JM, Best WR, Kern Jr F, et al. National Cooperative Crohn's Disease Study: results of drug treatment. Gastroenterology. 1979;77(4 Pt 2):847–69.
3. Singleton JW, Hanauer SB, Gitnick GL, Peppercorn MA, Robinson MG, Wruble LD, et al. Mesalamine capsules for the treatment of active Crohn's disease: results of a 16-week trial. Pentasa Crohn's Disease Study Group. Gastroenterology. 1993; 104(5):1293–301.
4. Hanauer SB, Stromberg U. Oral Pentasa in the treatment of active Crohn's disease: a meta-analysis of double-blind, placebo-controlled trials. Clin Gastroenterol Hepatol. 2004;2(5):379–88.
5. Lim WC, Hanauer S. Aminosalicylates for induction of remission or response in Crohn's disease. Cochrane Database System Rev. 2010(12):CD008870.
6. Ford AC, Kane SV, Khan KJ, Achkar JP, Talley NJ, Marshall JK, et al. Efficacy of 5-aminosalicylates in Crohn's disease: systematic review and meta-analysis. Am J Gastroenterol. 2011;106(4):617–29.
7. Box SA, Pullar T. Sulphasalazine in the treatment of rheumatoid arthritis. Br J Rheumatol. 1997;36(3): 382–6.
8. Navarro F, Hanauer SB. Treatment of inflammatory bowel disease: safety and tolerability issues. Am J Gastroenterol. 2003;98(12 Suppl):S18–23.
9. Muller AF, Stevens PE, McIntyre AS, Ellison H, Logan RF. Experience of 5-aminosalicylate nephrotoxicity in the United Kingdom. Aliment Pharmacol Ther. 2005;21(10):1217–24.
10. Sutherland L, Singleton J, Sessions J, Hanauer S, Krawitt E, Rankin G, et al. Double blind, placebo controlled trial of metronidazole in Crohn's disease. Gut. 1991;32(9):1071–5.
11. Prantera C, Zannoni F, Scribano ML, Berto E, Andreoli A, Kohn A, et al. An antibiotic regimen for the treatment of active Crohn's disease: a randomized, controlled clinical trial of metronidazole plus ciprofloxacin. Am J Gastroenterol. 1996;91(2):328–32.
12. Rutgeerts P, Hiele M, Geboes K, Peeters M, Penninckx F, Aerts R, et al. Controlled trial of metronidazole treatment for prevention of Crohn's recurrence after ileal resection. Gastroenterology. 1995;108(6):1617–21.
13. Bernstein LH, Frank MS, Brandt LJ, Boley SJ. Healing of perineal Crohn's disease with metronidazole. Gastroenterology. 1980;79(2):357–65.
14. Brandt LJ, Bernstein LH, Boley SJ, Frank MS. Metronidazole therapy for perineal Crohn's disease: a follow-up study. Gastroenterology. 1982;83(2): 383–7.
15. Thia KT, Mahadevan U, Feagan BG, Wong C, Cockeram A, Bitton A, et al. Ciprofloxacin or metronidazole for the treatment of perianal fistulas in patients with Crohn's disease: a randomized, double-blind, placebo-controlled pilot study. Inflamm Bowel Dis. 2009;15(1):17–24.
16. Dewint P, Hansen BE, Verhey E, Oldenburg B, Hommes DW, Pierik M, et al. Adalimumab combined with ciprofloxacin is superior to adalimumab monotherapy in perianal fistula closure in Crohn's disease: a randomised, double-blind, placebo controlled trial (ADAFI). Gut. 2014;63(2):292–9.
17. West RL, van der Woude CJ, Hansen BE, Felt-Bersma RJ, van Tilburg AJ, Drapers JA, et al. Clinical and endosonographic effect of ciprofloxacin on the treatment of perianal fistulae in Crohn's disease with infliximab: a double-blind placebo-controlled study. Aliment Pharmacol Ther. 2004; 20(11–12):1329–36.
18. Jigaranu AO, Nedelciuc O, Blaj A, Badea M, Mihai C, Diculescu M, et al. Is rifaximin effective in maintaining remission in Crohn's disease? Dig Dis. 2014;32(4):378–83.
19. Prantera C, Lochs H, Campieri M, Scribano ML, Sturniolo GC, Castiglione F, et al. Antibiotic treatment of Crohn's disease: results of a multicentre, double blind, randomized, placebo-controlled trial with rifaximin. Aliment Pharmacol Ther. 2006;23(8):1117–25.
20. Prantera C, Lochs H, Grimaldi M, Danese S, Scribano ML, Gionchetti P. Rifaximin-extended intestinal release induces remission in patients with moderately active Crohn's disease. Gastroenterology. 2012;142(3):473–81.e4.
21. Khan KJ, Ullman TA, Ford AC, Abreu MT, Abadir A, Marshall JK, et al. Antibiotic therapy in inflammatory bowel disease: a systematic review and meta-analysis. Am J Gastroenterol. 2011;106(4):661–73.
22. Malchow H, Ewe K, Brandes JW, Goebell H, Ehms H, Sommer H, et al. European Cooperative Crohn's Disease Study (ECCDS): results of drug treatment. Gastroenterology. 1984;86(2):249–66.
23. Hayashi R, Wada H, Ito K, Adcock IM. Effects of glucocorticoids on gene transcription. Eur J Pharmacol. 2004;500(1–3):51–62.
24. Faubion Jr WA, Loftus Jr EV, Harmsen WS, Zinsmeister AR, Sandborn WJ. The natural history of corticosteroid therapy for inflammatory bowel disease: a population-based study. Gastroenterology. 2001;121(2):255–60.
25. Benchimol EI, Seow CH, Steinhart AH, Griffiths AM. Traditional corticosteroids for induction of remission in Crohn's disease. Cochrane Database System Rev. 2008(2):CD006792.
26. Ford AC, Bernstein CN, Khan KJ, Abreu MT, Marshall JK, Talley NJ, et al. Glucocorticosteroid therapy in inflammatory bowel disease: systematic review and meta-analysis. Am J Gastroenterol. 2011;106(4):590–9. quiz 600.
27. Lichtenstein GR, Feagan BG, Cohen RD, Salzberg BA, Diamond RH, Price S, et al. Serious infection and mortality in patients with Crohn's disease: more than 5 years of follow-up in the TREAT registry. Am J Gastroenterol. 2012;107(9):1409–22.
28. Curkovic I, Egbring M, Kullak-Ublick GA. Risks of inflammatory bowel disease treatment with glucocorticosteroids and aminosalicylates. Dig Dis. 2013;31(3–4):368–73.

29. Seow CH, Benchimol EI, Griffiths AM, Otley AR, Steinhart AH. Budesonide for induction of remission in Crohn's disease. Cochrane Database System Rev. 2008(3):CD000296.
30. Steinhart AH, Ewe K, Griffiths AM, Modigliani R, Thomsen OO. Corticosteroids for maintenance of remission in Crohn's disease. Cochrane Database System Rev. 2003(4):CD000301.
31. Benchimol EI, Seow CH, Otley AR, Steinhart AH. Budesonide for maintenance of remission in Crohn's disease. Cochrane Database System Rev. 2009(1): CD002913.
32. Lennard L. TPMT in the treatment of Crohn's disease with azathioprine. Gut. 2002;51(2):143–6.
33. Sparrow MP, Hande SA, Friedman S, Cao D, Hanauer SB. Effect of allopurinol on clinical outcomes in inflammatory bowel disease nonresponders to azathioprine or 6-mercaptopurine. Clin Gastroenterol Hepatol. 2007;5(2):209–14.
34. Govani SM, Higgins PD. Combination of thiopurines and allopurinol: adverse events and clinical benefit in IBD. J Crohns Colitis. 2010;4(4):444–9.
35. Brooke BN, Hoffmann DC, Swarbrick ET. Azathioprine for Crohn's disease. Lancet. 1969; 2(7621):612–4.
36. Present DH, Korelitz BI, Wisch N, Glass JL, Sachar DB, Pasternack BS. Treatment of Crohn's disease with 6-mercaptopurine. A long-term, randomized, double-blind study. N Engl J Med. 1980;302(18): 981–7.
37. Candy S, Wright J, Gerber M, Adams G, Gerig M, Goodman R. A controlled double blind study of azathioprine in the management of Crohn's disease. Gut. 1995;37(5):674–8.
38. Cosnes J, Bourrier A, Laharie D, Nahon S, Bouhnik Y, Carbonnel F, et al. Early administration of azathioprine vs conventional management of Crohn's disease: a randomized controlled trial. Gastroenterology. 2013;145(4):758–65.e2; quiz e14–5.
39. Panes J, Lopez-Sanroman A, Bermejo F, Garcia-Sanchez V, Esteve M, Torres Y, et al. Early azathioprine therapy is no more effective than placebo for newly diagnosed Crohn's disease. Gastroenterology. 2013;145(4):766–74.e1.
40. Rogler G, Sandborn WJ. Is there still a role for thiopurines in Crohn's disease? Gastroenterology. 2013;145(4):714–6.
41. Kariyawasam VC, Selinger CP, Katelaris PH, Jones DB, McDonald C, Barr G, et al. Early use of thiopurines or methotrexate reduces major abdominal and perianal surgery in Crohn's disease. Inflamm Bowel Dis. 2014;20(8):1382–90.
42. Chatu S, Subramanian V, Saxena S, Pollok RC. The role of thiopurines in reducing the need for surgical resection in Crohn's disease: a systematic review and meta-analysis. Am J Gastroenterol. 2014;109(1): 23–34. quiz 5.
43. Chaparro M, Ordas I, Cabre E, Garcia-Sanchez V, Bastida G, Penalva M, et al. Safety of thiopurine therapy in inflammatory bowel disease: long-term follow-up study of 3931 patients. Inflamm Bowel Dis. 2013;19(7):1404–10.
44. Hindorf U, Johansson M, Eriksson A, Kvifors E, Almer SH. Mercaptopurine treatment should be considered in azathioprine intolerant patients with inflammatory bowel disease. Aliment Pharmacol Ther. 2009;29(6):654–61.
45. Present DH, Meltzer SJ, Krumholz MP, Wolke A, Korelitz BI. 6-Mercaptopurine in the management of inflammatory bowel disease: short- and long-term toxicity. Ann Intern Med. 1989;111(8):641–9.
46. Kotlyar DS, Lewis JD, Beaugerie L, Tierney A, Brensinger CM, Gisbert JP, et al. Risk of lymphoma in patients with inflammatory bowel disease treated with azathioprine and 6-mercaptopurine: a meta-analysis. Clin Gastroenterol Hepatol. 2014. May 28 [Epub ahead of print].
47. Kandiel A, Fraser AG, Korelitz BI, Brensinger C, Lewis JD. Increased risk of lymphoma among inflammatory bowel disease patients treated with azathioprine and 6-mercaptopurine. Gut. 2005;54(8):1121–5.
48. Khan N, Abbas AM, Lichtenstein GR, Loftus Jr EV, Bazzano LA. Risk of lymphoma in patients with ulcerative colitis treated with thiopurines: a nationwide retrospective cohort study. Gastroenterology. 2013;145(5):1007–15.e3.
49. Kotlyar DS, Osterman MT, Diamond RH, Porter D, Blonski WC, Wasik M, et al. A systematic review of factors that contribute to hepatosplenic T-cell lymphoma in patients with inflammatory bowel disease. Clin Gastroenterol Hepatol. 2011;9(1):36–41.e1.
50. Ariyaratnam J, Subramanian V. Association between thiopurine use and nonmelanoma skin cancers in patients with inflammatory bowel disease: a meta-analysis. Am J Gastroenterol. 2014;109(2):163–9.
51. Genestier L, Paillot R, Fournel S, Ferraro C, Miossec P, Revillard JP. Immunosuppressive properties of methotrexate: apoptosis and clonal deletion of activated peripheral T cells. J Clin Invest. 1998; 102(2):322–8.
52. Feagan BG, Rochon J, Fedorak RN, Irvine EJ, Wild G, Sutherland L, et al. Methotrexate for the treatment of Crohn's disease. The North American Crohn's Study Group Investigators. N Engl J Med. 1995;332(5):292–7.
53. Feagan BG, Fedorak RN, Irvine EJ, Wild G, Sutherland L, Steinhart AH, et al. A comparison of methotrexate with placebo for the maintenance of remission in Crohn's disease. North American Crohn's Study Group Investigators. N Engl J Med. 2000;342(22):1627–32.
54. Arora S, Katkov W, Cooley J, Kemp JA, Johnston DE, Schapiro RH, et al. Methotrexate in Crohn's disease: results of a randomized, double-blind, placebo-controlled trial. Hepatogastroenterology. 1999;46(27):1724–9.
55. McDonald JW, Tsoulis DJ, Macdonald JK, Feagan BG. Methotrexate for induction of remission in refractory Crohn's disease. Cochrane Database System Rev. 2012;12:CD003459.

56. Seinen ML, Ponsioen CY, de Boer NK, Oldenburg B, Bouma G, Mulder CJ, et al. Sustained clinical benefit and tolerability of methotrexate monotherapy after thiopurine therapy in patients with Crohn's disease. Clin Gastroenterol Hepatol. 2013;11(6):667–72.
57. Terdiman JP, Gruss CB, Heidelbaugh JJ, Sultan S, Falck-Ytter YT. American Gastroenterological Association Institute guideline on the use of thiopurines, methotrexate, and anti-TNF-alpha biologic drugs for the induction and maintenance of remission in inflammatory Crohn's disease. Gastroenterology. 2013;145(6):1459–63.
58. Targan SR, Hanauer SB, van Deventer SJ, Mayer L, Present DH, Braakman T, et al. A short-term study of chimeric monoclonal antibody cA2 to tumor necrosis factor alpha for Crohn's disease. Crohn's Disease cA2 Study Group. N Engl J Med. 1997;337(15):1029–35.
59. Hanauer SB, Feagan BG, Lichtenstein GR, Mayer LF, Schreiber S, Colombel JF, et al. Maintenance infliximab for Crohn's disease: the ACCENT I randomised trial. Lancet. 2002;359(9317):1541–9.
60. Teshima CW, Thompson A, Dhanoa L, Dieleman LA, Fedorak RN. Long-term response rates to infliximab therapy for Crohn's disease in an outpatient cohort. Can J Gastroenterol. 2009;23(5): 348–52.
61. Sprakes MB, Ford AC, Warren L, Greer D, Hamlin J. Efficacy, tolerability, and predictors of response to infliximab therapy for Crohn's disease: a large single centre experience. J Crohns Colitis. 2012;6(2): 143–53.
62. Present DH, Rutgeerts P, Targan S, Hanauer SB, Mayer L, van Hogezand RA, et al. Infliximab for the treatment of fistulas in patients with Crohn's disease. N Engl J Med. 1999;340(18):1398–405.
63. Sands BE, Anderson FH, Bernstein CN, Chey WY, Feagan BG, Fedorak RN, et al. Infliximab maintenance therapy for fistulizing Crohn's disease. N Engl J Med. 2004;350(9):876–85.
64. Sands BE, Blank MA, Patel K, van Deventer SJ. Long-term treatment of rectovaginal fistulas in Crohn's disease: response to infliximab in the ACCENT II Study. Clin Gastroenterol Hepatol. 2004;2(10):912–20.
65. Lichtenstein GR, Yan S, Bala M, Blank M, Sands BE. Infliximab maintenance treatment reduces hospitalizations, surgeries, and procedures in fistulizing Crohn's disease. Gastroenterology. 2005;128(4): 862–9.
66. Hanauer SB, Sandborn WJ, Rutgeerts P, Fedorak RN, Lukas M, MacIntosh D, et al. Human anti-tumor necrosis factor monoclonal antibody (adalimumab) in Crohn's disease: the CLASSIC-I trial. Gastroenterology. 2006;130(2):323–33. quiz 591.
67. Colombel JF, Sandborn WJ, Rutgeerts P, Enns R, Hanauer SB, Panaccione R, et al. Adalimumab for maintenance of clinical response and remission in patients with Crohn's disease: the CHARM trial. Gastroenterology. 2007;132(1):52–65.
68. Schreiber S, Reinisch W, Colombel JF, Sandborn WJ, Hommes DW, Robinson AM, et al. Subgroup analysis of the placebo-controlled CHARM trial: increased remission rates through 3 years for adalimumab-treated patients with early Crohn's disease. J Crohns Colitis. 2013;7(3):213–21.
69. Colombel JF, Schwartz DA, Sandborn WJ, Kamm MA, D'Haens G, Rutgeerts P, et al. Adalimumab for the treatment of fistulas in patients with Crohn's disease. Gut. 2009;58(7):940–8.
70. Sandborn WJ, Rutgeerts P, Enns R, Hanauer SB, Colombel JF, Panaccione R, et al. Adalimumab induction therapy for Crohn disease previously treated with infliximab: a randomized trial. Ann Intern Med. 2007;146(12):829–38.
71. Sandborn WJ, Feagan BG, Stoinov S, Honiball PJ, Rutgeerts P, Mason D, et al. Certolizumab pegol for the treatment of Crohn's disease. N Engl J Med. 2007;357(3):228–38.
72. Schreiber S, Khaliq-Kareemi M, Lawrance IC, Thomsen OO, Hanauer SB, McColm J, et al. Maintenance therapy with certolizumab pegol for Crohn's disease. N Engl J Med. 2007;357(3): 239–50.
73. Schreiber S, Colombel JF, Bloomfield R, Nikolaus S, Scholmerich J, Panes J, et al. Increased response and remission rates in short-duration Crohn's disease with subcutaneous certolizumab pegol: an analysis of PRECiSE 2 randomized maintenance trial data. Am J Gastroenterol. 2010;105(7):1574–82.
74. Schreiber S, Lawrance IC, Thomsen OO, Hanauer SB, Bloomfield R, Sandborn WJ. Randomised clinical trial: certolizumab pegol for fistulas in Crohn's disease – subgroup results from a placebo-controlled study. Aliment Pharmacol Ther. 2011;33(2): 185–93.
75. Sandborn WJ, Abreu MT, D'Haens G, Colombel JF, Vermeire S, Mitchev K, et al. Certolizumab pegol in patients with moderate to severe Crohn's disease and secondary failure to infliximab. Clin Gastroenterol Hepatol. 2010;8(8):688–95.e2.
76. Gisbert JP, Panés J. Loss of response and requirement of infliximab dose intensification in Crohn's disease: a review. Am J Gastroenterol. 2009;104(3): 760–7.
77. Billioud V, Sandborn WJ, Peyrin-Biroulet L. Loss of response and need for adalimumab dose intensification in Crohn's disease: a systematic review. Am J Gastroenterol. 2011;106(4):674–84.
78. Ordás I, Feagan BG, Sandborn WJ. Therapeutic drug monitoring of tumor necrosis factor antagonists in inflammatory bowel disease. Clin Gastroenterol Hepatol. 2012;10(10):1079–87.
79. Rutgeerts P, Feagan BG, Lichtenstein GR, Mayer LF, Schreiber S, Colombel JF, et al. Comparison of scheduled and episodic treatment strategies of infliximab in Crohn's disease. Gastroenterology. 2004;126(2):402–13.
80. Mohan N, Edwards ET, Cupps TR, Oliverio PJ, Sandberg G, Crayton H, et al. Demyelination occurring

during anti-tumor necrosis factor alpha therapy for inflammatory arthritides. Arthritis Rheum. 2001;44(12):2862.
81. Chung ES, Packer M, Lo KH, Fasanmade AA, Willerson JT. Randomized, double-blind, placebo-controlled, pilot trial of infliximab, a chimeric monoclonal antibody to tumor necrosis factor-alpha, in patients with moderate-to-severe heart failure: results of the Anti-TNF Therapy Against Congestive Heart Failure (ATTACH) trial. Circulation. 2003;107(25):3133.
82. Vermeire S, Noman M, Van Assche G, Baert F, Van Steen K, Esters N, et al. Autoimmunity associated with anti-tumor necrosis factor alpha treatment in Crohn's disease: a prospective cohort study. Gastroenterology. 2003;125(1):32–9.
83. Cullen G, Kroshinsky D, Cheifetz AS, Korzenik JR. Psoriasis associated with anti-tumour necrosis factor therapy in inflammatory bowel disease: a new series and a review of 120 cases from the literature. Aliment Pharmacol Ther. 2011;34(11–12):1318–27.
84. Marehbian J, Arrighi HM, Hass S, Tian H, Sandborn WJ. Adverse events associated with common therapy regimens for moderate-to-severe Crohn's disease. Am J Gastroenterol. 2009;104(10):2524–33.
85. Lichtenstein GR, Feagan BG, Cohen RD, Salzberg BA, Diamond RH, Langholff W, et al. Drug therapies and the risk of malignancy in Crohn's disease: results from the TREAT Registry. Am J Gastroenterol. 2014;109(2):212–23.
86. Siegel CA, Marden SM, Persing SM, Larson RJ, Sands BE. Risk of lymphoma associated with combination anti-tumor necrosis factor and immunomodulator therapy for the treatment of Crohn's disease: a meta-analysis. Clin Gastroenterol Hepatol. 2009;7(8):874–81.
87. Caspersen S, Elkjaer M, Riis L, Pedersen N, Mortensen C, Jess T, et al. Infliximab for inflammatory bowel disease in Denmark 1999–2005: clinical outcome and follow-up evaluation of malignancy and mortality. Clin Gastroenterol Hepatol. 2008;6(11):1212–7. quiz 176.
88. Long MD, Herfarth HH, Pipkin CA, Porter CQ, Sandler RS, Kappelman MD. Increased risk for non-melanoma skin cancer in patients with inflammatory bowel disease. Clin Gastroenterol Hepatol. 2010;8(3):268–74.
89. Long MD, Martin CF, Pipkin CA, Herfarth HH, Sandler RS, Kappelman MD. Risk of melanoma and nonmelanoma skin cancer among patients with inflammatory bowel disease. Gastroenterology. 2012;143(2):390–9.e1.
90. Williams CJ, Peyrin-Biroulet L, Ford AC. Systematic review with meta-analysis: malignancies with anti-tumour necrosis factor-alpha therapy in inflammatory bowel disease. Aliment Pharmacol Ther. 2014;39(5):447–58.
91. Sandborn WJ, Colombel JF, Enns R, Feagan BG, Hanauer SB, Lawrance IC, et al. Natalizumab induction and maintenance therapy for Crohn's disease. N Engl J Med. 2005;353(18):1912–25.
92. Targan SR, Feagan BG, Fedorak RN, Lashner BA, Panaccione R, Present DH, et al. Natalizumab for the treatment of active Crohn's disease: results of the ENCORE Trial. Gastroenterology. 2007; 132(5):1672–83.
93. MacDonald JK, McDonald JW. Natalizumab for induction of remission in Crohn's disease. Cochrane Database System Rev. 2007(1):CD006097.
94. Kleinschmidt-DeMasters BK, Tyler KL. Progressive multifocal leukoencephalopathy complicating treatment with natalizumab and interferon beta-1a for multiple sclerosis. N Engl J Med. 2005;353(4):369–74.
95. Bloomgren G, Richman S, Hotermans C, Subramanyam M, Goelz S, Natarajan A, et al. Risk of natalizumab-associated progressive multifocal leukoencephalopathy. N Engl J Med. 2012;366(20): 1870–80.
96. Lichtenstein GR, Hanauer SB, Sandborn WJ. Risk of biologic therapy-associated progressive multifocal leukoencephalopathy: use of the JC virus antibody assay in the treatment of moderate-to-severe Crohn's disease. Gastroenterol Hepatol. 2012;8(11 Suppl 8):1–20.
97. Milch C, Wyant T, Xu J, Parikh A, Kent W, Fox I, et al. Vedolizumab, a monoclonal antibody to the gut homing alpha4beta7 integrin, does not affect cerebrospinal fluid T-lymphocyte immunophenotype. J Neuroimmunol. 2013;264(1–2):123–6.
98. Sandborn WJ, Feagan BG, Rutgeerts P, Hanauer S, Colombel JF, Sands BE, et al. Vedolizumab as induction and maintenance therapy for Crohn's disease. N Engl J Med. 2013;369(8):711–21.
99. Sands BE, Feagan BG, Rutgeerts P, Colombel JF, Sandborn WJ, Sy R, et al. Effects of vedolizumab induction therapy for patients with Crohn's disease in whom tumor necrosis factor antagonist treatment had failed. Gastroenterology. 2014;147(3): 618–27.e3.
100. Cosnes J, Cattan S, Blain A, Beaugerie L, Carbonnel F, Parc R, et al. Long-term evolution of disease behavior of Crohn's disease. Inflamm Bowel Dis. 2002;8(4):244–50.
101. Colombel JF, Sandborn WJ, Reinisch W, Mantzaris GJ, Kornbluth A, Rachmilewitz D, et al. Infliximab, azathioprine, or combination therapy for Crohn's disease. N Engl J Med. 2010;362(15):1383–95.
102. Feagan BG, McDonald JW, Panaccione R, Enns RA, Bernstein CN, Ponich TP, et al. Methotrexate in combination with infliximab is no more effective than infliximab alone in patients with Crohn's disease. Gastroenterology. 2014;146(3):681–8.e1.
103. Narula N, Peyrin-Biroulet L, Colombel JF. Combination therapy with methotrexate in inflammatory bowel disease: time to COMMIT? Gastroenterology. 2014;146(3):608–11.
104. Sands BE, Blank MA, Diamond RH, Barrett JP, Van Deventer SJ. Maintenance infliximab does not result in increased abscess development in fistulizing Crohn's disease: results from the ACCENT II study. Aliment Pharmacol Ther. 2006;23(8): 1127–36.

Medical Therapy: The Future 4

Joel Pekow and Russell D. Cohen

Introduction

It was not until 1998 that the first FDA-approved treatment for Crohn's disease (CD), infliximab, came on the market. Prior to this time, clinical evidence to support medical therapy for Crohn's disease centered around the 5-aminosalicylates (5-ASA) [1], corticosteroids [2, 3], and immunosuppressants (6-mercaptopurine, azathioprine [4], methotrexate [5], or cyclosporine [6]). Since the initial approval of infliximab 15 years ago, four additional biologic treatments have been approved for the treatment of Crohn's disease. These include two additional therapies targeting tumor necrosis factor α (TNFα), adalimumab and certolizumab pegol, and two therapies targeting integrins (natalizumab and vedolizumab). Although superior to placebo in the treatment of Crohn's disease, response rates to currently available therapies are modest. As such, future targeted therapies and tools to predict a given individuals response to medication are needed. This chapter will focus on trends in management of Crohn's disease and future treatment options in development.

J. Pekow, MD
Department of Gastroenterology, Hepatology, and Nutrition, University of Chicago, 900 East 57th Street, MB #9, Chicago, IL 60637, USA
e-mail: jpekow@medicine.bsd.uchicago.edu

R.D. Cohen, MD (✉)
Department of Medicine, Inflammatory Bowel Disease Center, The University of Chicago Medicine, 5841 S. Maryland, MC 4076, Chicago, IL 60637, USA
e-mail: rcohen@medicine.bsd.uchicago.edu

Goals of Therapy

It is common in patients with Crohn's disease to have a discordance between clinical symptoms and mucosal inflammation. This is reflected in data from the SONIC (Study of Biologic and Immunomodulator Naïve Patients in Crohn's Disease) trial in which half of the patients in clinical remission (defined as a Crohn's Disease Activity Index (CDAI) <150) had endoscopic evidence of inflammation [7]. As such, there has been a shift in clinical trials for Crohn's disease from reliance on subjective clinical scores to the use of objective markers of inflammation, including C-reactive protein (CRP), fecal calprotectin, endoscopic evaluation, and histologic scoring. This practice reflects acceptance that mucosal healing is associated with improved outcomes including less corticosteroid use, hospitalizations and surgeries, improved quality of life, as well as a decreased risk of colorectal cancer [8–10]. Furthermore, achieving mucosal healing on therapy is associated with sustained remission in several clinical trials [10–12]. Unfortunately, there is no standard definition for mucosal healing in Crohn's disease [13, 14]. In the SONIC and the EXTEND (Extend the Safety and Efficacy of Adalimumab Through Endoscopic Healing) trial,

A. Fichera and M.K. Krane (eds.), *Crohn's Disease: Basic Principles*,
DOI 10.1007/978-3-319-14181-7_4, © Springer International Publishing Switzerland 2015

mucosal healing was defined as the absence of mucosal ulcers at week 26 and week 12, respectively. However, this definition does not take into account other findings suggestive of active inflammation, such as erosions, granularity, and friability. Furthermore, partial mucosal healing has also been associated with improved long-term outcomes [15].

A second important development in treating Crohn's disease has been a change towards early initiation of an aggressive treatment approach. In a 2-year open randomized trial, 133 Crohn's patients naïve to corticosteroids, immunosuppressants, or biologics were blindly randomized to one of two groups. Group one received a "top-down" induction with three infusions of infliximab (weeks 0, 2, and 6) and initiation of daily azathioprine, followed by repeat infliximab infusions only as needed in the event of recurrent symptoms. Group two received a "step up" approach of corticosteroids, with relapse treated by further corticosteroids courses and subsequently with azathioprine, those failing or relapsing then went on to start infliximab (5 mg/kg). The top-down group who received early combined immunosuppression had increased mucosal healing, clinical remission, and steroid free remission [16].

The benefit of early introduction of a biologic in Crohn's disease was also shown in other studies. Post-hoc analysis from the PRECiSE 2 (Pegylated Antibody Fragment Evaluation in Crohn's Disease: Safety and Efficacy) randomized control maintenance trial with certolizumab pegol as well as the CHARM (Crohn's Trial of the Fully Human Antibody Adalimumab for Remission Maintenance) trials with adalimumab demonstrated that subjects who are early in their disease course have higher response rates than those who are in a later stage of their disease [17, 18]. Data from the SONIC trial, where anti-TNF and immunosuppressive naïve patients were randomized to infliximab, azathioprine, or the combination demonstrated that combination therapy was superior in patients relatively early in their disease course [19]. This is in contrast to data from the COMMIT (Combination of Maintenance Methotrexate-Infliximab Trial) trial, where no differences were seen in rate of treatment failure between patients who were randomized to infliximab with or without subcutaneous methotrexate [20]. Although the differences in outcomes between these two trials may also be explained by dissimilarities in study design and treatment groups, it is worth noting that subjects in the SONIC trial were substantially earlier in their disease course than those in the COMMIT trial (2.3 years vs. >9 years) [19, 20].

Targeted Pharmacological Therapy

Therapies Targeting Lymphocyte Homing, Adhesion, and Migration

In order for leukocytes to migrate into tissues, they traffic across the vascular wall through a series of maneuvers consisting of capturing, rolling, adhesion, and migration [21, 22]. The capturing of lymphocytes involves the interaction between L-selectins and P- and E-selectins [23]. Following capturing, secondary adhesion molecules expressed on lymphocytes, termed integrins, facilitate migration through an interaction with receptors expressed on the vascular endothelium. Several integrins participate in this mechanism. These include $\alpha_2\beta_2$ that is expressed on neutrophils and binds to ICAM-1 (Intercellular Adhesion Molecule 1), $\alpha_4\beta_1$ that is expressed on most leukocytes and binds to VCAM-1 (Vascular Cell Adhesion Molecule 1), $\alpha_4\beta_7$ that is expressed on gut specific lymphocytes and binds to MADCAM-1 (Mucosal Vascular Addressin Cell Adhesion Molecule 1), and $\alpha_E\beta_7$ which is expressed on intraepithelial lymphocytes and binds to E-cadherin on epithelial cells [24–26]. Thus, β_7 containing integrins as well as the C–C chemokine receptor 9 (CCR-9) interacting with chemokine (C–C motif) ligand 25 (CCL25) facilitates homing of lymphocytes to the gut [27, 28]. Because of the central role they play in trafficking lymphocytes to areas of inflammation, several pharmacological treatments have been developed to target receptors involved in lymphocyte homing, adhesion, and migration.

Natalizumab, a monoclonal antibody directed against the α_4 integrin on leukocytes, was the first anti-adhesion molecule to be tested in Crohn's disease. Clinical trials have demonstrated that natalizumab is effective for the induction and maintenance of remission in patients with Crohn's disease [29–32]. These trials did reveal two important aspects regarding the therapeutic mechanism of natalizumab. First, there did not appear to be a dose response to natalizumab as seen with anti-TNF inhibitor therapy. Second, response and remission rates with natalizumab induction therapy were modest compared to placebo, although maintenance of remission rates was more robust. Widespread use of natalizumab has been limited secondary to safety concerns related to reactivation of the JC virus resulting in progressive multifocal leukoencephalopathy (PML) in rare cases [33, 34]. The occurrence of PML in JC treated patients reflects natalizumab's lack of gut specificity through targeting α_4 integrin [35].

Vedolizumab, a monoclonal antibody directed against $\alpha_4\beta_7$ integrin complex, was approved by the FDA in 2014 for the treatment of both UC and CD. Clinical trials in UC demonstrated that vedolizumab is effective for both the induction and maintenance of remission as well as mucosal healing in UC [36, 37]. Although an initial phase II trial of vedolizumab in active CD did not reach its primary endpoint of clinical response at day 57, there was a suggestion of a dose-dependent response with vedolizumab [38]. A subsequent larger phase III trial, however, showed improved clinical response and remission in CD patients treated with vedolizumab compared to placebo [39]. A second phase III randomized control trial with vedolizumab focusing on patients who previously failed anti-TNF therapy demonstrated significantly increased remission rates at week 10, but not at week 6, in those treated with vedolizumab [40]. Importantly, there were no reported cases of PML in the vedolizumab treated patients in these studies which is in agreement with mechanistic studies that demonstrate $\alpha_4\beta_7$ selectivity to the gut, as well as reports that vedolizumab treatment does not affect cerebrospinal fluid T cell phenotypes [41].

In addition to natalizumab and vedolizumab, several biologics targeting the adhesion pathway are currently in development. This includes etrolizumab, a humanized monoclonal antibody that targets $\alpha_4\beta_7$ and $\alpha_E\beta_7$. A phase II trial of induction therapy with etrolizumab demonstrated significant remission rates in patients with UC at week 10. Larger phase III trials in UC with etrolizumab are ongoing (ClinicalTrials.gov identifier NCT02163759, NCT02171429, NCT02136069, NCT02165215, NCT02100696) with plans to begin phase III trials in Crohn's disease. Similar to vedolizumab, AMG 181 is a monoclonal antibody that binds to the alpha-4-beta-7 heterodimer [42]. The antibody is being studied as a subcutaneous injection in a phase II trial in patients with moderate to severe Crohn's disease (NCT01696396). A monoclonal antibody targeting MAdCAM-1 was also developed (PF-00547659) [43]. Although an initial randomized, double-blind, placebo-controlled trial did not demonstrate statistically significant differences in clinical response, clinical remission, or endoscopic remission, there were trends in response to all three parameters and significant reductions in fecal calprotectin [44]. Phase II trials in Crohn's disease and ulcerative colitis with this monoclonal antibody are currently ongoing (NCT01276509, NCT01620255).

AJM300 is a unique oral compound targeting α_4 integrins. Two randomized control trials of AJM300 in CD and UC were presented at Digestive Disease week in 2009 and 2014, respectively [45, 46]. Although the study in CD did not meet the primary endpoints, there were differences in CDAI decreases following AJM300 treatment in those with a CDAI $\geq$ 200 at baseline [45]. A second trial of AJM300 in 102 Japanese patients with moderately active UC demonstrated significance in clinical response, remission, and mucosal healing at week 8 [46].

CCX282-B is a selective antagonist of CCR9. In the PROTECT-1 (Prospective Randomized Oral-Therapy Evaluation in Crohn's disease) trial, CCX282-B demonstrated efficacy at week 12 in both 70 point CDAI response with 500 mg daily compared to placebo (61 % vs. 47 %, $p=0.039$) and 100 point CDAI response at 500 mg daily compared to placebo (55 % vs. 40 %, $p=0.029$). In addition, maintenance of remission was higher in subjects who received the treatment (47 % vs. 31 %, $p=0.011$) at week 36 [47]. Phase III trials to investigate this compound were initiated although terminated early secondary to a lack of efficacy and increased serious adverse events (SAEs), including 2 cardiac SAEs in subjects who received 500 mg of the medication.

BMS-936557 is a monoclonal antibody to interferon-γ-inducible protein 10 (IP-10), a chemokine that plays a key role in inflammatory and epithelial cell migration. A phase II randomized study of BMS-936557 given intravenously every other week in patients with active UC did not reach the primary endpoints of clinical response at day 57. However, subgroup analysis revealed that subjects with a higher steady-state concentration of the drug were significantly more likely to achieve clinical response and histological improvement [48]. A phase II study examining induction and maintenance of remission of BMS-93557 in subjects with moderate to severe Crohn's disease is ongoing (NCT01466374).

IL12/23 Inhibitors

Interleukin (IL)-12 and IL-23 play a key role in the T cell immune response [49]. Genome-wide association studies suggest that multiple genes in the IL-12/23 signaling pathway have an association with Crohn's disease [50]. IL-12 is expressed on antigen presenting cells, and has two subunits, p35 and p40. These subunits bind to the receptors, IL-12β1 (p40) and IL-12β2 (p35) initiating a signaling cascade. This intracellular signaling shifts cell differentiation to a Th1 phenotype [51]. IL-23 also consists of two subunits, the IL-12p40 bound to p19. The p19 binds to IL-23 receptor (IL23R) and induce a TH17 response, promoting inflammation [52].

The first drug to target this pathway was ustekinumab, an IgG1 monoclonal antibody targeting the common p40 subunit of IL-12 and IL-23 which inhibits it from binding to IL-12β1. Randomized, placebo-controlled studies have demonstrated the effectiveness of ustekinumab in the treatment of plaque psoriasis and psoriatic arthritis [53–55]. In Crohn's disease, a phase IIa multicenter, double-blinded, placebo-controlled crossover study examined ustekinumab in two groups. Group 1 ($n=104$) included patients with moderate to severe Crohn's disease who were given either subcutaneous ustekinumab 90 mg weekly at weeks 0–3 and placebo at weeks 8–11, placebo at weeks 0–3, and subcutaneous ustekinumab at weeks 8–11, intravenous ustekinumab 4.5 mg/kg at week 0 and placebo at week 8, or IV placebo at week 0 and intravenous ustekinumab 4.5 mg/kg at week 8. Group 2 ($n=27$) were primary or secondary nonresponders to anti-TNF agents and were randomized to receive open-label ustekinumab either subcutaneous 90 mg at week 0–3 or a single dose of 4.5 mg/kg given intravenously. Although the study did not reach its primary endpoint, which was clinical response (CDAI decrease of ≥70) at week 8 (49 % vs. 40 %, $p=0.34$), response rates at 4 and 6 weeks were significantly higher in the ustekinumab group. Further, the study demonstrated a significant response in anti-TNF nonresponders and in those who lost response (43 % with subcutaneous dosing and 54 % with IV dosing) [56]. A follow-up phase IIb randomized control trial in patients resistant to anti-TNF therapy evaluated induction and maintenance of ustekinumab [57]. In the study, 526 subjects were randomized to receive 1, 3, or 6 mg of intravenous ustekinumab or placebo. Patients who responded to induction therapy were further randomized to receive 90 mg of subcutaneous ustekinumab or placebo at weeks 8 and 16 with efficacy assessed at week 22. The proportion of patients who had ≥100 point decrease in CDAI at week 6 were 36.6, 34.1, 39.7, and 23.5 % for the 1 mg/kg, 3 mg/kg, 6 mg, and placebo doses respectively. In addition, maintenance therapy with ustekinumab 90 mg was associated with a higher rate of clinical remission at week 22 than placebo (41.7 % vs. 27.4 %). A phase III trial examining induction treatment with 6 mg/kg intravenous vs. 130 mg intravenous vs. placebo was recently completed in patients who were intolerant or failed anti-TNF therapy (NCT01369329), and a similar study in patients who are not intolerant and have not failed anti-TNF therapy is ongoing (NCT01369342). A follow-up study, examining maintenance dosing with 90 mg of ustekinumab given subcutaneously is ongoing (NCT01369355).

Two monoclonal antibodies to IL-23 are also currently in clinical trials investigating their efficacy in Crohn's disease. A phase II trial in patients with moderate to severe Crohn's disease is studying both intravenous and subcutaneous medi-2070 (NCT01714726). BI-655066 is a monoclonal antibody targeting the p19 subunit of IL-23 and is currently being investigated in a phase II trial in patients with moderate to severe Crohn's disease (NCT02031276).

JAK Inhibitors

Numerous cytokines direct intracellular signaling pathways through induction of the Janus Kinase/signal transducer and activator or transcription (JAK/STAT) pathway. There are four JAK proteins (JAK1, JAK2, JAK3, and tyrosine kinase 2 [TYK2]) and seven STAT proteins (1, 2, 3, 4, 5a, 5b, 6). Binding of cytokines to their transmembrane receptors results in dimerization of the receptor subunits and recruitment of JAKs. This recruitment results in phosphorylation of JAKs, the receptor chains, and STAT. STATs bind to phosphorylated tyrosine residues on the receptor. Following phosphorylation, they dimerize and translocate to the nucleus resulting in transcriptional regulation as shown in Fig. 4.1 [58, 59]. Previous Genome-Wide Association Studies (GWAS) in Crohn's disease have demonstrated an association with JAK2, TYK2, and STAT3 [60, 61]. Further supporting the role of the JAK/STAT pathway in IBD are studies which delineate the role of the pathway in T cell differentiation [62, 63]. In addition, several reports have demonstrated activation of STAT3 in IBD [64, 65].

Tofacitinib is an oral selective JAK inhibitor, which inhibits JAK 1 and 3 with reduced inhibition of JAK2 and TYK2. Tofacitinib has demonstrated efficacy in patients with moderate to severe rheumatoid arthritis and is currently FDA approved for that indication at a dose of 5 mg bid [66]. Clinical trials in rheumatoid arthritis (RA) have demonstrated superiority of tofacitinib to methotrexate and adalimumab [67, 68]. Studies have also demonstrated efficacy of tofacitinib in early phase clinical trials in the treatment of psoriasis and prevention of kidney allograft rejection [69, 70].

In patients with moderate to severe ulcerative colitis, a phase II trial demonstrated response rates at week 8 with 0.5, 3, 10, and 15 mg of 32 % ($p=0.39$), 48 % ($p=0.55$), 61 % ($p=0.1$), and 78 % ($p<0.001$), respectively, compared to placebo (42 %). Clinical remission was seen in 13 % ($p=0.76$), 33 % ($p=0.01$), 48 % ($p<0.001$), and 41 % (<0.001), respectively, compared to placebo (10 %). It is worth noting that a dose-dependent increase in LDL and HDL cholesterol was seen in this study. In addition three subjects in the study who were on 10 mg or 15 mg doses developed absolute neutrophil counts <1,500 cells/m^3 [71]. Phase III studies evaluate the efficacy of tofacitinib 10 mg bid vs. placebo in the induction of remission (NCT01465763) and 5 mg bid vs. 10 mg bid vs. placebo on the maintenance of remission in UC are ongoing (NCT01457574).

A phase II study was also conducted in subjects with moderate to severe Crohn's disease comparing 1, 5, or 15 mg bid compared to placebo. Although there were no differences in clinical remission or response at week 4, subjects who received 15 mg bid did have reductions in CRP and fecal calprotectin indicating biological activity [72]. As such, the lack of difference in response and remission rates may be explained by the high placebo response rates (47.1 %), small sample size, or short follow-up interval in this trial. Phase II studies to investigate tofacitinib 5 mg bid and 10 mg bid compared to placebo for induction and maintenance therapy in moderate to severe Crohn's disease are underway (NCT01393626 and NCT01393899). In addition, a clinical trial is currently enrolling subjects to examine the efficacy of GLPG0634, a selective inhibitor of JAK1, in patients with endoscopic evidence of active Crohn's disease (NCT02049618) [73].

IL-6 Signaling Blockade

Interleukin-6 (IL-6) is upregulated in mucosa with active inflammation from patients with Crohn's disease, and blocking IL-6 signaling attenuates colitis in murine models [74–76]. IL-6

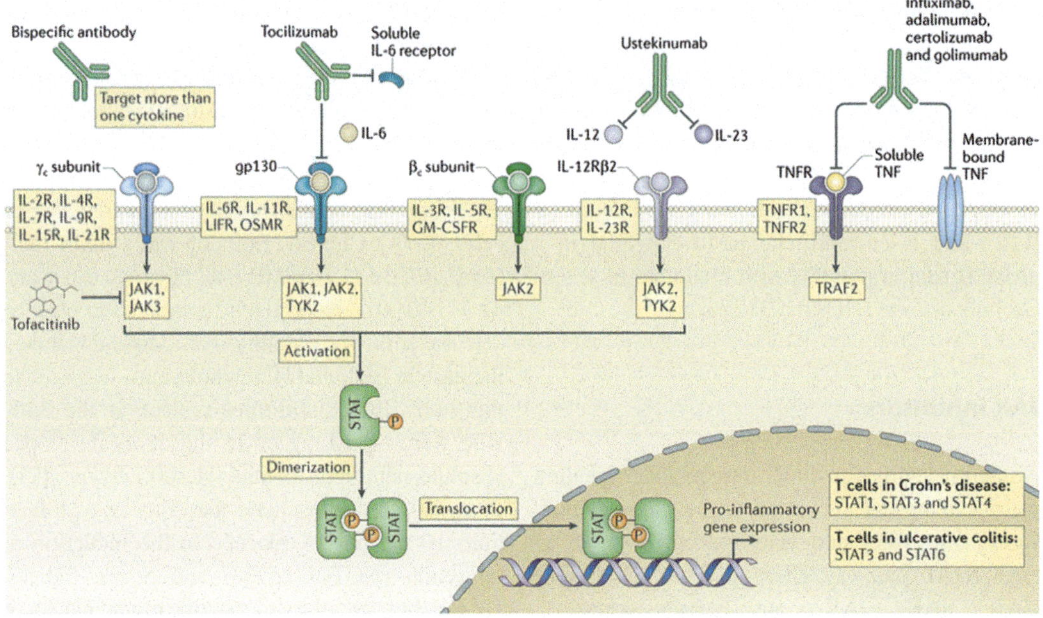

Fig. 4.1 Potential therapies in IBD targeting cytokine signaling and Janus kinase (JAK)–signal transducer and activator of transcription (STAT) signaling pathways. Reprinted with permission from Macmillan Publishers Ltd. Nature Reviews Immunology Neurath, M.F Cytokines in Inflammatory Bowel Disease; 14(5) 329–42. Copyright 2014

binds to both membrane bound and soluble IL-6 receptor (IL6R). The IL-6/IL6R complex attaches to the transmembrane glycoprotein, gp130, activating several intracellular pathways involved in inflammation, including JAK1-STAT3 as shown in Fig. 4.1. Because gp130 is expressed on several cell types, IL-6 has pluripotent activities. Tocilizumab is a humanized antibody to the IL-6 receptor which has demonstrated efficacy in rheumatoid arthritis, juvenile arthritis, and Castleman's disease [77–80]. In 2004, a randomized placebo-controlled trial in active Crohn's demonstrated that 80 % of the patients randomized to treatment with 8 mg/kg of the monoclonal antibody had a clinical response at 12 weeks compared to 31 % of those who received placebo ($p=0.019$) [81]. However, only two of ten patients treated with tocilizumab went into remission, and there were no differences in endoscopic or histologic appearance between the groups. Although tocilizumab has not been studied further in Crohn's disease, a second monoclonal antibody, PF-04236921 was subsequently developed. A phase II trial of PF-04236921 in patients with Crohn's disease who have failed anti-TNF therapy is ongoing (NCT01287897).

A list of targeted therapies in development for Crohn's disease is listed in Table 4.1.

Biosimilars

TNF-α is a proinflammatory cytokine overexpressed in tissue from patients with active inflammation with Crohn's disease [82]. There are currently three therapies that target TNF-α approved for the treatment of Crohn's disease in the USA: infliximab, adalimumab, and certolizumab pegol. All three therapies have demonstrated effectiveness in clinical trials in Crohn's disease [83–90]. An additional monoclonal antibody against TNFα, golimumab, is marketed for

Table 4.1 Targeted pharmacological agents currently in phase II and III trials for Crohn's disease

Name	Target	Route of administration	FDA approved for alternative indication	Phase of current clinical trial in Crohn's disease
Therapies targeting lymphocyte homing, adhesion, and migration				
Etrolizumab	$\alpha_4\beta_E/\alpha_4\beta_7$	SC	No	III
AMG181	$\alpha_4\beta_7$	SC	No	II
PF-00547659	MAdCAM-1	SC	No	II
AJM300	α_4	PO	No	IIa completed
CCX282-B	CCR9	PO	No	III
BMS-936557	IP-10	IV	No	II
IL-12/IL23 inhibitors				
Ustekinumab	IL-12/IL-23	IV/SC	Yes	III
Medi-2070	IL-23	IV/SC	No	II
BI-655066	IL-23	SC	No	II
JAK inhibitors				
Tofacitinib	JAK1/JAK2	PO	Yes	II
GLPG0634	JAK1	PO	No	II
Therapies targeting IL-6 signaling				
PF-04236921	IL-6	SC	No	II
Therapies targeting NKG2D				
NN01420-0002	NKG2D	SC	No	II
Therapies targeting IL-21 signaling				
NNC00114-0006	IL-21	IV	No	II

ulcerative colitis [91, 92]. Although not approved for the treatment of Crohn's disease, golimumab has also shown efficacy in other inflammatory conditions, including rheumatoid arthritis, psoriatic arthritis, and ankylosing spondylitis. As patents on these biologic therapies will be expiring in upcoming years, there is great interest in duplicating the effectiveness of these medications through development of biosimilars.

"Biosimilar" medications are treatments which are comparable to another biological medication that is already available for use. In contrast to small molecules for which generics can be developed, biologic therapies have high complexity and require a living organism for development. As such, biologics may have altered efficacy secondary to the manufacturing process. In order for a biosimilar to be approved, both the FDA and European Medicines Agency (EMA) require that a biologic be comparable in efficacy, quality, and safety to a reference medication. Although there are no studies comparing the effectiveness of these medications in IBD, there was a recently published randomized double-blind trial comparing infliximab to an infliximab biosimilar, CT-P13, in patients with ankylosing spondylitis and rheumatoid arthritis that demonstrated comparable efficacy with similar immunogenicity [93, 94]. Two manufacturers of CT-P13, Hospira and Celtrion, which produce the biosimilars Inflectra and Remsima, respectively, have been approved by the EMA. An additional Remicade biosimilar developed by Samsung Bioepis, SB2, is being studied in a phase III trial compared to Remicade in patients with rheumatoid arthritis (NC01936181). There are also several Humira biosimilars in development including GP2017 (Sandoz), SP5 (Samsung Bioepis), CHS-1420 (Coherus), ABP 501 (Amgen), PF 06410293 (Pfizer), BI 695501 (Boehringer Ingelheim), and others. Trials are underway comparing the effectiveness of GP2017 in plaque psoriasis (NCT02016105) as well as BI-695501 and SP5 in rheumatoid arthritis compared to Humira (NCT02137226, NCT02167139).

Stem Cell Therapy

Several observational series have demonstrated a benefit from hematopoietic stem cell transplantation (HSCT) in patients with refractory Crohn's disease [95–99]. A phase I study of autologous HSCT in 12 subjects with refractory Crohn's disease demonstrated sustained clinical remission in 11 of 12 patients as defined by a CDAI ≤ 150. Of these 11 patients, only 1 patient developed recurrence with a median follow-up of 18.5 months [99]. A second case series by the same group reported longer term follow-up in 24 patients with relapse free survival, defined as not starting medical therapy for Crohn's disease, as 91 % at 1 year, 63 % at 2 years, 57 % at 3 years, 39 % at 4 years, and 19 % at 5 years [98]. A third case series of four patients treated with autologous hematopoietic stem cell transplant reported clinical remission in all 4 patients at 3 months with 3 of 4 patients maintaining endoscopic and clinical remission with a median follow-up of 16.5 months [97]. More recently, a phase I/II trial of autologous peripheral blood stem cell transplantation in refractory Crohn's disease reported similar results with five of nine subjects in the cohort exhibiting mucosal healing after a mean period of 9.1 months [96]. It should be noted in this series that in six patients who had disease recurrence in follow-up and treated with immunosuppressive therapy, only one was subsequently started on anti-TNF treatment, potentially indicating improved responsiveness to immunosuppressive agents post HSCT.

Although these small trials have demonstrated the effectiveness of HSCT in Crohn's disease, the risks associated with myeloablation limit its use. Alternatives to HSCT are use of human placenta-derived stem cells and mesenchymal stromal cells (MSCs). A phase I trial of two infusions of human placenta-derived cells in treatment resistant Crohn's disease demonstrated clinical efficacy in all six subjects who received a low-dose infusions and two of six subjects who received a higher dose. The group who received the lower dose, however, did have lower CDAI scores and CRP at baseline. A phase II trial of human placenta-derived cells is currently investigating their efficacy in moderate to severe Crohn's disease (NCT01155362).

Mesenchymal stem cells (MSCs) are multipotent adult stem cells thought to lack immunogenicity. MSC treatment in refractory graft-vs-host disease demonstrated effectiveness in phase I and II studies, although a larger unpublished phase III trial failed to meet the primary end point at 28 days [100, 101]. Phase I and II trials investigating the use of adipose-derived MSC injection into complex perianal fistulas in patients with Crohn's disease have shown benefit [102, 103]. In a phase II trial, injection of adipose-derived MSC plus fibrin glue resulted in fistula healing in 71 % of patients compared to 16 % of patients who received fibrin glue alone ($p<0.001$) [103]. A phase III trial examining intralesional injection of adipose-derived MSC compared to placebo in patients with fistulizing Crohn's disease is ongoing (NCT01541579). In a phase II open-label study of MSC in 16 patients with anti-TNF refractory endoscopically active luminal Crohn's disease, median CDAI score decreased from 370 to 203 at 42 days ($p<0.0001$) with a decrease in CDAI after each infusion [104]. A phase III trial evaluating the effectiveness of MSC in patients with active luminal Crohn's disease refractory to biologic therapy, however, was recently terminated early secondary to flaws in trial design and a reported high placebo response rate (NCT00482092). Results from this study have not been published.

Therapies Aimed at Altering the Gut Microbiome

Several studies examining the gut microbiome demonstrate significant differences in the composition of enteric organisms in UC, CD, and normal controls [105–107]. In addition, enteric organisms can induce or protect the host from chronic inflammation in experimental models [108–111]. For this reason, there has been interest in altering the gut microbiome as a treatment for IBD with probiotics, prebiotics, antibiotics, or fecal microbiota transplant.

Antibiotics

The majority of trials regarding the use of antibiotics in Crohn's disease have focused on metronidazole and ciprofloxacin. Although several studies have demonstrated improvement in symptoms with treatment with ciprofloxacin and metronidazole, the benefit is modest and their long-term use is limited by side-effects [112–115]. Recently, rifaximin-extended intestinal release, a minimally absorbed broad-spectrum oral antibiotic, was studied in a 12-week randomized control trial in moderately active Crohn's disease [116]. Patients who received 800 mg bid had increased in clinical remission compared to placebo, although no benefit was seen with 400 mg bid or 1,200 mg bid. Two studies examining 800 mg of rifaximin delayed release with or without dose adjustment compared to placebo in the treatment of active Crohn's disease were recently initiated (NCT02240108, NCT02240121).

It has long been hypothesized that a specific bacteria is the cause of Crohn's disease. In 1984, Chiodini and colleagues isolated *Mycobacterium avium* subsp. *paratuberculosis* (MAP) from two patients with Crohn's disease. In this publication, mice that were inoculated with the bacteria developed granulomas in the liver and spleen and a goat inoculated with the species developed granulomatous disease in the distal small bowel [117]. Since that time, there have been several reports of *M. avium* subsp. *paratuberculosis* identified in a high percentage of patients with Crohn's disease [118–121]. However, many studies have refuted these findings [122–126]. In the largest controlled study to examine the effects of antimycobacterial therapy in the treatment of Crohn's disease, Selby and colleagues randomized 213 patients with Crohn's disease to a 16-week taper of prednisone plus either 2 years of treatment with clarithromycin 750 mg/day, rifabutin 450 mg/day, and clofazimine 50 mg/day or placebo. Although there were significantly more subjects in remission at week 16 who received the antibiotic therapy than placebo, the benefit was not seen in follow-up at 1, 2, or 3 years [127]. There were several confounders in this trial which may have led to a null result including the fact that MAP was not tested at baseline, there was an error in some of the clofazimine tablets gelatin coating where many patients may not have received the intended dose for up to 10 months, and subjects in the trial on the control arm could continue on mesalamine and immunomodulator therapy. A phase III trial using 5 RHB-104 capsules (clarithromycin 95 mg, rifabutin 45 mg, and clofazimine 10 mg) in subjects with moderate to severe Crohn's disease is currently underway to further investigate the effectiveness of antimycobacterial treatment (NCT01951326).

Fecal Microbiota Transplant

There has been extensive research recently at reestablishing a healthy microbial composition in the gut as a treatment for patients with Crohn's disease. Numerous studies have examined different probiotics for this purpose. Although there have been several published "positive" trials with various probiotic regimens, there has not been a consistent benefit seen in treating patients with Crohn's disease with probiotics overall [116]. For this reason, there has been significant interest in performing fecal microbiota transplantation (FMT) in IBD, which populates the recipient with polymicrobial species from a healthy individual rather than treating with a single organism as occurs with probiotic treatment.

FMT has garnered significant interest supported by recent evidence of the effectiveness of FMT in *Clostridium difficile* infection [128]. Several published and unpublished case reports and series have reported on the potential benefit of FMT in IBD [129–131]. Cui and colleagues recently published a pilot study where 30 subjects with refractory Crohn's disease with a single FMT by gastroscope from subject identified donors. The authors reported 60 % of patients were in clinical remission at 1 month which was sustained at 6 months [132]. At Digestive Disease week in 2014, two studies reported on FMT in patients with Crohn's disease. Wu and colleagues presented a case series of 10 pediatric Crohn's disease patients treated with FMT by nasogastric tube after a bowel cleanout, 3 days of rifaximin, and 1 day of omeprazole. Seven patients from this cohort were in remission 2 weeks post FMT and five were in remission 6 weeks post FMT. Although mean fecal calprotectin level decreased post-transplant, it remained elevated despite the reported clinical improvement (614±621 mcg/g at week 0, 496±533 mcg/g at week 2, and 430±378 mcg/g at week 6) [133]. A second study in adults with active CD described 4-week follow-up of eight patients treated with FMT by colonoscopic delivery in a prospective open-label trial. The authors reported a significant decrease in Harvey Bradshaw index, Short Inflammatory Bowel Disease Questionnaire (SIBDQ) scores, and CRP at 4 weeks. Five of eight patients were in clinical remission at week 4. There were no SAEs reported in the preliminary analysis [134]. Long-term follow-up and endoscopic evaluation of these patients is ongoing. In addition, several additional trials examining the effectiveness of FMT in Crohn's disease are under way (NCT01793831, NCT02199561, NCT02097797, NCT02033408).

Conclusion

Increased understanding of mechanisms of disease activity in IBD through preclinical and genetic association studies has led to the development of numerous novel therapeutic agents in Crohn's disease. Although these therapies are promising in regard to their therapeutic potential, less than half of the patients treated with the majority of these agents in early clinical trials achieve remission. Accordingly, there is a great need for future research to optimize response rates through monitoring of drug levels, studying the use of combination of these agents in Crohn's disease, as well as identifying patients who are most likely to respond prior to initiation of therapy. As technologies to easily obtain large-scale genomic data advance, there will be an increasing focus on using gene expression, genetic, metabolites, and microbiota data to predict response to therapy. This personalized approach to the treatment of Crohn's disease coupled with an increasing number of effective therapies is likely to greatly improve overall response rates to medical therapy while minimizing toxicity.

References

1. Winship DH, Summers RW, Singleton JW, Best WR, Becktel JM, Lenk LF, et al. National Cooperative Crohn's Disease Study: study design and conduct of the study. Gastroenterology. 1979; 77(4 Pt 2):829–42.
2. Jones JH, Lennard-Jones JE. Corticosteroids and corticotrophin in the treatment of Crohn's disease. Gut. 1966;7(2):181–7.
3. Cooke WT, Fielding JF. Corticosteroid or corticotrophin therapy in Crohn's disease (regional enteritis). Gut. 1970;11(11):921–7.
4. O'Donoghue DP, Dawson AM, Powell-Tuck J, Bown RL, Lennard-Jones JE. Double-blind withdrawal trial of azathioprine as maintenance treatment for Crohn's disease. Lancet. 1978;2(8097):955–7.
5. Feagan BG, Rochon J, Fedorak RN, Irvine EJ, Wild G, Sutherland L, et al. Methotrexate for the treatment of Crohn's disease. The North American Crohn's Study Group Investigators. N Engl J Med. 1995;332(5):292–7.
6. Brynskov J, Freund L, Rasmussen SN, Lauritsen K, de Muckadell OS, Williams N, et al. A placebo-controlled, double-blind, randomized trial of cyclosporine therapy in active chronic Crohn's disease. N Engl J Med. 1989;321(13):845–50.
7. Peyrin-Biroulet L, Reinisch W, Colombel JF, Mantzaris GJ, Kornbluth A, Diamond R, et al. Clinical disease activity, C-reactive protein normalisation and mucosal healing in Crohn's disease in the SONIC trial. Gut. 2014;63(1):88–95.
8. Peyrin-Biroulet L, Ferrante M, Magro F, Campbell S, Franchimont D, Fidder H, et al. Results from the 2nd Scientific Workshop of the ECCO. I: impact of mucosal healing on the course of inflammatory bowel disease. J Crohns Colitis. 2011;5(5):477–83.
9. Casellas F, Barreiro de Acosta M, Iglesias M, Robles V, Nos P, Aguas M, et al. Mucosal healing restores normal health and quality of life in patients with inflammatory bowel disease. Eur J Gastroenterol Hepatol. 2012;24(7):762–9.
10. Froslie KF, Jahnsen J, Moum BA, Vatn MH, Group I. Mucosal healing in inflammatory bowel disease: results from a Norwegian population-based cohort. Gastroenterology. 2007;133(2):412–22.
11. Baert F, Moortgat L, Van Assche G, Caenepeel P, Vergauwe P, De Vos M, et al. Mucosal healing predicts sustained clinical remission in patients with early-stage Crohn's disease. Gastroenterology. 2010;138(2):463–8; quiz e10–1.
12. Hebuterne X, Lemann M, Bouhnik Y, Dewit O, Dupas JL, Mross M, et al. Endoscopic improvement of

mucosal lesions in patients with moderate to severe ileocolonic Crohn's disease following treatment with certolizumab pegol. Gut. 2013;62(2):201–8.

13. De Cruz P, Kamm MA, Prideaux L, Allen PB, Moore G. Mucosal healing in Crohn's disease: a systematic review. Inflamm Bowel Dis. 2013;19(2): 429–44.
14. Panaccione R, Colombel JF, Louis E, Peyrin-Biroulet L, Sandborn WJ. Evolving definitions of remission in Crohn's disease. Inflamm Bowel Dis. 2013;19(8):1645–53.
15. Schnitzler F, Fidder H, Ferrante M, Noman M, Arijs I, Van Assche G, et al. Mucosal healing predicts long-term outcome of maintenance therapy with infliximab in Crohn's disease. Inflamm Bowel Dis. 2009;15(9):1295–301.
16. D'Haens G, Baert F, van Assche G, Caenepeel P, Vergauwe P, Tuynman H, et al. Early combined immunosuppression or conventional management in patients with newly diagnosed Crohn's disease: an open randomised trial. Lancet. 2008;371(9613): 660–7.
17. Schreiber S, Colombel JF, Bloomfield R, Nikolaus S, Scholmerich J, Panes J, et al. Increased response and remission rates in short-duration Crohn's disease with subcutaneous certolizumab pegol: an analysis of PRECiSE 2 randomized maintenance trial data. Am J Gastroenterol. 2010;105(7):1574–82.
18. Schreiber S, Reinisch W, Colombel JF, Sandborn WJ, Hommes DW, Robinson AM, et al. Subgroup analysis of the placebo-controlled CHARM trial: increased remission rates through 3 years for adalimumab-treated patients with early Crohn's disease. J Crohns Colitis. 2013;7(3):213–21.
19. Colombel JF, Sandborn WJ, Reinisch W, Mantzaris GJ, Kornbluth A, Rachmilewitz D, et al. Infliximab, azathioprine, or combination therapy for Crohn's disease. N Engl J Med. 2010;362(15):1383–95.
20. Feagan BG, McDonald JW, Panaccione R, Enns RA, Bernstein CN, Ponich TP, et al. Methotrexate in combination with infliximab is no more effective than infliximab alone in patients with Crohn's disease. Gastroenterology. 2014;146(3):681–8. 3.
21. Navarro RF, Jalkanen ST, Hsu M, Soenderstrup-Hansen G, Goronzy J, Weyand C, et al. Human T cell clones express functional homing receptors required for normal lymphocyte trafficking. J Exp Med. 1985;162(3):1075–80.
22. Butcher EC, Picker LJ. Lymphocyte homing and homeostasis. Science. 1996;272(5258):60–6.
23. Kansas GS. Selectins and their ligands: current concepts and controversies. Blood. 1996;88(9):3259–87.
24. Eksteen B. Targeting of gut specific leucocyte recruitment in IBD by vedolizumab. Gut. 2015 Jan;64(1):8–10. doi: 10.1136/gutjnl-2014-307397. Epub 2014 Jun 19.
25. Marlin SD, Springer TA. Purified intercellular adhesion molecule-1 (ICAM-1) is a ligand for lymphocyte function-associated antigen 1 (LFA-1). Cell. 1987;51(5):813–9.
26. Cepek KL, Shaw SK, Parker CM, Russell GJ, Morrow JS, Rimm DL, et al. Adhesion between epithelial cells and T lymphocytes mediated by E-cadherin and the alpha E beta 7 integrin. Nature. 1994;372(6502):190–3.
27. Kunkel EJ, Campbell JJ, Haraldsen G, Pan J, Boisvert J, Roberts AI, et al. Lymphocyte CC chemokine receptor 9 and epithelial thymus-expressed chemokine (TECK) expression distinguish the small intestinal immune compartment: epithelial expression of tissue-specific chemokines as an organizing principle in regional immunity. J Exp Med. 2000;192(5):761–8.
28. Mora JR, Bono MR, Manjunath N, Weninger W, Cavanagh LL, Rosemblatt M, et al. Selective imprinting of gut-homing T cells by Peyer's patch dendritic cells. Nature. 2003;424(6944):88–93.
29. Gordon FH, Lai CW, Hamilton MI, Allison MC, Srivastava ED, Fouweather MG, et al. A randomized placebo-controlled trial of a humanized monoclonal antibody to alpha4 integrin in active Crohn's disease. Gastroenterology. 2001;121(2):268–74.
30. Ghosh S, Goldin E, Gordon FH, Malchow HA, Rask-Madsen J, Rutgeerts P, et al. Natalizumab for active Crohn's disease. N Engl J Med. 2003; 348(1):24–32.
31. Sandborn WJ, Colombel JF, Enns R, Feagan BG, Hanauer SB, Lawrance IC, et al. Natalizumab induction and maintenance therapy for Crohn's disease. N Engl J Med. 2005;353(18):1912–25.
32. Targan SR, Feagan BG, Fedorak RN, Lashner BA, Panaccione R, Present DH, et al. Natalizumab for the treatment of active Crohn's disease: results of the ENCORE Trial. Gastroenterology. 2007;132(5): 1672–83.
33. Kleinschmidt-DeMasters BK, Tyler KL. Progressive multifocal leukoencephalopathy complicating treatment with natalizumab and interferon beta-1a for multiple sclerosis. N Engl J Med. 2005;353(4):369–74.
34. Bloomgren G, Richman S, Hotermans C, Subramanyam M, Goelz S, Natarajan A, et al. Risk of natalizumab-associated progressive multifocal leukoencephalopathy. N Engl J Med. 2012;366(20): 1870–80.
35. Stuve O, Marra CM, Bar-Or A, Niino M, Cravens PD, Cepok S, et al. Altered CD4+/CD8+ T-cell ratios in cerebrospinal fluid of natalizumab-treated patients with multiple sclerosis. Arch Neurol. 2006;63(10):1383–7.
36. Feagan BG, Greenberg GR, Wild G, Fedorak RN, Pare P, McDonald JW, et al. Treatment of ulcerative colitis with a humanized antibody to the alpha4beta7 integrin. N Engl J Med. 2005;352(24):2499–507.
37. Feagan BG, Rutgeerts P, Sands BE, Hanauer S, Colombel JF, Sandborn WJ, et al. Vedolizumab as induction and maintenance therapy for ulcerative colitis. N Engl J Med. 2013;369(8):699–710.
38. Feagan BG, Greenberg GR, Wild G, Fedorak RN, Pare P, McDonald JW, et al. Treatment of active Crohn's disease with MLN0002, a humanized anti-

body to the alpha4beta7 integrin. Clin Gastroenterol Hepatol. 2008;6(12):1370–7.
39. Sandborn WJ, Feagan BG, Rutgeerts P, Hanauer S, Colombel JF, Sands BE, et al. Vedolizumab as induction and maintenance therapy for Crohn's disease. N Engl J Med. 2013;369(8):711–21.
40. Sands BE, Feagan BG, Rutgeerts P, Colombel JF, Sandborn WJ, Sy R, et al. Effects of vedolizumab induction therapy for patients with Crohn's disease in whom tumor necrosis factor antagonist treatment failed. Gastroenterology. 2014;147(3):618–27. 3.
41. Milch C, Wyant T, Xu J, Parikh A, Kent W, Fox I, et al. Vedolizumab, a monoclonal antibody to the gut homing alpha4beta7 integrin, does not affect cerebrospinal fluid T-lymphocyte immunophenotype. J Neuroimmunol. 2013;264(1–2):123–6.
42. Pan WJ, Hsu H, Rees WA, Lear SP, Lee F, Foltz IN, et al. Pharmacology of AMG 181, a human anti-alpha4 beta7 antibody that specifically alters trafficking of gut-homing T cells. Br J Pharmacol. 2013;169(1):51–68.
43. Pullen N, Molloy E, Carter D, Syntin P, Clemo F, Finco-Kent D, et al. Pharmacological characterization of PF-00547659, an anti-human MAdCAM monoclonal antibody. Br J Pharmacol. 2009; 157(2):281–93.
44. Vermeire S, Ghosh S, Panes J, Dahlerup JF, Luegering A, Sirotiakova J, et al. The mucosal addressin cell adhesion molecule antibody PF-00547,659 in ulcerative colitis: a randomised study. Gut. 2011;60(8):1068–75.
45. Takazoe M, Wanatabe M, Kawaguchi T, Matsumoto T, Oshitani N, Hiwatashi N, et al. Oral alpha-4 integrin inhibitor (AJM300) in patients with active Crohn's disease – a randomized, double-blind, placebo-controlled trial. Gastroenterology. 2009; 136(5, Suppl 1):A-181.
46. Watanabe M, Yoshimura N, Motoya S, Tominaga K, Iwakiri R, Watabe K, et al. AJM300, an oral α4 integrin antagonist, for active ulcerative colitis: a multicenter, randomized, double-blind, placebo-controlled phase 2A study. Gastroenterology. 2014;146(5, Suppl 1):S-82.
47. Keshav S, Vanasek T, Niv Y, Petryka R, Howaldt S, Bafutto M, et al. A randomized controlled trial of the efficacy and safety of CCX282-B, an orally-administered blocker of chemokine receptor CCR9, for patients with Crohn's disease. PLoS One. 2013;8(3):e60094.
48. Mayer L, Sandborn WJ, Stepanov Y, Geboes K, Hardi R, Yellin M, et al. Anti-IP-10 antibody (BMS-936557) for ulcerative colitis: a phase II randomised study. Gut. 2014;63(3):442–50.
49. Oppmann B, Lesley R, Blom B, Timans JC, Xu Y, Hunte B, et al. Novel p19 protein engages IL-12p40 to form a cytokine, IL-23, with biological activities similar as well as distinct from IL-12. Immunity. 2000;13(5):715–25.
50. Wang K, Zhang H, Kugathasan S, Annese V, Bradfield JP, Russell RK, et al. Diverse genome-wide association studies associate the IL12/IL23 pathway with Crohn disease. Am J Hum Genet. 2009;84(3):399–405.
51. Trinchieri G, Pflanz S, Kastelein RA. The IL-12 family of heterodimeric cytokines: new players in the regulation of T cell responses. Immunity. 2003;19(5):641–4.
52. Wilson NJ, Boniface K, Chan JR, McKenzie BS, Blumenschein WM, Mattson JD, et al. Development, cytokine profile and function of human interleukin 17-producing helper T cells. Nat Immunol. 2007;8(9):950–7.
53. Leonardi CL, Kimball AB, Papp KA, Yeilding N, Guzzo C, Wang Y, et al. Efficacy and safety of ustekinumab, a human interleukin-12/23 monoclonal antibody, in patients with psoriasis: 76-week results from a randomised, double-blind, placebo-controlled trial (PHOENIX 1). Lancet. 2008; 371(9625):1665–74.
54. Papp KA, Langley RG, Lebwohl M, Krueger GG, Szapary P, Yeilding N, et al. Efficacy and safety of ustekinumab, a human interleukin-12/23 monoclonal antibody, in patients with psoriasis: 52-week results from a randomised, double-blind, placebo-controlled trial (PHOENIX 2). Lancet. 2008;371(9625):1675–84.
55. Gottlieb A, Menter A, Mendelsohn A, Shen YK, Li S, Guzzo C, et al. Ustekinumab, a human interleukin 12/23 monoclonal antibody, for psoriatic arthritis: randomised, double-blind, placebo-controlled, crossover trial. Lancet. 2009;373(9664):633–40.
56. Sandborn WJ, Feagan BG, Fedorak RN, Scherl E, Fleisher MR, Katz S, et al. A randomized trial of ustekinumab, a human interleukin-12/23 monoclonal antibody, in patients with moderate-to-severe Crohn's disease. Gastroenterology. 2008;135(4):1130–41.
57. Sandborn WJ, Gasink C, Gao LL, Blank MA, Johanns J, Guzzo C, et al. Ustekinumab induction and maintenance therapy in refractory Crohn's disease. N Engl J Med. 2012;367(16):1519–28.
58. Aittomaki S, Pesu M. Therapeutic targeting of the Jak/STAT pathway. Basic Clin Pharmacol Toxicol. 2014;114(1):18–23.
59. Coskun M, Salem M, Pedersen J, Nielsen OH. Involvement of JAK/STAT signaling in the pathogenesis of inflammatory bowel disease. Pharmacol Res. 2013;76:1–8.
60. Ferguson LR, Han DY, Fraser AG, Huebner C, Lam WJ, Morgan AR, et al. Genetic factors in chronic inflammation: single nucleotide polymorphisms in the STAT-JAK pathway, susceptibility to DNA damage and Crohn's disease in a New Zealand population. Mutat Res. 2010;690(1–2):108–15.
61. Franke A, McGovern DP, Barrett JC, Wang K, Radford-Smith GL, Ahmad T, et al. Genome-wide meta-analysis increases to 71 the number of confirmed Crohn's disease susceptibility loci. Nat Genet. 2010;42(12):1118–25.
62. Durant L, Watford WT, Ramos HL, Laurence A, Vahedi G, Wei L, et al. Diverse targets of the transcription factor STAT3 contribute to T cell pathogenicity and homeostasis. Immunity. 2010;32(5):605–15.

63. Yang XO, Panopoulos AD, Nurieva R, Chang SH, Wang D, Watowich SS, et al. STAT3 regulates cytokine-mediated generation of inflammatory helper T cells. J Biol Chem. 2007;282(13):9358–63.
64. Lovato P, Brender C, Agnholt J, Kelsen J, Kaltoft K, Svejgaard A, et al. Constitutive STAT3 activation in intestinal T cells from patients with Crohn's disease. J Biol Chem. 2003;278(19):16777–81.
65. Mudter J, Weigmann B, Bartsch B, Kiesslich R, Strand D, Galle PR, et al. Activation pattern of signal transducers and activators of transcription (STAT) factors in inflammatory bowel diseases. Am J Gastroenterol. 2005;100(1):64–72.
66. Kremer JM, Bloom BJ, Breedveld FC, Coombs JH, Fletcher MP, Gruben D, et al. The safety and efficacy of a JAK inhibitor in patients with active rheumatoid arthritis: results of a double-blind, placebo-controlled phase IIa trial of three dosage levels of CP-690,550 versus placebo. Arthritis Rheum. 2009;60(7):1895–905.
67. Lee EB, Fleischmann R, Hall S, Wilkinson B, Bradley JD, Gruben D, et al. Tofacitinib versus methotrexate in rheumatoid arthritis. N Engl J Med. 2014;370(25):2377–86.
68. van Vollenhoven RF, Fleischmann R, Cohen S, Lee EB, Garcia Meijide JA, Wagner S, et al. Tofacitinib or adalimumab versus placebo in rheumatoid arthritis. N Engl J Med. 2012;367(6):508–19.
69. Ports WC, Khan S, Lan S, Lamba M, Bolduc C, Bissonnette R, et al. A randomized phase 2a efficacy and safety trial of the topical Janus kinase inhibitor tofacitinib in the treatment of chronic plaque psoriasis. Br J Dermatol. 2013;169(1):137–45.
70. Vincenti F, Tedesco Silva H, Busque S, O'Connell P, Friedewald J, Cibrik D, et al. Randomized phase 2b trial of tofacitinib (CP-690,550) in de novo kidney transplant patients: efficacy, renal function and safety at 1 year. Am J Transplant. 2012;12(9):2446–56.
71. Sandborn WJ, Ghosh S, Panes J, Vranic I, Su C, Rousell S, et al. Tofacitinib, an oral Janus kinase inhibitor, in active ulcerative colitis. N Engl J Med. 2012;367(7):616–24.
72. Sandborn WJ, Ghosh S, Panes J, Vranic I, Wang W, Niezychowski W, et al. A phase 2 study of tofacitinib, an oral Janus kinase inhibitor, in patients with Crohn's disease. Clin Gastroenterol Hepatol. 2014;12:1485–93.e2.
73. Van Rompaey L, Galien R, van der Aar EM, Clement-Lacroix P, Nelles L, Smets B, et al. Preclinical characterization of GLPG0634, a selective inhibitor of JAK1, for the treatment of inflammatory diseases. J Immunol. 2013;191(7):3568–77.
74. Hosokawa T, Kusugami K, Ina K, Ando T, Shinoda M, Imada A, et al. Interleukin-6 and soluble interleukin-6 receptor in the colonic mucosa of inflammatory bowel disease. J Gastroenterol Hepatol. 1999;14(10):987–96.
75. Zorzi F, Monteleone I, Sarra M, Calabrese E, Marafini I, Cretella M, et al. Distinct profiles of effector cytokines mark the different phases of Crohn's disease. PLoS One. 2013;8(1):e54562.
76. Atreya R, Mudter J, Finotto S, Mullberg J, Jostock T, Wirtz S, et al. Blockade of interleukin 6 trans signaling suppresses T-cell resistance against apoptosis in chronic intestinal inflammation: evidence in Crohn disease and experimental colitis in vivo. Nat Med. 2000;6(5):583–8.
77. Maini RN, Taylor PC, Szechinski J, Pavelka K, Broll J, Balint G, et al. Double-blind randomized controlled clinical trial of the interleukin-6 receptor antagonist, tocilizumab, in European patients with rheumatoid arthritis who had an incomplete response to methotrexate. Arthritis Rheum. 2006;54(9):2817–29.
78. Smolen JS, Beaulieu A, Rubbert-Roth A, Ramos-Remus C, Rovensky J, Alecock E, et al. Effect of interleukin-6 receptor inhibition with tocilizumab in patients with rheumatoid arthritis (OPTION study): a double-blind, placebo-controlled, randomised trial. Lancet. 2008;371(9617):987–97.
79. Yokota S, Imagawa T, Mori M, Miyamae T, Aihara Y, Takei S, et al. Efficacy and safety of tocilizumab in patients with systemic-onset juvenile idiopathic arthritis: a randomised, double-blind, placebo-controlled, withdrawal phase III trial. Lancet. 2008;371(9617):998–1006.
80. Matsuyama M, Suzuki T, Tsuboi H, Ito S, Mamura M, Goto D, et al. Anti-interleukin-6 receptor antibody (tocilizumab) treatment of multicentric Castleman's disease. Intern Med. 2007;46(11):771–4.
81. Ito H, Takazoe M, Fukuda Y, Hibi T, Kusugami K, Andoh A, et al. A pilot randomized trial of a human anti-interleukin-6 receptor monoclonal antibody in active Crohn's disease. Gastroenterology. 2004;126(4):989–96. discussion 47.
82. Breese EJ, Michie CA, Nicholls SW, Murch SH, Williams CB, Domizio P, et al. Tumor necrosis factor alpha-producing cells in the intestinal mucosa of children with inflammatory bowel disease. Gastroenterology. 1994;106(6):1455–66.
83. van Dullemen HM, van Deventer SJ, Hommes DW, Bijl HA, Jansen J, Tytgat GN, et al. Treatment of Crohn's disease with anti-tumor necrosis factor chimeric monoclonal antibody (cA2). Gastroenterology. 1995;109(1):129–35.
84. Targan SR, Hanauer SB, van Deventer SJ, Mayer L, Present DH, Braakman T, et al. A short-term study of chimeric monoclonal antibody cA2 to tumor necrosis factor alpha for Crohn's disease. Crohn's Disease cA2 Study Group. N Engl J Med. 1997;337(15):1029–35.
85. Hanauer SB, Feagan BG, Lichtenstein GR, Mayer LF, Schreiber S, Colombel JF, et al. Maintenance infliximab for Crohn's disease: the ACCENT I randomised trial. Lancet. 2002;359(9317):1541–9.
86. Present DH, Rutgeerts P, Targan S, Hanauer SB, Mayer L, van Hogezand RA, et al. Infliximab for the treatment of fistulas in patients with Crohn's disease. N Engl J Med. 1999;340(18):1398–405.
87. Colombel JF, Sandborn WJ, Rutgeerts P, Enns R, Hanauer SB, Panaccione R, et al. Adalimumab for maintenance of clinical response and remission in

patients with Crohn's disease: the CHARM trial. Gastroenterology. 2007;132(1):52–65.
88. Hanauer SB, Sandborn WJ, Rutgeerts P, Fedorak RN, Lukas M, MacIntosh D, et al. Human anti-tumor necrosis factor monoclonal antibody (adalimumab) in Crohn's disease: the CLASSIC-I trial. Gastroenterology. 2006;130(2):323–33. quiz 591.
89. Schreiber S, Khaliq-Kareemi M, Lawrance IC, Thomsen OO, Hanauer SB, McColm J, et al. Maintenance therapy with certolizumab pegol for Crohn's disease. N Engl J Med. 2007;357(3):239–50.
90. Sandborn WJ, Feagan BG, Stoinov S, Honiball PJ, Rutgeerts P, Mason D, et al. Certolizumab pegol for the treatment of Crohn's disease. N Engl J Med. 2007;357(3):228–38.
91. Sandborn WJ, Feagan BG, Marano C, Zhang H, Strauss R, Johanns J, et al. Subcutaneous golimumab maintains clinical response in patients with moderate-to-severe ulcerative colitis. Gastroenterology. 2014;146(1):96–109. 1.
92. Sandborn WJ, Feagan BG, Marano C, Zhang H, Strauss R, Johanns J, et al. Subcutaneous golimumab induces clinical response and remission in patients with moderate-to-severe ulcerative colitis. Gastroenterology. 2014;146(1):85–95; quiz e14–5.
93. Yoo DH, Hrycaj P, Miranda P, Ramiterre E, Piotrowski M, Shevchuk S, et al. A randomised, double-blind, parallel-group study to demonstrate equivalence in efficacy and safety of CT-P13 compared with innovator infliximab when coadministered with methotrexate in patients with active rheumatoid arthritis: the PLANETRA study. Ann Rheum Dis. 2013;72(10):1613–20.
94. Park W, Hrycaj P, Jeka S, Kovalenko V, Lysenko G, Miranda P, et al. A randomised, double-blind, multicentre, parallel-group, prospective study comparing the pharmacokinetics, safety, and efficacy of CT-P13 and innovator infliximab in patients with ankylosing spondylitis: the PLANETAS study. Ann Rheum Dis. 2013;72(10):1605–12.
95. Hommes DW, Duijvestein M, Zelinkova Z, Stokkers PC, Ley MH, Stoker J, et al. Long-term follow-up of autologous hematopoietic stem cell transplantation for severe refractory Crohn's disease. J Crohns Colitis. 2011;5(6):543–9.
96. Hasselblatt P, Drognitz K, Potthoff K, Bertz H, Kruis W, Schmidt C, et al. Remission of refractory Crohn's disease by high-dose cyclophosphamide and autologous peripheral blood stem cell transplantation. Aliment Pharmacol Ther. 2012;36(8):725–35.
97. Cassinotti A, Annaloro C, Ardizzone S, Onida F, Della Volpe A, Clerici M, et al. Autologous haematopoietic stem cell transplantation without CD34+ cell selection in refractory Crohn's disease. Gut. 2008;57(2):211–7.
98. Burt RK, Craig RM, Milanetti F, Quigley K, Gozdziak P, Bucha J, et al. Autologous nonmyeloablative hematopoietic stem cell transplantation in patients with severe anti-TNF refractory Crohn disease: long-term follow-up. Blood. 2010;116(26):6123–32.
99. Oyama Y, Craig RM, Traynor AE, Quigley K, Statkute L, Halverson A, et al. Autologous hematopoietic stem cell transplantation in patients with refractory Crohn's disease. Gastroenterology. 2005;128(3):552–63.
100. Le Blanc K, Frassoni F, Ball L, Locatelli F, Roelofs H, Lewis I, et al. Mesenchymal stem cells for treatment of steroid-resistant, severe, acute graft-versus-host disease: a phase II study. Lancet. 2008;371(9624):1579–86.
101. Herrmann R, Sturm M, Shaw K, Purtill D, Cooney J, Wright M, et al. Mesenchymal stromal cell therapy for steroid-refractory acute and chronic graft versus host disease: a phase 1 study. Int J Hematol. 2012;95(2):182–8.
102. Garcia-Olmo D, Garcia-Arranz M, Herreros D, Pascual I, Peiro C, Rodriguez-Montes JA. A phase I clinical trial of the treatment of Crohn's fistula by adipose mesenchymal stem cell transplantation. Dis Colon Rectum. 2005;48(7):1416–23.
103. Garcia-Olmo D, Herreros D, Pascual I, Pascual JA, Del-Valle E, Zorrilla J, et al. Expanded adipose-derived stem cells for the treatment of complex perianal fistula: a phase II clinical trial. Dis Colon Rectum. 2009;52(1):79–86.
104. Forbes GM, Sturm MJ, Leong RW, Sparrow MP, Segarajasingam D, Cummins AG, et al. A phase 2 study of allogeneic mesenchymal stromal cells for luminal Crohn's disease refractory to biologic therapy. Clin Gastroenterol Hepatol. 2014;12(1):64–71.
105. Manichanh C, Rigottier-Gois L, Bonnaud E, Gloux K, Pelletier E, Frangeul L, et al. Reduced diversity of faecal microbiota in Crohn's disease revealed by a metagenomic approach. Gut. 2006;55(2):205–11.
106. Morgan XC, Tickle TL, Sokol H, Gevers D, Devaney KL, Ward DV, et al. Dysfunction of the intestinal microbiome in inflammatory bowel disease and treatment. Genome Biol. 2012;13(9):R79.
107. Gevers D, Kugathasan S, Denson LA, Vazquez-Baeza Y, Van Treuren W, Ren B, et al. The treatment-naive microbiome in new-onset Crohn's disease. Cell Host Microbe. 2014;15(3):382–92.
108. Llopis M, Antolin M, Carol M, Borruel N, Casellas F, Martinez C, et al. Lactobacillus casei downregulates commensals' inflammatory signals in Crohn's disease mucosa. Inflamm Bowel Dis. 2009;15(2):275–83.
109. Stepankova R, Powrie F, Kofronova O, Kozakova H, Hudcovic T, Hrncir T, et al. Segmented filamentous bacteria in a defined bacterial cocktail induce intestinal inflammation in SCID mice reconstituted with CD45RBhigh CD4+ T cells. Inflamm Bowel Dis. 2007;13(10):1202–11.
110. Devkota S, Wang Y, Musch MW, Leone V, Fehlner-Peach H, Nadimpalli A, et al. Dietary-fat-induced taurocholic acid promotes pathobiont expansion and colitis in Il10−/− mice. Nature. 2012;487(7405):104–8.
111. Mazmanian SK, Round JL, Kasper DL. A microbial symbiosis factor prevents intestinal inflammatory disease. Nature. 2008;453(7195):620–5.

112. Ursing B, Alm T, Barany F, Bergelin I, Ganrot-Norlin K, Hoevels J, et al. A comparative study of metronidazole and sulfasalazine for active Crohn's disease: the cooperative Crohn's disease study in Sweden. II. Result. Gastroenterology. 1982;83(3):550–62.
113. Steinhart AH, Feagan BG, Wong CJ, Vandervoort M, Mikolainis S, Croitoru K, et al. Combined budesonide and antibiotic therapy for active Crohn's disease: a randomized controlled trial. Gastroenterology. 2002;123(1):33–40.
114. Prantera C, Zannoni F, Scribano ML, Berto E, Andreoli A, Kohn A, et al. An antibiotic regimen for the treatment of active Crohn's disease: a randomized, controlled clinical trial of metronidazole plus ciprofloxacin. Am J Gastroenterol. 1996;91(2):328–32.
115. Colombel JF, Lemann M, Cassagnou M, Bouhnik Y, Duclos B, Dupas JL, et al. A controlled trial comparing ciprofloxacin with mesalazine for the treatment of active Crohn's disease. Groupe d'Etudes Therapeutiques des Affections Inflammatoires Digestives (GETAID). Am J Gastroenterol. 1999;94(3):674–8.
116. Prantera C, Lochs H, Grimaldi M, Danese S, Scribano ML, Gionchetti P, et al. Rifaximin-extended intestinal release induces remission in patients with moderately active Crohn's disease. Gastroenterology. 2012;142(3):473–81. 3.
117. Chiodini RJ, Van Kruiningen HJ, Thayer WR, Merkal RS, Coutu JA. Possible role of mycobacteria in inflammatory bowel disease. I. An unclassified *Mycobacterium* species isolated from patients with Crohn's disease. Dig Dis Sci. 1984;29(12):1073–9.
118. Sanderson JD, Moss MT, Tizard ML, Hermon-Taylor J. *Mycobacterium paratuberculosis* DNA in Crohn's disease tissue. Gut. 1992;33(7):890–6.
119. Schwartz D, Shafran I, Romero C, Piromalli C, Biggerstaff J, Naser N, et al. Use of short-term culture for identification of *Mycobacterium avium* subsp. *paratuberculosis* in tissue from Crohn's disease patients. Clin Microbiol Infect. 2000;6(6):303–7.
120. Sechi LA, Mura M, Tanda F, Lissia A, Solinas A, Fadda G, et al. Identification of *Mycobacterium avium* subsp. *paratuberculosis* in biopsy specimens from patients with Crohn's disease identified by in situ hybridization. J Clin Microbiol. 2001;39(12):4514–7.
121. Bull TJ, McMinn EJ, Sidi-Boumedine K, Skull A, Durkin D, Neild P, et al. Detection and verification of *Mycobacterium avium* subsp. *paratuberculosis* in fresh ileocolonic mucosal biopsy specimens from individuals with and without Crohn's disease. J Clin Microbiol. 2003;41(7):2915–23.
122. Rowbotham DS, Mapstone NP, Trejdosiewicz LK, Howdle PD, Quirke P. *Mycobacterium paratuberculosis* DNA not detected in Crohn's disease tissue by fluorescent polymerase chain reaction. Gut. 1995; 37(5):660–7.
123. Al-Shamali M, Khan I, Al-Nakib B, Al-Hassan F, Mustafa AS. A multiplex polymerase chain reaction assay for the detection of *Mycobacterium paratuberculosis* DNA in Crohn's disease tissue. Scand J Gastroenterol. 1997;32(8):819–23.
124. Frank TS, Cook SM. Analysis of paraffin sections of Crohn's disease for *Mycobacterium paratuberculosis* using polymerase chain reaction. Mod Pathol. 1996;9(1):32–5.
125. Dumonceau JM, Van Gossum A, Adler M, Fonteyne PA, Van Vooren JP, Deviere J, et al. No *Mycobacterium paratuberculosis* found in Crohn's disease using polymerase chain reaction. Dig Dis Sci. 1996;41(2):421–6.
126. Kanazawa K, Haga Y, Funakoshi O, Nakajima H, Munakata A, Yoshida Y. Absence of *Mycobacterium paratuberculosis* DNA in intestinal tissues from Crohn's disease by nested polymerase chain reaction. J Gastroenterol. 1999;34(2):200–6.
127. Selby W, Pavli P, Crotty B, Florin T, Radford-Smith G, Gibson P, et al. Two-year combination antibiotic therapy with clarithromycin, rifabutin, and clofazimine for Crohn's disease. Gastroenterology. 2007;132(7):2313–9.
128. van Nood E, Vrieze A, Nieuwdorp M, Fuentes S, Zoetendal EG, de Vos WM, et al. Duodenal infusion of donor feces for recurrent Clostridium difficile. N Engl J Med. 2013;368(5):407–15.
129. Anderson JL, Edney RJ, Whelan K. Systematic review: faecal microbiota transplantation in the management of inflammatory bowel disease. Aliment Pharmacol Ther. 2012;36(6):503–16.
130. Zhang FM, Wang HG, Wang M, Cui BT, Fan ZN, Ji GZ. Fecal microbiota transplantation for severe enterocolonic fistulizing Crohn's disease. World J Gastroenterol. 2013;19(41):7213–6.
131. Kao D, Hotte N, Gillevet P, Madsen K. Fecal microbiota transplantation inducing remission in Crohn's colitis and the associated changes in fecal microbial profile. J Clin Gastroenterol. 2014;48(7):625–8.
132. Cui B, Feng Q, Wang H, Wang M, Peng Z, Li P, et al. Fecal microbiota transplantation through mid-gut for refractory Crohn's disease: safety, feasibility and efficacy trial results. J Gastroenterol Hepatol. 2015;30:51–8.
133. Suskind D, Wahbeh G, Vendetoulli H, Singh N, Miller S. Fecal microbial transplant in pediatric Crohn's disease. Gastroenterology. 2014;146(5):S-834.
134. Vaughn BP, Gevers D, Ting A, Korzenik JR, Robson SC, Moss AC. Fecal microbiota transplantation induces early improvement in symptoms in patients with active Crohn's disease. Gastroenterology. 2014;146(5):S-591-S5-2.

Diagnostic Fluoroscopy for Imaging Crohn's Disease

5

Michael F. McNeeley, Malak Itani, and Charles A. Rohrmann Jr.

Introduction

With the advent of cross-sectional imaging modalities such as computed tomography (CT) and magnetic resonance (MR) imaging, the role of contrast fluoroscopy in evaluating Crohn's disease has evolved. Because of its limited utility for assessing extraluminal disease, fluoroscopy has been largely supplanted by these advanced techniques. However, because of its superior spatial resolution and capacity for dynamic and real-time evaluation of the alimentary tract, contrast fluoroscopy remains an invaluable tool for the gastrointestinal radiologist and referring clinician. In particular, fluoroscopy (when used with enteric contrast agents) provides considerable value for delineating complications of Crohn's disease such as fistulae, strictures, and altered motility, while simultaneously offering a nuanced view of the mucosal relief.

This chapter provides an overview of the fluoroscopic evaluation of Crohn's disease. Particular emphasis will be placed on the information that is required by clinicians in order to request the appropriate examination and to guide the consulting radiologist in tailoring its performance. Additionally, an overview of the early and advanced radiologic manifestations of Crohn's disease will be provided so that the clinician may gain the maximal value from the radiologist's report.

Planning the Examination

When requesting a fluoroscopic examination of the alimentary tract, it is important to convey certain information to the consulting radiologist so that the examination is tailored to address the clinical need. At a minimum, the request should include: a precise statement of the clinical question; a focused patient history including current symptoms and prior surgeries, if applicable; and whether or not enteric perforation is clinically suspected. Additionally, if the patient is known to be at risk for aspiration, is incapable of tolerating oral intake, or has other potentially relevant conditions (e.g., fulminant colitis that would preclude rectal catheterization), then such information should be conveyed to the radiologist.

Plain Radiographs

The initial phase of any fluoroscopic examination of the gastrointestinal tract should consist of one or more radiographs of the abdomen. Although

M.F. McNeeley, MD (✉) • M. Itani, MD
C.A. Rohrmann Jr., MD (✉)
Department of Radiology, University of Washington Hospitals, 1959 Pacific Avenue, NE, Seattle, WA 98195, USA
e-mail: mcneeley@u.washington.edu; rohrmann@u.washington.edu

A. Fichera and M.K. Krane (eds.), *Crohn's Disease: Basic Principles*,
DOI 10.1007/978-3-319-14181-7_5, © Springer International Publishing Switzerland 2015

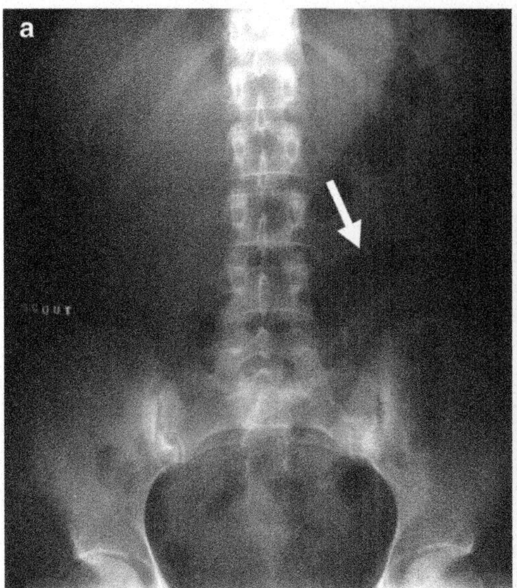

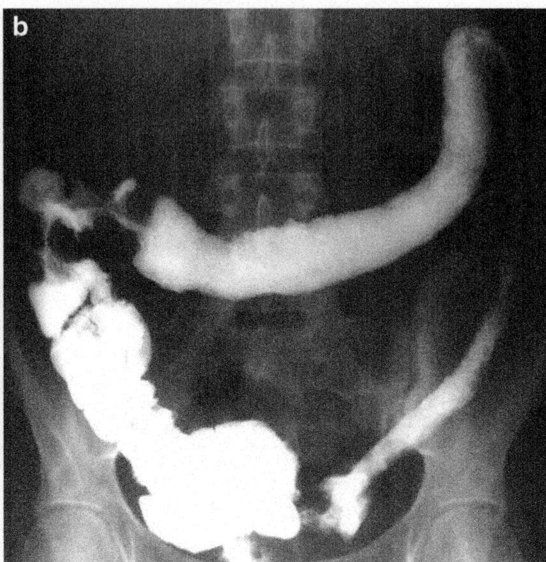

Fig. 5.1 Importance of plain film inspection. 43-year-old woman with diarrhea. (**a**) Plain film of the abdomen demonstrates sclerosis of both sacroiliac joints with ill-defined margins of both the iliac and sacral sides of the joint. The patient is known to have Crohn's disease of the colon diagnosed by rectal biopsy. Also note the abnormal colon contour (*arrow*). (**b**) Single contrast barium enema delineates the extent of disease with marked mucosal irregularities and diffuse narrowing of the left hemicolon, most pronounced along the descending and sigmoid colon

plain radiography is not a reliable means of assessing for bowel inflammation, several important pieces of information can be obtained. First, the presence of any residual enteric contrast agents from prior exams must be accounted for. Second, a survey for intestinal obstruction (which may infer stricture), pneumoperitoneum (which may infer perforation/fistulization), displaced bowel loops (which may infer extraluminal disease such as creeping fat, mesenteric phlegmon, or abscess) will help to tailor the fluoroscopic phase of the exam. Lastly, the presence of sacroiliitis, renal calculi, and other potential extraintestinal manifestations of inflammatory bowel disease should be noted (Fig. 5.1).

Selection of Contrast Agent

Enteric contrast agents for fluoroscopy can be broadly classified as agents based on barium sulfate and those based on iodine. When there is no clinical suspicion for free perforation, barium-based agents are preferred due to their superior coating of mucosal surfaces and their high radiographic conspicuity in the abdomen. However, when a perforated viscous is suspected (e.g., as in the setting of fistulizing Crohn's disease), an iodine-based agent is employed, so as to avoid the morbidity associated with barium leakage into the peritoneal cavity. Moreover, barium can be retained indefinitely when extravasated into the peritoneum or interstitium, thereby compromising the quality of any subsequent fluoroscopic or CT examinations. On the other hand, barium is safe when aspirated into the lungs, as opposed to iodinated contrast agents, which can cause pulmonary edema and/or pneumonitis (Fig. 5.2).

Upper GI Series

Fluoroscopic evaluation of the esophagus, stomach, and duodenum (commonly referred to as the "upper GI series") via double-contrast technique can be a useful adjunct to upper endoscopy when evaluating the mucosa of patients with inflammatory bowel disease. In this protocol, the patient first ingests a packet of effervescent granules in order to distend the upper alimentary tract with carbon dioxide gas. This is followed by several

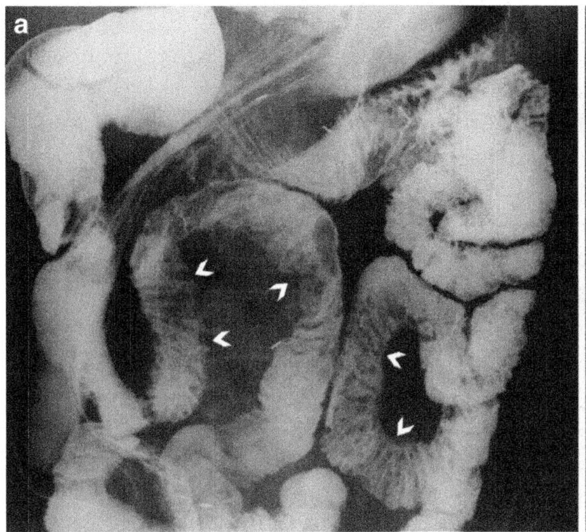

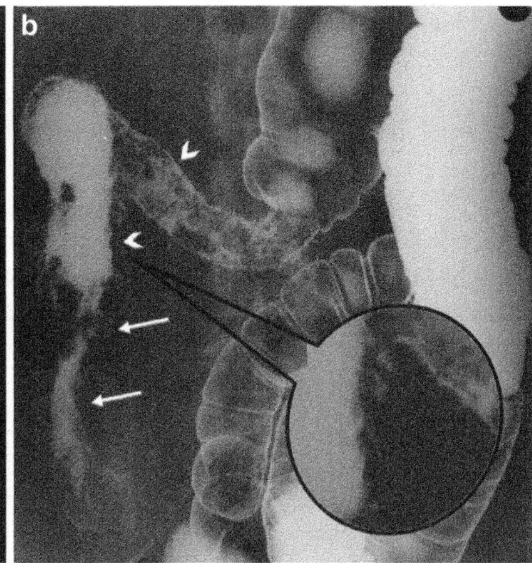

Fig. 5.2 Inflammatory polyps in active Crohn's disease. (**a**) 32-year-old woman with Crohn's disease, status post partial colectomy with ileocolic anastomosis 5 years previously, now presenting with abdominal pain and distention. Multiple nodular filling defects are present in the small bowel (*arrowheads*), consistent with inflammatory polyps. Also note the loop separation in the central abdomen reflecting mesenteric fibrofatty proliferation. (**b**) Active Crohn's disease in the terminal ileum and proximal colon. 24-year-old woman with cramping pain and diarrhea. Double contrast enema demonstrates diffusely diseased terminal ileum (*arrows*) and right colon with abrupt transition to a normal left colon. There are multiple colonic pseudopolyps, as well as linear and irregular deep mucosal ulcers (*arrowheads*)

large swallows of high-density (250 % weight/volume) barium sulfate suspension.

Initial upright images of the esophagus are obtained with the patient standing in a left-posterior oblique (LPO) position (in order to prevent radiographic overlap of the esophagus and vertebral column). Then, the examination table is tilted horizontally, so that the patient comes to rest on his or her left side. The patient is instructed to roll counterclockwise by 360° in order to coat the gastric mucosa with barium, then guided into the supine and bilateral oblique positions for spot imaging of the gastric and duodenal anatomy. The protocol may be enhanced with additional spot views and/or cinematic loop acquisitions as necessary to depict any abnormalities detected during the study.

Small Bowel Follow-Through

In this examination, the patient ingests approximately 700–750 mL of medium-density (60 % weight/volume) barium sulfate suspension (or less, if the study immediately follows an upper GI series) and is monitored with serial overhead radiographic images as the contrast column transits through the small bowel to reach the colon. As the contrast column advances, periodic inspection of individual barium-filled bowel loops is performed with manual compression. Manual compression, in which a radiolucent paddle or spoon is pressed on the abdomen to separate overlapping bowel loops for fluoroscopic interrogation, may be performed using a quadrant-screening approach or may be reserved for suspicious segments detected during the exam. Any focal abnormalities are documented with magnified spot images; any disorders of motility are documented with cinematic loop acquisitions.

In a comparison of MR enterography, CT enterography, and fluoroscopic small bowel follow-through for imaging Crohn's disease, Lee et al. [1] found no significant differences in sensitivity for detecting active terminal ileitis (67–89 %, $p>0.05$). However, small bowel follow-through was of limited utility for detecting extraluminal manifestations of disease (sensitivity of 32–37 %) and demonstrated only moderate interobserver agreement ($\kappa=0.542$) as opposed to substantial agreement for MR enterography ($\kappa=0.718$) and near-perfect agreement for CT enterography ($\kappa=0.812$). Nonetheless, because of the complement of anatomic and function information it provides, the small bowel follow-through remains a staple technique for imaging small bowel disease.

Enteroclysis

In enteroclysis, fluoroscopic or cross-sectional imaging of the small bowel is preceded by the administration of an enteric contrast via a nasoduodenal or nasojejunal catheter. Either barium sulfate or methylcellulose-based agents may be used for single-contrast imaging, or they may be combined with each other (or with carbon dioxide gas) for double-contrast imaging.

Double-contrast enteroclysis with barium is a highly reliable radiologic method of evaluating for small bowel mucosal disease [2], with a similar diagnostic yield to capsule endoscopy [3] and the potential to improve the diagnostic yield of double balloon endoscopy [4]. However, despite its diagnostic utility, enteroclysis is often reserved for special circumstances due to the need for transnasal intubation as well as considerable patient discomfort that generally requires the use of conscious sedation. With regard to Crohn's disease, the situations for which enteroclysis is particularly suited include the evaluation of occult intestinal bleeding, the differentiation of fibrous strictures from transient inflammatory stenosis, and the preoperative assessment of disease extent [5].

Retrograde Enema Per Ileostomy

For patients who have undergone surgical repair of Crohn's disease requiring the formation of an ileostomy, the radiologist has the option of performing a retrograde fluoroscopic evaluation of the small bowel as either a substitute for, or supplement to, the anterograde techniques described above. Because of its capacity for optimal ileal distention, retrograde studies are particularly useful for defining the intestinal anatomy and detecting any abnormalities prior to ileostomy takedown [6].

The retrograde ileostomy enema is typically performed using a soft, 18–24 French catheter with an inflatable balloon or a cone-shaped tip. Although some authors [6–8] recommend gentle inflation of the balloon inside the stoma, in our institution this is rarely done. Rather, the catheter tip is placed carefully into the stoma as the balloon is inflated externally, coated with a lubricant, and held firmly against the stoma by the patient's gloved hand. In our experience, this precaution minimizes the risk of disrupting the stoma or damaging the distal ileum; exceptions are made when studying an ileostomy that is double-barreled or is vented distally (as by a second stoma).

As dilute barium suspension is instilled under gravity assistance, the patient is turned into a steep lateral decubitus position so that the stoma may be imaged in profile as the distal loop traverses the anterior abdominal wall; images are obtained both pre- and post-evacuation. Additional oblique images and spot compression views are obtained as indicated. Using similar techniques, Kessler et al. [6] described a positive predictive value of 96 %, and negative predictive value of 86 % for detecting abnormalities in the small bowel.

Fistulogram

Enterocutaneous fistulae may be well delineated by administering a contrast agent via the cutaneous sinus. In this setting, a small caliber (8 French) malleable Foley-type catheter is inserted at the site of oozing. To minimize the leakage of contrast onto the skin (which could confound the evaluation of subcutaneous disease), the retention balloon may be inflated externally and held against the skin by the patient's gloved hand. Alternatively, if the subcutaneous tract or cavity is large enough to accommodate the inflated retention balloon, then this may be performed interiorly. A small amount (approximately 10 mL) of water-soluble iodinated contrast is injected via the catheter. A magnified spot image is then taken with the patient in lateral decubitus position to delineate the cutaneous tract in profile. Additional contrast is then slowly injected as the patient is imaged in various projections as necessary to delineate all sites of enteric communication and extraluminal extension. If a small bowel follow-through is to be performed during the same visit, the fistulogram should always be performed first, since a hairline fistula and sinus tract may be obscured by superimposed intraluminal contrast.

Barium Enema

Although involvement of the colonic mucosa by Crohn's disease is usually established colonoscopically, the findings can also be well depicted via barium enema. Double-contrast imaging, which entails the rectal administration of barium and then air, provides superior evaluation of the mucosa when compared to single-contrast techniques [9, 10].

When a barium enema is requested, the radiologist should investigate the reason for the examination, the patient's fitness for participation in the exam, and the severity of the patient's disease. At the authors' institution, barium enemas are not performed in any patient with toxic megacolon or fulminant colitis due to the risk of perforation and bacteremia. Similarly, the barium enema is avoided in patients who have undergone colonoscopic biopsy within 48 h.

Before performing a barium enema, the radiologist should ensure that the patient has undergone a mechanical bowel preparation (as by per oral magnesium citrate) and is in a fasting state. Following a digital rectal examination, a lubricated rectal catheter is inserted. Once the rectum has been outlined with contrast, a retention balloon may be inflated gently. Upon filling of the descending colon, the patient is rolled by 360° and placed into a prone position to fill the transverse colon. Subsequently, air is insufflated per rectum. The patient is then turned into a right lateral decubitus position, then supine to outline the ascending colon and hepatic flexure.

Radiologic Manifestations of Crohn's Disease

The fluoroscopic manifestations of Crohn's disease depend upon a host of factors including the acuity and severity of inflammation, the region of bowel involved, and underlying dysfunction from prior insult. The abnormalities may be organic (e.g., fold thickening) or functional (e.g., spasm); fluoroscopy can be used to differentiate these etiologies.

Early Intestinal Mucosal Manifestations of Crohn's Disease

The initial phase of intestinal involvement by Crohn's disease may be depicted fluoroscopically as morphologic changes in mucosal relief, alterations of intestinal fold pattern, and loss of mucosal integrity.

Normally, the intestinal mucosal villi are arranged with a density of 3–7 villi per mm^2 [5]. Early in the inflammatory process, the villi may become variably edematous or atrophied, causing the intervillous spaces to become irregular. This results in a coarsened and granular appearance of the mucosa on double contrast fluoroscopy, with a reticular pattern of irregular radiolucent foci ranging from 0.5 to 1.0 mm in diameter [5, 8]. Although commonly seen in early Crohn's disease, this pattern may also be seen in the setting of infection (e.g., Yersiniosis), ischemia, and other inflammatory conditions (e.g., radiation enteritis).

Lymphatic congestion and inflammatory exudate may result in smooth or nodular thickening of the valvulae conniventes. Subsequently, valvular fusion or morphologic distortion may develop. While also nonspecific, these fold changes are commonly seen in early Crohn's disease and often occur in close proximity to more advanced lesions [5].

Aphthous mucosal lesions are an early manifestation of inflammation and consist of tiny erosions superimposed on hyperplastic lymphoid follicles [8]. Radiographically, aphthous lesions are a 1–2 mm collection of contrast within a shallow erosion surrounded by a 5–15 mm radiolucent halo of elevated edematous tissue (Fig. 5.3). Aphthous lesions may be seen in any portion of the alimentary tract and occur in a host of inflammatory and infectious conditions. However, they are most common in the small intestine and may be present in as many as 52.5 % of patients with Crohn's disease [5].

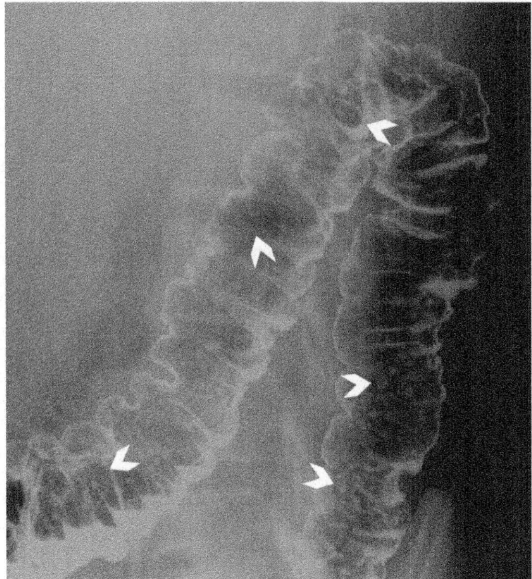

Fig. 5.3 Aphthous lesions. 34-year-old woman with diarrhea. Double contrast barium enema demonstrates diffuse aphthae throughout the colon (*arrowheads*) manifesting as shallow erosions surrounded by a zone of edema

Mucosal hypersecretion may result in the dilution and/or flocculation of the intraluminal contrast column. Flocculation, which refers to the woolly or cloud-like aggregation of enteric contrast, is less commonly seen with modern contrast agents due to the inclusion of stabilizing additives that prevent the barium particles from clumping [11].

Advanced Intestinal Mucosal Manifestations of Crohn's Disease

As mucosal erosions progress, they may develop into convex ulcerations atop mounds of edematous mucosa. With continued progression the following changes may be seen [5]: the ulcers take on a linear conformation, typically only 1–2 mm wide and extending up to 15 cm in length. Typically, they form along the mesenteric margin, coursing parallel to the intestinal long axis; the subjacent mesentery becomes thickened and rigid due to transmural inflammation. The antimesenteric side is often free of ulcerations; because it maintains its pliability, the antimesenteric side may appear sacculated when compared to the contracted and rigid mesenteric side (Fig. 5.4).

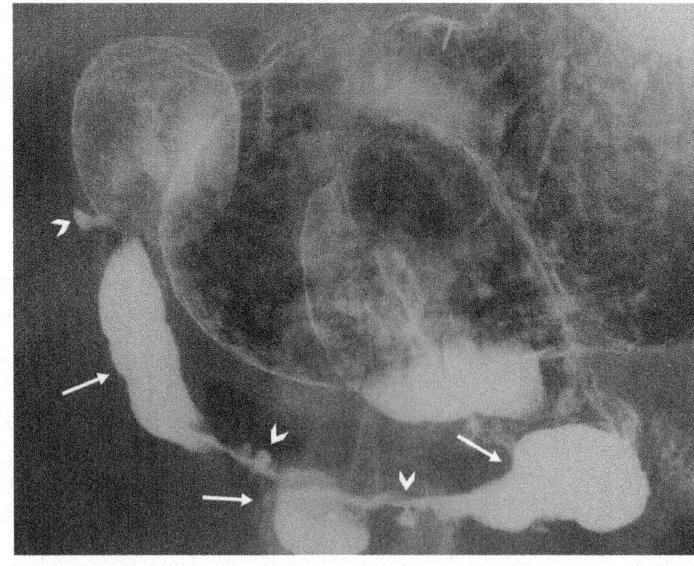

Fig. 5.4 Crohn's disease of the duodenum, with sacculations. 30-year-old woman with diarrhea. Upper GI study demonstrates a diffusely diseased duodenum with areas of focal dilation (*arrows*) consistent with sacculations. Additionally, there are several ulcers (*arrowheads*) and discontinuous segments of focal narrowing

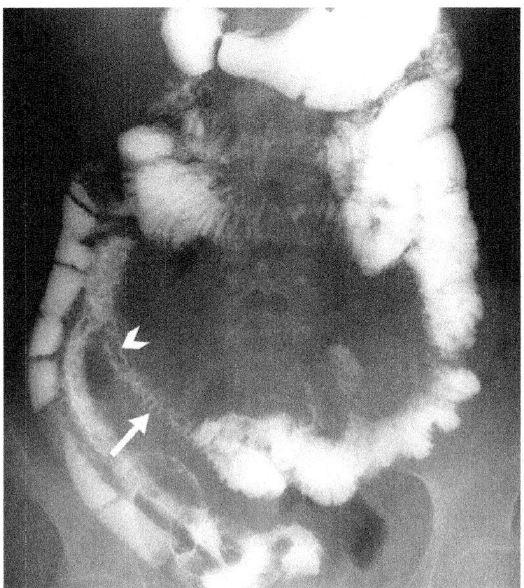

Fig. 5.5 Crohn's ileitis with cobblestone configuration. 23-year-old woman with chronic diarrhea, malnourishment, and evidence of enteric blood loss. Small bowel follow-through shows loop separation due to severe mural edema as well as transverse (*arrowhead*) and linear (*arrow*) ulcerations involving the distal ileum. The coexistence of pseudopolyps produces the characteristic cobblestone appearance

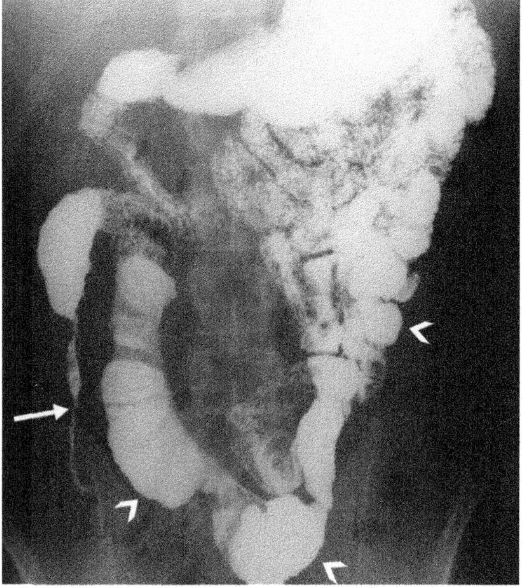

Fig. 5.6 Frayed string appearance. 22-year-old woman with chronic diarrhea diagnosed with Crohn's disease. Small bowel follow-through shows contrast traversing a diffusely narrowed segment of distal ileum, resembling the appearance of a frayed string (*arrow*). Note the eccentric involvement of the bowel wall, with sacculations along the antimesenteric margin (*arrowheads*)

However, in time, the disease will progress transaxially to involve the mucosa circumferentially.

As deep longitudinal, oblique, and transverse linear ulcers intersect, broad areas of mucosal denudation are seen. Extant islands of edematous mucosa, commonly referred to as "pseudopolyps," may mimic the appearance of nodules protruding beyond the mucosal surface (Fig. 5.2b). Pseudopolyps should be distinguished from true inflammatory polyps, which occur when focal inflammatory cellular infiltrate and edema cause the involved mucosa to project above the level of the neighboring mucosa [12]. On contrast fluoroscopy, inflammatory polyps will appear as multiple small, rounded luminal filling defects (Fig. 5.2a) [13].

The coexistence of regional mucosal denudation and pseudopolyps gives rise to the characteristic "cobblestone" appearance of advanced Crohn's disease (Fig. 5.5). On contrast fluoroscopy, cobblestoning appears as large and irregular regions of mucosal ulceration with interspersed pseudopolyps of variable size and shape. The involved segment of bowel may demonstrate reduced pliability and luminal narrowing [5, 8].

Fibroinflammatory Stenosis in Advanced Crohn's Disease

Intestinal pliability may be compromised in advanced Crohn's disease by any combination of fibrosis, inflammatory infiltration, and spasm. Because inflammatory stenosis and spasm may be amenable to medical therapy, whereas fibrous stricture generally requires surgical repair, the radiologist is often called upon to help distinguish between these entities.

On contrast fluoroscopy, both inflammatory stenosis and fibrous stricture will appear as luminal narrowing; the classic "string sign" describes a thin column of intraluminal barium within the narrowed segment of bowel that resembles a frayed string (Fig. 5.6). The key to differentiating

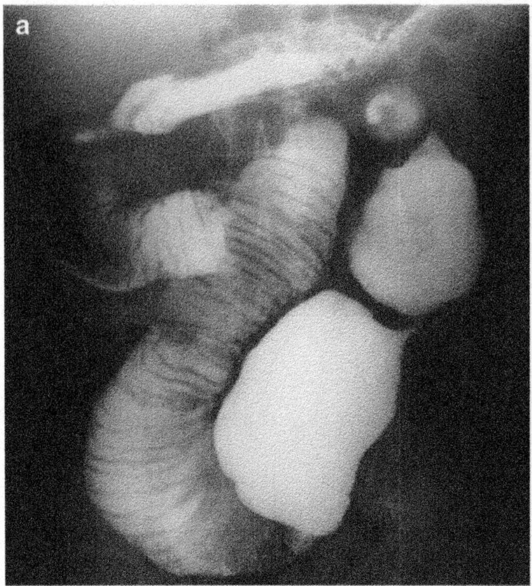

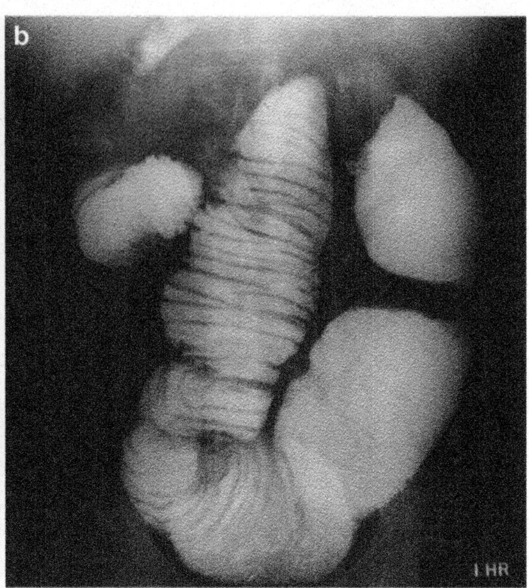

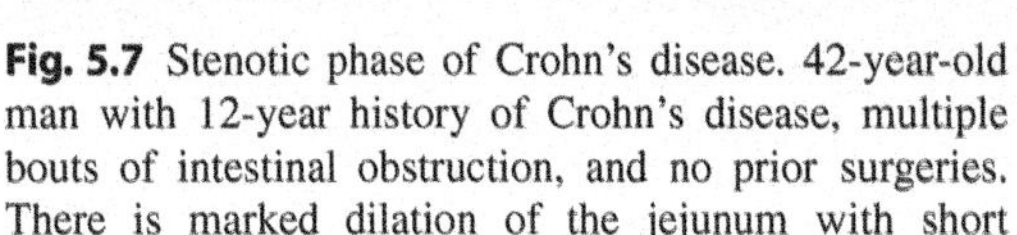

Fig. 5.7 Stenotic phase of Crohn's disease. 42-year-old man with 12-year history of Crohn's disease, multiple bouts of intestinal obstruction, and no prior surgeries. There is marked dilation of the jejunum with short segments of stenosis. Images taken at (**a**) 30 min and (**b**) 1 h post-ingestion show marked hypomotility due to severe stricturing and near-obstruction

stricture from other causes of luminal narrowing is the careful monitoring of luminal distensibility during enteroclysis or small bowel follow-through with paddle compression, glucagon, and/or metoclopramide administration: in fibrous stricture, luminal distensibility is lost (Fig. 5.7); in spasm, distensibility is preserved; in inflammatory stenosis, distensibility should remain at least partially intact. When significant inflammation is present, wall thickening may be appreciable as abnormal separation of bowel loops. When the narrowing is due to spasm, the diameter of the lumen will vary during real-time fluoroscopic monitoring.

Mesenteric Involvement and Perforating Disease

Although plain radiographs and contrast fluoroscopy are relatively insensitive for detecting extraenteric manifestations of inflammatory bowel disease, inflammatory mesenteric infiltration and/or "creeping fat" may be suspected when contrast-filled bowel loops appear abnormally separated (Figs. 5.2 and 5.5). In contrast, reactive fibrosis in the mesentery may result in kinking and fixation of the neighboring small bowel loops. Of note, these findings are nonspecific and may seen in variety of infiltrative and fibrotic conditions, respectively.

The presence of fistulae and/or sinus tracts from transmural Crohn's disease may be depicted by contrast fluoroscopy as extension of contrast agent beyond the expected boundaries of the intestinal lumen. In the case of fistulization, the tract may communicate between two epithelium-lined organs, in which case it is termed an "internal" fistula (Fig. 5.8), or it may communicate with the skin surface, in which case it is termed an "external" fistula (Fig. 5.9). Sinus tracts, on the other hand, generally terminate in a blind-ending fashion.

Roughly 20 % of patients with Crohn's disease will eventually develop an abscess. Typically, these abscesses are a consequence of perforating disease but they also may occur as a complication of colonoscopy or surgery. Barium studies are of limited sensitivity for detecting extraluminal disease [1], but may demonstrate extraluminal contrast agent, extraluminal gas, and/or displacement of edematous bowel loops (Fig. 5.10).

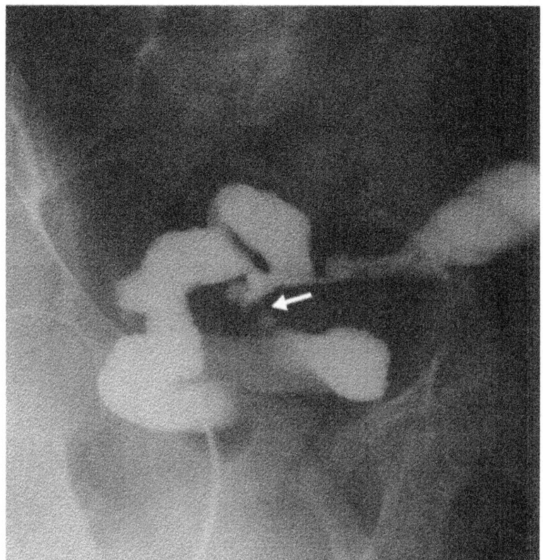

Fig. 5.8 Colovesical internal fistula. 52-year-old woman with diffuse Crohn's disease status post multiple prior small bowel resections resulting in short bowel syndrome. This image from a single contrast barium retrograde rectal enema demonstrates a narrowed and irregular rectosigmoid colon, with a fistula communicating from the inferior aspect of the sigmoid colon to the bladder (*arrow*)

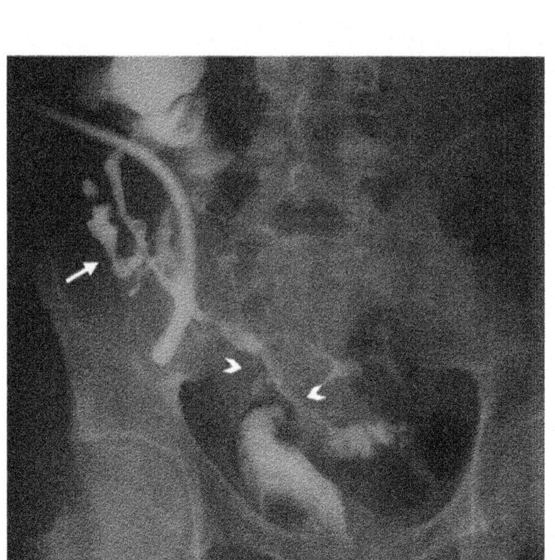

Fig. 5.9 Fistulogram. 20 mL of water-soluble iodinated contrast was injected through a percutaneous tube into a fistulous tract. It demonstrates ramifying fistulae, communicating with the distal ileum (*arrows*) and the rectosigmoid (*arrowheads*)

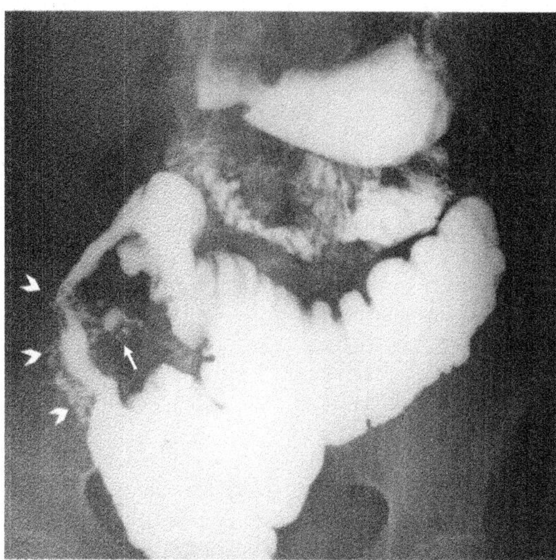

Fig. 5.10 Terminal ileal deep ulcers and abscess formation. This 25-year-old woman with Crohn's ileocolitis underwent ileocecal resection 4 years prior to this study. The patient presented with a non-resolving right lower quadrant mass for over a year. Small bowel follow-through shows active inflammation involving the distal ileum just proximal to the ileocolic anastomosis. There are deep ulcers (*arrowheads*) with medial perforation into an abscess demonstrated by irregular collections of contrast material (*arrow*)

Summary

Although advanced imaging techniques such as CT and MR have become the mainstay of imaging Crohn's disease, diagnostic fluoroscopy remains an invaluable component of the surgeons' and radiologists' repertoire for evaluating complex patients with Crohn's disease. Because the exact protocol for fluoroscopic evaluation of the alimentary tract is customized to address the clinical question, clear communication between the clinician and radiologist is necessary to achieve an optimal diagnostic result.

References

1. Lee SS, Kim AY, Yang SK, Chung JW, Kim SY, Park SH, et al. Crohn disease of the small bowel: comparison of CT enterography, MR enterography, and small-bowel follow-through as diagnostic techniques. Radiology. 2009;251(3):751–61.

2. Maglinte DD, Kohli MD, Romano S, Lappas JC. Air (CO2) double-contrast barium enteroclysis. Radiology. 2009;252(3):633–41.
3. Rajesh A, Sandrasegaran K, Jennings SG, Maglinte DD, McHenry L, Lappas JC, et al. Comparison of capsule endoscopy with enteroclysis in the investigation of small bowel disease. Abdom Imaging. 2009;34(4):459–66.
4. Matsumoto T, Esaki M, Yada S, Jo Y, Moriyama T, Iida M. Is small-bowel radiography necessary before double-balloon endoscopy? AJR Am J Roentgenol. 2008;191(1):175–81.
5. Herlinger H, Maglinte DDT, Birnbaum BA, Herlinger H. Clinical imaging of the small intestine. 2nd ed. New York: Springer; 1999. p. 259–82.
6. Kessler JM, Levine MS, Rubesin SE, Rombeau JL, Laufer I. Accuracy of retrograde ileostomy radiographic examination for detecting small-bowel abnormalities. AJR Am J Roentgenol. 2008;190(2):353–60.
7. Levine MS, Ramchandani P, Rubesin SE. Practical fluoroscopy of the GI and GU tracts. New York: Cambridge University Press; 2012. p. 117–55.
8. Freeny PC, Stevenson GW. Margulis and Burhenne's alimentary tract radiology. 5th ed. St. Louis: Mosby; 1994. p. 564–600.
9. Sahani DV, Samir A. Abdominal imaging. Maryland Heights: Saunders; 2011. p. 413–23.
10. Ott DJ. Accuracy of double-contrast barium enema in diagnosing colorectal polyps and cancer. Semin Roentgenol. 2000;35(4):333–41.
11. Gourtsoyiannis NC. Radiological imaging of the small intestine. Berlin: Springer; 2002. p. 340.
12. Buck JL, Dachman AH, Sobin LH. Polypoid and pseudopolypoid manifestations of inflammatory bowel disease. Radiographics. 1991;11(2):293–304.
13. Nolan DJ, Piris J. Crohn's disease of the small intestine: a comparative study of the radiological and pathological appearances. Clin Radiol. 1980;31(5):591–6.

Diagnostics: Body Imaging

6

Sachin S. Kumbhar, Ryan B. O'Malley, Manjiri K. Dighe, and Neeraj Lalwani

Abbreviations

ACR	American College of Radiology
ADC	Apparent diffusion coefficient
CD	Crohn's disease
CT(E)	Computed tomography (enterography)
DWI	Diffusion weighted imaging
FOV	Field of vision
GIT	Gastrointestinal tract
MR(E)	Magnetic resonance (enterography)
SSFP	Steady state free precession
SSFSE	Single shot fast spin echo
UC	Ulcerative colitis
US	Ultrasound

Introduction

Diagnosis of Crohn's disease (CD) relies on a combination of endoscopy, imaging, and pathologic examination. Imaging is used to suggest the diagnosis of CD, document the distribution of disease, assess activity, and detect complications. Imaging is also useful to suggest alternate diagnoses in patients suspected of having CD.

Traditionally, enteroclysis and barium follow through of the small bowel have been used to image patients with CD. However, these studies fail to detect extraluminal pathology and offer limited sensitivity due to overlapping of bowel loops. Cross-sectional imaging techniques such as computed tomography (CT) and magnetic resonance (MR) enterography are now more commonly employed in the evaluation of CD.

The American College of Radiology (ACR) Appropriateness Criteria® has deemed CT enterography (CTE) to be the preferred investigation for Crohn's disease, and MR enterography (MRE) is deemed equivalent to CTE in most of the clinical settings [1]. The choice of investigation varies with the institutional preferences and resources.

An ideally performed enterography study provides exquisite details of the intestine. However, like any other investigations both CT/MR enterography have their own limitations and pitfalls. Signs of very early (mucosal) disease, and subtle lesions or mural inflammation may be overlooked on both studies. Moreover, some findings like mural hyperenhancement without skip areas remain nonspecific. Rectal involvement may be difficult to differentiate from any other inflammatory disease or cancer.

Radiation exposure with CTE remains the major concern. Most of the patients with Crohn's disease are young and undergo multiple imaging

S.S. Kumbhar, MD • R.B. O'Malley, MD
M.K. Dighe, MD
Department of Radiology, University of Washington, 1959 NE Pacific Street, BB308, Seattle, WA 98195, USA
e-mail: skumbhar@uw.edu; ryanomal@uw.edu; dighe@uw.edu

N. Lalwani, MD (✉)
Department of Radiology, University of Washington, 325 9th Avenue, Box 359728, Seattle, WA 98104-2499, USA
e-mail: neerajl@u.washington.edu

A. Fichera and M.K. Krane (eds.), *Crohn's Disease: Basic Principles*,
DOI 10.1007/978-3-319-14181-7_6,

studies during their lifetime and cumulative radiation dose can be substantial. Increased radiation dose predisposes them to radiation induced cancers. Investigations without radiation exposure are therefore preferred to image these patients.

MR has recently emerged as the preferred investigation to evaluate inflammatory bowel disease due to the lack of radiation and high accuracy. It offers equivalent sensitivity to CTE with several distinct advantages, including better delineation between acute and chronic disease, superior assessment of perianal disease, and the ability to dynamically image bowel peristalsis. However the high cost of MR equipment and lack of availability and expertise may prove to be prohibitive.

Imaging Techniques

The following essentials should be met while performing a high quality enterography examination on CT or MR: (1) appropriately distended intestinal lumen with large volumes of neutral oral contrast, (2) rapid intravenous contrast exploiting the luminal and mural details in "enteric phase" (45–50 s delay), (3) pharmacological manipulation to decrease peristalsis, and (4) multiplanar reconstruction.

Ideally, a fasting state for 4 h before the examination is recommended. CTE takes less than 10 min to acquire all images, whereas MRE may take 30–45 min depending on the protocol. The patient may resume their normal diet and activities after the study is completed.

Oral Contrast

Oral contrast is used to distend the small bowel so that it can be adequately evaluated.

VoLumen (0.1 % wt/vol barium sulfate suspension) (Bracco Diagnostics, Inc., Princeton, NJ) is widely used for this purpose. Other available options may include methylcellulose, water, mannitol, and sorbitol. To achieve optimal bowel distension, the patient should drink 500 ml of VoLumen 2 h before, 500 ml 1 h before, and 500 ml 30 min before the exam.

Diluted 0.1 % wt/vol barium sulfate suspension provides a negative luminal contrast on CTE. However, it acts like a biphasic agent on MR and demonstrates high signal on T2-weighted images and low signal on T1-weighted images [2]. As such, biphasic oral contrast material serves as a positive contrast agent on T2-weighted images for detection of fold thickening while, as a positive contrast agent on post-contrast T1-weighted images, and does not obscure subtle mucosal enhancement of the GIT [2].

To minimize degradation of images by peristalsis, 0.5 mg Glucagon can be administered intramuscularly 10 min before beginning the exam and 0.5 mg intravenously 10 min before injecting gadolinium for the dynamic phase acquisition. Alternatively, Scopolamine (Hyoscine) can be used for the same purpose.

Patient Position

Prone positioning for enterography is believed to result in better distension of the bowel lumen and greater separation of bowel loops. It also decreases the number of sections required to image the bowel during a coronal acquisition, resulting in decreased scan time and hence, better images [2]. However, a prone position is inconvenient or impossible for some patients, including acutely ill patients, patients with stomas and those with entero-cutaneous fistulae. One study that compared the prone versus supine position of patients in MR imaging of the small bowel found significantly better distension of the small bowel with prone imaging, but no significant difference in detection of small bowel pathologies in the two positions, suggesting that either position can be utilized reliably [3].

CTE Protocol

CTE is globally performed to diagnose and stage Crohn's disease. Combination of oral and IV contrast and multiplanar reconstruction renders outstanding tissue detail and visualization of enhancing small bowel wall and inflammation. Appropriate windowing [liver-type (W215, L135) or "enterographic type" settings (W430, L155)] have been recommended while interpreting CTEs to avoid errors and pitfalls [4]. Moreover, meticulous technique and timing are mandatory to perform high quality examinations. Thin (≤3 mm) images are preferred to reconstruct multiplanar images. Contrast enhanced images can be acquired in enteric (45–50 s delayed) phase, when peak small bowel enhancement is achieved [5, 6]. To obtain high quality coronal images a minimal detector configuration (<1 mm) is recommended. Automatic exposure control and lower tube voltages can be used to decrease radiation dosage [7].

MRE Protocol

MRE has gained tremendous popularity as an investigation of choice to evaluate small bowel pathologies and evolved as a preferred investigation to evaluate Crohn's disease in the last decade [8]. MRE protocol varies from institution to institution; a combination of axial and coronal T1- and T2-weighted sequences with and without fat suppression should be used for MR imaging of CD. Cine loops, steady state free precession (SSFP), and diffusion weighted imaging are often used to complement T1- and T2-weighted sequences. Coronal images should utilize a large field of view (FOV) so as to include the entire bowel. Fat suppressed T1-weighted images should be obtained after injection of gadolinium to detect bowel wall hyperenhancement.

Steady state free precession images: Fast gradient echo sequences employing steady state free precession (SSFP) are an important component of MR enterography, typically obtained both in the coronal and axial planes. This sequence is acquired very rapidly during a single breath-hold, thus minimizing motion artifacts and optimizing contrast between the distended bowel lumen and bowel wall [9]. However, SSFP sequences contain mixed T1/T2 signal, which limits their assessment for bowel wall and mesenteric edema. Another disadvantage is the presence of the black boundary artifact, which may obscure small lesions and preclude assessment of true bowel wall thickness [9]. The single shot fast spin echo (SSFSE) sequence is also an ultrafast acquisition in which the entire abdomen is acquired in a single excitation pulse. This is done by applying a series of 180° pulses after the initial 90° excitation pulse. As with SSFP sequence, SSFSE sequence also provides rapid images and has lesser susceptibility artifact [10].

T2-weighted images: Although more susceptible to motion artifact, T2-weighted sequences can depict bowel wall and mesenteric edema, bowel wall thickening, mucosal ulcerations, and fluid collections [2]. Utilizing fat suppression also allows for differentiation of bowel wall edema of acute disease from fatty infiltration seen in chronic disease, as the former does not demonstrate suppression on fat saturated images, while the latter does [2].

Diffusion weighted images: Diffusion weighted imaging (DWI) relies on the Brownian motion of water to provide a valuable complementary means for assessing for the presence of inflammation. Free breathing diffusion sequences are often acquired at three different *b* values (0, 100 and 800 s/mm^2). In order to image both the abdomen and pelvis, images are obtained in two different acquisitions [11].

Cine loops: For cine imaging, T2 weighted SSFSE images are obtained in the same coronal plane one after the other in a sequential manner from anterior to posterior. These images help differentiate peristalsis from focal bowel strictures. It is also possible to differentiate between inflammatory narrowing and fibrotic narrowing using cine imaging. A fibrotic stenosis will be of a persistently narrow caliber, while in the case of inflammatory stenosis, the degree of narrowing will vary with peristalsis [8]. The balanced SSFSE sequence can be used to perform cine imaging. It has a high signal-to-noise ratio and a mixed T1 and T2 weighted contrast. This sequence is acquired in the form of different coronal slabs to encompass the entire bowel. Multiple images are acquired of each slab so that they can be viewed one after the other to provide a cine loop [12, 13].

Dynamic gadolinium enhanced images: Coronal and axial spoiled gradient echo T1-weighted images should be obtained with fat suppression after intravenous injection of gadolinium [13]. This sequence allows for detection of hyperenhancing bowel, mesenteric hypervascularity, or rim-enhancing fluid collections [14].

CTE Versus MRE

Selection of an appropriate imaging investigation remains controversial, and a great number of variables are considered before an investigation is selected. Both CTE and MRE perform similarly in evaluating Crohn's disease. MRE is the modality of choice when imaging perianal fistula or assessing response to therapy. Moreover, MRE can be a viable alternative to CTE when impairment of renal function, contrast allergy, or pregnancy is a concern. CTE remains the investigation of choice if there is concern of sepsis or patients with history of claustrophobia or implantable devices. In general, CTE is preferred by certain institutions because it is readily available and costs less than MRE. However, increasing availability of MRE, better (or at least similar) diagnostic performance, and lack of radiation make MRE a preferred investigation in general. In our institution, almost all patients (with a few exceptions) with Crohn's disease are evaluated with MREs.

Imaging Features

CD can involve any part of the GIT, but the most common site is the terminal ileum near the ileocecal (IC) junction. Skip lesions may be seen in CD, with a segment of normal bowel intervening between segments of inflamed bowel, which can be a key feature distinguishing CD from UC. MR features can differ in acute and chronic disease. However, an overlap of acute and chronic imaging features is not uncommon [15].

Acute Disease

A number of intra- and extra-luminal findings are characteristic of active disease. Mucosal inflammation may cause ulcerations, which may be aphthoid, transverse, or longitudinal. A combination of transverse and longitudinal ulcers produces the characteristic "cobblestone" pattern described in CD [14]. The early disease often requires a dedicated mucosal study with proper bowel distension. However, CT scan is often normal when disease is confined to the mucosa. Inflammatory and post-inflammatory pseudopolyps may be seen on CT or MR.

On MRE, ulcers are best detected on the balanced SSFP sequence, as the hyperintense fluid in the ulcer lumen contrasts well against the hypointense bowel wall. Linear ulcers appear as high intensity linear areas in the bowel wall. Cobblestoning caused by a combination of linear and transverse ulcers may also be best depicted on this sequence [16]. Mucosal inflammation may manifest as mucosal hyperenhancement relative to the submucosa and also compared to adjacent normal bowel loops.

When the inflammation extends transmurally, there is thickening of the bowel wall greater than 3 mm. However, the small bowel must be well distended for accurate evaluation of the wall thickness [17].

As described earlier, the T2-weighted sequences should be used to measure bowel wall thickness rather than SSFP sequence due to the presence of the black border artifact in the latter sequence. In isolation, wall thickening is nonspecific and may reflect inflammatory edema, fibrosis, or fatty infiltration. These are differentiated on MRE based upon the signal intensity characteristics of the bowel wall on all of the pulse sequences.

Bowel wall edema is indicative of active inflammation in the bowel wall and manifests on T2-weighted sequences as high signal intensity in the normally hypointense bowel wall (Fig. 6.1). This signal is not suppressed on fat saturated T2 weighted images and usually becomes more conspicuous (Fig. 6.2). Hence, the fat saturated T2-weighted sequence may be used to differentiate edema from fatty infiltration [18]. An actively inflamed bowel wall has increased cellularity due to infiltration by inflammatory cells. As a result, DWI demonstrates restricted diffusion in actively inflamed bowel segments (Fig. 6.3). Furthermore, quantitative apparent diffusion coefficient (ADC) values have been shown to be significantly lower in actively inflamed bowel compared to normal

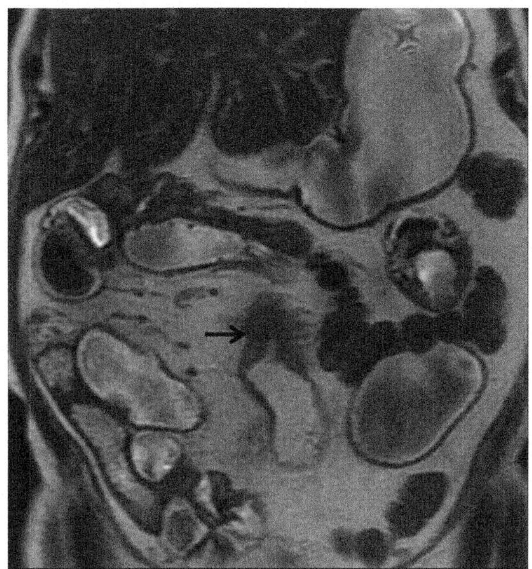

Fig. 6.1 Acute bowel wall edema. T2 weighted coronal image shows bowel wall thickening with T2 intermediate signal in the bowel wall (*arrow*)

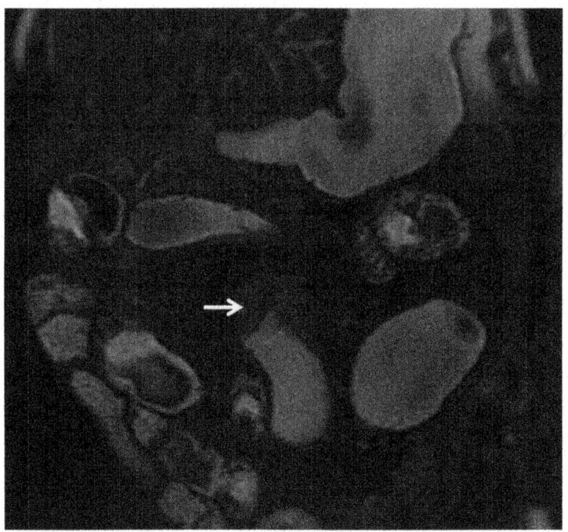

Fig. 6.2 Acute bowel wall edema. T2 weighted fat saturated coronal image of same patient as figure shows persistence of hyperintense signal in the bowel wall (*arrow*) with fat suppression indicating that it is due to edema rather than fat infiltration

bowel loops [11]. For both adult and pediatric patients, restricted diffusion in the bowel wall has been shown to correlate well with traditional MR enterography findings of active inflammation [19]. DWI has also been shown to be more sensitive than dynamic contrast enhanced MR imaging in differentiating inflamed small bowel from normal bowel in CD, highlighting its key

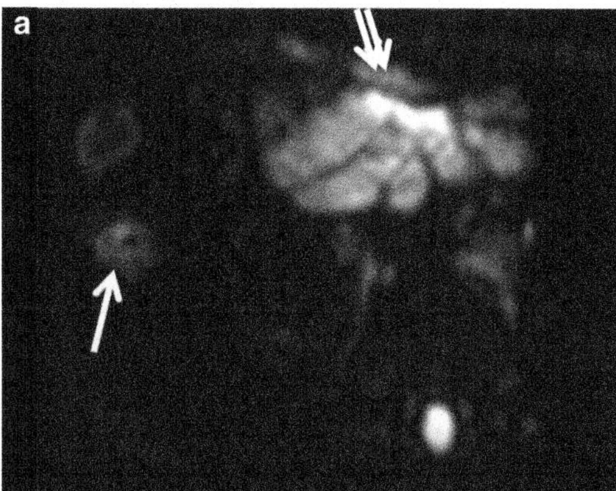

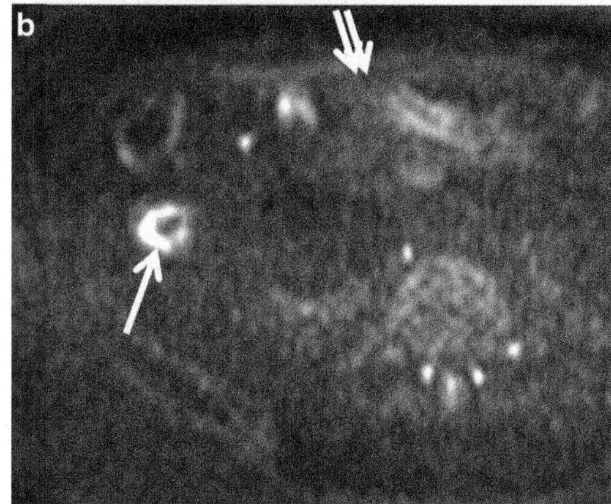

Fig. 6.3 Restricted diffusion. Diffusion weighted axial images with a b value of 0 s/mm^2 (**a**) and 800 s/mm^2 (**b**) demonstrate restricted diffusion in the terminal ileum (*arrows*) evident as increased hyperintense signal with a b value of 800 s/mm^2. In contrast, signal of fluid in normal bowel loops (*double arrows*) is suppressed with b value of 800 s/mm^2

role in the MRE examination and also offering significant potential value for patients who cannot receive intravenous contrast [11].

Characteristic bowel wall enhancement patterns are observed in CD. Enhancement of bowel loops suspected to be involved should be compared with adjacent bowel loops which are normal in appearance.

Mucosal hyperenhancement is visualized in active disease (Fig. 6.4). Another pattern that may be visualized in active disease is mural stratification or the so-called target or double halo pattern of enhancement, which is created by enhancement of the mucosal and muscular layers with an intervening non-enhancing submucosal layer (Fig. 6.5) [20].

Good distension of the bowel is essential for accurate assessment of wall enhancement as collapsed loops of bowel may both mask and mimic disease [21].

For inflamed segments of bowel, corresponding changes are also visualized in its mesentery. This includes mesenteric edema and engorgement of mesenteric vessels [20]. Mesenteric edema implies active inflammation with high signal intensity on T2-weighted images (Fig. 6.6) [20]. Mesenteric edema often coexists with other signs of active disease, such as the "comb sign," mural stratification, and bowel wall edema. The "comb sign" refers to the increased vascularity in the small bowel mesentery supplying the affected segment of the bowel [18, 22] and is best appreciated on SSFP and contrast enhanced T1-weighted images (Fig. 6.4 and 6.7). Prominent or enlarged lymph nodes may also be seen in the mesentery, often demonstrating prominent enhancement on post-contrast images in active disease (Fig. 6.8) [23].

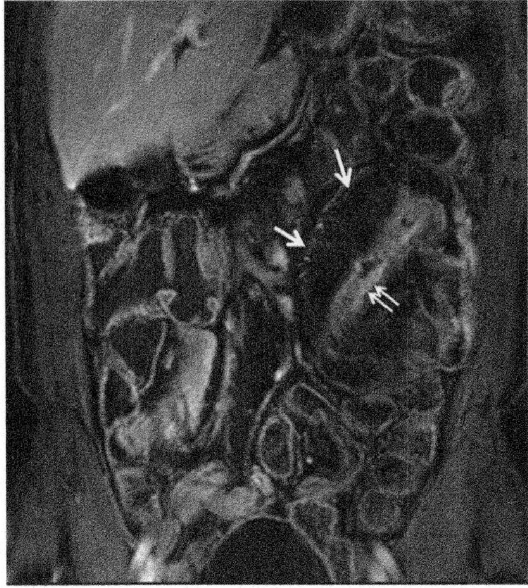

Fig. 6.4 Mucosal enhancement. Post gadolinium T1 weighted coronal image shows mucosal enhancement of the small bowel (*double arrows*) seen in acute CD. Also seen is increased vascularity in the mesentery supplying this segment of small bowel, i.e. combs sign (*arrows*)

Chronic Disease

The differentiation of acute and chronic disease is important, as the management differs markedly. While acute disease is treated medically, surgery is often required in chronic disease, particularly in the context of strictures and obstruction [8]. Chronically fibrotic bowel may appear thickened, but lack the T2 hyperintensity and mesenteric hypervascularity seen in acutely inflamed bowel [18]. Reduced motility of the involved segment might be appreciated on cine MR images. Sometimes, bowel wall thickening

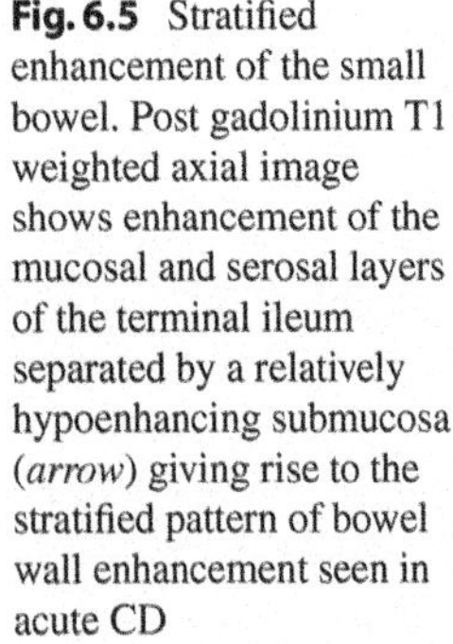

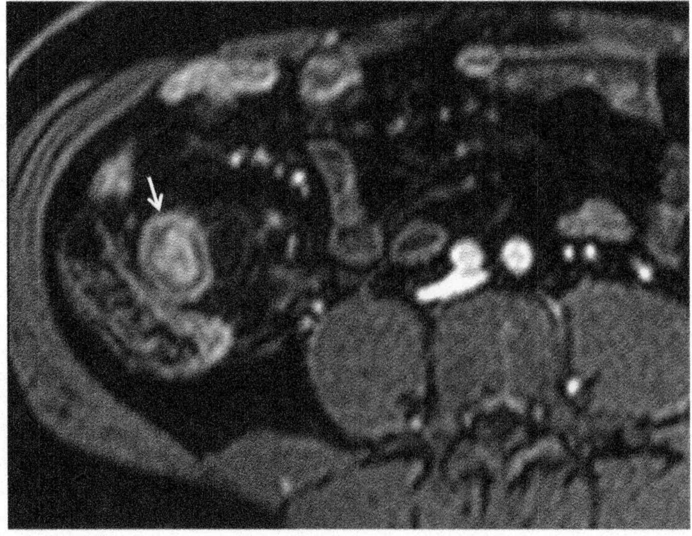

Fig. 6.5 Stratified enhancement of the small bowel. Post gadolinium T1 weighted axial image shows enhancement of the mucosal and serosal layers of the terminal ileum separated by a relatively hypoenhancing submucosa (*arrow*) giving rise to the stratified pattern of bowel wall enhancement seen in acute CD

may be due to acute or chronic inflammation. In these cases, there is intense mucosal enhancement with relatively non-enhancing submucosa and muscularis layers. The T2 signal in the bowel wall is decreased [24]. In chronic disease, there may be deposition of fat tissue in the segment of bowel involved by CD. However, this finding is not specific to CD, as it may be seen in many other diseases and even in normal individuals [2]. Fatty infiltration of the bowel may mimic acute bowel wall edema, as both of these appear hyperintense on T2 weighted images. However, these can be easily differentiated on fat saturated T2 weighted sequences [18]. Chronic fibrostenotic disease may be characterized by a stratified or homogenous transmural pattern of enhancement [8].

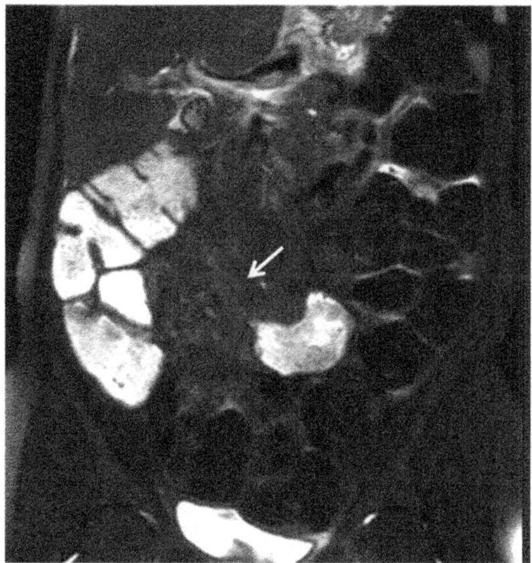

Fig. 6.6 Mesenteric edema in acute CD. Fat saturated T2 weighted coronal image demonstrates T2 hyperintense signal in the mesentery (*arrow*) that represents mesenteric edema

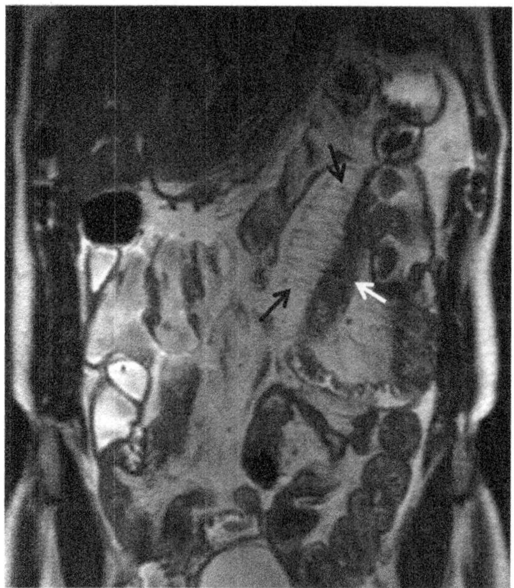

Fig. 6.7 Combs sign of acute CD. T2 weighted coronal image demonstrates prominence of mesenteric vessels (combs sign) (*black arrow*) in the mesentery supplying an involved segment of small bowel (*white arrow*)

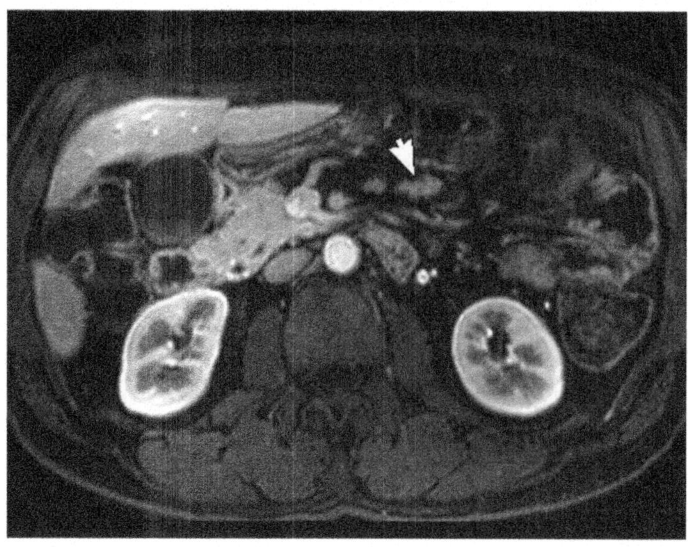

Fig. 6.8 Mesenteric lymphadenopathy. Post gadolinium T1 weighted axial image shows an enhancing enlarged mesenteric lymph node (*arrow*). These are seen in acute CD

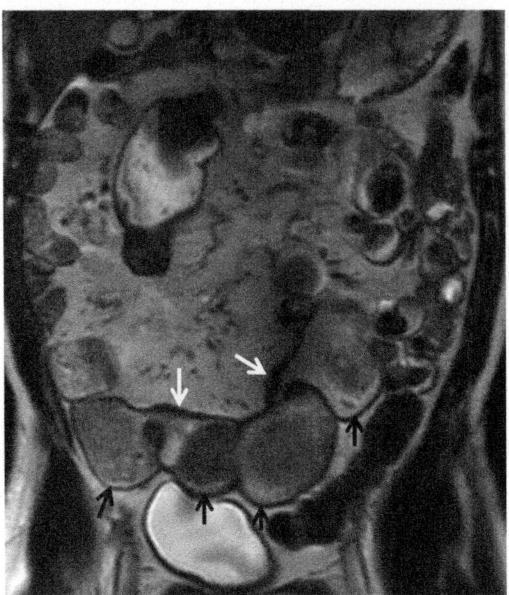

Fig. 6.9 Pseudosacculations. T2 weighted coronal image shows asymmetric small bowel wall thickening involving the mesenteric side of the bowel (*white arrows*) with resultant formation of pseudosacculations on the antimesenteric side (*black arrows*)

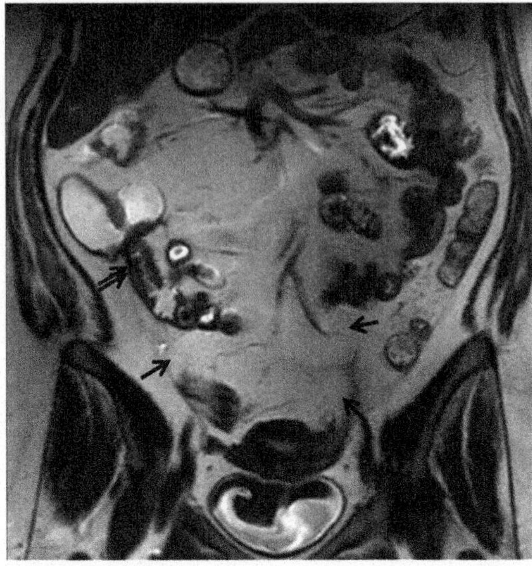

Fig. 6.10 Mesenteric fat proliferation. T2 weighted coronal image shows excessive amount of mesenteric fat (*arrows*) seen in chronic CD. Also seen is bowel wall thickening (*double arrows*) of the neoterminal ileum adjacent to the ileocolic anastomosis. This represents postoperative recurrence of CD

Fibrosis in the bowel wall develops in chronic disease. If there is sparing of the antimesenteric bowel, asymmetric fibrotic shortening of the mesenteric bowel wall may cause formation of pseudodiverticula or pseudosacculations [8] due to asymmetric fibrosis of the mesenteric part of the small bowel circumference, with relative sparing of the antimesenteric portion (Fig. 6.9). Progressive shortening of the length of the small bowel segments on the mesenteric side results in abnormal ballooning of the uninvolved antimesenteric side [25]. These are called pseudodiverticula because they contain all of the layers of the bowel wall, unlike true diverticula visualized in the colon, which are comprised of only the mucosal layer.

Fibrofatty proliferation in the mesentery is visualized in long-standing disease (Fig. 6.10). It produces a mass effect on the mesenteric vasculature and the bowel loops and sometimes completely surrounds the bowel circumference. Fibrofatty proliferation is considered to be a specific finding of CD [2, 25].

Complications

Luminal narrowing and intestinal obstruction may be seen in both acute and chronic CD and can be a result of bowel wall thickening, inflammatory edema, or fibrosis [2]. A stricture refers to narrowing of the caliber of the bowel lumen, which can be secondary to acute edema or chronic fibrosis. This is an important distinction as inflammatory strictures are managed medically while strictures that are predominantly fibrotic are managed surgically. Both inflammatory and fibrotic strictures can be complicated by small bowel obstruction if the bowel proximal to the stricture dilates to more than 3 cm in diameter and there is decompressed bowel distal to the stricture (Fig. 6.11) [8, 26]. A definite transition zone may or may not be visualized.

Bowel inflammation may itself extend out of the bowel wall in the form of fistulae and sinuses, which is referred to as penetrating disease. Fistulae may connect one loop of bowel with another (interloop) or may communicate with the external skin surface, urinary bladder, or vagina (Fig. 6.12) whereas sinuses are blind ending tracts. Sinuses and fistula tracts both appear hyperintense linear or curvilinear tracts on T2-weighted images and enhance on post gadolinium images [18]. Other complications of CD include bowel perforation, which can lead to phlegmon (Fig. 6.13) or abscess formation. Abscesses appear as rim-enhancing collections containing fluid and air. It is important to identify abscesses, as they are a contraindication to anti-tumor necrosis factor therapy and may require surgical or percutaneous drainage [8]. CTE remains the investigation of choice if a perforation or abscess is suspected in the clinical settings of sepsis (Fig. 6.14). Perianal disease is common in patients with CD and includes fistula in ano and perianal abscess (Fig. 6.15) [27]. Perianal fistulas may be intersphincteric, transphincteric, or extrasphincteric and have similar imaging characteristics as fistulas described above. MRE is the investigation of choice to evaluate perianal fistulas.

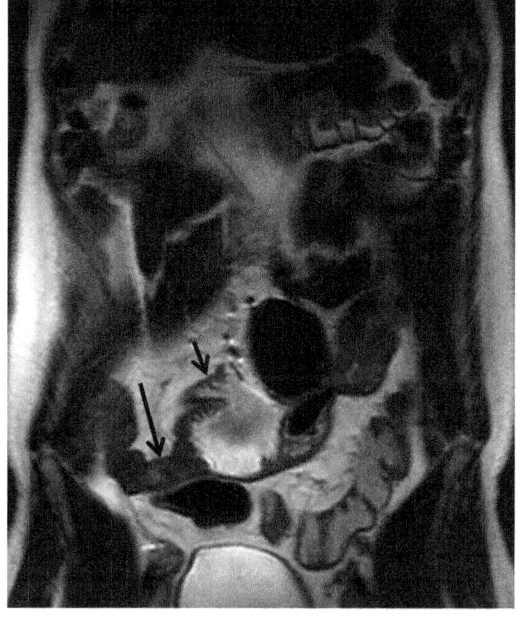

Fig. 6.11 CD with bowel stricture and intestinal obstruction. T2 weighted coronal image shows T2 intermediate small bowel wall thickening resulting in a stricture formation (*long arrow*). There is resultant dilatation of the proximal bowel (*short arrow*) indicating obstruction

Impact on Patient Care

Crohn's disease activity index (CDAI) has a poor correlation with endoscopic disease activity [28], and the addition of enterography (CTE/MRE) can significantly impact patient management and clinical decisions.

Patients with high clinical suspicion of Crohn's disease but normal findings on ileocolonoscopy may benefit from CT/MR enterography to identify enteric inflammation proximal to terminal ileum. Additionally, enterography may

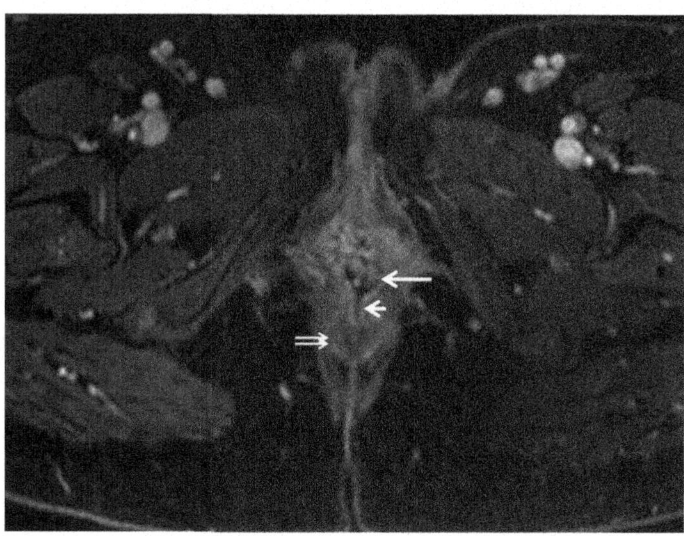

Fig. 6.12 Rectovaginal fistula. Post gadolinium T1 weighted axial image demonstrates enhancing tract of rectovaginal fistula (*short arrow*) connecting the vagina (*long arrow*) and the rectum (*double arrows*)

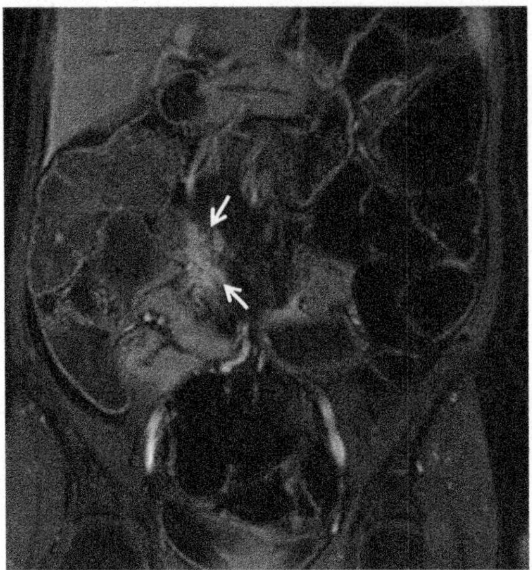

Fig. 6.13 Mesenteric phlegmon. Post gadolinium T1 weighted coronal image shows enhancing soft tissue in the mesentery (*arrow*). This represents a mesenteric phlegmon

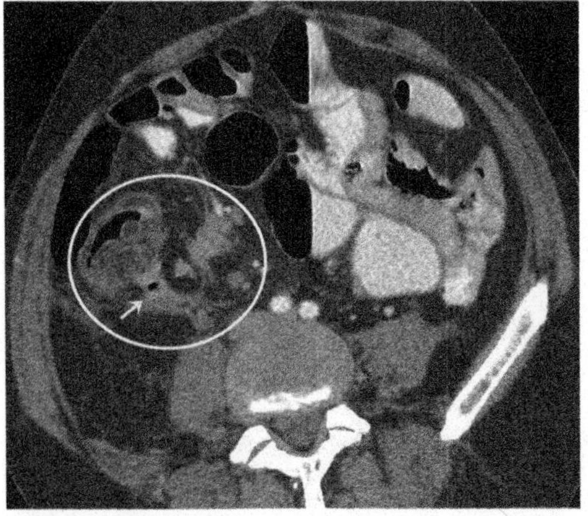

Fig. 6.14 Perforation. Post-contrast axial CT image through right lower quadrant showing microperforation (*arrow*). Note the inflammatory changes in the surrounding and thickened terminal ileum (*circle*)

even depict active ileal disease even though mucosa is found normal on ileoscopy [29, 30].

It has been shown that the CTE may alter the decision to initiate steroids and likelihood of benefit in 61 % of the patients [31]. MRE can be used to monitor disease activity or to assess the effectiveness of treatment or interventions [32, 33].

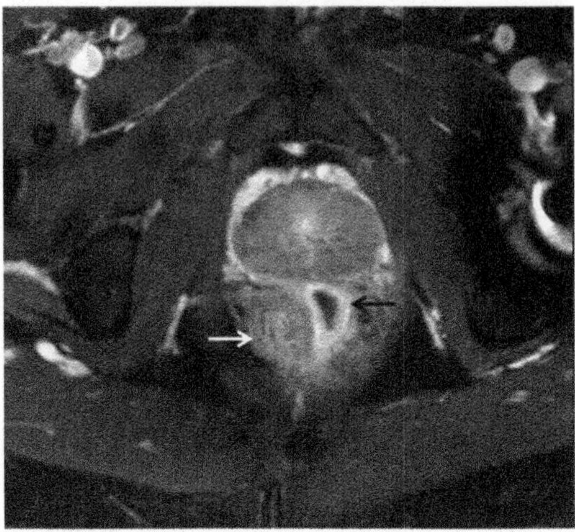

Fig. 6.15 Perianal abscess. Post gadolinium T1 weighted axial image demonstrated rim-enhancing collection (*black arrow*) adjacent to the anal canal (*white arrow*). This represents a perianal abscess

Conclusion

CD can affect any part of the GIT, with the terminal ileum being the most commonly affected site. MR Imaging represents an increasingly employed imaging modality in the management of this disease. Optimal bowel distension is the cornerstone for adequate evaluation of the disease. MRI can detect the changes of acute and chronic CD, both within the bowel and in the mesentery. It can also be used to detect complications of the disease.

References

1. Huprich JE, Rosen MP, Fidler JL, Gay SB, Grant TH, Greene FL, et al. ACR Appropriateness Criteria® on Crohn's disease. J Am Coll Radiol. 2010;7(2):94–102.
2. Tolan DJ, Greenhalgh R, Zealley IA, Halligan S, Taylor SA. MR enterographic manifestations of small bowel Crohn disease. Radiographics. 2010;30(2):367–84. PMID: 20228323.
3. Cronin CG, Lohan DG, Mhuircheartaigh JN, McKenna D, Alhajeri N, Roche C, et al. MRI small-bowel follow-through: prone versus supine patient positioning for best small-bowel distention and lesion detection. AJR Am J Roentgenol. 2008;191(2):502–6. PMID: 18647923.
4. Gollub M. Small-bowel imaging: pitfalls in computed tomography enterography/enteroclysis. In: Hodler J,

Zollikofer CL, Von Schulthess GK, editors. Diseases of the abdomen and pelvis 2010–2013. Milan: Springer; 2010. p. 28–31.
5. Schindera ST, Nelson RC, DeLong DM, Jaffe TA, Merkle EM, Paulson EK, et al. Multi-detector row CT of the small bowel: peak enhancement temporal window—initial experience. Radiology. 2007;243(2): 438–44. PMID: 17384239.
6. Vandenbroucke F, Mortele KJ, Tatli S, Pelsser V, Erturk SM, De Mey J, et al. Noninvasive multidetector computed tomography enterography in patients with small-bowel Crohn's disease: is a 40-second delay better than 70 seconds? Acta Radiol. 2007;48(10):1052–60. PMID: 17963078.
7. Kambadakone AR, Prakash P, Hahn PF, Sahani DV. Low-dose CT examinations in Crohn's disease: impact on image quality, diagnostic performance, and radiation dose. AJR Am J Roentgenol. 2010;195(1):78–88. PMID: 20566800.
8. Griffin N, Grant LA, Anderson S, Irving P, Sanderson J. Small bowel MR enterography: problem solving in Crohn's disease. Insights Imaging. 2012;3(3):251–63. PMID: 22696087. PMCID: 3369125.
9. Sinha R, Verma R, Verma S, Rajesh A. MR enterography of Crohn disease: part 1, rationale, technique, and pitfalls. AJR Am J Roentgenol. 2011;197(1):76–9. PMID: 21701013.
10. Elmouglu MCA. Patient positioning, and protocols. MRI handbook: MR physics. New York City: Springer Science and Business Media; 2011.
11. Oto A, Kayhan A, Williams JT, Fan X, Yun L, Arkani S, et al. Active Crohn's disease in the small bowel: evaluation by diffusion weighted imaging and quantitative dynamic contrast enhanced MR imaging. J Magn Reson Imaging. 2011;33(3):615–24. PMID: 21563245.
12. Scheffler K, Lehnhardt S. Principles and applications of balanced SSFP techniques. Eur Radiol. 2003;13(11):2409–18. PMID: 12928954.
13. Chavhan GB, Babyn PS, Walters T. MR enterography in children: principles, technique, and clinical applications. Indian J Radiol Imaging. 2013;23(2):173–8. PMID: 24082485. PMCID: 3777330.
14. Furukawa A, Saotome T, Yamasaki M, Maeda K, Nitta N, Takahashi M, et al. Cross-sectional imaging in Crohn disease. Radiographics. 2004;24(3):689–702. PMID: 15143222.
15. Herrmann K. Diseases of the small bowel, including the duodenum—MRI. In: Hodler J, Zollikofer CL, Von Schulthess GK, editors. Diseases of the abdomen and pelvis 2010–2013. Milan: Springer; 2010. p. 32–6.
16. Prassopoulos P, Papanikolaou N, Grammatikakis J, Rousomoustakaki M, Maris T, Gourtsoyiannis N. MR enteroclysis imaging of Crohn disease. Radiographics. 2001;21 Spec No:S161–72. PMID: 11598255.
17. Cronin E. Prednisolone in the management of patients with Crohn's disease. Br J Nurs. 2010;19(21):1333–6. PMID: 21355357.
18. Ramalho M, Heredia V, Cardoso C, Matos AP, Palas J, De Freitas J, et al. Magnetic resonance imaging of small bowel Crohn's disease. Acta Med Port. 2012;25(4):231–40. PMID: 23079251.
19. Ream JM, Dillman JR, Adler J, Khalatbari S, McHugh JB, Strouse PJ, et al. MRI diffusion-weighted imaging (DWI) in pediatric small bowel Crohn disease: correlation with MRI findings of active bowel wall inflammation. Pediatr Radiol. 2013;43(9):1077–85. PMID: 23949929.
20. Sinha R, Verma R, Verma S, Rajesh A. MR enterography of Crohn disease: part 2, imaging and pathologic findings. AJR Am J Roentgenol. 2011;197(1):80–5. PMID: 21701014.
21. Florie J, Wasser MN, Arts-Cieslik K, Akkerman EM, Siersema PD, Stoker J. Dynamic contrast-enhanced MRI of the bowel wall for assessment of disease activity in Crohn's disease. AJR Am J Roentgenol. 2006;186(5):1384–92. PMID: 16632735.
22. Madureira AJ. The comb sign. Radiology. 2004;230(3):783–4. PMID: 14990842.
23. Herraiz Hidalgo L, Alvarez Moreno E, Carrascoso Arranz J, Cano Alonso R, Martínez de Vega Fernández V. Magnetic resonance enterography: review of the technique for the study of Crohn's disease. Radiología. 2011;53(5):421–33 (English edition).
24. Kitazume Y, Satoh S, Hosoi H, Noguchi O, Shibuya H. Cine magnetic resonance imaging evaluation of peristalsis of small bowel with longitudinal ulcer in Crohn disease: preliminary results. J Comput Assist Tomogr. 2007;31(6):876–83. PMID: 18043349.
25. Hidalgo M, Cabrero Gomez F, de la Fuente Simon F. Crohn disease. Comments on 43 surgical cases. Rev Esp Enferm Apar Dig. 1985;67(1):3–14. PMID: 3883447. Enfermedad de Crohn. Comentario sobre 43 casos intervenidos.
26. Nicolaou S, Kai B, Ho S, Su J, Ahamed K. Imaging of acute small-bowel obstruction. AJR Am J Roentgenol. 2005;185(4):1036–44. PMID: 16177429.
27. Haggett PJ, Moore NR, Shearman JD, Travis SP, Jewell DP, Mortensen NJ. Pelvic and perineal complications of Crohn's disease: assessment using magnetic resonance imaging. Gut. 1995;36(3):407–10. PMID: 7698701. PMCID: 1382455.
28. Jones J, Loftus Jr EV, Panaccione R, Chen LS, Peterson S, McConnell J, et al. Relationships between disease activity and serum and fecal biomarkers in patients with Crohn's disease. Clin Gastroenterol Hepatol. 2008;6(11):1218–24. PMID: 18799360.
29. Siddiki HA, Fidler JL, Fletcher JG, Burton SS, Huprich JE, Hough DM, et al. Prospective comparison of state-of-the-art MR enterography and CT enterography in small-bowel Crohn's disease. AJR Am J Roentgenol. 2009;193(1):113–21. PMID: 19542402.
30. Samuel S, Bruining DH, Loftus Jr EV, Becker B, Fletcher JG, Mandrekar JN, et al. Endoscopic skipping of the distal terminal ileum in Crohn's disease can lead to negative results from ileocolonoscopy.

Clin Gastroenterol Hepatol. 2012;10(11):1253–9. PMID: 22503995.

31. Higgins PD, Caoili E, Zimmermann M, Bhuket TP, Sonda LP, Manoogian B, et al. Computed tomographic enterography adds information to clinical management in small bowel Crohn's disease. Inflamm Bowel Dis. 2007;13(3):262–8. PMID: 17206719.
32. Makanyanga JC, Taylor SA. Current and future role of MR enterography in the management of Crohn disease. Am J Roentgenol. 2013;201(1):56–64.
33. Leyendecker JR, Bloomfeld RS, DiSantis DJ, Waters GS, Mott R, Bechtold RE. MR enterography in the management of patients with Crohn disease. Radiographics. 2009;29(6):1827–46. PMID: 19959524.

Diagnostics: Endoluminal

7

Scott David Lee, Kindra Clark-Snustad, and Jessica Fisher

Crohn's Disease Diagnostics

Endoluminal Evaluation

The initial diagnosis and subsequent evaluation of inflammatory bowel disease (IBD) require multiple diagnostic modalities. However, endoscopic evaluation is still considered the gold standard diagnostic test. Endoscopic evaluation includes colonoscopy, esophagogastroduodenoscopy (EGD), enteroscopy, and capsule endoscopy. IBD encompasses Crohn's disease (CD), ulcerative colitis (UC), and IBD unclassified (IBDU). Colonoscopy with ileoscopy is essential in the vast majority of CD cases for diagnosis and ongoing evaluation. EGD, enteroscopy, and capsule endoscopy are used in specific groups of patients with CD. The role of endoluminal diagnostic studies in the initial diagnosis and subsequent evaluation of CD will be discussed in detail in this chapter.

S.D. Lee, MD (✉)
Division of Gastroenterology, Clinical Inflammatory Bowel Disease Program, University of Washington, 1959 NE Pacific Street, Seattle, WA 98195, USA
e-mail: ScottL@medicine.washington.edu

K. Clark-Snustad, DNP, ARNP
Inflammatory Bowel Disease Research Program, University of Washington, 1959 NE Pacific Street AA103, Seattle, WA 98195, USA
e-mail: KClark-Snustad@medicine.washington.edu

J. Fisher
Division of Gastroenterology, University of Washington, 1959 NE Pacific Street, Box 356424, Seattle, WA 98195, USA
e-mail: JFisher@medicine.washington.edu

Initial Diagnosis

IBD is generally divided into Crohn's disease (CD) and ulcerative colitis (UC). While IBD may be evaluated with multiple methods of testing, only endoscopic evaluation allows both direct visualization of the gastrointestinal mucosal and permits histologic assessment via biopsy collection with the exception of capsule endoscopy which does not allow for biopsy collection. Procedures including colonoscopy, ileoscopy, esophagogastroduodenoscopy (EGD), enteroscopy, and WCE enable assessment of distinct regions of the digestive tract, and while colonoscopy with ileoscopy is the gold standard for diagnosis of IBD in the majority of patients, EGD, enteroscopy, and WCE may be helpful for the initial diagnosis of IBD in select populations.

Colonoscopy with Ileoscopy

Role/Indication

Colonoscopy with ileoscopy (ileocolonoscopy) enables assessment of the colonic mucosa through direct endoscopic visualization, allowing evaluation of disease severity, extent, and histologic assessment [1]. Ileocolonoscopy is essential in

A. Fichera and M.K. Krane (eds.), *Crohn's Disease: Basic Principles*,
DOI 10.1007/978-3-319-14181-7_7, © Springer International Publishing Switzerland 2015

the initial diagnosis of CD and helpful in differentiating CD, UC, and other pathology that can present with similar clinical findings to IBD.

The primary initial role of ileocolonoscopy in CD is to establish the diagnosis by ruling out other causes of symptoms, and differentiating CD from UC. Ileocolonoscopy with biopsies is the gold standard for diagnosis of CD, and should be performed in the vast majority of patients with suspected CD [2–4]. Identifying terminal ileitis is important for accurate initial CD diagnosis; intubation of the terminal ileum should always be attempted during the initial assessment of suspected CD, and is possible in 95 % of patients with UC and 75 % of patients with CD [3, 5, 6]. Biopsies during the initial ileocolonoscopy should always be obtained from the terminal ileum and throughout the colon even if the mucosa appears normal.

Contraindications and Complications

Potential complications of ileocolonoscopy include perforation, bleeding, and rarely, postpolypectomy syndrome and infection. Additionally, complications related to sedation and preparation are possible. Perforation is the most serious complication, with a high morbidity and potential need for surgery and colostomy [3].

In stable patients with IBD, rates of endoscopy-related complications are similar to the general population, most commonly bleeding and perforation. A 2013 study evaluating 685 patients with IBD suggests that overall rates of endoscopy-related complications for IBD patients are 1.17 %, compared to 0.96 % in the general population. This same study identifies the lifetime risk of complication in IBD patients undergoing screening colonoscopy as 12.7 %, compared to 2.0 % in non-IBD patients [7]. In the general population, the incidence of hemorrhage from diagnostic colonoscopy is 0.02 %, and 1.61 % with polypectomy, and the overall rate of perforation is 0.045 % [3, 8]. In one example, Rubin et al. (1999) report no episodes of bleeding, perforation, postpolyectomy fever, or mortality in a series of 151 colonoscopies and 70 polypectomies in patients with IBD [3, 8]. The incidence of complications has decreased over time, presumably due to advancements in colonoscopy technology as well as improved training of endoscopists [3].

In hospitalized IBD patients, the risk of endoscopy-related complication is also similar to non-IBD patients. A large retrospective study reports colonoscopy perforation rates for hospitalized patients with IBD as 1 % compared to 0.6 % in non-IBD patients [9]. Certain risk factors for perforation in severe colitis have been identified and include female gender, older age, and performing endoscopic dilation [9, 10]. Minimizing air insufflation and avoiding advancing the scope in a tortuous colon can help reduce risk of complications [10]. Certain populations of IBD patients, including those with severe, fulminant colitis or those with stricture formation, are at increased risk of complications [3]. Although the risk of complication is higher, colonoscopy may still be performed safely, and endoscopic evaluation may provide essential information that will affect both surgical and medical management. However, in emergency settings where surgery is indicated urgently (e.g., uncontrollable hemorrhage, toxic megacolon, or bowel perforation) endoscopy often plays a limited role as it will not affect the immediate management of this group of patients [3].

In general, endoscopic evaluation can be performed safely and plays a pivotal role in the diagnosis and management in the vast majority of IBD patients. Endoscopic evaluation in specific scenarios such as complete obstruction from strictures or toxic colitis carries higher risks and is unlikely to change a patient's management as urgent surgical intervention is often warranted. In these patients careful consideration should be taken prior to performing ileocolonoscopy, and the study should be performed only if the procedure is likely to change the management.

Mucosal Appearance and Distribution

Although the typical endoscopic appearance of CD is described as patchy disease affecting any part of the gastrointestinal tract, endoscopic findings in CD vary greatly depending on disease activity and duration [5, 10]. Classically, CD presents as sections of inflamed mucosa separated by areas of normal tissue (skip areas) [5].

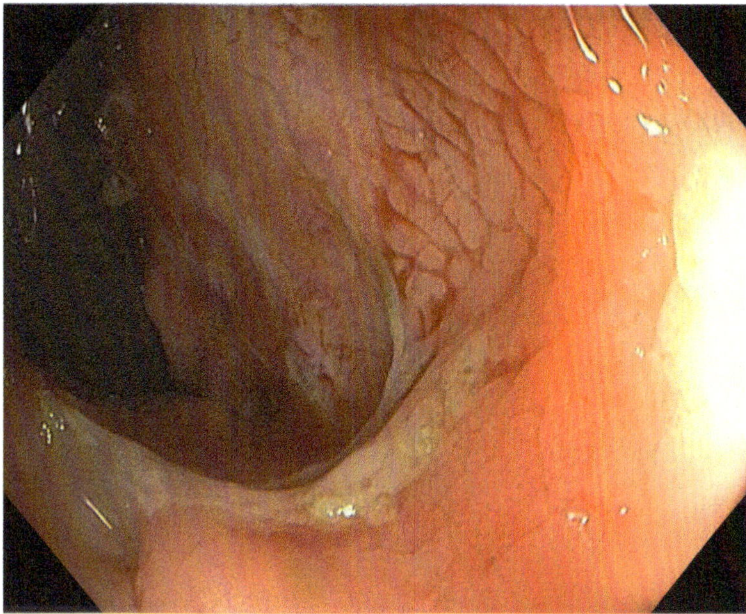

Fig. 7.1 Rectal erosions due to mild Crohn's disease as seen on retroflexion during colonoscopy

The inflammation in CD often presents on the anti-mesenteric side of the colon, and does not generally extend circumferentially [5]. In early disease, lesions present as small, punched out ulcers surrounded by healthy mucosa (Fig. 7.1). The pathogenesis of early lesions involves submucosal lymphoid follicle expansion that occurs before lesions are visualized [3, 5]. These findings are consistent with mild disease. In moderate CD, stellate (star) ulcers form as small aphthous lesions coalesce to create larger ulcers (Fig. 7.2). Submucosal edema and tissue damage can cause mucosal cobblestoning, which occurs when overlapping linear and transverse ulcers are superimposed on relatively normal mucosa (Fig. 7.3) [5]. In severe CD, deep serpiginous ulcers (Fig. 7.4) and large linear ulcers (bear claw) (Fig. 7.5) may be appreciated. The continuous pattern of inflammation in severe CD may be difficult to differentiate from UC, where inflammatory changes are continuous [5]. In up to 50 % of patients with colonic CD, the rectum is spared [10, 11]. Inflammatory pseudopolyps may be seen in CD, a finding that is also consistent with UC [5, 12] (Fig. 7.6). The afore described mucosal findings are the typical findings in CD patients, but they are all nonspecific and can be found in other disease states. Additionally, CD patients may have other mucosal findings not described above.

Disease Extent and Severity (Classification)

Classification of disease extent and severity facilitates assessment of disease prognosis, selection of appropriate medical or surgical interventions, and determination of cancer risk. It also allows clinicians to appropriately counsel patients regarding disease risk and management choices [3, 13]. Additionally, changes in endoscopic activity as a therapeutic endpoint has gained favor in recent years, making endoscopic scoring a growing tenet of clinical care [14]. In the basic sciences, classification aids researchers to better understand the pathophysiology of the various manifestations of IBD [13].

Although multiple endoscopic scores have been developed and used in clinical practice in attempts to more uniformly and objectively quantitate disease extent and severity, the Crohn's disease endoscopic index of severity (CDEIS), the simple endoscopic score for Crohn's disease (SES-CD), and the Rutgeerts' score are the only scores that have been validated [2, 15].

The CDEIS, developed in the 1980s, classifies disease extent according to the location and type

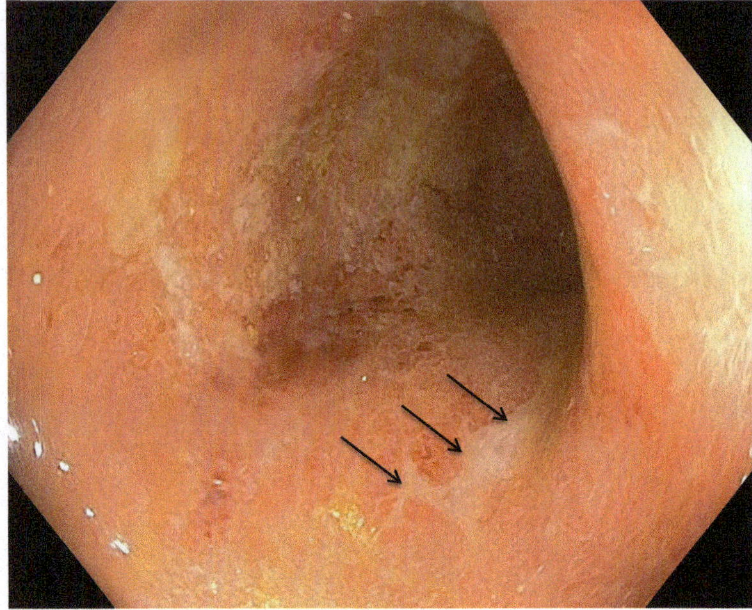

Fig. 7.2 Crohn's disease of moderate severity in the rectum. Note the stellate ulcer (*black arrows*), exudate, and friable mucosa

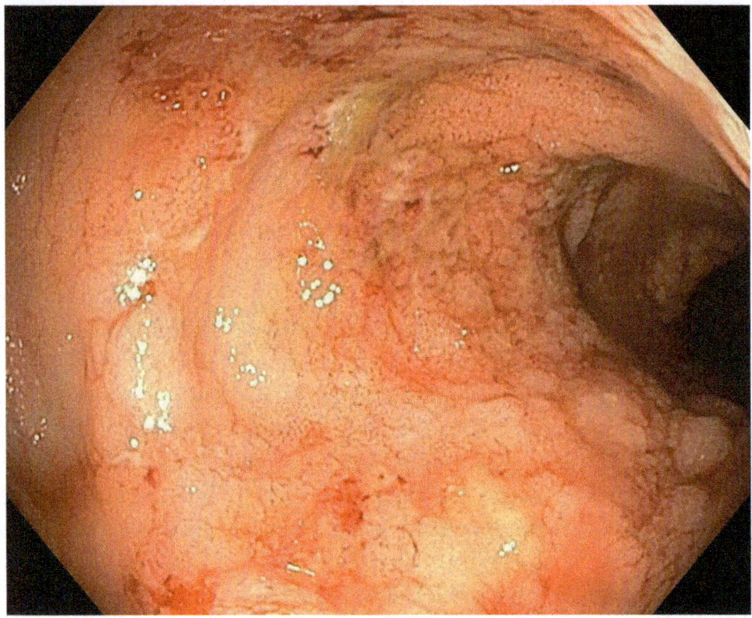

Fig. 7.3 Mucosal cobblestoning due to Crohn's disease as seen on colonoscopy

of lesions present in the gastrointestinal tract. Specifically, the CDEIS describes lesions as deep ulceration, superficial ulceration, surface involvement, or ulcerated surface, and also categorizes the location of lesions in the rectum, sigmoid and descending colon, transverse colon, ascending colon, and ileum. Scores range from 0 to 44, and authors recommend that values less than 6 be defined as endoscopic remission, values less than 4 be defined as complete endoscopic remission, and a decrease of 6 or greater points qualify as endoscopic response in CD [10, 15, 16] (Table 7.1).

Because the CDEIS requires tedious classification of endoscopic findings, some clinicians prefer the SES-CD, a simplified scoring system developed by Daperno et al. [14]. The SES-CD was

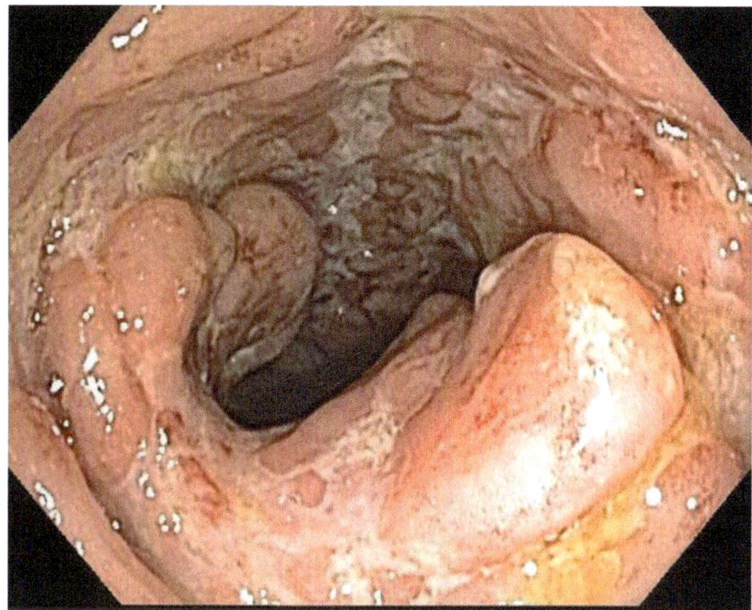

Fig. 7.4 Linear and serpiginous ulcers due to severe Crohn's disease as seen on colonoscopy

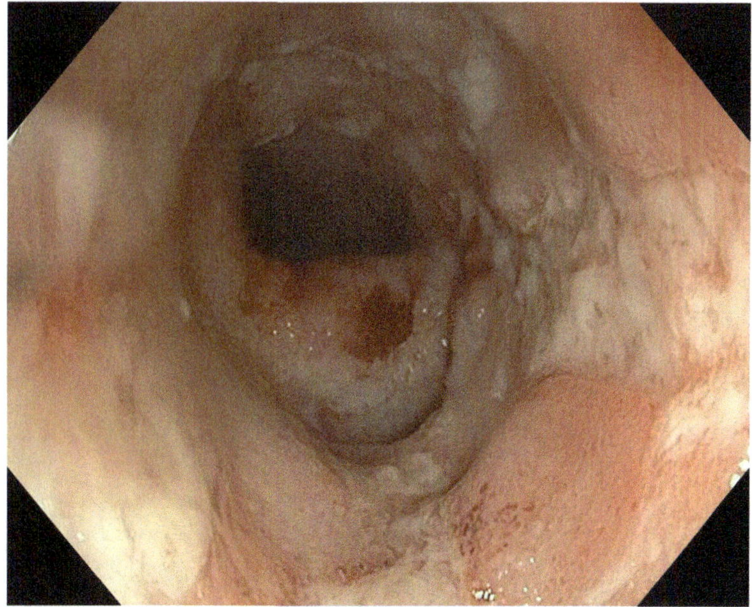

Fig. 7.5 Large linear ulcer due to Crohn's disease as seen on colonoscopy

found to have superior interobserver consistency compared to the CDEIS, and also correlates with clinical symptoms and CRP [10, 14] (Table 7.2).

To classify disease extent and severity in the post-surgical patient with IBD, the Rutgeerts' score is commonly used. This scoring system quantifies the occurrence of inflammation, aphthous ulcers, and strictures, and also documents the extent of disease involvement in the colon and terminal ileum [10, 18] (Table 7.3).

One limitation of the above scores is that none include classification of upper gastrointestinal (UGI) involvement. Endoscopic scores after medical treatment have been shown to predict sustained remission [19] and are also predictive of need for colectomy [20]. Postoperatively, the

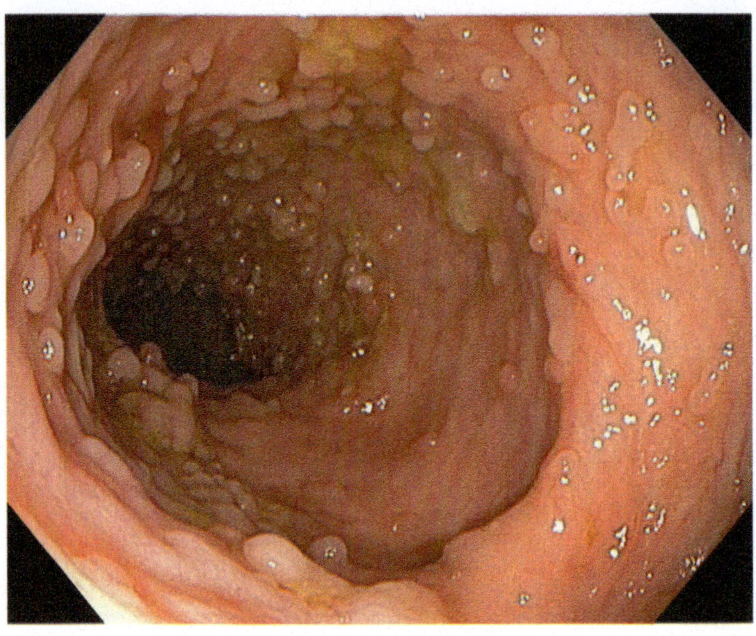

Fig. 7.6 Inflammatory pseudopolyps in the colon resulting from chronic inflammation due to Crohn's disease

Table 7.1 Crohn's disease endoscopic index of severity (CDEIS) [16]

	Ileum	Sigmoid and left colon	Transverse colon	Right colon	Rectum	Totals
Deep ulceration 0 = absent 12 = present						Total of line 1 =
Superficial ulceration 0 = absent 6 = present						Total of line 2 =
Surface involved by disease (cm)						Total of line 3 =
Surface involved by ulcerations (cm)						Total of line 4 =
Total of lines 1 through 4 = **(A)** =						
Number of segments explored (1–5) = **(n)** =						
Total **A/n** = **(B)** =						
If ulcerated stenosis present anywhere add 3 = **(C)** =						
If non-ulcerated stenosis present anywhere add 3 = **(D)** =						
Total B + C + D = (CDEIS score) =						

Rutgeerts' score has been shown to correlate with the likelihood of clinically significant recurrent CD. However, the endoscopic scores in general have not been found to predict clinical response to therapy or reliably predict disease prognosis [5, 16].

In recent efforts to quantify interobserver agreement in endoscopic scoring, interobserver agreement for both gastroenterologists experienced with endoscopic scoring systems and inexperienced gastroenterologists was good for CDEIS and SES-CD scoring systems, and fair for the Rutgeerts' score, while interobserver agreement for the Mayo score was poor [14].

Regarding classification of CD, in 2005 a working group of gastroenterologists developed

Table 7.2 Simple endoscopic score for Crohn's disease (SES-CD) [17]

	Ileum	Right colon	Transverse colon	Left colon	Rectum	Total
Presence and size of ulcers (0–3)						
Extent of ulcerated surface (0–3)						
Extent of affected surface (0–3)						
Presence and type of narrowings (0–3)						
Total =						

Table 7.3 Rutgeers' endoscopic score: postoperative recurrence in the terminal ileum in patients with CD [18]

Endoscopic score	Endoscopic findings
0	No lesions
1	Less than 5 aphthous lesions
2	Greater than 5 aphthous lesions with normal mucosa between lesions or skip areas of larger lesions or lesions confined to the ileocolonic anastomosis (i.e., less than 1 cm in length)
3	Diffuse aphthous ileitis with diffusely inflamed mucosa
4	Diffuse inflammation with larger ulcers, nodules, and/or narrowing

the Montreal classification to categorize patients with IBD according to clinical, serological, and genetic parameters. The classification system catalogues disease according to age of onset (A), disease location (L), and disease behavior (B) [21]. One study by Magro et al. reports that patient stratification according to the Montreal Classification may help identify disease phenotypes that require specific therapies; however, the predictive value of the Montreal Classification requires further investigation [22].

Biopsy Collection During Colonoscopy

Biopsy collection is an integral part of the initial diagnosis of CD, given that colonoscopy with multiple biopsies is the gold standard for diagnosis of CD [2–4].

During endoscopic evaluation, sampling from the entire colon provides more accurate pathologic diagnosis than limited biopsy collection [23]. Importantly, even with normal appearing mucosa, histologic changes associated with active disease may be present. For this reason it is important that biopsy specimens be collected from inflamed as well as normal appearing mucosa, particularly from the terminal ileum to evaluate for small bowel disease [5, 24]. Ideally, biopsy sampling should include at least two biopsies from the terminal ileum, cecum, ascending colon, transverse colon, descending colon, sigmoid colon, and rectum [2, 10]. Optimal biopsy collection is important; Bentley et al. describe that expert pathologists correctly diagnose 64 % of IBD cases when provided with a full series of biopsies as compared to 24 % of correctly diagnosed IBD cases when only a rectal biopsy is provided [23].

Differential Diagnosis in Colonoscopy

As the endoscopic findings of CD are nonspecific, differentiating IBD from other disorders is essential, especially as infectious diarrhea commonly presents with rectal bleeding [5, 10]. Other diagnoses in the differential include ischemia, diverticulitis, neoplasia, radiation enteritis, and drug-induced colitis. Treatments for all of these are vastly different making it critical to distinguish CD from other causes that can symptomatically present and endoscopically appear similar to CD.

Infection

A thorough evaluation of clinical history, stool studies, and endoscopy with biopsies is important to differentiate IBD from other causes. Various studies have reported that patients with suspected IBD may in fact have an infectious cause of symptoms. IBD with super-infection is also not uncommon [3, 25]. The majority of currently available medical therapies for IBD are relatively contraindicated in patients with active infections, thus ruling out an infectious etiology is critical prior to starting IBD specific therapy, with the exception of mesalamine products, as this class of therapy is unlikely to result in complications when given to patients with active infection. One prospective study of patients with suspected IBD showed that up to 1/3 of patients were diagnosed with an infectious cause [5, 10, 25]. However, another study reports that 20 % of IBD patients may have positive stool studies, suggesting that infection and IBD may occur concurrently, or that infection may precipitate disease exacerbation [3, 26].

Specific infections that present with mucosal and histologic findings similar to IBD include salmonellosis, shigellosis, campylobacteriosis, tuberculosis (TB), *Escherichia coli* infection, yersiniosis, *Clostridium difficile* infection, gonorrhea, *Klebsiella* infection, chlamydiosis, syphilis, schistosomiasis, amebiasis, herpes simplex, cytomegalovirus (CMV), and certain fungi [10]. While infectious colitis more often presents with continuous inflammation, TB, CMV, and yersiniosis may present with discrete ulcers with normal appearing mucosa adjacent to the ulcers, similar to CD [10, 27]. Additionally, infection with *Yersinia*, *Salmonella*, and TB may present with isolated ileitis, much like some presentations of CD [10, 27]. Endoscopic findings more characteristic of infection include yellowish, thick, and creamy exudate, and intensely erythematous surface mucosa [3]. Differentiation of IBD and intestinal TB may be particularly challenging, but findings including longitudinal or transverse ulcers, cobblestone appearance, fixed-open ileocecal valve, and more severe inflammation in terminal ileitis than in the cecum favor, but are not definitive for a diagnosis of CD [10, 28]. CMV is particularly important to rule out, especially in more severe disease. One study of rectal biopsy results from 62 patients with severe IBD reports that 36 % had super-infection with CMV [29]. Conclusively differentiating infectious entero-colitides from IBD can be difficult as the endoscopic findings can be similar and the clinical history, microbiology results, and biopsy should always be evaluated in conjunction with the endoscopic findings [3, 5].

If an infectious pathogen is identified, even in situations thought to be super-infection rather than the primary etiology of the patient's findings, the infectious pathogen needs to be treated and removed from the differential diagnosis prior to initiating CD specific medication. Essentially all CD specific medications currently available cause varying degrees of immune suppression and therefore are relatively contraindicated in a patient with a suspected or verified infectious pathogen.

Ischemia

Ischemic colitis occurs when blood flow to the bowel is interrupted, causing colonic inflammation and mesenteric ischemia. Endoscopically, ischemic colitis presents with loss of vascularity, erythema, granularity, confluent ulceration, serpiginous ulceration, longitudinal ulceration, friability, and submucosal hemorrhage [10, 30]. Segments of acutely ischemic mucosa may be abruptly demarcated from healthy tissue [3]. Most commonly affected areas correspond with areas along the border of colonic tissue supplied by the superior and inferior mesenteric arteries, with corresponding endoscopic involvement of the cecum and splenic flexure [10]. Ischemic colitis rarely presents as pancolitis, and often spares the rectal area where redundant blood supply is protective [10, 30]. Histologic evaluation of ischemic areas will reveal iron-laden macrophages and submucosal fibrosis [10, 31].

Diverticulitis

Diverticular disease of the colon may occasionally mimic IBD presenting with segmental colitis in areas with diverticula, often referred to as segmental colitis associated with diverticulosis (SCAD). However, multiple findings are suggestive of a diagnosis of diverticulitis. Muscular hypertrophy is more characteristic of diverticulitis, and is an uncommon finding in IBD. Additionally, the individual orifices of diverticula are usually appreciated on endoscopy, and biopsy of erythematous regions does not reveal inflammation [3].

Radiation Enteritis

Radiation therapy may cause injury to the gastrointestinal tract, the effects of which are dependent on the volume of irradiated tissue as well as the total dose of radiation [10, 32]. Chronic radiation injury may present endoscopically as stricture formation, while acute radiation injury more likely presents with friability, granularity, pallor, erythema, and prominent submucosal telangiectasias [10, 33]. The most common location of radiation injury is in the proximal rectum and distal sigmoid, although affected regions may vary according to the pattern of irradiation [3]. While the findings can be similar to IBD, patients will clearly have an antecedent history of significant radiation exposure to the affected area of bowel.

Drug-Induced Colitis

A variety of medications may cause drug-induced colitis, nonsteroidal anti-inflammatory drugs (NSAID) being the most common offenders [10]. Endoscopic findings include inflammation, erosions, ulcerations, stricture formation, and rarely, neoplastic-like masses [10, 34]. Follow-up endoscopy may be helpful to evaluate the colonic mucosa after the offending agent has been discontinued. Additionally, the use of sodium based bowel preparation and NSAIDs may cause mucosal changes similar to IBD, and it is recommended that these be avoided prior to diagnostic colonoscopy [35, 36].

Differentiating UC and CD

Certain disease characteristics help to classify IBD into CD and UC; however, significant overlap in disease presentation may complicate definitive diagnosis [2, 5]. While select endoscopic findings may favor one disease over the other, no endoscopic finding is specific only to UC or CD [2]. Endoscopy alone is limited in its ability to positively differentiate between the two conditions; however, obtaining detailed information from an initial ileocolonoscopy is important given that once therapy is initiated, certain discriminating factors may be obscured because of mucosal improvement or healing [35, 37] (Table 7.4).

Table 7.4 Differentiating ulcerative colitis (UC) and Crohn's disease (CD) [5]

CD	UC
Rectum often spared	Rectum involved
Skip areas of disease involvement	Confluent, continuous disease involvement
Disease presentation on anti-mesenteric side of the colon more common	Circumferential disease presentation more common
Aphthous ulcers	Loss of vascular markings
Cobblestoning more common	Diffuse erythema
Linear or serpiginous ulcers	Mucosal granularity (wet sandpaper)
Fistulizing disease	Fistulizing disease rare
Terminal ileal disease	No disease in terminal ileum
Upper GI involvement more common	Upper GI involvement less common

As discussed earlier, the endoscopic presentation of CD changes according to disease activity and duration [5]. Early CD presents as skip areas with small aphthous ulcers surrounded by healthy mucosa that may occur anywhere in the gastrointestinal tract. Comparatively, the inflammatory changes in early UC characteristically present above the anorectal junction and extend proximally. The pattern of inflammation in UC is confluent and continuous, and appears as diffuse erythema and vascular congestion [3, 10]. In UC, progressive edema results in a fine granular appearance of the colon mucosa that is friable and bleeds easily with contact [3]. Additionally, the inflammatory pattern in CD tends to appear on the anti-mesenteric side of the colon, whereas UC presents circumferentially [5].

Moderate CD presents with larger lesions due to the coalescence of smaller aphthous ulcers, and then as cobblestoning when submucosal edema and tissue damage progress. Cobblestoning is more often seen in CD than in UC; however, cobblestoning may also be present in severe UC [5]. In moderate UC, inflammation presents as small surface ulcers that also coalesce and may form large linear lesions known as "bear claw" ulcers. Mucosal ulceration may cause spontaneous bleeding [3]. In severe CD, deep serpiginous and large linear ulcers occur. In moderate to severe CD, the classical skip lesions maybe less appreciated due to coalescence, and differentiating CD from UC is more difficult [3, 5].

Lesions more characteristic of UC include erosions and microulcerations within a granular mucosa [10, 38]. Findings more consistent with CD include rectal sparing, UGI tract involvement, involvement of the terminal ileum, and anal or perianal disease; however, these characteristics are not exclusive to CD [35].

In up to 50 % of patients with colonic CD, the rectum can be spared [10, 11]. However, this characteristic remains an imperfect indicator of disease. Although rectal involvement is classically observed in UC, endoscopists have reported rectal sparing in about 32 % of UC patients [39, 40]. Additionally, various studies have suggested that pediatric patients with UC may present with rectal sparing. An analysis of 898 pediatric patients with UC reports 5 % presented with rectal sparing, and the occurrence of rectal sparing is inversely associated with age [39, 41, 42].

UGI tract involvement may occur in up to 13 % of CD patients, and evidence of disease in the UGI tract on initial evaluation with EGD may support a diagnosis of CD [35, 43, 44]. In a study by Lemberg et al., 25 children with IBD unclassified (IBDU) pancolitis were eventually diagnosed with CD based on EGD results [10, 45]. UGI involvement, however, does not definitely point to CD. Four percent of pediatric patients with UC were reported to have UGI involvement in a study of 898 patients, as compared to 22 % of pediatric patients diagnosed with CD [41]. In the absence of *Helicobacter pylori*, UGI lesions including focally active gastritis have been described as more characteristic of CD [2, 46]. However, this finding has been reported in UC as well, making differentiation difficult [2].

Classically, the terminal ileum is not involved in UC, and terminal ileitis is more characteristic of CD. However, studies have described that 10 % of cases of active pancolitis present with a finding of ileitis termed backwash ileitis, described as mild inflammation in the distal terminal ileum without ulceration [2, 3, 47]. Differentiating the two can prove challenging, and some researchers propose that any evidence of inflammation in the terminal ileum should support a diagnosis of CD. Others report that although differentiation is difficult, characteristics more consistent with CD include discrete ulcers, strictures of the terminal ileum or ileocecal valve, transmural ileal inflammation with granulomas and neural hyperplasia, extensive small bowel disease, jejunitis, proximal ileitis separated by skip areas, more inflammatory activity in the terminal ileal biopsies on pathology, and mucous gland metaplasia of the ileal mucosa [3, 10, 12, 35, 47–49]. Terminal ileitis may also be a result of infection, malignancy, radiation, vasculitis, or autoimmune disease [50]. One retrospective study showed that 68 % of patients with terminal ileitis had histologic confirmation; however, one third of patients in this study had no evidence of inflammation on histology [50].

While histologic evaluation of endoscopic biopsies can help differentiate between CD and UC, interobserver variation in the classification of IBD is common, and it is thought to be impossible to distinguish between the two diseases in approximately 10–20 % of cases [51]. A study by Farmer et al. describes that diagnosis by both board certified pathologists and specialized gastrointestinal pathologists differed significantly from the initial clinical diagnosis. Gastrointestinal pathologist's diagnoses differed from the initial diagnosis in 45 % of surgical specimens and 54 % of biopsies [10, 51].

Despite efforts to differentiate between CD and UC with endoscopy, clinical history, serologic markers, and radiologic imaging, definitive diagnosis is not always possible and 4–6 % of patients carry the diagnosis of IBDU. This seems more common in pediatric populations [10, 52, 53]. Although differentiation is difficult, definitive diagnosis of UC is essential prior to curative surgery. A prospective study by Murrell et al. identified that as many as 12 % of patients who underwent surgery following initial diagnosis of either UC or IBDU were subsequently diagnosed as having CD [10, 54]. As curative surgery in UC carries significant risk of morbidity and is an irreversible intervention, careful, extensive evaluation should occur prior to planned curative surgery to try to distinguish between CD and UC.

Role of Esophagogastroduodenoscopy (EGD) in IBD

Crohn's disease can affect any portion of the gut, from mouth to anus, although the most commonly affected areas are the terminal ileum and colon. In adults, colonoscopy with ileoscopy is generally adequate for diagnosis of CD versus UC in patients with IBD presenting with lower GI symptoms. Estimates regarding prevalence of upper GI tract involvement in CD range from 16 to 51 % [55–58], although precise definitions of upper GI involvement vary widely between studies, with some including only patients with macroscopic findings [55], and others including all patients with histologic evidence of CD [56–58].

In adult patients with UGI symptoms (nausea, vomiting, gastroesophageal reflux disease, early satiety, dyspepsia, and dysphagia), iron-deficiency anemia, vitamin B12 deficiency, or indeterminate colitis, EGD may be helpful to rule out CD involvement of the upper GI tract versus other etiologies such as celiac disease, *H. pylori* gastritis, viral infection, eosinophilic enteritis, or atrophic gastritis. Since NSAIDs can induce ulcerations of the stomach and small bowel, as with other endoscopic evaluation, EGD should be performed once the patient has been off all NSAIDs for a minimum of 4 weeks whenever possible. In patients who are immunosuppressed, viral etiologies such as CMV and HSV should be entertained, with biopsies obtained both for histology and viral culture.

We also advocate for EGD prior to elective colectomy in patients with ulcerative colitis or indeterminate colitis, since up to 17 % of patients undergoing total colectomy with ileal pouch-anal anastomosis (IPAA) are later diagnosed with CD [59].

Macroscopic findings consistent with upper GI Crohn's lesions may range from subtle to severe, consisting of aphthae, ulcerations, erosions, strictures, erythema, and edema (Figs. 7.7, 7.8, 7.9, and 7.10). Biopsies of the stomach and duodenum should be obtained in these patients with upper GI symptoms with particular attention paid to findings of granulomas, focal or patchy chronic inflammation, focal crypt distortion, and irregular villous architecture [55], eosinophils, intraepithelial lymphocytes, and *Helicobacter pylori* infection.

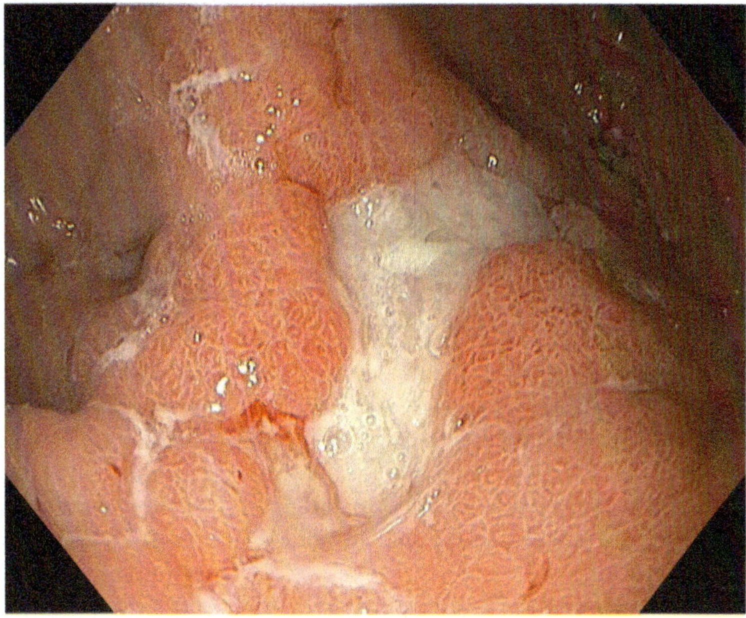

Fig. 7.7 Gastric ulcer due to upper gastrointestinal Crohn's disease

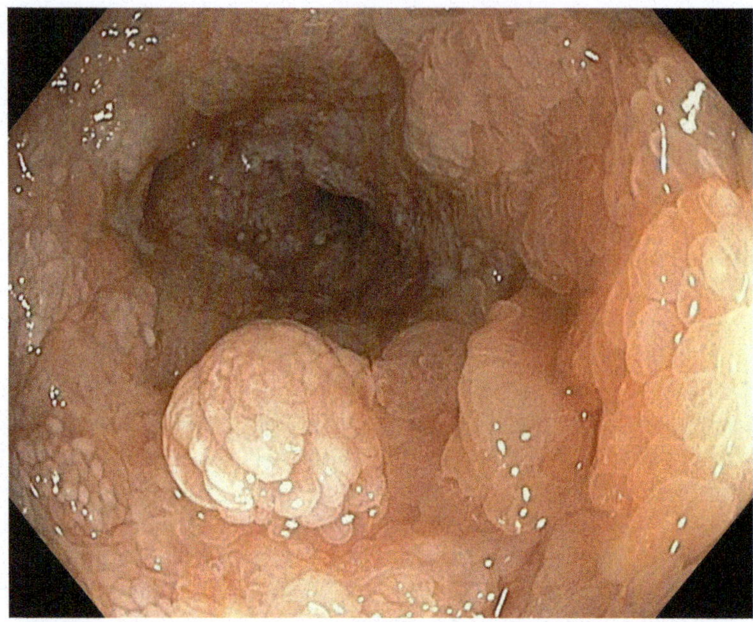

Fig. 7.8 Duodenal stricture due to Crohn's disease in the upper gastrointestinal tract

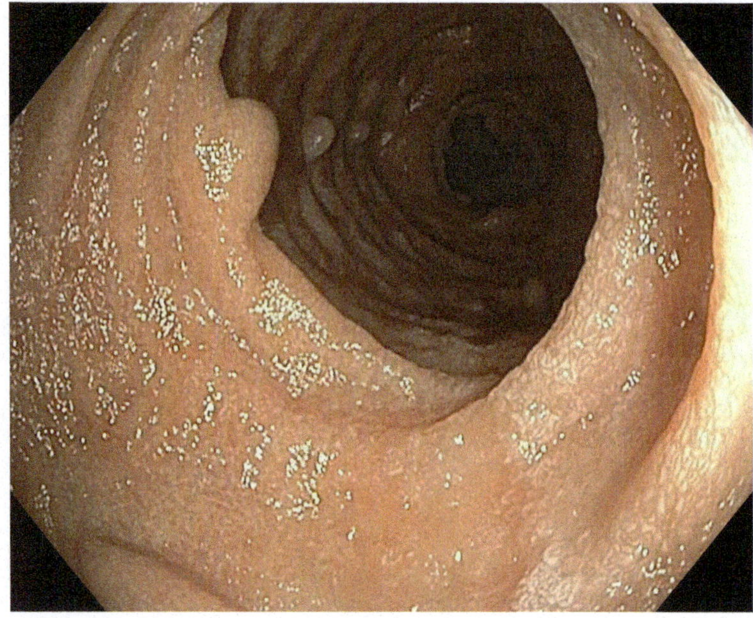

Fig. 7.9 Inflammatory pseudopolyps in the duodenum due to upper gastrointestinal Crohn's disease

In children, UC and CD can present with overt and classic symptoms such as bloody diarrhea and abdominal pain, or may be more subtle. Some children may present with failure to thrive or other symptoms related to malnutrition or anemia, or it may be difficult to obtain a detailed history of symptoms. Additionally, since many endoscopic evaluations in pediatric cases utilize general anesthesia, it is generally preferable not to have the patient undergo anesthesia multiple times, and therefore it is considered standard of care to perform both EGD and colonoscopy in patients in whom there is concern for IBD. This standard is not only to establish a diagnosis of CD versus UC, but also to rule out other etiologies such as celiac disease,

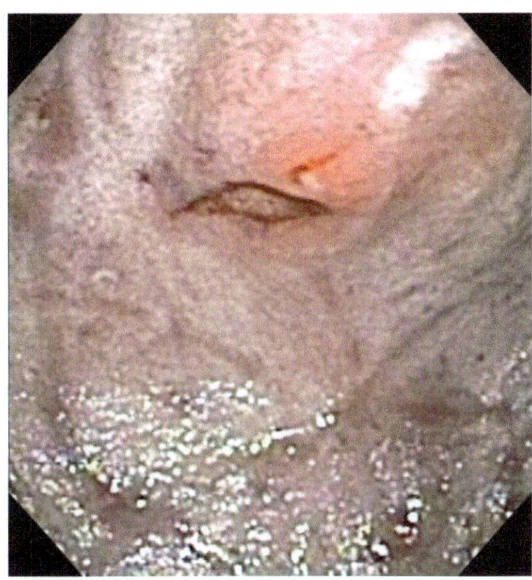

Fig. 7.10 Duodenal ulcer due to Crohn's disease in the upper GI tract

which can present with growth failure or other vague symptoms.

While there are no guidelines regarding when or where to biopsy during EGD in Crohn's patients, we generally recommend biopsies of any abnormal appearing mucosa in the esophagus, stomach, or duodenum. If there is suspicion for celiac disease, 4–6 biopsies should be obtained from the duodenal bulb and more distal duodenum. For nonspecific symptoms without overt mucosal abnormalities, it is reasonable to biopsy the stomach to evaluate for the presence of *H. pylori* gastritis. If there are changes consistent with viral infections, such as esophageal ulcers in a patient on immunosuppression, biopsies should be obtained of the ulcer perimeter and base and sent for viral culture [60].

Role of Capsule Endoscopy in the Evaluation of Crohn's Disease

Capsule endoscopy is a relatively new tool for evaluation of the mucosa in IBD. Since the introduction of the first capsule endoscopy in 2001 [61], the technology has evolved rapidly, with significant improvement in image quality and even adjustments in how rapidly images are obtained based on the rate of transit through the bowel. Additionally, capsule endoscopy is generally quite safe in most patient populations. Small bowel capsule endoscopy (SBCE) is most commonly used to evaluate for bleeding source in cases of iron-deficiency anemia or obscure overt GI bleeding when EGD and colonoscopy are unrevealing. Recently, a colon capsule was approved by the Food and Drug Administration for colorectal cancer (CRC) screening in cases where colonoscopy could not be completed [62], and is being evaluated as a potential tool for assessing disease state in ulcerative colitis [63].

Here we will focus on use of SBCE in the evaluation of suspected or confirmed IBD. In IBD, the primary value is for assessment of the small bowel in suspected CD in cases where findings on traditional endoscopy or imaging do not explain the entire clinical picture, or for restaging known small bowel CD (i.e., assessing response to therapy). SBCE has the advantage of being non-invasive, with excellent diagnostic yield in the assessment of the small bowel mucosa. In a meta-analysis comparing diagnostic yield of SBCE to small bowel follow-through (SBFT), colonoscopy with ileoscopy, CT enterography, push enteroscopy, and MRI, SBCE was found to be superior to all other modalities for diagnosis of non-stricturing small bowel CD [64].

In addition to its utility in the initial diagnosis of CD, SBCE also has the potential to complement traditional endoscopy to guide therapy in patients undergoing medical or surgical treatment for CD. For example, over the last several years the value of mucosal healing in response to medical therapies has come to light [65, 66]. The goal for treatment of patients with CD is no longer simply resolution of symptoms, but lack of endoscopic and histologic inflammation. Because biopsies are necessary to fully assess mucosal healing, capsule endoscopy is not adequate for definitive assessment of treatment response, but may be a useful less invasive method of assessing for endoscopic improvement, particularly in patients with small bowel CD out of the reach of traditional endoscopy [67]. Additionally, capsule endoscopy may be used for assessment of early disease recurrence after surgical intervention in cases where colonoscopy with ileoscopy is not possible or visualization of more proximal small bowel is needed to guide decisions regarding postoperative medical therapies [68].

Differential Diagnosis of Lesions Seen by SBCE

As with traditional endoscopy, findings of small bowel CD by SBCE may range from subtle (erythema, edema, aphthae, fissuring, villous atrophy) to severe (large ulcerations, strictures, fistulas). However, these findings are not specific to CD. In fact, approximately 9 % of healthy patients may have small bowel mucosal breaks without CD [69]. Other potential etiologies for small bowel lesions seen on SBCE include medication toxicity (especially NSAID-induced enteritis), autoimmune conditions (celiac sprue, Behcet's), malignancy, infection, ischemia, or radiation enteritis. Since SBCE is limited by the lack of biopsy capability, it is important to evaluate for these other etiologies with clinical history, laboratory testing, and other diagnostic techniques such as cross-sectional imaging when necessary. Mergener et al. proposed an algorithm to establish adequate pretest probability to justify the use of SBCE for suspected small bowel Crohn's [70] (Fig. 7.11).

Scoring Disease Activity with SBCE

There are two validated scoring systems for assessing CD extent and severity using SBCE [71–74]. The Lewis score [71] assesses villous appearance (normal versus edematous) and ulcerations (single, few [2–7], or multiple ≥8) in each tertile of the small bowel, as well as the presence of stenosis anywhere in the small bowel (single/multiple; ulcerated/non-ulcerated; traversed/not traversed). The tertiles are determined by dividing the small bowel transit time by three. A score <135 is considered normal or clinically insignificant inflammation; 135–790 mild inflammation; and >790 moderate to severe inflammation (Table 7.5). The scoring index is now included in the PillCam™ (RAPID) capsule endoscopy software to allow for ease of use and standardization [67].

The second validated scoring system is the capsule endoscopy Crohn's disease activity index (CECDAI, or Niv score) [72]. The CECDAI evaluates inflammation (A), extent of disease (B), and stricture (C), in both the proximal (1) and distal (2) portions of the small bowel. The score is calculated using a simple formula: CECDAI=([A1×B1]+C1)+([A2×B2]+C2) [74] (Fig. 7.12). Only the most severe lesion is used to determine the score for each segment. A score of 0 is normal, and a score of 26 represents severe disease.

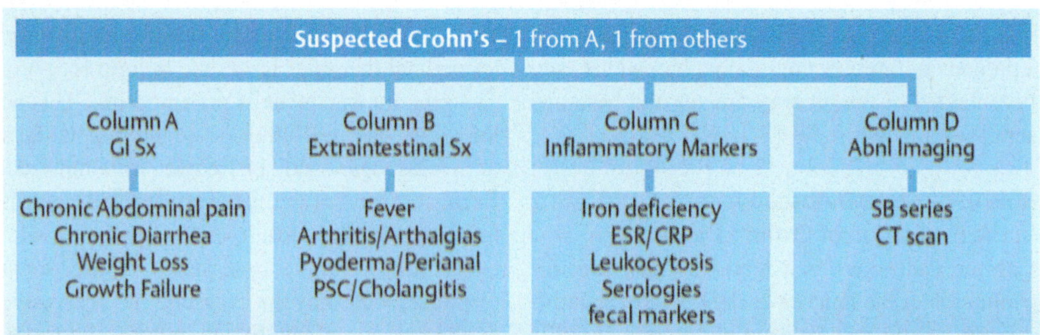

Fig. 7.11 Guideline to define suspected Crohn's disease [70]. *Sx* symptoms and signs, *PSC* primary sclerosing cholangitis, *ESR* erythrocyte sedimentation rate, *CRP* C-reactive protein, *Abnl* abnormal, *SB* small bowel, *CT* computed tomography

Table 7.5 Parameters and weightings for the capsule endoscopy scoring index [73]

Parameters	Number	Longitudinal extent	Descriptors
First tertile			
Villous appearance	Normal—0 Edematous—1	Short segment—8 Long segment—12 Whole tertile—20	Single—1 Patchy—14 Diffuse—17
Ulcer	None—0 Single—3 Few—5 Multiple—10	Short segment—5 Long segment—10 Whole tertile—15	<1/4—9 1/4–1/2—12 >1/2—18
Second tertile			
Villous appearance	Normal—0 Edematous—1	Short segment—8 Long segment—12 Whole tertile—20	Single—1 Patchy—14 Diffuse—17
Ulcer	None—0 Single—3 Few—5 Multiple—10	Short segment—5 Long segment—10 Whole tertile—15	<1/4—9 1/4–1/2—12 >1/2—18
Third tertile			
Villous appearance	Normal—0 Edematous—1	Short segment—8 Long segment—12 Whole tertile—20	Single—1 Patchy—14 Diffuse—17
Ulcer	None—0 Single—3 Few—5 Multiple—10	Short segment—5 Long segment—10 Whole tertile—15	<1/4—9 1/4–1/2—12 >1/2—18
Stenosis-rated for whole study			
Stenosis	None—0 Single—14 Multiple—20	Ulcerated—24 Non-ulcerated—2	Traversed—7 Not traversed—10

Complications and Contraindications to Capsule Endoscopy

The main risk with capsule endoscopy is capsule retention. Capsule retention is generally defined as a situation where the capsule will not pass through the bowel without medical, endoscopic, or surgical intervention [75]. Capsule retention usually does not lead to bowel obstruction or even symptoms, although the potential for these certainly exists. Capsule retention may occur in the case of luminal narrowing for any reason, including Crohn's stricture, NSAID stricture, tumor, surgical anastomotic stricture, or radiation enteritis. Capsule retention has been reported to occur in 5–13 % of patients with known CD [67].

Capsules may become retained proximal to any narrowing in the bowel, whether this is from inflammation, fibrosis, or a combination of the two. In cases of CD, the approach we recommend is optimization of medical therapy for 8-12 weeks prior to performing capsule endoscopy in whom there is concern for stenosis. With this approach, we feel that the inflammatory component should be well treated, and therefore any narrowing of the bowel which causes capsule retention requiring surgery is in an area of the bowel that was not amenable to medical therapy anyway. Patients with CD undergoing SBCE should be informed about the risk of capsule retention with potential need for surgery or endoscopy for removal, as well as symptoms of small bowel obstruction which should prompt them to return for evaluation.

Alternatively, a soluble "patency capsule" has been developed for use in patients with suspected stenosis prior to capsule endoscopy to assess luminal patency [76]. The patency capsule is the same size as the functional capsule

A. Inflammation score
0 = None
1 = Mild to moderate edema/hyperemia/denudation
2 = Severe edema/hyperemia/denudation
3 = Bleeding, exudate, aphthae, erosion, small ulcer (<0.5 cm)
4 = Moderate ulcer (0.5 – 2 cm), pseudo polyp
5 = Large ulcer (>2 cm)
B. Extent of disease score
0 = No disease – normal examination
1 = Focal disease (single segment is involved)
2 = Patchy disease (2 – 3 segments are involved)
3 = Diffuse disease (more than 3 segments are involved)
C. Stricture score
0 = None
1 = Single-passed
2 = Multiple-passed
3 = Obstruction (non-passage)
Segmental score (proximal or distal) = (A × B) + C
Total score = proximal ([A × B] + C) + distal ([A × B] + C)

Fig. 7.12 Capsule endoscopy Crohn's disease activity index: scoring system worksheet [74]

endoscopy, but the exterior is composed of wax plugs and cellophane, with a 2 × 10 mm radio-opaque tag inside the capsule. The capsule is swallowed by the patient, and an X-ray is performed 30 hours after ingestion to determine if the capsule is retained. The capsule begins to dissolve at 30 h, and all are completely dissolved by 36–72 h.

Patient Preparation for Capsule Endoscopy

Quality of visualization and potentially diagnostic yield of SBCE appear to be improved with the use of bowel lavage and antifoaming agents based on a recent meta-analysis [70]. However, the optimal timing and dosages of these agents has not been determined. It appears that 2 L of polyethylene glycol (PEG) is equally effective as 4 L. The addition of simethicone also improves quality of visualization. Studies of the use of prokinetic agents have had variable results, although in a recent meta-analysis they did not improve the completion rate in SBCE. In our practice, we recommend a clear liquid diet and consumption of 2 L of PEG the evening prior to morning capsule placement. Patients should then be NPO after midnight, and should swallow the capsule in the morning with 12 ounces of water mixed with 300 mg of simethicone. The patient may then consume a clear liquid diet beginning 2 h after capsule placement and resume a regular diet 4 h after placement. In patients with concern for slow gastric emptying or swallowing difficulties, we recommend that the capsule be placed in the duodenum endoscopically. If endoscopic placement is not feasible, it may be helpful to use a prokinetic agent in cases of delayed gastric emptying.

Enteroscopy/Device Assisted Enteroscopy

Small bowel disease has been reported in 10–30 % of patients with CD, and up to 20 % may have disease that is isolated to the small bowel [77, 78]. Other studies argue that SBCE revealed disease in the proximal small bowel in greater than 50 % of CD patients, and that 30 %

of patients newly diagnosed with CD may have disease limited to the small bowel beyond the reach of ileocolonoscopy [55, 79]. It is likely that technical and diagnostic limitations result in an underestimate of isolated small bowel CD [77]. Because CD involvement of the small bowel may correlate with a higher rate of complications including stricture and fistula formation, it is important to identify those patients who may benefit from more aggressive therapy [77, 80].

While colonoscopy is capable of visualizing the colon and terminal ileum, and EGD assesses the UGI tract and duodenum, a large portion of the small intestine remains unseen. Enteroscopy permits evaluation and biopsy collection from previously unreachable regions of small bowel [5, 35]. In initial diagnosis of CD, enteroscopy is most helpful when other diagnostics are inconclusive and histologic analysis of the small bowel would change treatment decisions [81, 82].

Enteroscopy and device assisted enteroscopy (DAE) includes various endoscopic methods for evaluating the small bowel: push enteroscopy, double balloon enteroscopy (DBE), single balloon enteroscopy (SBE), and spiral enteroscopy (SE). These methods access the small bowel by either enterograde (oral) or retrograde (anal) approach, permitting assessment of the small bowel, collection of biopsies, and enteroscopic intervention (e.g., dilation) [83]. Although enteroscopy is a helpful tool in small bowel CD, results should be interpreted in the context of clinical findings and other diagnostic results, and it is recommended that other evaluations such as colonoscopy, EGD and imaging be considered before enteroscopy [77].

Role/Indication

Push Enteroscopy and DAE

Traditional push enteroscopy was developed in the 1980s and involves inserting an enteroscope or a pediatric or adult colonoscopy in the proximal jejunum. Push enteroscopy is generally utilized to treat proximal small bowel pathology, and complication rates for the procedure are reported as 1 % [84].

DAE including DBE, SBE, and SE have improved the reach of enteroscopes allowing assessment and treatment of more distal disease. DBE may be performed with an enterograde or retrograde approach. The technique uses two balloons, the first of which attaches to the enteroscope tip. After the scope is inserted into the bowel, the overtube balloon is inflated and used to anchor the tip in place. The scope is then pulled back to fold the small bowel behind the balloon. Using repetitive cycles of balloon inflation and deflation, the scope is advanced into the small bowel [84]. One study of 37 patients suggests that the overall yield of DBE is about 60 %, but yield varies according to indication (40 % in obscure bleeding and 100 % in strictures) [84, 85]. A 2008 meta-analysis revealed that diagnostic yield is similar in DBE and SBCE. The study reports the diagnostic yield of DBE as 60 % in small bowel disease and 18 % in CD, while the diagnostic yield of SBCE is 57 % in small bowel disease and 16 % in CD [15, 86]. Another study of 44 patients found that DBE identified more aphthae, erosions, and small ulcers in the ileum than radiologic studies [87]. This could be significant as radiologic findings are thought to precede endoscopic findings by 1–7 years, which may permit earlier diagnosis and a better indicator of mucosal healing [84, 88, 89].

DBE is likely most useful after initial assessment with small bowel cross-sectional imaging and/or SBCE for the indication of diagnosing small bowel CD, collecting small bowel biopsies, or assessing a suspicious lesion [15, 84, 90]. Consideration should also be given to the location of the lesion in question and the expertise of available endoscopists [83, 90, 91]. DBE may be less useful in patients with tortuous anatomy in whom the procedure would be technically difficult and complication rates higher [84]. Additionally, DBE balloons are made from latex, thus the procedure is contraindicated in patients with serious latex allergy [88]. In DBE, complications are rare, and occur in less than 1 % of patients. Complications of DBE include pancreatitis (0.3 %), bleeding (0.2 %), and aspiration pneumonia [84, 92]. Overall complication rates for patients with CD are not higher, although a history of CD or gastrointestinal surgery increases the risk of perforation [15, 90]. A 2008 study of 2,478 DBE procedures reported a complication rate that was ten times as high as conventional colonoscopy with the most common complications being post-procedure abdominal pain, bleeding, and perforation [15, 93]. SBE, introduced in 2007, utilizes a similar technique as DBE, but in SBE the tip of the enteroscope is used as an anchor thus avoiding the need for a second balloon [84].

The most recent advancement in DAE, spiral enteroscopy (SE), was developed in 2008. The SE device consists of an overtube with a soft, raised helix that allows simpler and faster evaluation of the small bowel [84, 94]. SE uses clockwise rotation to advance the scope into the small bowel, minimizing twisting of the intestines. Although SE allows rapid advancement and facilitates therapeutic intervention, it has only been demonstrated safely in retrograde, whereas DBE may be administered retrograde or antegrade. Complications are similar to other DAE techniques, and include perforation and pancreatitis [84]. A review of 2,950 patients treated with SE reported a severe complication rate of 0.3 % and a perforation rate of 0.4 % [84, 95]. A 2013 multicenter study found that SE appears as safe as DBE, and that the diagnostic and therapeutic yield is comparable; however, no studies have looked specifically at patients with IBD [96].

Although DAE is helpful in specific situations, it is a more invasive, costly and time-consuming test, and is not recommended as first line evaluation of small bowel CD [83, 90].

Evaluation After Initial Diagnosis

For patients with an established diagnosis of CD, endoscopy still plays a critical role in ongoing evaluation of CD for adequate response to therapy, complications of disease and therapy, therapeutic intervention, and cancer screening. As with the initial diagnosis of CD, endoscopy in established patients is still critical and is the best currently available modality for ongoing evaluation of CD as it is the most sensitive diagnostic test, allows for biopsies, and is typically the only intervention other than surgery that allows for therapeutic intervention for certain complications associated with CD. The remainder of this chapter will review the role and utility of endoscopy in patients with established CD.

Colonoscopy

Role/Indication

Colonoscopy continues to play a central role in the evaluation of patients with an established diagnosis of CD, especially given that mucosal healing has become a key outcome in assessing the efficacy of therapies [1]. Ileocolonoscopy is indicated in a variety of settings in the care of patients with CD, including restaging disease activity; evaluating for disease activity and alternate etiologies in patients with worsening symptoms; dysplasia surveillance in appropriate patients; and therapeutic interventions such as stricture dilation. Ileocolonoscopy is also helpful preoperatively to establish if patients have evidence of disease activity that warrants further medical optimization and postoperatively to assess for recurrence and risk stratify for the need to initiate or continue postoperative medical therapy. In patients who have undergone colectomy with J-pouch formation, pouchoscopy is the best test to evaluate patients with clinical symptoms that are more severe than expected postoperatively to differentiate pouchitis, pouch structural abnormalities versus CD as the etiology for symptoms [2, 5, 10, 29, 35, 97, 98].

Restaging Disease, Response to Therapy

While clinical exacerbation of symptoms often indicates increasing inflammatory activity, clinical symptoms do not reliably correlate with disease severity, and symptom scores do not consistently match endoscopic evaluation or mucosal healing [99]. Endoscopic evaluation can more objectively evaluate the extent and severity of active inflammatory disease, thus guiding therapeutic decision-making. Additionally, during symptom flares, it is essential to rule out other causes of exacerbation such as CMV or *Clostridium difficile* infection [5, 29]. Ileocolonoscopy with biopsy is critical to differentiate infectious causes of disease exacerbation and prevent changes in treatment that do not reflect inadequate response or loss of response to medical therapy. Prior to any significant changes to medical therapy, we recommend that patients with disease that is evaluable by ileocolonoscopy undergo endoscopic evaluation with biopsies.

Mucosal Healing

Since the development of anti-tumor necrosis factor alpha (TNFα) and other biologic agents, mucosal healing has become an important indicator of treatment success [3, 35, 65]. Although no definition has been validated, the term 'mucosal healing' commonly refers to the absence of visible ulcers on endoscopy [1]. This definition, however, does not consider improvement or grading of mucosal healing [100]. In CD, mucosal healing has been described using the CDEIS in a number of clinical trials. Endoscopic remission has been described as CDEIS less than 6, and endoscopic response as CDEIS less than 5. Others have assigned values less than 3 to complete endoscopic remission [1, 15]. In a post hoc analysis of the SONIC trial, researchers defined mucosal healing and endoscopic response as a decrease in the SES-CD or CDEIS of at least 50 % from baseline at week 26 of treatment. They identified that patients meeting this criteria were more likely to be in corticosteroid free clinical remission at week 50 [101]. Importantly, no consistent endoscopic scoring value has been agreed upon.

Recent studies have focused on the utility of mucosal healing as a sign of effective medical therapy that may predict disease prognosis. Studies suggest that mucosal healing may correlate with a reduction in hospitalizations and surgical interventions, a decrease in the risk of clinical relapse, and a reduction in the risk of CRC [49, 66, 77, 102–104]. In one study, Baert et al. report that 70.8 % of patients with an SES-CD of zero at 2 years after initial diagnosis were in steroid free remission at years 3 and 4 [19]. Another study looking at 71 patients with CD treated with infliximab shows that in those patients who had responded to therapy at 3 months, 77 % maintained response at 12 months, suggesting that early endoscopic healing may predict sustained response. Ninety percent of patients with complete mucosal healing at the 3 month post-treatment endoscopy had sustained response at 12 months [105]. Overall, mucosal healing appears to be a good indicator of disease prognosis, but further study is needed to define mucosal healing, to recommend frequency of endoscopic evaluation, and to confirm how treatment decisions should change based on endoscopic healing [15]. At the current time without more definitive data with regard to the implications of mucosal disease activity, we recommend including the distribution and severity of endoscopic mucosal disease activity with laboratory, radiographic, and clinical symptoms to choose if modification to a patient's current medical therapy is warranted.

Preoperative Colonoscopy

Preoperative colonoscopy may provide useful information regarding the extent of disease in both planned partial colectomy and the vitality of a planned primary anastomosis [5]. Often planned partial colectomy or TI resection is secondary to a fibro-stenotic segment that is not amenable to medical therapy. However, such patients can have areas distinct from the fibro-stenotic area that has active inflammation. Preoperatively we recommend that medical therapy be optimized to try and achieve mucosal healing in areas with active inflammation to decrease the likelihood that these segments would require resection during the planned surgery, to decrease the possibility that a primary anastomosis cannot be performed due to active disease and to decrease the possibility that a primary anastomosis will have complications such as leaks or rapid stenosis from active CD. Preoperative endoscopy can also provide endoscopic dilation of any strictures that may not require resection, such as an anal stricture. This can allow for both salvage of the segment with a stricture and ensure that the upstream primary anastomosis does not leak due to downstream obstruction. Pre-operative sigmoidoscopy may also aid surgical decision-making when surgical correction of perianal CD is considered. For patients with CD undergoing resection of only small bowel, ileocolonoscopy primarily adds an assessment of colonic disease and evaluation of any possible colonic neoplasm [5].

Postoperative Colonoscopy

In patients with CD, postoperative ileocolonoscopy with biopsy is helpful to assess postoperative recurrence of disease at the anastomosis [5, 8]. Active CD recurs at the surgical anastomosis within 1 year in 70–90 % of CD patients, and an estimated 50 % of patients with recurrence and inadequate medical therapy will require anastomotic revision [5, 6, 8]. Evaluation with ileocolonoscopy may be helpful to identify these patients, particularly to rule out disease recurrence in cases where modifying CD therapy would not treat the problem. Postoperative medical therapy has been considered to reduce rates of disease recurrence; however, there are currently no endoscopic indicators as to which patients may benefit from treatment [5, 106]. Currently, endoscopic evaluation 6–12 months after surgery is recommended [2, 81].

In addition to the evaluation for disease recurrence, ileocolonoscopy allows the differentiation of symptoms from active disease recurrence versus other etiologies such as bile acid malabsorption or bacterial overgrowth which can be common in patients after ileal resection. In patients with no clinical symptoms, laboratory abnormalities such as anemia or elevated CRP, we would recommend if a Rutgeerts score of greater than 2 is identified that patients be considered for initiation of postoperative medical therapy. For those patients with clear signs of clinical disease activity based on other evaluation, we still recommend evaluation with ileocolonoscopy prior to initiation of medical therapy to assess pre-treatment disease activity and to insure there are no infectious etiologies such as *C. difficile* or CMV.

For patients who are considered high risk and require ongoing postoperative medical therapy regardless of endoscopic findings, such as those with two or more surgeries in 5 years, greater than three lifetime surgeries, or patients with disease pre-operatively involving areas that are not resected, we still recommend evaluation with ileocolonoscopy postoperatively to assess for adequate mucosal healing.

Pouchitis vs. Active IBD

Pouchitis is an inflammatory condition that occurs in the ileal pouch reservoir in an IPAA, which may present with diffuse erythema, friability, granularity, exudates, erosions, and/or ulcerations [107, 108]. Twenty-three to forty-six percent of patients with IPAA develop pouchitis, and the endoscopic differences between pouchitis and IBD are not specific [2, 109]. Pouch disease activity indices may help diagnose the condition, and biopsies should be taken, even in normal appearing mucosa, to rule out active inflammation of CD as well as dysplasia [107]. In the absence of an alternative etiology, the finding of endoscopic or histologic inflammatory changes in the neo-terminal ileum (neo-TI) upstream of the J-pouch is often representative that the patient has CD, and we recommend that all patients undergoing endoscopy for evaluation of their J-pouch have biopsies taken in the neo-TI, the J-pouch and just upstream of the dentate line (this will be discussed further in sections below with regard to colon cancer screening).

Interventional Endoscopy

CD patients have a high risk of stricture formation with 10 % developing colonic and 25 % developing small bowel strictures [81, 110]. Strictures, either inflammatory or fibrotic, may occur at bowel anastomoses, de novo, or in the ileal pouch [111, 112]. While inflammatory strictures may respond to medical therapy, surgery is required in a reported 64 % of patients [111, 113]. Fibrotic strictures are best treated with intestinal resection or strictureplasty [114]. Due to the significant operative recurrence rate (34 % according to one study), and the potential for short bowel syndrome, the decision to treat strictures surgically should take into account clinical and prognostic factors [111, 115]. Interventional endoscopy with balloon dilation is a reasonable option for many CD patients with symptomatic fibrotic strictures [2]. Recommendations suggest that localized, ileocecal CD with obstructive symptoms, but no

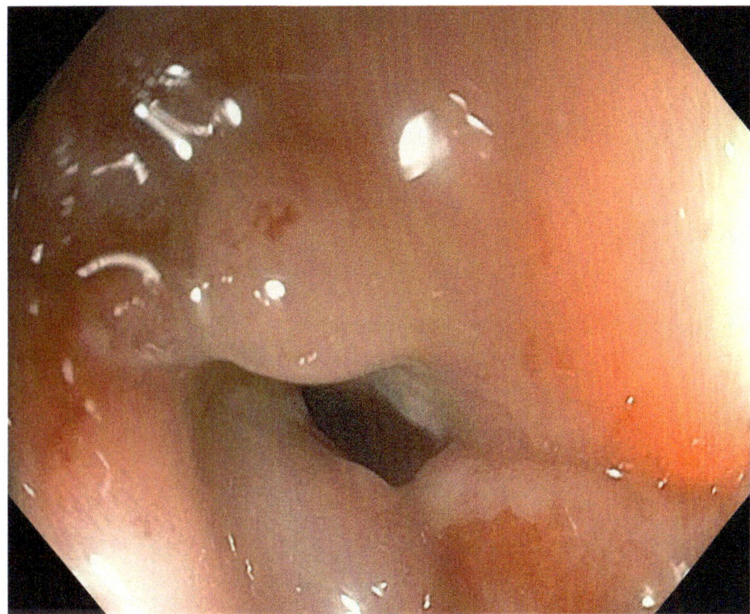

Fig. 7.13 Ascending colon stricture due to Crohn's disease. The stricture did not allow passage of the pediatric colonoscope (12 mm). It was biopsied to rule out malignancy, and then dilated with a through-the-scope (TTS) balloon

significant evidence of active inflammation, should be treated by surgery. Alternatively, short stricture, as well as recurrence of stricture post-surgery would benefit from balloon dilation [2, 15] (Figs. 7.13, 7.14, and 7.15).

Prior to balloon dilation, lesions should be evaluated with cross-sectional imaging to identify the location, number, activity, and extension of strictures, as well as the presence of fistulas or abscesses [15]. Strictures measuring 4 cm or less have been associated with better outcomes. Strictures may recur post dilation, and as many as 50 % of patients will require repeat dilation over 5 years [2]. Results from multiple studies suggest that endoscopic balloon dilation is effective and safe. A systematic review showed that 58 % of patients underwent successful dilation, with 22 % of patients requiring repeat dilation, and 19 % requiring multiple endoscopic interventions [15, 116]. Another systematic review reported that 90 % of cases ended with successful dilation, with 27 % of patients requiring surgery after 21 months [15, 117].

Major complications of endoscopic balloon dilation include perforation and bleeding, and complication rates in reviewed studies ranged from 2 to 3 % [15, 116–118]. Of the modifiable risk factors, smoking seems to be linked with worse outcomes, specifically with regard to stricture recurrence post dilation [92, 111].

Intra-lesional steroid injections have been used by some to prevent recurrence, but studies have yet to definitely show benefit from this practice and some studies have suggested a worse outcome in those who underwent injection compared to those who did not during dilation [79, 119].

Enteroscopy

Role/Indication

Enteroscopy may be useful to specifically evaluate occult gastrointestinal bleeding or suspicious small bowel lesions, or for dilation of fibrotic strictures, however at this time it likely has little place in routine evaluation of small bowel CD, unless intervention or biopsy is required.

Intraoperative Enteroscopy

Intraoperative enteroscopy can be utilized in specific situations by specialized practitioners, to guide surgery intraoperatively, and also to evaluate lesions that exist deep in the small bowel, out of reach of other forms of endoscopy and enteroscopy [84, 120, 121]. Complications

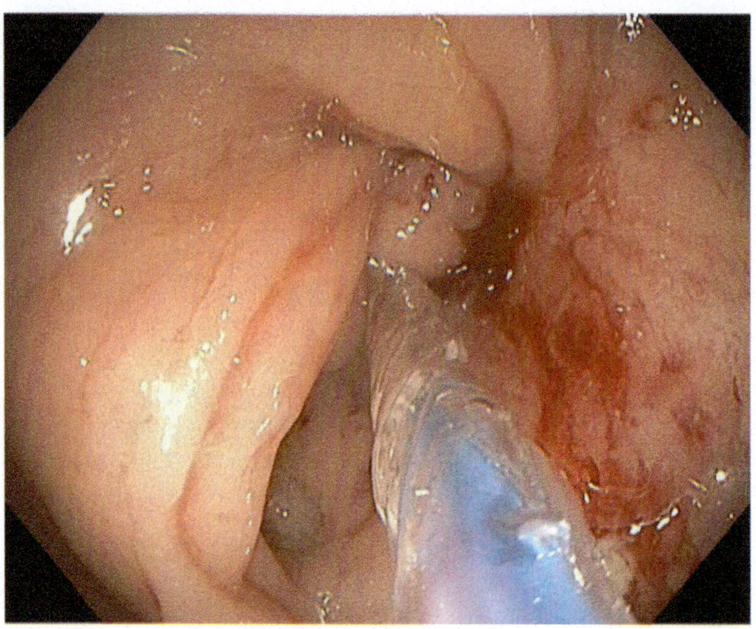

Fig. 7.14 Stricture with wire-guided balloon dilator in place prior to inflation

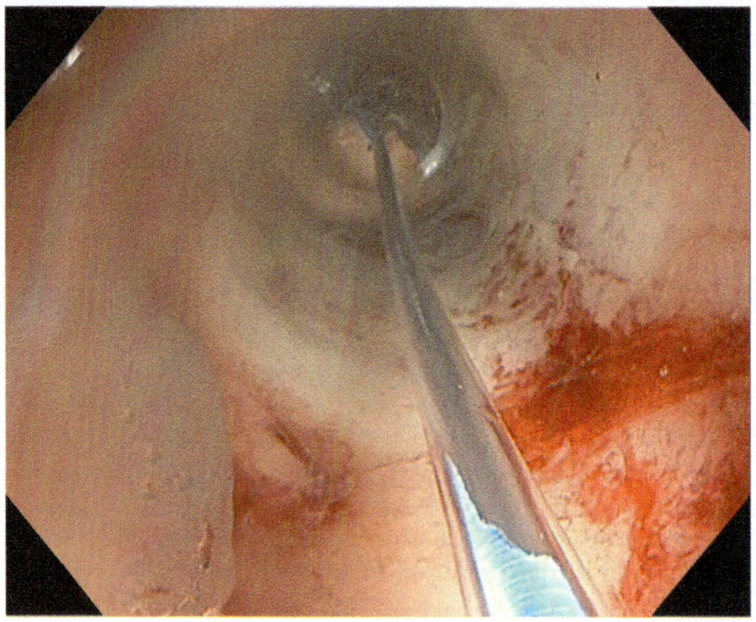

Fig. 7.15 Stricture during balloon inflation

may include prolonged postoperative ileus, air embolism, and multi-organ failure, although studies evaluating the diagnostic yield and safety of intraoperative enteroscopy in CD are limited [84, 121–123].

CRC Surveillance for Patients with Crohn's Disease

Risk of CRC in IBD

Compared with the general population, there is an increased risk of development of CRC in patients with ulcerative colitis and Crohn's colitis

(RR 2.75 UC; 2.64 CD) [124]. The risk of developing CRC correlates directly with the degree of histologic and endoscopic inflammation, extent of colonic involvement, disease duration, presence of family history of sporadic CRC, and presence of primary sclerosing cholangitis (PSC). Proctitis alone does not increase the risk of CRC, but involvement of at least 1/3 of the colon appears to be associated with cancer development [125–128]. It is estimated that patients with IBD-related colitis have up to a 1 in 5 chance of developing CRC after 30 years of disease [129]. For these reasons, it is crucial to establish which patients are at increased risk of CRC and perform appropriate surveillance based on patient risk factors.

Data comparing Crohn's colitis to UC has shown essentially equivalent risk of development of malignancy [124]. Therefore, recommendations for cancer surveillance in the setting of IBD-related colitis are the same regardless of whether CD or UC is the underlying disease. Surveillance strategy should be primarily based on the aforementioned risk factors rather than an individual's diagnosis of CD vs. UC [128]. The risk of developing CRC rises significantly after 8 years of IBD-related colitis, with most cancers arising in the setting of pancolitis. Patients with disease limited to the rectum or rectosigmoid are not felt to have increased risk of CRC, and risk is intermediate in patients with left-sided disease (to the splenic flexure). Disease extent is defined by the most extensive histologic, rather than endoscopic, inflammation [130]. Therefore it is important to obtain biopsies of the right colon, left colon, and rectum during staging colonoscopy regardless of endoscopic involvement, since signs of microscopic inflammation may extend beyond the endoscopically visible area of inflammation.

Utility of Surveillance Colonoscopy

The benefit of surveillance colonoscopy in the IBD population is supported by a recent retrospective study which found that the incidence of CRC was significantly higher (2.7 %) in IBD patients without a colonoscopy within the previous 36 months compared with IBD patients who had colonoscopy in the prior 36 months (1.6 %) (odds ratio [OR], 0.56; 95 % CI 0.39–0.80). Additionally, patients with CRC with recent colonoscopy had a reduced mortality rate when compared with those without colonoscopy in the previous 36 months (OR, 0.34; 95 % CI 0.12–0.95) [131].

Because the risk of developing CRC increases with long-standing inflammation, it is generally recommended that patients undergo surveillance colonoscopy beginning 8 years after IBD diagnosis or IBD symptom onset for restaging and to determine surveillance needs. In UC, colonic strictures, shortened colon, and pseudopolyps are associated with increased risk of cancer, likely due to the fact that these features typically signify long-standing inflammation [132]. It is unclear if these features are also associated with increased risk of CRC in Crohn's patients, since the findings of strictures and colonic shortening may simply be due to the transmural nature of the underlying disease process. The finding of a colonic stricture especially in UC should always be evaluated to definitively rule out a neoplasm.

Significance of DALMs, Flat Dysplasia, and Sporadic Adenomas

The goal of surveillance colonoscopy in IBD patients is early detection of dysplasia so that appropriate management may be implemented to prevent development of CRC. The endoscopist should assess for abnormal appearing mucosa such as polyps, strictures, carpet-like masses, or plaques, which may indicate DALMs (dysplasia-associated lesion or mass), flat dysplasia, or sporadic adenomas. DALMs are typically endoscopically indistinguishable from sporadic adenomas, but DALMs arise in areas with adjacent invisible dysplasia in an area of active or quiescent inflammation. Therefore, the determination of DALM versus sporadic adenoma is a histologic diagnosis based on the presence or absence of dysplasia in the surrounding mucosa. The distinction between flat dysplasia, DALM, and adenoma is crucial because flat dysplasia and DALMs frequently warrant surgical resection in the form of colectomy, whereas sporadic adenomas are not associated with synchronous or metachronous CRC and therefore may be removed endoscopically and require similar follow-up to sporadic adenomas in non-IBD patients. To distinguish these entities, we recommend endoscopic removal of the visible portion of the lesion followed by biopsies of the surrounding tissue for assessment for surrounding dysplasia. The lesion and the biopsies should then be submitted to the pathologist in separate bottles. In some cases, especially in cases of flat dysplasia or sessile serrated adenomas, it may be difficult or impossible to visualize the borders of the lesion with white light endoscopy. In these cases, we feel that the use of narrow-band imaging or dye spray (methylene blue or indigo carmine) may be helpful to ensure that as much of the lesion as possible is removed. It is frequently also appropriate to tattoo the area to aid in endoscopic re-assessment or surgical planning [35]. The diagnosis of dysplasia should be confirmed by an expert GI pathologist [133].

Use of Flow Cytometry and Other Biomarkers

The detection of abnormal DNA ploidy is frequently helpful in determining surveillance intervals and probability of dysplasia in cases of indeterminate histology. Abnormal DNA content is associated with up to 6.6-fold increased risk of advanced neoplasia [134]. We recommend obtaining one biopsy every 10 cm for flow cytometry at the time of random surveillance biopsies. The presence of abnormal DNA content should prompt increase in frequency of surveillance to at least once per year. We typically treat the finding of ploidy similar to indefinite for dysplasia or low-grade dysplasia (LGD).

Management of Dysplasia

Dysplastic lesions arising outside the area of inflammation, if completely excised, may be managed as sporadic adenomas. In cases of high-grade flat dysplasia, colectomy is recommended because of the unacceptably high risk of synchronous CRC in at least 42 % of cases [135, 136]. The management of LGD is more controversial, with wide variations in reports of synchronous CRC and progression to CRC amongst various studies, partly because of significant heterogeneity with regard to the definition of DALMs. One meta-analysis assessing outcomes in cases of LGD found a ninefold risk of developing CRC and a 12-fold risk of developing any advanced lesion [137]. Based on the available data, the AGA has proposed an algorithm in which all patients with flat high-grade dysplasia undergo colectomy, and those with LGD either are managed with colectomy or close interval follow-up examination. In cases of indefinite dysplasia, colonoscopy should be repeated within 3–12 months depending on the pathologic findings (see figure). Those with no dysplasia should undergo repeat colonoscopy in 1–2 years [128, 138] (Fig. 7.16).

In practice, the decision of whether to proceed with total colectomy in patients with CD and dysplasia or CRC is frequently more complicated than in patients with UC. In CD, a total colectomy necessitates an ileostomy with risk of complications such as peristomal disease recurrence, stricture, and poor wound healing. Therefore we recommend an informed and multidisciplinary discussion with the patient, pathologist, and surgeon to determine appropriate individualized management. In patients with rectal sparing, it may be appropriate to consider ileorectal anastomosis as total colectomy with J-pouch formation is relatively contraindicated in CD. If undertaken, careful ongoing close surveillance of the rectum and anastomosis is required in the post-operative period.

Special Populations

Primary Sclerosing Cholangitis

Patients with IBD and PSC have approximately fourfold increased risk of CRC when compared with patients with UC alone [139], and the increased risk persists even after liver transplantation [140]. Therefore, patients with UC or Crohn's colitis are advised to begin annual surveillance colonoscopies at the time of initial diagnosis of PSC, to be continued indefinitely even after liver transplantation [141]. Additionally, since PSC is strongly associated with IBD,

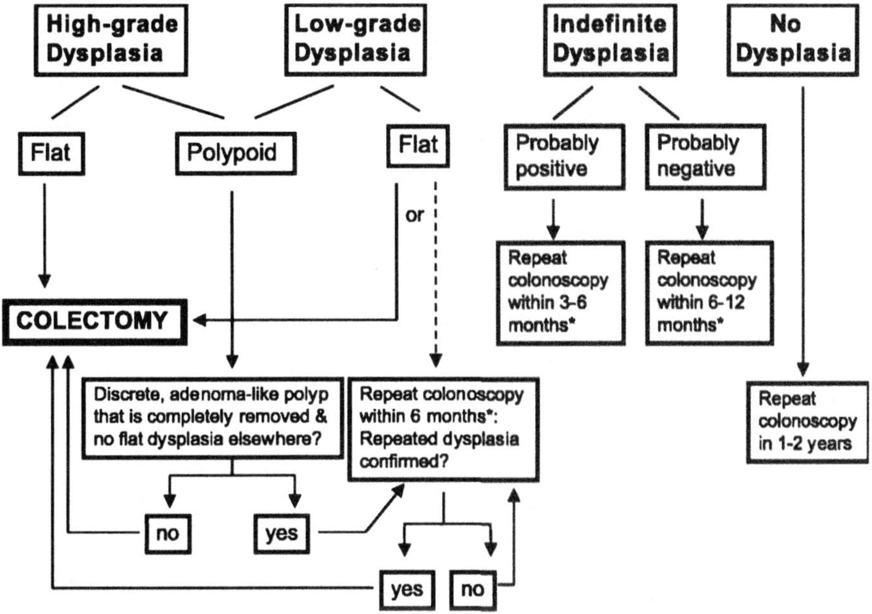

Fig. 7.16 Algorithm for the management of colonic dysplasia in IBD [127]

patients newly diagnosed with PSC but without a diagnosis of IBD should undergo colonoscopy with random biopsies to evaluate for endoscopic and histologic changes consistent with IBD, even without symptoms suggestive of IBD [141].

Ileal Pouch-Anal Anastomosis

Total colectomy with IPAA is usually performed in patients with familial adenomatous polyposis syndrome (FAP), or in UC patients with medically refractory colitis, dysplasia, or localized CRC. Additionally, patients thought to have UC who undergo total colectomy with IPAA may subsequently have their diagnosis changed to Crohn's disease in up to 12 % of cases [54]. Although the dysplasia risk of the ileal pouch mucosa generally appears to be low [142], there are certain high-risk features that warrant endoscopic pouch surveillance. These features include PSC, atrophic pouch mucosa, and presence of dysplasia in the original colectomy specimen [143–145]. Ileal pouch-rectal anastomosis is also considered a high-risk feature, although even in the ideal situation of hand-sewn anal anastomosis there is risk of retained rectal mucosa [145], and as such we recommend surveillance pouchoscopy with particular attention and biopsies at the anal anastomosis to evaluate for evidence of retained rectal mucosa and associated dysplasia annually in patients with an IPAA.

Techniques for Surveillance

The optimal technique for surveillance colonoscopy has been a topic of debate over the last several years [146]. It is generally accepted that simple optical inspection with white light endoscopy, while important, is not adequate for surveillance because up to 23 % of neoplastic areas are macroscopically invisible [147]. Therefore colonoscopy with careful visual inspection of the mucosa and targeted and random biopsies, or chromoendoscopy with targeted biopsies, are acceptable alternatives.

When using traditional endoscopy, biopsies should be performed in a 4-quadrant fashion every 10 cm with a total of at least 33 biopsies in patients with pancolitis, along with targeted biopsies of any suspicious lesions (Figs. 7.17, 7.18, 7.19, and 7.20). Some guidelines also suggest more extensive sampling of the left colon and

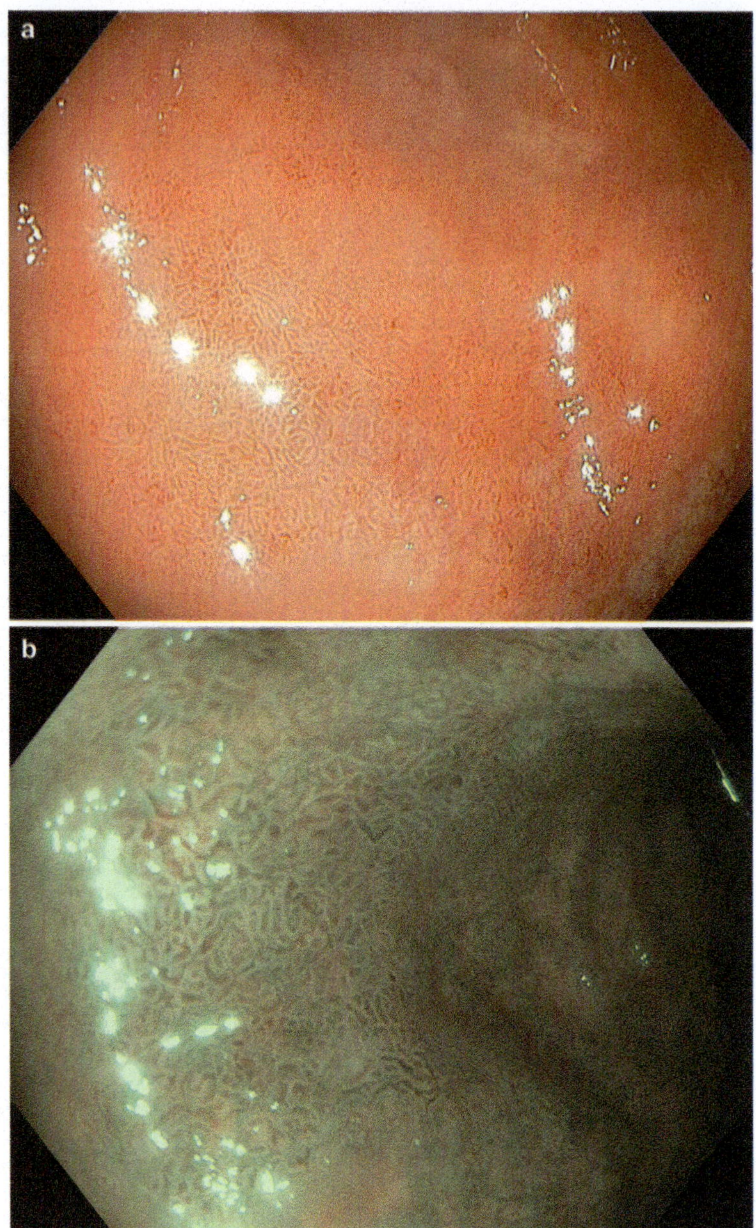

Fig. 7.17 (**a**) Visible low-grade dysplasia in the colon. (**b**) The same area of low-grade dysplasia, highlighted with narrow-band imaging (NBI)

rectum since inflammation tends to be more severe in the left colon [128]. Targeted biopsies should also be performed of strictures and mucosal abnormalities, and should be labeled and submitted to the pathologist in a separate jar. In addition to removal of DALMs whenever possible, biopsies should be obtained of the remaining mucosa surrounding the area to ensure complete removal of any dysplastic tissue. Biopsies should be placed in separate jars and labeled as to location (i.e., "80 cm," "70 cm," "raised lesion at 65 cm," "60 cm," etc.).

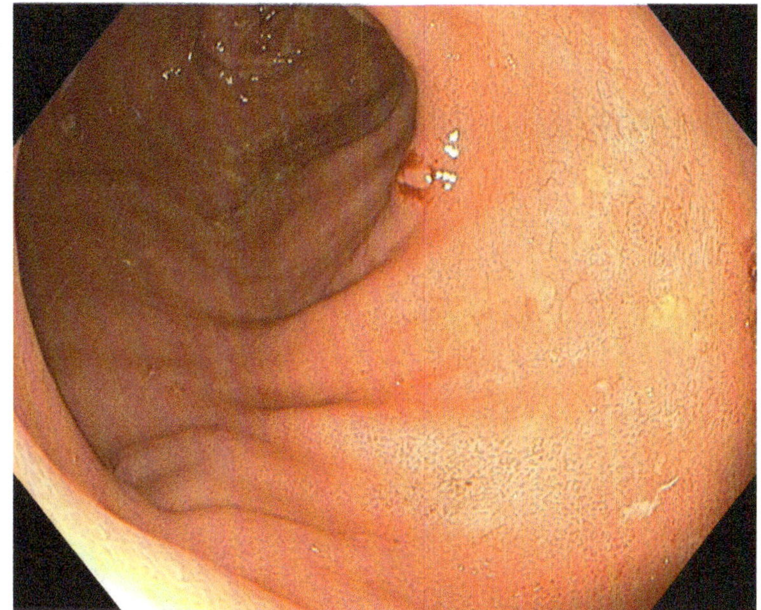

Fig. 7.18 Visible high-grade dysplasia in Crohn's colitis

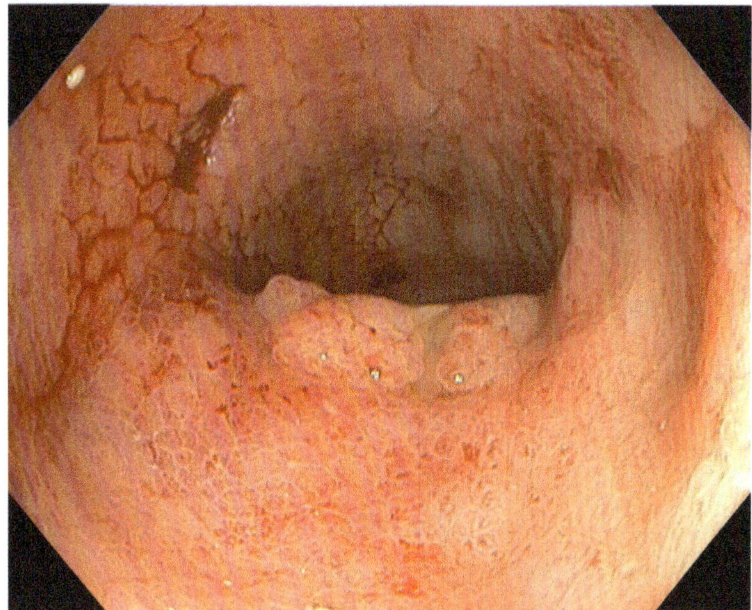

Fig. 7.19 Sporadic adenocarcinoma in a patient with Crohn's colitis

Chromoendoscopy by an endoscopist trained in the technique is an acceptable alternative to white light endoscopy with random biopsies and may be superior to the traditional method of surveillance for the detection of dysplasia, although the effect of chromoendoscopy versus traditional surveillance colonoscopy with biopsies on long-term outcomes has not been evaluated. In the case of chromoendoscopy, random biopsies are not required but removal of suspicious lesions is necessary [128].

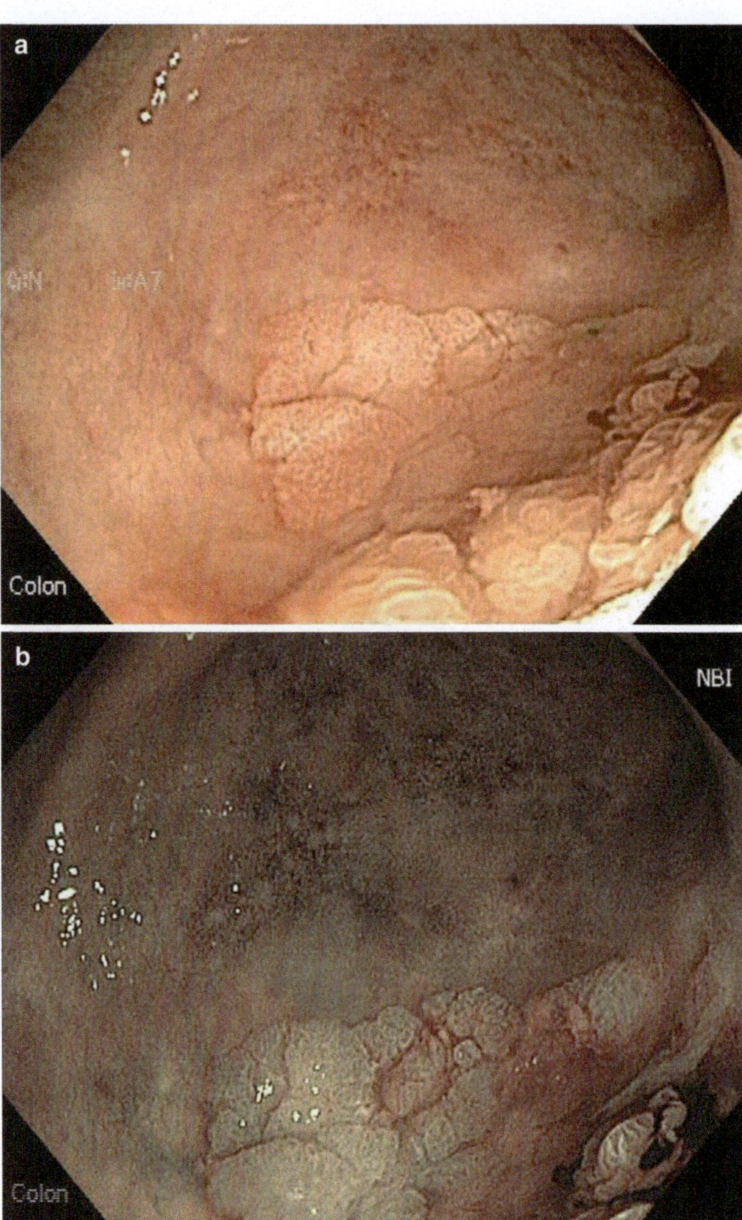

Fig. 7.20 (**a**) Dysplasia-associated lesion or mass (DALM). (**b**) DALM, with mucosal abnormality highlighted by NBI

References

1. Kim YG, Jang BI. The role of colonoscopy in inflammatory bowel disease. Clin Endosc. 2013;46(4):317–20.
2. Annese V, Daperno M, Rutter MD, Amiot A, Bossuyt P, East J, et al. European evidence based consensus for endoscopy in inflammatory bowel disease. J Crohns Colitis. 2013;7(12):982–1018.
3. Chutkan RK. Colonoscopy in inflammatory bowel disease. Gastrointest Endosc Clin N Am. 2002;12(3): 463–83.
4. Mitros FA. The biopsy in evaluating patients with inflammatory bowel disease. Med Clin North Am. 1980;64(6):1037–57.
5. Lee SD, Cohen RD. Endoscopy in inflammatory bowel disease. Gastroenterol Clin North Am. 2002; 31(1):119–32.

6. Waye JD. Endoscopy in inflammatory bowel disease. Med Clin North Am. 1990;74(1):51–65.
7. Ferreira J, Akbari M, Gashin L, Cullen G, Moss A, Leffler DA, et al. Prevalence and lifetime risk of endoscopy-related complications among patients with inflammatory bowel disease. Clin Gastroenterol Hepatol. 2013;11(10):1288–93.
8. Rubin PH, Friedman S, Harpaz N, Goldstein E, Weiser J, Schiller J, et al. Colonoscopic polypectomy in chronic colitis: conservative management after endoscopic resection of dysplastic polyps. Gastroenterology. 1999;117(6):1295–300.
9. Navaneethan U, Parasa S, Venkatesh PG, Trikudanathan G, Shen B. Prevalence and risk factors for colonic perforation during colonoscopy in hospitalized inflammatory bowel disease patients. J Crohns Colitis. 2011; 5(3):189–95.
10. Chan G, Fefferman DS, Farrell RJ. Endoscopic assessment of inflammatory bowel disease: colonoscopy/esophagogastroduodenoscopy. Gastroenterol Clin North Am. 2012;41(2):271–90.
11. Fujimura Y, Kamoi R, Iida M. Pathogenesis of aphthoid ulcers in Crohn's disease: correlative findings by magnifying colonoscopy, electron microscopy, and immunohistochemistry. Gut. 1996;38:724–32.
12. Jevon GP, Ravikumara M. Endoscopic and histologic findings in pediatric inflammatory bowel disease. Gastroenterol Hepatol. 2010;6(3):174–80.
13. Satsangi J, Silverberg MS, Vermeire S, Colombel JF. The Montreal classification of inflammatory bowel disease: controversies, consensus, and implications. Gut. 2006;55(6):749–53.
14. Daperno M, Comberlato M, Bossa F, Biancone L, Bonanomi AG, Cassinotti A, et al. Inter-observer agreement in endoscopic scoring systems: preliminary report of an ongoing study from the Italian group for inflammatory bowel disease (IG-IBD). Dig Liver Dis. 2014;46(11):969–73.
15. Peyrin-Biroulet L, Bonnaud G, Bourreille A, Chevaux JB, Faure P, Filippi J, et al. Endoscopy in inflammatory bowel disease: recommendations from the IBD Committee of the French Society of Digestive Endoscopy (SFED). Endoscopy. 2013;45(11): 936–43.
16. Groupe D'etudes Therapeutiques Des Affections Inflammatoires D. Development and validation of an endoscopic index of the severity for Crohn's disease: a prospective multicentre study. Gut. 1989;30:983–9.
17. Daperno M, D'Haens G, Van Assche G, Baert F, Bulois P, Maunoury V, et al. Development and validation of a new, simplified endoscopic activity score for Crohn's disease: the SES-CD. Gastrointest Endosc. 2004;60(4):505–12.
18. Rutgeerts P, Geboes K, Vantrappen G, Beyls J, Kerremans R, Hiele M. Predictability of the postoperative course of Crohn's disease. Gastroenterology. 1990;99(4):956–63.
19. Baert F, Moortgat L, Van Assche G, Caenepeel P, Vergauwe P, De Vos M, et al. Mucosal healing predicts sustained clinical remission in patients with early-stage Crohn's disease. Gastroenterology. 2010; 138(2):463–8; quiz e10–1.
20. Allez M, Lemann M, Bonnet J, Cattan P, Jian R, Modigliani R. Long term outcomes of patients with active Crohn's disease exhibiting extensive and deep ulcerations at colonoscopy. Am J Gastroenterol. 2002;97(4):947–53.
21. Silverberg MS, Satsangi J, Ahmad T, Arnott ID, Bernstein CN, Brant SR, et al. Toward an integrated clinical, molecular and serological classification of inflammatory bowel disease: report of a Working Party of the 2005 Montreal World Congress of Gastroenterology. Can J Gastroenterol (Journal canadien de gastroenterologie). 2005;19(Suppl A): 5a–36a.
22. Magro F, Portela F, Lago P, Ramos de Deus J, Vieira A, Peixe P, et al. Crohn's disease in a southern European country: Montreal classification and clinical activity. Inflamm Bowel Dis. 2009;15(9):1343–50.
23. Bentley E, Jenkins D, Campbell F, Warren B. How could pathologists improve the initial diagnosis of colitis? Evidence from an international workshop. J Clin Pathol. 2002;55:955–60.
24. Quinn PG, Binion DG, Connors PJ. The role of endoscopy in inflammatory bowel disease. Med Clin North Am. 1994;78(6):1331–52.
25. Tedesco F, Hardin R, Harper R, Edwards B. Infectious colitis endoscopically simulating inflammatory bowel disease: a prospective evaluation. Gastrointest Endosc. 1983;29(3):195–7.
26. Schumacher G, Killberg B, Sandstedt B, Jorup C, Grillner L, Ljunch A, et al. A prospective study of first attacks of inflammatory bowel disease and non-relapsing colitis. Scand J Gastroenterol. 1993;28(12): 1077–85.
27. Surawicz CM. What's the best way to differentiate infectious colitis (acute self-limited colitis) from IBD? Inflamm Bowel Dis. 2008;14 Suppl 2:S157–8.
28. Li X, Liu X, Zou Y, Ouyang C, Wu X, Zhou M, et al. Predictors of clinical and endoscopic findings in differentiating Crohn's disease from intestinal tuberculosis. Dig Dis Sci. 2011;56(1):188–96.
29. Cottone M, Pietrosi G, Martorana G, Casà A, Pecoraro G, Oliva L, et al. Prevalence of cytomegalovirus infection in severe and refractory ulcerative and Crohn's colitis. Am J Gastroenterol. 2001;96(3):773–5.
30. Lozano-Maya M, Ponferrada-Diaz A, Gonzalez-Asanza C, Nogales-Rincon O, Senent-Sanchez C, Perez-de-Ayala V, et al. Usefulness of colonoscopy in ischemic colitis. Rev Esp Enferm Dig. 2010;102(8):478–83.
31. Toursarkissian B, Thompson RW. Ischemic colitis. Surg Clin North Am. 1997;77(2):461–70.
32. Kennedy GD, Heise CP. Radiation colitis and proctitis. Clin Colon Rectal Surg. 2007;20(1):64–72.
33. Hovdenak N, Fajardo LF, Hauer-Jensen M. Acute radiation proctitis: a sequential clinicopathologic study during pelvic radiotherapy. Int J Radiat Oncol Biol Phys. 2000;48(4):1111–7.
34. Margolius DM, Cataldo TE. Nonsteroidal anti-inflammatory drug colopathy mimicking malignant

masses of the colon: a report of three cases and review of the literature. Am Surg. 2010;76(11):1282–6.

35. Leighton JA, Shen B, Baron TH, Adler DG, Davila R, Egan JV, et al. ASGE guideline: endoscopy in the diagnosis and treatment of inflammatory bowel disease. Gastrointest Endosc. 2006;63(4):558–65.
36. Rejchrt S, Bures J, Siroky M, Kopacova M, Slezak L, Langr F. A prospective, observational study of colonic mucosal abnormalities associated with orally administered sodium phosphate for colon cleansing before colonoscopy. Gastrointest Endosc. 2004;59(6):651–4.
37. Kim B, Barnett JL, Kleer CG, Appelman HD. Endoscopic and histological patchiness in treated ulcerative colitis. Am J Gastroenterol. 1999;94(11): 3258–62.
38. Pera A, Bellando P, Caldera D, Ponti V, Astegiano M, Barletti C, et al. Colonoscopy in inflammatory bowel disease. Diagnostic accuracy and proposal of an endoscopic score. Gastroenterology. 1987;92(1):181–5.
39. DeRoche TC, Xiao SY, Liu X. Histological evaluation in ulcerative colitis. Gastroenterol Rep. 2014;2(3): 178–92.
40. Price AB, Morson BC. Inflammatory bowel disease: the surgical pathology of Crohn's disease and ulcerative colitis. Hum Pathol. 1975;6(1):7–29.
41. Levine A, de Bie CI, Turner D, Cucchiara S, Sladek M, Murphy MS, et al. Atypical disease phenotypes in pediatric ulcerative colitis: 5-year analyses of the EUROKIDS registry. Inflamm Bowel Dis. 2013;19(2): 370–7.
42. Rajwal SR, Puntis JW, McClean P, Davison SM, Newell SJ, Sugarman I, et al. Endoscopic rectal sparing in children with untreated ulcerative colitis. J Pediatr Gastroenterol Nutr. 2004;38(1):66–9.
43. Witte AM, Veenendaal RA, Van Hogezand RA, Verspaget HW, Lamers CB. Crohn's disease of the upper gastrointestinal tract: the value of endoscopic examination. Scand J Gastroenterol Suppl. 1998;225: 100–5.
44. Wagtmans MJ, van Hogezand RA, Griffioen G, Verspaget HW, Lamers CB. Crohn's disease of the upper gastrointestinal tract. Neth J Med. 1997;50(2): S2–7.
45. Lemberg DA, Clarkson CM, Bohane TD, Day AS. Role of esophagogastroduodenoscopy in the initial assessment of children with inflammatory bowel disease. J Gastroenterol Hepatol. 2005;20(11):1696–700.
46. Oberhuber G, Puspok A, Oesterreicher C, Novacek G, Zauner C, Burghuber M, et al. Focally enhanced gastritis: a frequent type of gastritis in patients with Crohn's disease. Gastroenterology. 1997;112(3):698–706.
47. Kirshner J. Endoscopy in inflammatory bowel disease. Inflammatory bowel disease. 5th ed. Baltimore, MD: Williams and Wilkins; 2000. p. 453–77.
48. Goldstein N, Dulai M. Contemporary morphologic definition of backwash ileitis in ulcerative colitis and features that distinguish it from Crohn disease. Am J Clin Pathol. 2006;126(3):365–76.
49. Rutgeerts P, Feagan BG, Lichtenstein GR, Mayer LF, Schreiber S, Colombel JF, et al. Comparison of scheduled and episodic treatment strategies of infliximab in Crohn's disease. Gastroenterology. 2004;126(2): 402–13.
50. Zafar S, Trevatt A, Joshi A, Besherdas K. Terminal ileitis at endoscopy in clinical practice: is it always due to Crohn's disease. Gut. 2014;63 Suppl 1:A1–288.
51. Farmer M, Petras RE, Hunt LE, Janosky JE, Galandiuk S. The importance of diagnostic accuracy in colonic inflammatory bowel disease. Am J Gastroenterol. 2000;95(11):3184–8.
52. Prenzel F, Uhlig HH. Frequency of indeterminate colitis in children and adults with IBD - a metaanalysis. J Crohns Colitis. 2009;3(4):277–81.
53. Zhou N, Chen WX, Chen SH, Xu CF, Li YM. Inflammatory bowel disease unclassified. J Zhejiang Univ Sci B. 2011;12(4):280–6.
54. Murrell ZA, Melmed GY, Ippoliti A, Vasiliauskas EA, Dubinsky M, Targan SR, et al. A prospective evaluation of the long-term outcome of ileal pouch-anal anastomosis in patients with inflammatory bowel disease-unclassified and indeterminate colitis. Dis Colon Rectum. 2009;52(5):872–8.
55. Annunziata ML, Caviglia R, Papparella LG, Cicala M. Upper gastrointestinal involvement of Crohn's disease: a prospective study on the role of upper endoscopy in the diagnostic work-up. Dig Dis Sci. 2012;57(6):1618–23.
56. Sakuraba A, Iwao Y, Matsuoka K, Naganuma M, Ogata H, Kanai T, et al. Endoscopic and pathologic changes of the upper gastrointestinal tract in Crohn's disease. BioMed Res Int. 2014;2014:610767.
57. Lenaerts C, Roy CC, Vaillancourt M, Weber AM, Morin CL, Seidman E. High incidence of upper gastrointestinal tract involvement in children with Crohn disease. Pediatrics. 1989;83(5):777–81.
58. Oberhuber G, Hirsch M, Stolte M. High incidence of upper gastrointestinal tract involvement in Crohn's disease. Virchows Arch. 1998;432(1):49–52.
59. Yu CS, Pemberton JH, Larson D. Ileal pouch-anal anastomosis in patients with indeterminate colitis: long-term results. Dis Colon Rectum. 2000;43(11):1487–96.
60. Sharaf RN, Shergill AK, Odze RD, Krinsky ML, Fukami N, Jain R, et al. Endoscopic mucosal tissue sampling. Gastrointest Endosc. 2013;78(2):216–24.
61. Iddan G, Meron G, Glukhovsky A, Swain P. Wireless capsule endoscopy. Nature. 2000;405(6785):417.
62. Food and Drug Administration, HHS. Medical devices; gastroenterology-urology devices; classification of the colon capsule imaging system. Final order. Fed Regist. 2014;79(95):28401–4.
63. San Juan-Acosta M, Caunedo-Alvarez A, Arguelles-Arias F, Castro-Laria L, Gomez-Rodriguez B, Romero-Vazquez J, et al. Colon capsule endoscopy is a safe and useful tool to assess disease parameters in patients with ulcerative colitis. Eur J Gastroenterol Hepatol. 2014;26(8):894–901.
64. Triester SL, Leighton JA, Leontiadis GI, Gurudu SR, Fleischer DE, Hara AK, et al. A meta-analysis of the yield of capsule endoscopy compared to other diagnostic modalities in patients with non-stricturing

small bowel Crohn's disease. Am J Gastroenterol. 2006;101(5):954–64.
65. D'Haens G, Van Deventer S, Van Hogezand R, Chalmers D, Kothe C, Baert F, et al. Endoscopic and histological healing with infliximab anti-tumor necrosis factor antibodies in Crohn's disease: a European multicenter trial. Gastroenterology. 1999;116(5): 1029–34.
66. Schnitzler F, Fidder H, Ferrante M, Noman M, Arijs I, Van Assche G, et al. Mucosal healing predicts long-term outcome of maintenance therapy with infliximab in Crohn's disease. Inflamm Bowel Dis. 2009;15(9): 1295–301.
67. Kopylov U, Seidman EG. Role of capsule endoscopy in inflammatory bowel disease. World J Gastroenterol. 2014;20(5):1155–64.
68. Pons Beltran V, Nos P, Bastida G, Beltran B, Arguello L, Aguas M, et al. Evaluation of postsurgical recurrence in Crohn's disease: a new indication for capsule endoscopy? Gastrointest Endosc. 2007;66(3): 533–40.
69. Lewis Jr P, Tinsley A, Lewis B. Capsule endoscopy in healthy individuals. In: Abstract Presented at the American Gastroenterological Association; 2012.
70. Mergener K, Ponchon T, Gralnek I, Pennazio M, Gay G, Selby W, et al. Literature review and recommendations for clinical application of small-bowel capsule endoscopy, based on a panel discussion by international experts. Consensus statements for small-bowel capsule endoscopy, 2006/2007. Endoscopy. 2007; 39(10):895–909.
71. Lewis BS. Expanding role of capsule endoscopy in inflammatory bowel disease. World J Gastroenterol. 2008;14(26):4137–41.
72. Gal E, Geller A, Fraser G, Levi Z, Niv Y. Assessment and validation of the new capsule endoscopy Crohn's disease activity index (CECDAI). Dig Dis Sci. 2008;53(7):1933–7.
73. Gralnek IM, Defranchis R, Seidman E, Leighton JA, Legnani P, Lewis BS. Development of a capsule endoscopy scoring index for small bowel mucosal inflammatory change. Aliment Pharmacol Ther. 2008; 27(2):146–54.
74. Niv Y, Ilani S, Levi Z, Hershkowitz M, Niv E, Fireman Z, et al. Validation of the capsule endoscopy Crohn's disease activity index (CECDAI or Niv score): a multicenter prospective study. Endoscopy. 2012;44(1): 21–6.
75. Cave D, Legnani P, de Franchis R, Lewis BS. ICCE consensus for capsule retention. Endoscopy. 2005; 37(10):1065–7.
76. Hartmann D. Capsule endoscopy and Crohn's disease. Dig Dis. 2011;29 Suppl 1:17–21.
77. Schulz C, Monkemuller K, Salheiser M, Bellutti M, Schutte K, Malfertheiner P. Double-balloon enteroscopy in the diagnosis of suspected isolated Crohn's disease of the small bowel. Dig Endosc. 2014;26(2):236–42.
78. Molinie F. Opposite evolution in incidence of Crohn's disease and ulcerative colitis in Northern France (1988–1999). Gut. 2004;53(6):843–8.
79. Carter D, Eliakim R. Current role of endoscopy in inflammatory bowel disease diagnosis and management. Curr Opin Gastroenterol. 2014;30(4):370–7.
80. Oostenbrug LE, van Dullemen HM, te Meerman GJ, Jansen PL, Kleibeuker JH. Clinical outcome of Crohn's disease according to the Vienna classification: disease location is a useful predictor of disease course. Eur J Gastroenterol Hepatol. 2006;18(3):255–61.
81. Eliakim R, Carter D. Endoscopic assessment of the small bowel. Dig Dis. 2013;31(2):194–8.
82. Leighton JA. The role of endoscopic imaging of the small bowel in clinical practice. Am J Gastroenterol. 2011; 106(1):27–36; quiz 7.
83. Tontini GE, Vecchi M, Neurath MF, Neumann H. Review article: newer optical and digital chromoendoscopy techniques vs dye-based chromoendoscopy for diagnosis and surveillance in inflammatory bowel disease. Aliment Pharmacol Ther. 2013;38(10):1198–208.
84. Tharian B, Caddy G, Tham TC. Enteroscopy in small bowel Crohn's disease: a review. World J Gastrointest Endosc. 2013;5(10):476–86.
85. Manes G, Imbesi V, Ardizzone S, Cassinotti A, Pallotta S, Porro GB. Use of double-balloon enteroscopy in the management of patients with Crohn's disease: feasibility and diagnostic yield in a high-volume centre for inflammatory bowel disease. Surg Endosc. 2009;23(12):2790–5.
86. Pasha SF, Leighton JA, Das A, Harrison ME, Decker GA, Fleischer DE, et al. Double-balloon enteroscopy and capsule endoscopy have comparable diagnostic yield in small-bowel disease: a meta-analysis. Clin Gastroenterol Hepatol. 2008;6(6):671–6.
87. Oshitani N, Yukawa T, Yamagami H, Inagawa M, Kamata N, Watanabe K, et al. Evaluation of deep small bowel involvement by double-balloon enteroscopy in Crohn's disease. Am J Gastroenterol. 2006; 101(7):1484–9.
88. Semrad CE. Role of double balloon enteroscopy in Crohn's disease. Gastrointest Endosc. 2007;66 Suppl 3:S94–5.
89. Pimentel M, Chang M, Chow EJ, Tabibzadeh S, Kirit-Kiriak V, Targan SR, et al. Identification of a prodromal period in Crohn's disease but not ulcerative colitis. Am J Gastroenterol. 2000;95(12):3458–62.
90. Bourreille A, Ignjatovic A, Aabakken L, Loftus Jr EV, Eliakim R, Pennazio M, et al. Role of small-bowel endoscopy in the management of patients with inflammatory bowel disease: an international OMED-ECCO consensus. Endoscopy. 2009;41(7):618–37.
91. Neumann H, Fry LC, Neurath MF. Review article on current applications and future concepts of capsule endoscopy. Digestion. 2013;87(2):91–9.
92. Gustavsson A, Magnuson A, Blomberg B, Andersson M, Halfvarson J, Tysk C. Endoscopic dilation is an efficacious and safe treatment of intestinal strictures in Crohn's disease. Aliment Pharmacol Ther. 2012;36(2):151–8.
93. Jarbandhan S-VA. Double balloon endoscopy associated pancreatitis: a description of six cases. World J Gastroenterol. 2008;14(5):720.

94. Lenz P, Domagk D. Double- vs single-balloon vs spiral enteroscopy. Best Pract Res Clin Gastroenterol. 2012;26(3):303–13.
95. Akerman PA, Agrawal D, Chen W, Cantero D, Avila J, Pangtay J. Spiral enteroscopy: a novel method of enteroscopy by using the endo-ease discovery SB overtube and a pediatric colonoscope. Gastrointest Endosc. 2009;69(2):327–32.
96. Rahmi G, Samaha E, Vahedi K, Ponchon T, Fumex F, Filoche B, et al. Multicenter comparison of double-balloon enteroscopy and spiral enteroscopy. J Gastroenterol Hepatol. 2013;28(6):992–8.
97. Carbonnel F, Lavergne A, Lemann M, Bitoun A, Valleur P, Hautefeuille P, et al. Colonoscopy of acute colitis. A safe and reliable tool for assessment of severity. Dig Dis Sci. 1994;39(7):1550–7.
98. Rutgeerts P, Sandborn WJ, Feagan BG, Reinisch W, Olson A, Johanns J, et al. Infliximab for induction and maintenance therapy for ulcerative colitis. N Engl J Med. 2005;353(23):2462–76.
99. Landi B, Anh TN, Cortot A, Soule JC, Rene E, Gendre JP, et al. Endoscopic monitoring of Crohn's disease treatment: a prospective, randomized clinical trial. The Groupe d'Etudes Therapeutiques des Affections Inflammatoires Digestives. Gastroenterology. 1992;102(5):1647–53.
100. Mazzuoli S, Guglielmi FW, Antonelli E, Salemme M, Bassotti G, Villanacci V. Definition and evaluation of mucosal healing in clinical practice. Dig Liver Dis. 2013;45(12):969–77.
101. Ferrante M, Colombel JF, Sandborn WJ, Reinisch W, Mantzaris GJ, Kornbluth A, et al. Validation of endoscopic activity scores in patients with Crohn's disease based on a post hoc analysis of data from SONIC. Gastroenterology. 2013; 145(5):978–86 e5.
102. Froslie KF, Jahnsen J, Moum BA, Vatn MH. Mucosal healing in inflammatory bowel disease: results from a Norwegian population-based cohort. Gastroenterology. 2007;133(2):412–22.
103. Ardizzone S, Maconi G, Russo A, Imbesi V, Colombo E, Bianchi Porro G. Randomised controlled trial of azathioprine and 5-aminosalicylic acid for treatment of steroid dependent ulcerative colitis. Gut. 2006;55(1):47–53.
104. Actis GC, Pellicano R, David E, Sapino A. Azathioprine, mucosal healing in ulcerative colitis, and the chemoprevention of colitic cancer: a clinical-practice-based forecast. Inflamm Allergy Drug Targets. 2010;9(1):6–9.
105. af Bjorkesten CG, Nieminen U, Turunen U, Arkkila PE, Sipponen T, Farkkila MA. Endoscopic monitoring of infliximab therapy in Crohn's disease. Inflamm Bowel Dis. 2011;17(4):947–53.
106. Rutgeerts P, Geboes K, Vantrappen G, Kerremans R, Coenegrachts JL, Coremans G. Natural history of recurrent Crohn's disease at the ileocolonic anastomosis after curative surgery. Gut. 1984;25(6): 665–72.
107. Shen B, Achkar JP, Lashner BA, Bevins CL, Brzezinski A, Ormsby AH, et al. Endoscopic and histologic evaluation together with symptom assessment are required to diagnose pouchitis. Gastroenterology. 2001;121(2):261–7.
108. Moskowitz RL, Shepherd NA, Nicholls RJ. An assessment of inflammation in the reservoir after restorative proctocolectomy with ileoanal ileal reservoir. Int J Color Dis. 1986;1(3):167–74.
109. Fazio VW, Ziv Y, Church JM, Oakley JR, Lavery IC, Milsom JW, et al. Ileal pouch-anal anastomoses complications and function in 1005 patients. Ann Surg. 1995;222(2):120–7.
110. Goldberg HI, Caruthers Jr SB, Nelson JA, Singleton JW. Radiographic findings of the national cooperative Crohn's disease study. Gastroenterology. 1979;77(4 Pt 2):925–37.
111. Modha K, Navaneethan U. Advanced therapeutic endoscopist and inflammatory bowel disease: dawn of a new role. World J Gastroenterol. 2014;20(13): 3485–94.
112. Lichtenstein GR, Olson A, Travers S, Diamond RH, Chen DM, Pritchard ML, et al. Factors associated with the development of intestinal strictures or obstructions in patients with Crohn's disease. Am J Gastroenterol. 2006;101(5):1030–8.
113. Samimi R, Flasar MH, Kavic S, Tracy K, Cross RK. Outcome of medical treatment of stricturing and penetrating Crohn's disease: a retrospective study. Inflamm Bowel Dis. 2010;16(7):1187–94.
114. Vrabie R, Irwin GL, Friedel D. Endoscopic management of inflammatory bowel disease strictures. World J Gastrointest Endosc. 2012;4(11):500–5.
115. Dietz DW, Laureti S, Strong SA, Hull TL, Church J, Remzi FH, et al. Safety and longterm efficacy of strictureplasty in 314 patients with obstructing small bowel Crohn's disease. J Am Coll Surg. 2001; 192(3):330–7; discussion 7–8.
116. Hassan C, Zullo A, De Francesco V, Ierardi E, Giustini M, Pitidis A, et al. Systematic review: endoscopic dilatation in Crohn's disease. Aliment Pharmacol Ther. 2007;26(11–12):1457–64.
117. Wibmer AG, Kroesen AJ, Grone J, Buhr HJ, Ritz JP. Comparison of strictureplasty and endoscopic balloon dilatation for stricturing Crohn's disease—review of the literature. Int J Color Dis. 2010;25(10): 1149–57.
118. Thienpont C, D'Hoore A, Vermeire S, Demedts I, Bisschops R, Coremans G, et al. Long-term outcome of endoscopic dilatation in patients with Crohn's disease is not affected by disease activity or medical therapy. Gut. 2010;59(3):320–4.
119. East JE, Brooker JC, Rutter MD, Saunders BP. A pilot study of intrastricture steroid versus placebo injection after balloon dilatation of Crohn's strictures. Clin Gastroenterol Hepatol. 2007;5(9):1065–9.
120. Douard R, Wind P, Panis Y, Marteau P, Bouhnik Y, Cellier C, et al. Intraoperative enteroscopy for diagnosis and management of unexplained gastrointestinal bleeding. Am J Surg. 2000;180(3):181–4.
121. Kopacova M, Bures J, Vykouril L, Hladik P, Simkovic D, Jon B, et al. Intraoperative enteroscopy: ten years' experience at a single tertiary center. Surg Endosc. 2007;21(7):1111–6.

122. Monsanto P, Almeida N, Lerias C, Figueiredo P, Gouveia H, Sofia C. Is there still a role for intraoperative enteroscopy in patients with obscure gastrointestinal bleeding? Rev Esp Enferm Dig. 2012;104(4):190–6.
123. Bonnet S, Douard R, Malamut G, Cellier C, Wind P. Intraoperative enteroscopy in the management of obscure gastrointestinal bleeding. Dig Liver Dis. 2013;45(4):277–84.
124. Bernstein CN, Blanchard JF, Kliewer E, Wajda A. Cancer risk in patients with inflammatory bowel disease: a population-based study. Cancer. 2001; 91(4):854–62.
125. Rutter M, Saunders B, Wilkinson K, Rumbles S, Schofield G, Kamm M, et al. Severity of inflammation is a risk factor for colorectal neoplasia in ulcerative colitis. Gastroenterology. 2004;126(2):451–9.
126. Gupta RB, Harpaz N, Itzkowitz S, Hossain S, Matula S, Kornbluth A, et al. Histologic inflammation is a risk factor for progression to colorectal neoplasia in ulcerative colitis: a cohort study. Gastroenterology. 2007; 133(4):1099–105; quiz 340–1.
127. Itzkowitz SH, Yio X. Inflammation and cancer IV. Colorectal cancer in inflammatory bowel disease: the role of inflammation. Am J Physiol Gastrointest Liver Physiol. 2004;287(1):G7–17.
128. Farraye FA, Odze RD, Eaden J, Itzkowitz SH. AGA technical review on the diagnosis and management of colorectal neoplasia in inflammatory bowel disease. Gastroenterology. 2010;138(2):746–74, 74.e1–4; quiz e12–3.
129. Eaden JA, Abrams KR, Mayberry JF. The risk of colorectal cancer in ulcerative colitis: a meta-analysis. Gut. 2001;48(4):526–35.
130. Mathy C, Schneider K, Chen YY, Varma M, Terdiman JP, Mahadevan U. Gross versus microscopic pancolitis and the occurrence of neoplasia in ulcerative colitis. Inflamm Bowel Dis. 2003;9(6):351–5.
131. Ananthakrishnan AN, Cagan A, Cai T, Gainer VS, Shaw SY, Churchill S, et al. Colonoscopy is associated with a reduced risk for colon cancer and mortality in patients with inflammatory bowel diseases. Clin Gastroenterol Hepatol; 2014.
132. Rutter M, Bernstein C, Matsumoto T, Kiesslich R, Neurath M. Endoscopic appearance of dysplasia in ulcerative colitis and the role of staining. Endoscopy. 2004;36(12):1109–14.
133. Itzkowitz SH, Present DH. Consensus conference: colorectal cancer screening and surveillance in inflammatory bowel disease. Inflamm Bowel Dis. 2005;11(3):314–21.
134. Gerrits MM, Chen M, Theeuwes M, van Dekken H, Sikkema M, Steyerberg EW, et al. Biomarker-based prediction of inflammatory bowel disease-related colorectal cancer: a case-control study. Cell Oncol (Dordr). 2011;34(2):107–17.
135. Bernstein CN, Shanahan F, Weinstein WM. Are we telling patients the truth about surveillance colonoscopy in ulcerative colitis? Lancet. 1994;343(8889): 71–4.
136. Rutter MD, Saunders BP, Wilkinson KH, Rumbles S, Schofield G, Kamm MA, et al. Thirty-year analysis of a colonoscopic surveillance program for neoplasia in ulcerative colitis. Gastroenterology. 2006;130(4):1030–8.
137. Thomas T, Abrams KA, Robinson RJ, Mayberry JF. Meta-analysis: cancer risk of low-grade dysplasia in chronic ulcerative colitis. Aliment Pharmacol Ther. 2007;25(6):657–68.
138. Itzkowitz SH, Harpaz N. Diagnosis and management of dysplasia in patients with inflammatory bowel diseases. Gastroenterology. 2004;126(6): 1634–48.
139. Soetikno RM, Lin OS, Heidenreich PA, Young HS, Blackstone MO. Increased risk of colorectal neoplasia in patients with primary sclerosing cholangitis and ulcerative colitis: a meta-analysis. Gastrointest Endosc. 2002;56(1):48–54.
140. Singh S, Edakkanambeth Varayil J, Loftus Jr EV, Talwalkar JA. Incidence of colorectal cancer after liver transplantation for primary sclerosing cholangitis: a systematic review and meta-analysis. Liver Transpl. 2013;19(12):1361–9.
141. Chapman R, Fevery J, Kalloo A, Nagorney DM, Boberg KM, Shneider B, et al. Diagnosis and management of primary sclerosing cholangitis. Hepatology. 2010;51(2):660–78.
142. Borjesson L, Willen R, Haboubi N, Duff SE, Hulten L. The risk of dysplasia and cancer in the ileal pouch mucosa after restorative proctocolectomy for ulcerative proctocolitis is low: a long-term term follow-up study. Colorectal Dis. 2004;6(6):494–8.
143. Kariv R, Remzi FH, Lian L, Bennett AE, Kiran RP, Kariv Y, et al. Preoperative colorectal neoplasia increases risk for pouch neoplasia in patients with restorative proctocolectomy. Gastroenterology. 2010;139(3):806–12, 12.e1–2.
144. Das P, Johnson MW, Tekkis PP, Nicholls RJ. Risk of dysplasia and adenocarcinoma following restorative proctocolectomy for ulcerative colitis. Colorectal Dis. 2007;9(1):15–27.
145. Scarpa M, van Koperen PJ, Ubbink DT, Hommes DW, Ten Kate FJ, Bemelman WA. Systematic review of dysplasia after restorative proctocolectomy for ulcerative colitis. Br J Surg. 2007;94(5):534–45.
146. Collins PD, Mpofu C, Watson AJ, Rhodes JM. Strategies for detecting colon cancer and/or dysplasia in patients with inflammatory bowel disease. Cochrane Database Syst Rev. 2006; (2):CD000279.
147. Rutter MD, Saunders BP, Wilkinson KH, Kamm MA, Williams CB, Forbes A. Most dysplasia in ulcerative colitis is visible at colonoscopy. Gastrointest Endosc. 2004;60(3):334–9.

Ultrasound

8

Emma Calabrese and Francesca Zorzi

Abbreviations

CD	Crohn's disease
CEUS	Contrast-enhanced ultrasonography
IBD	Inflammatory bowel disease
PEG	Polyethylene glycol
SICUS	Small intestine contrast ultrasonography
TPUS	Transperineal ultrasound
US	Ultrasonography

Crohn's disease (CD) is a trans-mural, progressive disease leading to irreversible bowel damage characterized by stenosis of the intestinal lumen and penetrating lesions such as fistulas and abscesses. Assessment of intestinal lesion pattern by cross-sectional imaging techniques is essential for a proper management plan of CD patients.

Most published studies have found bowel ultrasonography (US) to be a useful tool in the management of CD. The most important application of bowel US is in follow-up of patients already diagnosed with CD, to assess the site and the extent of the lesions and to ensure early detection of complications, particularly abscesses and strictures.

E. Calabrese, MD, PhD (✉) • F. Zorzi, MD, PhD
Gastroenterology Unit, Department of Systems Medicine, University of Rome Tor Vergata, Via Montpelier 1, 00133 Rome, Italy
e-mail: emma.calabrese@uniroma2.it; emmac@libero.it

Ultrasound Equipment and Technology

Bowel US in inflammatory bowel disease (IBD) requires high-frequency (5–17 MHz) linear probes that offer detailed spatial resolution of the intestinal wall, essential for the assessment of wall thickness and discrimination of the wall layers. A disadvantage of this high-resolution transducer is the reduced penetration depth that may not be sufficient in obese or muscular patients. In these cases, a conventional 3.75 MHz convex probe may be used.

Over the past few years, the technical evolution of US equipment combined with the use of color or power Doppler imaging and intravenous contrast-enhanced US (CEUS) has provided detailed information on mural and extra-intestinal vascularity, which reflects inflammatory disease activity. The second generation echo-signal enhancer SonoVue® (Bracco) is injected as a bolus in units of 1.2–4.5 mL into an antecubital vein, immediately followed by injection of 10 mL of normal saline solution (0.9 % NaCl). For each examination, a recording is begun a few seconds before the intravenous administration of the contrast agent, and continuous imaging is performed for 40 s.

The use of oral contrast agents, such as polyethylene glycol (PEG) solution, has been proposed as a way to improve the detection of CD lesions using small intestine contrast ultrasonography (SICUS). From a practical point of view, use of an

A. Fichera and M.K. Krane (eds.), *Crohn's Disease: Basic Principles*,
DOI 10.1007/978-3-319-14181-7_8, © Springer International Publishing Switzerland 2015

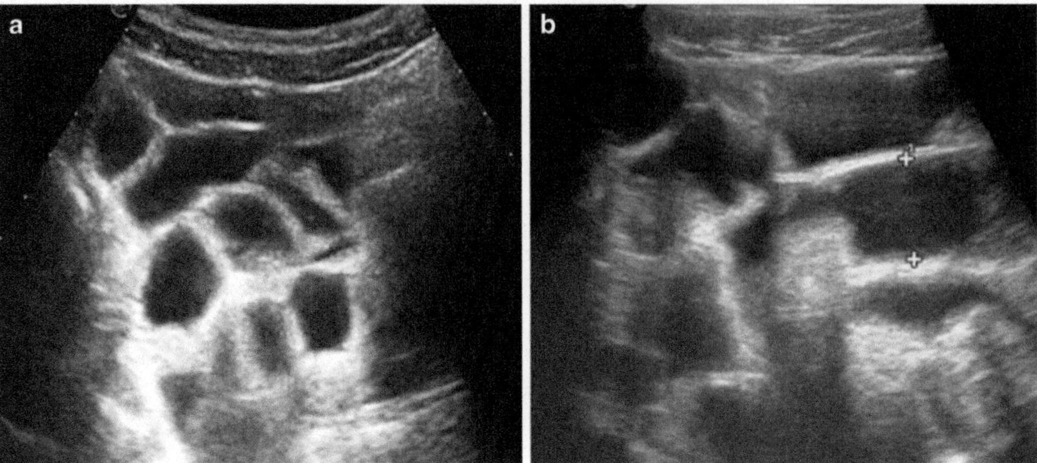

Fig. 8.1 Small intestine contrast ultrasonography (SICUS): in *panel A* normal appearance of ileal loops; in *panel B* normal bowel wall (<3 mm) and normal lumen diameter (<25 mm) of the ileum

oral contrast agent does not alter the procedure greatly; the same equipment is used with the addition of 375–800 mL of oral contrast fluid and the procedure duration ranges from 25 to 60 min. The oral contrast agent passes from the stomach to the duodenum, jejunum, and ileum, distending the intestinal loops and removing gas, and thus enhancing the sequential visualization of the entire gut and improving the sonographic examination of the morphologic and functional aspects of the bowel wall, such as thickening, echo pattern, valvulae conniventes, and enhancing contraction and relaxation (Fig. 8.1).

Early Evaluation of Patients with Suspected CD

In Europe bowel US is now becoming the first-line imaging procedure in patients with suspected CD for early diagnosis and several studies have evaluated the accuracy of bowel US in the diagnosis of IBD. Prospective studies, performed in unselected groups of patients, have shown that bowel US may diagnose CD with a sensitivity ranging from 67 to 96 % and specificity ranging from 79 to 100 % [1–10]. In a recent study, Castiglione et al. showed that bowel US has 94 % sensitivity and 97 % specificity in comparison with MR-Enterography (96 and 94 %) in detecting small bowel CD lesions [11]. Most of the results were obtained from studies that included patients with a previous diagnosis of CD but lacked a control population; thus, it is difficult to draw conclusions about true sensitivity and specificity of bowel US. These methodological problems were evaluated by Fraquelli et al. [12]. In their meta-analysis, in which only five case-control and two cohort studies were ultimately considered from an initial 44 full-text studies identified, the impact of different cut-off values of bowel wall thickening (3 mm vs. 4 mm) in determining the presence of CD was evaluated. The authors concluded that, using a cut-off level of 3 mm as normal, sensitivity and specificity were 88 % and 93 %, respectively. In contrast, when a cut-off level of 4 mm was used, the sensitivity was 75 % and specificity 97 %. The meta-analysis conducted by Horsthuis et al. compared bowel US with MRI, scintigraphy, CT, and positron emission tomography, based on predefined reference standard, in the diagnosis of IBD [13]. No significant differences in diagnostic accuracy among the imaging techniques were observed. The authors concluded that because patients with IBD often needed frequent re-evaluation of disease status, use of a diagnostic modality that does not involve the use of ionizing radiation is preferable. In a recent systematic review, Panes et al. confirmed that bowel US is an accurate technique for diagnosis of suspected CD (sensitivity 84 %, specificity 92 %) [14]. However, the results showed that bowel US has, even in expert hands, significant rates of false-positive and false-negative findings. Thickening of the bowel walls is not specific for CD, and found also in infectious, neoplastic, and other inflammatory diseases [15].

Sonographic visualization of the small bowel can be improved by filling the bowel with an oral contrast agent [16]. Isotonic anechoic electrolyte solutions containing PEG, which is used for bowel cleansing before colonoscopy, are now considered the contrast media of choice. PEG is ingested in variable amounts, ranging from 250 to 800 mL, after an overnight fast. If distention and visualization of the bowel are not adequate, further aliquots of PEG can be used because it does not appear to affect the luminal diameter or the wall thickness at any level of the small bowel in healthy controls [20]. Bowel examination can be performed immediately, starting to scan continuously after the ingestion of PEG, and then repeated at 20 min intervals until the contrast agent is seen to flow through the terminal ileum into the cecum. Because of the small amount of fluid ingested (usually no more than 500 mL) and its palatability, this procedure has been reported to be well accepted and safe. None of the studies have reported significant side effects or major complaints during or immediately after PEG ingestion. The use of PEG appears to reduce intra-observer variability between sonographers and to increase sensitivity in the detection of small bowel lesions in CD patients, in defining disease extent, lesion site, and bowel complications of CD; thus, it has value in the early diagnosis and in the follow-up of CD [18, 19]. The accuracy of bowel US in detecting and localizing CD lesions within the bowel has been assessed in several studies [9, 21, 22]. Most of these studies agreed in reporting the highest sensitivity (approximately 90 %) of bowel US in detecting ileal lesions but less accuracy in lesions located in the upper small bowel and rectum. The accuracy of detection of CD lesions in the proximal small bowel can be significantly improved with the use of oral contrast agents, whereas the sensitivity in detecting ileal and colonic lesions is comparable between conventional and oral contrast US [18]. With regard to accuracy in assessing the extent of small bowel involved, different authors have shown that the extent of pathologically thickened bowel wall is significantly correlated with the extent of ileal CD, as measured by X-ray, CT-enteroclysis, and surgery [21, 23]. The use of oral contrast agents has been proved to be of value in accurately defining the extent of diseased ileal walls, significantly increasing the correlation between the sonographic and radiographic extent of ileal disease and reducing interobserver variability in defining such evaluations [17, 18]. These findings suggest that SICUS may be used as an alternative technique to invasive procedures to assess ileal lesions and monitor their progression of CD over time.

CEUS is a new sensitive technique to visualize micro-perfusion and has been shown to be superior to conventional color or power Doppler imaging in determining tumor vascularity [24]. Currently, the clinical value of CEUS in IBD is not well defined. Most studies on CEUS have been feasibility or pilot studies. In a small study with histologically confirmed CD and bowel wall thickness >5 mm, contrast enhancement was observed after a mean of 13.4 s (±4.2 s; range, 7–19 s) with a maximum vascularity after 30 s [25]. Migaleddu et al. [26] evaluated the diagnostic accuracy of bowel US, Color-Doppler, and CEUS in the evaluation of inflammatory activity in patients with CD. CEUS parameters as bowel wall thickness perfusion (trans-mural starting from the sub-mucosa or starting from extra-visceral vessels) were identified as a qualitative method indicating inflammatory activity but these parameters are subjective and less standardized [26].

Diagnosis of Complications in CD

Bowel stenosis can be detected by bowel US as thickened bowel walls associated with a narrowed lumen and increased lumen diameter of the proximal loop greater than 25 mm. Stenoses are often associated with liquid and gas entering

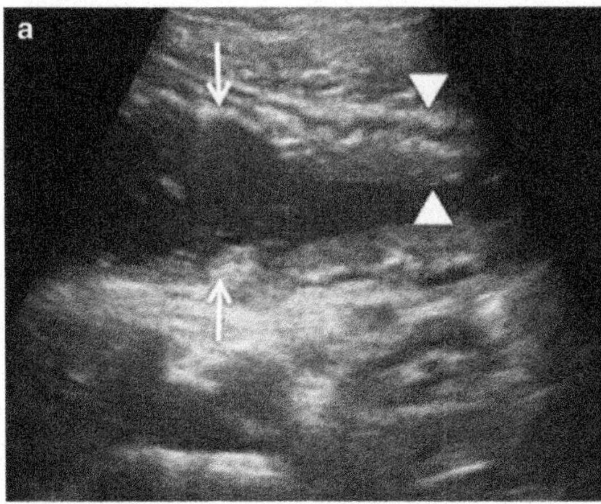

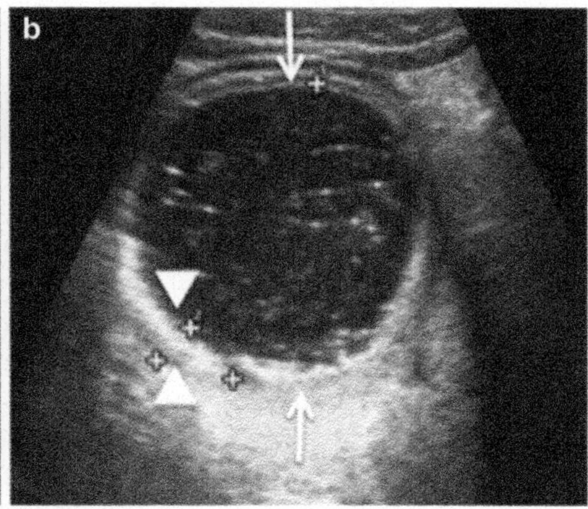

Fig. 8.2 In *panel A*, small intestine contrast ultrasonography showed stenosis of the ileum (*white arrowheads* indicate *bowel wall thickness*) with prestenotic dilation (*white arrows*) and in *panel B* small bowel loop dilation (*white arrowheads* indicate *bowel wall thickness* and *white arrows dilation*) in a 20-year-old CD patient

the lumen, and increased peristalsis. Bowel US currently diagnoses stenosis in 70–79 % of unselected CD patients and in >90 % of those with severe bowel stenoses needing surgery, with false-positive diagnoses limited to 7 % [19, 27, 28]. The use of PEG leads to a significantly greater accuracy of bowel US in detecting the presence and the number of stenosis (Fig. 8.2). SICUS detected at least one or two stenoses in >10 % and >20 % more patients, respectively, in comparison with bowel US, resulting in a sensitivity of approximately 90 % for detection of a single stenosis and >75 % for detection of multiple stenoses [18, 19].

Several prospective studies have evaluated the role of bowel US in determining the presence of internal fistulae using surgical-pathological findings as the reference standard [27–30]. In one study, Gasche et al. reported a sensitivity of 87 % and a specificity of 90 % for bowel US in the detection of internal fistulae [27]. In the other prospective study, Maconi et al. determined the accuracy of bowel US and X-ray studies for detecting internal fistulae to be comparable, with a sensitivity of 71.4 % for US and 69.6 % for X-ray, and specificity of 95.8 % for both techniques. Maconi et al. showed also that the combination of these two techniques significantly improved preoperative diagnostic performance (sensitivity 97.4 % and specificity 90 %), with bowel US being more accurate in detecting entero-mesenteric fistulae while X-ray studies were superior in the diagnosis of entero-enteric fistulae [29]. In a recent study conducted by Pallotta et al., SICUS identified fistulas in 27/28 patients and excluded in 19/21 patients (96 % sensitivity, 90.5 % specificity) using surgery as the gold standard [28].

CT and MRI are considered to be non-surgical gold standard for the diagnosis of CD related abscesses [31]. However, bowel US is also considered as a first-line procedure mainly because it is simple to use. Different studies have prospectively assessed the accuracy of bowel US in the detection of intra-abdominal abscesses, showing a mean sensitivity and specificity of 91.5 % and 93 %, respectively [27, 29, 32]. In these studies, bowel US showed a higher sensitivity in the detection of superficial intra-peritoneal abscesses, whereas the diagnosis of deep pelvic or retroperitoneal abscesses was more difficult due to the presence of overlying bowel gas (Fig. 8.3). Pallotta et al. showed that intra-abdominal abscesses were correctly detected in 10/10 patients and excluded in 37/39 patients (100 % sensitivity, 95 % specificity, $k=0.89$) by SICUS [28].

The detection of vascular signals by power-Doppler US around—but not within—the lesions may help to differentiate intra-abdominal abscesses from inflammatory masses. The latter,

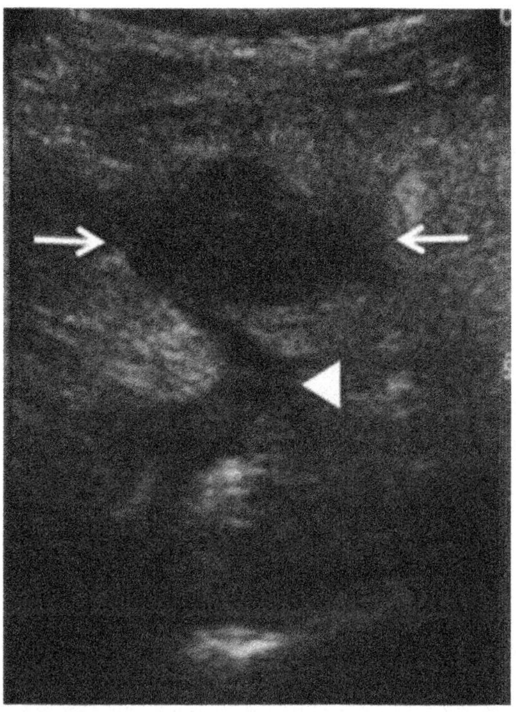

Fig. 8.3 Bowel ultrasonography showed small abscess (*white arrows*) and fistulas (*white arrowhead*) in the right lower quadrant near the terminal ileum in a 40-year-old CD patient

in fact, usually appear as mesenteric masses with increased color signals inside them, whereas abscesses present as fluid collections with a peripheral flow [30, 33]. Inflammatory masses and intra-abdominal abscesses, identified or suspected at US, may also be distinguished or confirmed using CEUS [33]. The use of intravenous contrast-enhancing agents by increasing the number and intensity of the color signals not only in lesions with previously detected vascularity on power-Doppler US, but also in some lesions showing no vascularity at the baseline examination (Fig. 8.4) facilitates the diagnosis of inflammatory masses in doubtful cases and characterizes abdominal masses of 1 cm or more, being even more accurate than CT. Findings emerging from one retrospective study from Ripolles et al. showed that the assessment of vascularity within intra-abdominal masses may distinguish inflammatory masses and abscesses though this must be confirmed by further studies [34].

Postoperative Follow-Up of CD Recurrence

The sensitivity of bowel US in identifying endoscopic recurrence after ileocolonic resection has been investigated in three studies, showing 79–82 % sensitivity [35–37]. The use of PEG solution increased the sensitivity of bowel US for assessing CD recurrence in patients under regular follow-up after ileocolonic resection [38–41]. In our series, bowel US showed a high sensitivity (92.5 %), positive predictive value (94 %), and accuracy (87.5 %) for detecting CD recurrence lesions using ileocolonoscopy as the gold standard [40].

In this setting SICUS provides higher accuracy than bowel US as well as proving predictive value on the risk of recurrence. Pallotta et al. demonstrated that in patients undergoing ileal resection for CD, SICUS accurately detects initial and minimal lesions of CD recurrence at the anastomosis level and the severity of the post-surgical recurrence by assessing both thickness of ileocolonic anastomosis and extent of intramural lesions of neo-terminal ileum [41]. Use of SICUS in CD postoperative setting is advisable given the large number of endoscopic and radiographic investigations to which these patients are submitted during the course of their disease.

Assessment of CD Activity

The assessment of inflammatory activity in CD is mainly based on clinical and laboratory data that not entirely satisfactory and sufficient in order to monitor and adjust therapy. Therefore direct evaluation of inflammatory activity in CD by bowel US has been suggested, to date the role of bowel US in the assessment of CD activity remains controversial. Attempts have been made to correlate wall thickness with disease activity particularly with the Crohn's disease activity index (CDAI). Maconi et al. showed that the degree of bowel wall thickening and extent of the thickened bowel wall on US showed a significant but weak direct correlation between these features and clinical

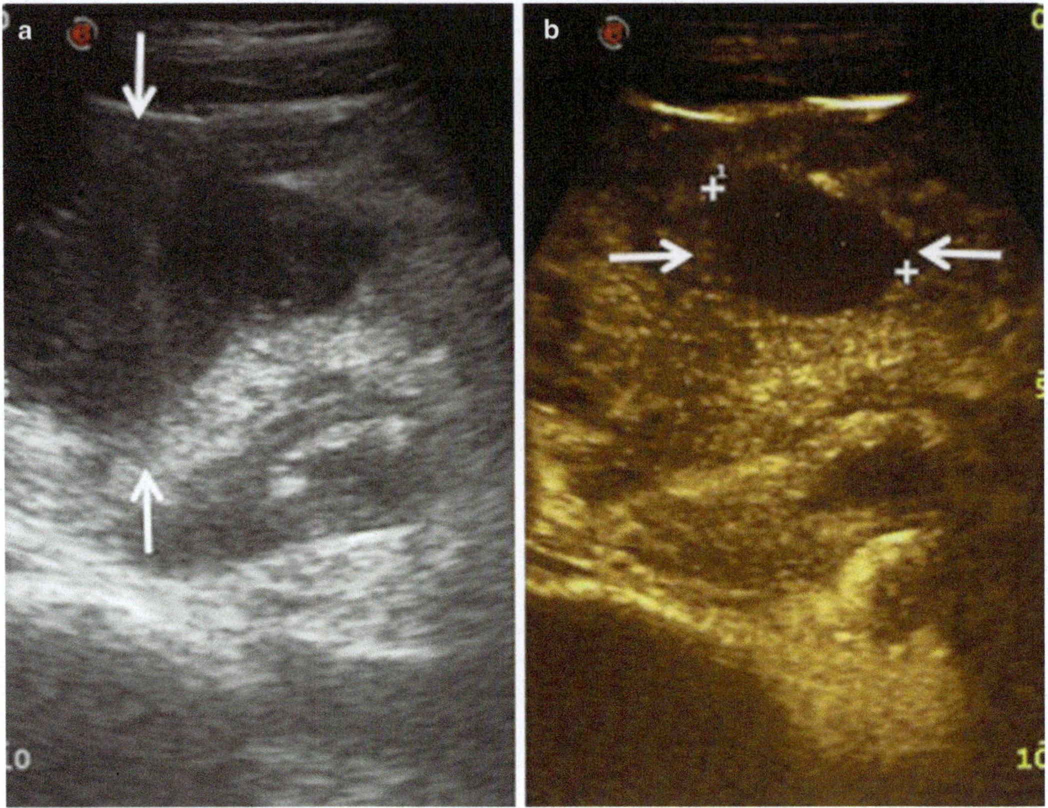

Fig. 8.4 In *panel A*, bowel ultrasonography showed a 3 cm mass (*white arrows*) in the right lower quadrant in a 22-year-old female with ileocolonic CD. In *panel B*, the use of intravenous contrast-enhancing agent (SonoVue®, Bracco) allows for the differentiation between inflammatory masses and abscesses. No vascular lesion representing an abscess was detected by CEUS in the large inflammatory mass (*white arrows*)

and biochemical parameters [21]. In a large series of patients, Hirche et al. showed that bowel wall thickness was significantly higher compared to normal (4.9 ± 2.7 mm versus <2.0 mm) and greater in active (CDAI > 150) than in inactive disease (CDAI < 150): 5.8 ± 2.9 mm versus 4.3 ± 2.2 mm ($p < 0.0001$) [42]. Furthermore a significant correlation was found between maximum bowel wall thickness and disease activity score in children and young adults [43]. The echopattern of bowel wall in defining CD activity has been investigated in a Japanese study comparing US images and in vitro histopathological findings of resected bowel specimens. The authors demonstrated that the loss of stratification (hypoechoic echopattern) and the degree of maximum bowel wall thickness correlated with the severity of inflammation [44]. Moreover different studies evaluated the relationship between bowel US and disease severity assessed by endoscopy and histological finding show a good correlation between US findings and CD activity assessed by endoscopy [45–47].

Also the vascularity of the bowel walls assessed by power-Doppler US has been evaluated as a quantitative method for determining CD activity. Vascularity within the bowel wall has been evaluated using a subjective scoring system according to the semi-quantitative intensity of color signals and/or by the analysis of Doppler curves (measurement of resistive index) obtained from vessels detected within the bowel wall. In most studies, no correlation between US parameters and clinical or biochemical activity was observed, while vascularity evaluations and endoscopic/radiological activity often correlated [45, 48–53].

To increase the sensitivity of Doppler US in detecting vascularity of the diseased bowel wall, US intravenous contrast agents have been introduced. Despite some positive findings, the effectiveness of intravenous contrast agents in detection and assessment of bowel US activity of CD remains controversial [26, 54, 55]. Migaleddu et al. reported in a prospective study that CEUS showed 93.5 % sensitivity, 93.7 % specificity, and 93.6 overall accuracy in detecting inflammatory activity, calculated using endoscopy/biopsy as the gold standard. The linear correlation coefficient for CEUS versus CDAI was 0.74 ($p < 0.0001$) [26]. In a prospective study, Ripolles et al. reported sensitivity and specificity of 96 % and 73 %, respectively, in the prediction of moderate or severe grade of inflammation at CEUS using endoscopy as the gold standard [55]. In another study one hundred and four consecutive patients with CD were prospectively examined using CEUS with respect to the disease activity index [54]. It was found that the pattern of contrast enhancement and the ratio of enhanced to entire wall thickness had a positive predictive value of 63.0 % and 58.6 %, respectively, in distinguishing active from inactive disease. Some authors postulated that CEUS can also provide prognostic data concerning relapse and/or response to therapy.

Perianal Disease

Transperineal ultrasound (TPUS) is a simple, non-invasive and low-cost ultrasonographic technique, which can be usefully employed to study the pelvis and perianal inflammatory diseases in static and dynamic evaluations [56–60]. TPUS can be performed with patient in the left lateral position by placing the transducer on the perineum, with the probe directly above the anus. Several studies showed that TPUS is accurate in detecting the number of perianal fistulas and abscesses with results comparable to that of pelvic MRI and EUS [58, 61–63], and it can also provide a correct classification of perianal fistulas according to the Park's classification with sensitivity greater than 85 % [63, 64]. It can also be useful in patients with anal stenosis, in children and patients where for different reasons, radiographic cross-sectional imaging modalities are contraindicated or not appropriate [60]. However, despite the obvious advantages of the TPUS, it is not widely used in the detection of perianal fistulae and abscesses.

Limits of Bowel US

Limitations of bowel US have been identified in several studies. Bowel US is associated with a significant rate of false-negative results even in the hands of experienced operators, for example in obese patients. Bowel US has no multi-planar capabilities, as with CT and MR enterography/enteroclysis [14, 65, 66]. Inter-observer agreement between sonographers with various degrees of experience in bowel US, and its learning curve, needs to be investigated further. Preliminary result from an Italian study evaluated whether bowel US signs used in CD can be standardized and showed a fair to good reproducibility among six sonographers. In particular bowel wall thickness, the most relevant parameter for CD detection, showed an excellent reproducibility [67]. Further studies will imply the assessment, in a larger sample of patients, of the inter-observer agreement among different operators.

References

1. Hollerbach S, Geissler A, Schiegl H, et al. The accuracy of abdominal ultrasound in the assessment of bowel disorders. Scand J Gastroenterol. 1998;33:1201–8.
2. Sonnenberg A, Erckenbrecht J, Peter P, et al. Detection of Crohn's disease by ultrasound. Gastroenterology. 1982;83:430–4.
3. Pera A, Cammarota T, Comino E, et al. Ultrasonography in the detection of Crohn's disease and in the differential diagnosis of inflammatory bowel disease. Digestion. 1988;41:180–4.
4. Hata J, Haruma K, Suenaga K, et al. Ultrasonographic assessment of inflammatory bowel disease. Am J Gastroenterol. 1992;87:443–7.
5. Sheridan MB, Nicholson DA, Martin DF. Transabdominal ultrasonography as the primary investigation in patients with suspected Crohn's disease or recurrence: a prospective study. Clin Radiol. 1993;48:402–4.

6. Bozkurt T, Richter F, Lux G. Ultrasonography as a primary diagnostic tool in patients with inflammatory disease and tumors of the small intestine and large bowel. J Clin Ultrasound. 1994;22:85–91.
7. Solvig J, Ekberg O, Lindgren S, et al. Ultrasound examination of the small bowel: comparison with enteroclysis in patients with Crohn disease. Abdom Imaging. 1995;20:323–6.
8. Astegiano M, Bresso F, Cammarota T, et al. Abdominal pain and bowel dysfunction: diagnostic role of intestinal ultrasound. Eur J Gastroenterol Hepatol. 2001;13:927–31.
9. Parente F, Greco S, Molteni M, et al. Role of early ultrasound in detecting inflammatory intestinal disorders and identifying their anatomical location within the bowel. Aliment Pharmacol Ther. 2003;18: 1009–16.
10. Rispo A, Imbriaco M, Celentano L, et al. Noninvasive diagnosis of small bowel Crohn's disease: combined use of bowel sonography and Tc-99 m-HMPAO leukocyte scintigraphy. Inflamm Bowel Dis. 2005;11: 376–82.
11. Castiglione F, Mainenti PP, De Palma GD, et al. Noninvasive diagnosis of small bowel Crohn's disease: direct comparison of bowel sonography and magnetic resonance enterography. Inflamm Bowel Dis. 2013;19:991–8.
12. Fraquelli M, Colli A, Casazza G, et al. Role of US in detection of Crohn disease: meta-analysis. Radiology. 2005;236:95–101.
13. Horsthuis K, Bipat S, Bennink RJ, et al. Inflammatory bowel disease diagnosed with US, MR, scintigraphy, and CT: meta-analysis of prospective studies. Radiology. 2008;247:64–79.
14. Panes J, Bouzas R, Chaparro M, et al. Systematic review: the use of ultrasonography, computed tomography and magnetic resonance imaging for the diagnosis, assessment of activity and abdominal complications of Crohn's disease. Aliment Pharmacol Ther. 2011;34:125–45.
15. Truong M, Atri M, Bret PM, et al. Sonographic appearance of benign and malignant conditions of the colon. AJR Am J Roentgenol. 1998;170:1451–5.
16. Pallotta N, Baccini F, Corazziari E. Ultrasonography of the small bowel after oral administration of anechoic contrast solution. Lancet. 1999;353:985–6.
17. Pallotta N, Tomei E, Viscido A, et al. Small intestine contrast ultrasonography: an alternative to radiology in the assessment of small bowel disease. Inflamm Bowel Dis. 2005;11:146–53.
18. Calabrese E, La Seta F, Buccellato A, et al. Crohn's disease: a comparative prospective study of transabdominal ultrasonography, small intestine contrast ultrasonography, and small bowel enema. Inflamm Bowel Dis. 2005;11:139–45.
19. Parente F, Greco S, Molteni M, et al. Oral contrast enhanced bowel ultrasonography in the assessment of small intestine Crohn's disease. A prospective comparison with conventional ultrasound, X ray studies, and ileocolonoscopy. Gut. 2004;53:1652–7.
20. Pallotta N, Baccini F, Corazziari E. Small intestine contrast ultrasonography. J Ultrasound Med. 2000; 19:21–6.
21. Maconi G, Parente F, Bollani S, et al. Abdominal ultrasound in the assessment of extent and activity of Crohn's disease: clinical significance and implication of bowel wall thickening. Am J Gastroenterol. 1996;91:1604–9.
22. Parente F, Maconi G, Bollani S, et al. Bowel ultrasound in assessment of Crohn's disease and detection of related small bowel strictures: a prospective comparative study versus x ray and intraoperative findings. Gut. 2002;50:490–5.
23. Calabrese E, Zorzi F, Onali S, et al. Accuracy of small-intestine contrast ultrasonography, compared with computed tomography enteroclysis, in characterizing lesions in patients with Crohn's disease. Clin Gastroenterol Hepatol. 2013;11:950–5.
24. Strobel D, Raeker S, Martus P, et al. Phase inversion harmonic imaging versus contrast-enhanced power Doppler sonography for the characterization of focal liver lesions. Int J Colorectal Dis. 2003;18:63–72.
25. Kratzer W, Schmidt SA, Mittrach C, et al. Contrast-enhanced wideband harmonic imaging ultrasound (SonoVue): a new technique for quantifying bowel wall vascularity in Crohn's disease. Scand J Gastroenterol. 2005;40:985–91.
26. Migaleddu V, Scanu AM, Quaia E, et al. Contrast-enhanced ultrasonographic evaluation of inflammatory activity in Crohn's disease. Gastroenterology. 2009;137:43–52.
27. Gasche C, Moser G, Turetschek K, et al. Transabdominal bowel sonography for the detection of intestinal complications in Crohn's disease. Gut. 1999;44:112–7.
28. Pallotta N, Vincoli G, Montesani C, et al. Small intestine contrast ultrasonography (SICUS) for the detection of small bowel complications in Crohn's disease: a prospective comparative study versus intraoperative findings. Inflamm Bowel Dis. 2012;18:74–84.
29. Maconi G, Sampietro GM, Parente F, et al. Contrast radiology, computed tomography and ultrasonography in detecting internal fistulas and intra-abdominal abscesses in Crohn's disease: a prospective comparative study. Am J Gastroenterol. 2003;98:1545–55.
30. Neye H, Ensberg D, Rauh P, et al. Impact of high-resolution transabdominal ultrasound in the diagnosis of complications of Crohn's disease. Scand J Gastroenterol. 2010;45:690–5.
31. Van Assche G, Dignass A, Panes J, et al. The second European evidence-based consensus on the diagnosis and management of Crohn's disease: definitions and diagnosis. J Crohns Colitis. 2010;4:7–27.
32. Maconi G, Bollani S, Bianchi PG. Ultrasonographic detection of intestinal complications in Crohn's disease. Dig Dis Sci. 1996;41:1643–8.
33. Rapaccini GL, Pompili M, Orefice R, et al. Contrast-enhanced power Doppler of the intestinal wall in the evaluation of patients with Crohn disease. Scand J Gastroenterol. 2004;39:188–94.

34. Ripolles T, Martinez-Perez MJ, Paredes JM, et al. Contrast-enhanced ultrasound in the differentiation between phlegmon and abscess in Crohn's disease and other abdominal conditions. Eur J Radiol. 2013;82:e525–31.
35. DiCandio G, Mosca F, Campatelli A, et al. Sonographic detection of postsurgical recurrence of Crohn disease. AJR Am J Roentgenol. 1986;146:523–6.
36. Andreoli A, Cerro P, Falasco G, et al. Role of ultrasonography in the diagnosis of postsurgical recurrence of Crohn's disease. Am J Gastroenterol. 1998;93: 1117–21.
37. Rispo A, Bucci L, Pesce G, et al. Bowel sonography for the diagnosis and grading of postsurgical recurrence of Crohn's disease. Inflamm Bowel Dis. 2006;12:486–90.
38. Biancone L, Calabrese E, Petruzziello C, et al. Wireless capsule endoscopy and small intestine contrast ultrasonography in recurrence of Crohn's disease. Inflamm Bowel Dis. 2007;13:1256–65.
39. Castiglione F, Bucci L, Pesce G, et al. Oral contrast-enhanced sonography for the diagnosis and grading of postsurgical recurrence of Crohn's disease. Inflamm Bowel Dis. 2008;14:1240–5.
40. Calabrese E, Petruzziello C, Onali S, et al. Severity of postoperative recurrence in Crohn's disease: correlation between endoscopic and sonographic findings. Inflamm Bowel Dis. 2009;15:1635–42.
41. Pallotta N, Giovannone M, Pezzotti P, et al. Ultrasonographic detection and assessment of the severity of Crohn's disease recurrence after ileal resection. BMC Gastroenterol. 2010;10:69.
42. Hirche TO, Russler J, Schroder O, et al. The value of routinely performed ultrasonography in patients with Crohn disease. Scand J Gastroenterol. 2002;37: 1178–83.
43. Haber HP, Busch A, Ziebach R, et al. Bowel wall thickness measured by ultrasound as a marker of Crohn's disease activity in children. Lancet. 2000; 355:1239–40.
44. Hata J, Haruma K, Yamanaka H, et al. Ultrasonographic evaluation of the bowel wall in inflammatory bowel disease: comparison of in vivo and in vitro studies. Abdom Imaging. 1994;19:395–9.
45. Haber HP, Busch A, Ziebach R, et al. Ultrasonographic findings correspond to clinical, endoscopic, and histologic findings in inflammatory bowel disease and other enterocolitides. J Ultrasound Med. 2002;21:375–82.
46. Bremner AR, Griffiths M, Argent JD, et al. Sonographic evaluation of inflammatory bowel disease: a prospective, blinded, comparative study. Pediatr Radiol. 2006;36:947–53.
47. Pascu M, Roznowski AB, Muller HP, et al. Clinical relevance of transabdominal ultrasonography and magnetic resonance imaging in patients with inflammatory bowel disease of the terminal ileum and large bowel. Inflamm Bowel Dis. 2004;10:373–82.
48. Yekeler E, Danalioglu A, Movasseghi B, et al. Crohn disease activity evaluated by Doppler ultrasonography of the superior mesenteric artery and the affected small-bowel segments. J Ultrasound Med. 2005; 24:59–65.
49. Scholbach T, Herrero I, Scholbach J. Dynamic color Doppler sonography of intestinal wall in patients with Crohn disease compared with healthy subjects. J Pediatr Gastroenterol Nutr. 2004;39:524–8.
50. Neye H, Voderholzer W, Rickes S, et al. Evaluation of criteria for the activity of Crohn's disease by power Doppler sonography. Dig Dis. 2004;22:67–72.
51. Heyne R, Rickes S, Bock P, et al. Non-invasive evaluation of activity in inflammatory bowel disease by power Doppler sonography. Z Gastroenterol. 2002; 40:171–5.
52. Esteban JM, Maldonado L, Sanchiz V, et al. Activity of Crohn's disease assessed by colour Doppler ultrasound analysis of the affected loops. Eur Radiol. 2001;11:1423–8.
53. Spalinger J, Patriquin H, Miron MC, et al. Doppler US in patients with Crohn disease: vessel density in the diseased bowel reflects disease activity. Radiology. 2000;217:787–91.
54. Serra C, Menozzi G, Labate AM, et al. Ultrasound assessment of vascularization of the thickened terminal ileum wall in Crohn's disease patients using a low-mechanical index real-time scanning technique with a second generation ultrasound contrast agent. Eur J Radiol. 2007;62:114–21.
55. Ripolles T, Martinez MJ, Paredes JM, et al. Crohn disease: correlation of findings at contrast-enhanced US with severity at endoscopy. Radiology. 2009;253: 241–8.
56. Kleinubing Jr H, Jannini JF, Malafaia O, et al. Transperineal ultrasonography: new method to image the anorectal region. Dis Colon Rectum. 2000;43: 1572–4.
57. Stewart LK, McGee J, Wilson SR. Transperineal and transvaginal sonography of perianal inflammatory disease. AJR Am J Roentgenol. 2001;177:627–32.
58. Wedemeyer J, Kirchhoff T, Sellge G, et al. Transcutaneous perianal sonography: a sensitive method for the detection of perianal inflammatory lesions in Crohn's disease. World J Gastroenterol. 2004;10:2859–63.
59. Bonatti H, Lugger P, Hechenleitner P, et al. Transperineal sonography in anorectal disorders. Ultraschall Med. 2004;25:111–5.
60. Kim IO, Han TI, Kim WS, et al. Transperineal ultrasonography in imperforate anus: identification of the internal fistula. J Ultrasound Med. 2000;19: 211–6.
61. Zbar AP, Oyetunji RO, Gill R. Transperineal versus hydrogen peroxide-enhanced endoanal ultrasonography in never operated and recurrent cryptogenic fistula-in-ano: a pilot study. Tech Coloproctol. 2006; 10:297–302.
62. Domkundwar SV, Shinagare AB. Role of transcutaneous perianal ultrasonography in evaluation of fistulas in ano. J Ultrasound Med. 2007;26:29–36.
63. Maconi G, Ardizzone S, Greco S, et al. Transperineal ultrasound in the detection of perianal and rectovaginal

fistulae in Crohn's disease. Am J Gastroenterol. 2007;102:2214–9.
64. Maconi G, Tonolini M, Monteleone M, et al. Transperineal perineal ultrasound versus magnetic resonance imaging in the assessment of perianal Crohn's disease. Inflamm Bowel Dis. 2013;19:2737–43.
65. Fiorino G, Bonifacio C, Peyrin-Biroulet L, et al. Prospective comparison of computed tomography enterography and magnetic resonance enterography for assessment of disease activity and complications in ileocolonic Crohn's disease. Inflamm Bowel Dis. 2011;17:1073–80.
66. Maccioni F, Viscido A, Broglia L, et al. Evaluation of Crohn disease activity with magnetic resonance imaging. Abdom Imaging. 2000;25:219–28.
67. Fraquelli M, Sarno A, Girelli C, et al. Reproducibility of bowel ultrasonography in the evaluation of Crohn's disease. Dig Liver Dis. 2008;40:860–6.

9 Diagnostics: The Future

Joseph H. Yacoub and Aytekin Oto

Abbreviations

ADC	Apparent diffusion coefficient
ASIR	Adaptive statistical iterative reconstruction
bSSFP	Balanced steady state free precession
CD	Crohn's disease
CEUS	Contrast-enhanced ultrasound
CNR	Contrast to noise ratio
DCE-MRI	Dynamic contrast-enhanced magnetic resonance imaging
DWI	Diffusion weighted imaging
FBP	Filtered back projection
FDG-PET	Flouro-deoxy-glucose positron emission tomography
MI	Motility index
MT	Magnetization transfer
SSFSE	Single shot fast spin echo
SNR	Signal to noise ratio

J.H. Yacoub, MD
Department of Radiology, Loyola University Chicago, Stritch School of Medicine, 2160 S. 1st Avenue, Maywood, IL 60153, USA
e-mail: jyacoub@lumc.edu

A. Oto, MD (✉)
Department of Radiology, University of Chicago, 5841 S. Maryland Avenue, MC 2026, Chicago, IL 60637, USA
e-mail: aoto@radiology.bsd.uchicago.edu

Introduction

The imaging of Crohn's disease (CD) has evolved rapidly in past two decades improving noninvasive assessment of the disease and its complications, however, there remain major opportunities for imaging to play an even bigger role in clinical decision making. One such opportunity is the differentiation of active inflammation that will be responsive to medical therapy from fibrostenotic disease that requires surgical intervention. Another opportunity is assessing and monitoring response to therapy. In response to these clinical needs, there are emerging new imaging methods. New imaging techniques are moving beyond anatomic imaging to provide functional and histologic information about tissue compositions and inflammation. Emerging techniques are increasingly becoming more quantitative. In addition, there is increased awareness of radiation exposure that brings attention to radiation reduction techniques or imaging techniques that do not expose the patients to the ionizing radiation. In this chapter, we will discuss advances in MR enterography, CT enterography, PET imaging, and ultrasound of Crohn's disease. We will discuss the most recent advances that are being applied clinically, as well as novel techniques that are not yet ready for clinical application.

A. Fichera and M.K. Krane (eds.), *Crohn's Disease: Basic Principles*,
DOI 10.1007/978-3-319-14181-7_9, © Springer International Publishing Switzerland 2015

Advances in MR Enterography

High Resolution MR Images

Single shot fast spin echo (SSFSE) and balanced steady state free precession (bSSFP) are the workhorses of the MR enterography protocol. While these are very fast sequences with a reasonable spatial resolution, there is room for improvement on the spatial resolution. Higher resolution could offer more detailed assessment of the diseased bowel loops particularly of the mucosal changes that remain practically out of reach of the standard MR enterography protocol. By focusing the imaging on the segments of bowel with suspected active disease, it would be possible to obtain higher resolution images that can offer better evaluation of subtle disease. Sinha et al. [1] described an imaging protocol in which the radiologist evaluated the standard MR sequences to select bowel segments for further, high resolution evaluation. The selected segments would then be imaged with fat suppressed bSSFP and SSFSE sequences with a small field of view and higher resolution. The images were aligned parallel and perpendicular to that bowel segment and obtained with contiguous thin 2–3 mm sections. Multi-planar and endoluminal views could then be reconstructed. Using this technique, the diagnostic confidence was increased by depicting aphthous ulcers and transmural and mesenteric changes. This technique can allow for more accurate characterization and classification of CD. In a subsequent study [2], the authors added high resolution bSSFP sequences obtained in each of the four abdominal quadrants to the standard protocol. This added only 3 min to the length of the study. Furthermore, the standard images were also reviewed by the radiologists to select potential other segments for further evaluation. Using this protocol they reported higher accuracy of the high resolution MR enterography in the diagnosis of bowel ulceration, fistulae, and abscesses [2].

3Tesla MR Imaging

High magnetic field imaging is becoming more clinically plausible with increasing availability of 3T MRI in many centers. MR enterography with 3T MRI offers benefits that are of particular relevance in bowel imaging. Compared to 1.5T MRI, 3T MRI increases the signal to noise ratio (SNR) by about 1.7–1.8-fold [3, 4] which can translate into improving the special resolution or reducing the scan time. Contrast to noise ratio (CNR) is also increased which translated into increased conspicuity of enhancing structure and lesions, as well as decrease in the amount of Gadolinium needed. In addition, fat suppression in 3T can be more homogeneous than in 1.5T. The use of parallel acquisition techniques further improves the SNR and temporal resolution and mitigates some of the disadvantages of 3T imaging.

Studies have demonstrated feasibility of performing high quality MR enterography on 3T [5, 6] and have shown strong correlation between MRI findings and endoscopic activity in ileocolonic disease [7] and in terminal ileitis [8]. In a more recent study, 3T MR imaging was equally accurate to 1.5T MR imaging in evaluating ileocolonic CD and was superior in detecting mucosal ulcers [9]. The mean length of the examination was 30 min for the 1.5T MR and 20 min for the 3T MR.

3T MR in body imaging has traditionally posed technical challenges, many of which have been tackled successfully in the recent literature. 3T MR imaging results in increasing artifacts and increasing energy deposition [3, 4, 10]. Three commonly encountered artifacts in 3T imaging are B1-inhomogeneity artifact (also referred to as standing wave artifact or dielectric effect), chemical shift artifact of the first type, and susceptibility artifact (Fig. 9.1). The challenges have been mitigated by the use of parallel imaging as well as the use of torso coils instead of body coils. Additional specific solutions for specific artifacts have also been proposed including dielectric pads and adjusting the sequence parameters.

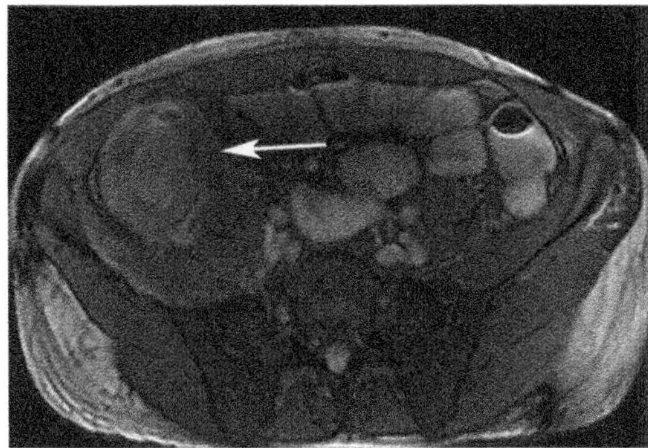

Fig. 9.1 bSSFP image obtained on a 3T MRI scanner demonstrating abnormal ascending colon in the right lower quadrant (*arrow*)

The bSSFP sequence remains to be the sequence that poses the greatest challenge in 3T imaging of the bowel, particularly when applying fat suppression. In a continuing effort to resolve these problems a modified form of bSSFP has been presented to optimize abdominal imaging at 3T with fat suppression [11]. Using this modified sequence, known as alternating TR-SSFP, the authors were able to obtain a fat suppressed high contrast 3D-isotropic abdominal image within a single breath-hold. Similar ongoing advances in pulse sequence design, parallel imaging, and coil design will continue to promise improved MR imaging of the abdomen at higher magnetic field strength.

Dynamic Contrast-Enhanced Magnetic Resonance Imaging

Dynamic contrast-enhanced magnetic resonance imaging (DCE-MRI) is a technique used to assess tissue perfusion by repeatedly scanning the organ of interest before, during and after the infusion of contrast (Fig. 9.2). The images acquired can visually demonstrate the uptake of contrast in the tissue highlighting areas of altered perfusion. More importantly the images are analyzed in various ways to extract parameters that indicate regions of altered perfusion and draw conclusion about underlying disease processes. These parameters can also be used for quantitative assessment of tissue perfusion, which is a growing aspect of quantitative imaging and quantitative assessment of treatment response (Fig. 9.3). The use of DCE-MRI is mostly popular in oncologic imaging such as breast and prostate cancer. Active inflammation is also another cause of increased tissue perfusion, which makes this technique of interest in the imaging of CD. Actively inflamed bowel segments demonstrate increased enhancement [12–16] with an early hyperenhancement that increases over time till a plateau is reached [17–20] (Fig. 9.4). Actively inflamed bowel has also been observed to display a different enhancement pattern than inactive disease [18, 21, 22]. Using DCE-MRI, these altered patterns of enhancement can be detected and used to assess disease activity and extent. Studies have shown a correlation between dynamic enhancement parameters such as peak uptake and slope of enhancement curve and the clinical activity of the disease [17] and the inflammatory activity on biopsy [23, 24]. The parameters that describe the enhancement curve (signal vs. time) are referred to as semi-quantitative parameters. These parameters describe the pattern of enhancement, which can be compared with other segments of bowel. The exact values of these parameters, however, can't be compared across patients and studies. More recently a new set of parameters have been described which are more quantitative and at least theoretically can be replicated across studies and across patients. Quantitative DCE-MRI analysis has been applied to MR enterography yielding early promising results. In quantitative analysis, pharmacokinetic models are used to convert the signal intensity to tissue concentration of Gadolinium and calculate parameters that reflect the tissue perfusion. The inflamed bowel segments have been shown to demonstrate faster K^{trans} values and larger V_e values [20]. K^{trans} is the transfer constant between the intravascular to the extravascular extracellular space. V_e is the volume of the extravascular extracellular space per unit volume of tissue (Fig. 9.5). In addition to distinguishing areas of active inflammation, these semi-quantitative and quantitative parameters have the potential to monitor response to treatment. More efforts to standardize image acquisition and analysis and more

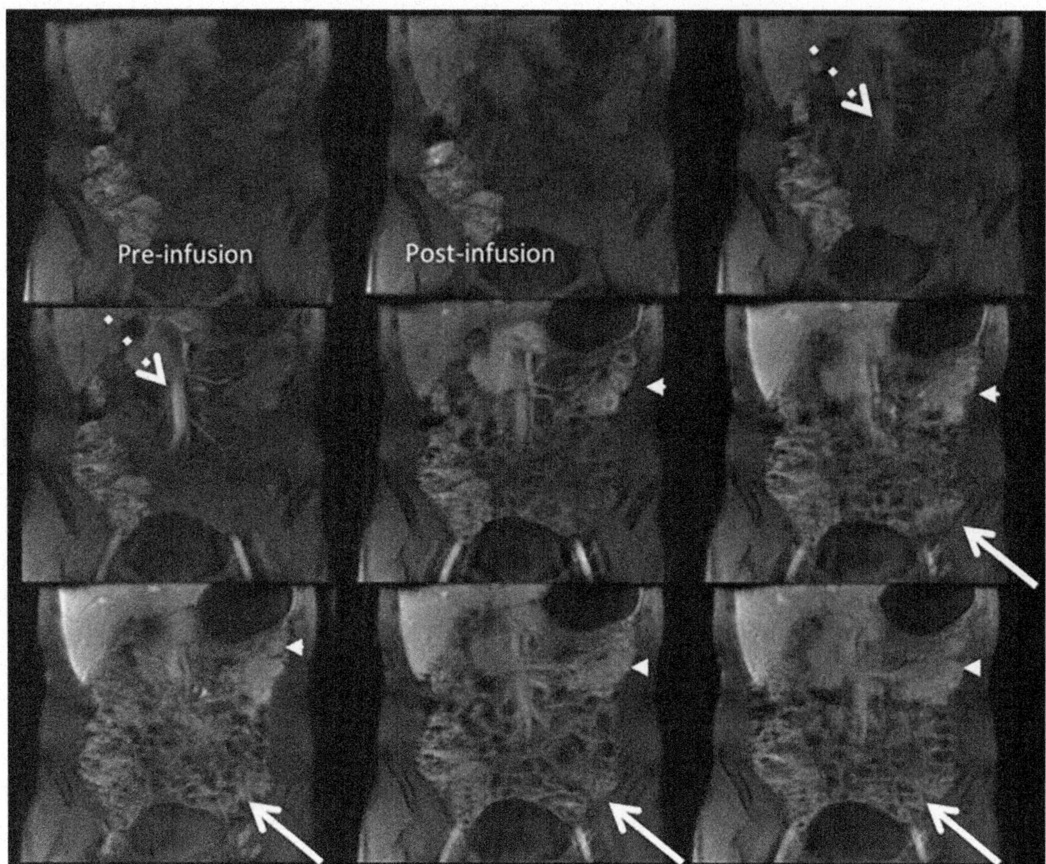

Fig. 9.2 Dynamic contrast enhanced images of small bowel in a normal patient. This patient had 90 post-contrast phases through the entire small bowel segment. Nine representative images are shown here for illustration, the first of which is before the start of the infusion. Arterial enhancement is seen in the aorta (*dashed arrow*) shortly after infusion of contrast followed by enhancement of the jejunum (*arrow head*) followed by enhancement of ileum (*solid arrow*)

studies to confirm the clinical utility of these parameters are needed. Acquisition of DCE-MRI is within the reach of most radiology practices but require a high degree of MRI expertise, however, the software packages commercially available for analysis are not optimized for bowel imaging making the application of this technique limited to research at the time.

Diffusion Weighted Imaging

Diffusion weighted imaging (DWI) is an MRI sequence where the signal intensity reflects the degree of restricted motion of water molecules; a phenomenon that is most notable in malignancies and inflammation. Much of the attention has been primarily focused on the role of DWI in evaluating patients with cancer. The increased cellularity of tumors leads to more restriction in the diffusion of the water molecules due to their interaction with intact cell membranes and entrapment within the intracellular compartment. DWI is sensitive to water molecules exhibiting restricted diffusion. A value known as "b-value" determines the relative contribution of non-restricted and restricted water molecules to the signal. The higher the b-value the lower the contribution from unrestricted water molecules to the signal and therefore the signal reflects the diffusion restriction. By imaging at least 2b-values, the apparent diffusion coefficient (ADC) can be calculated such that the

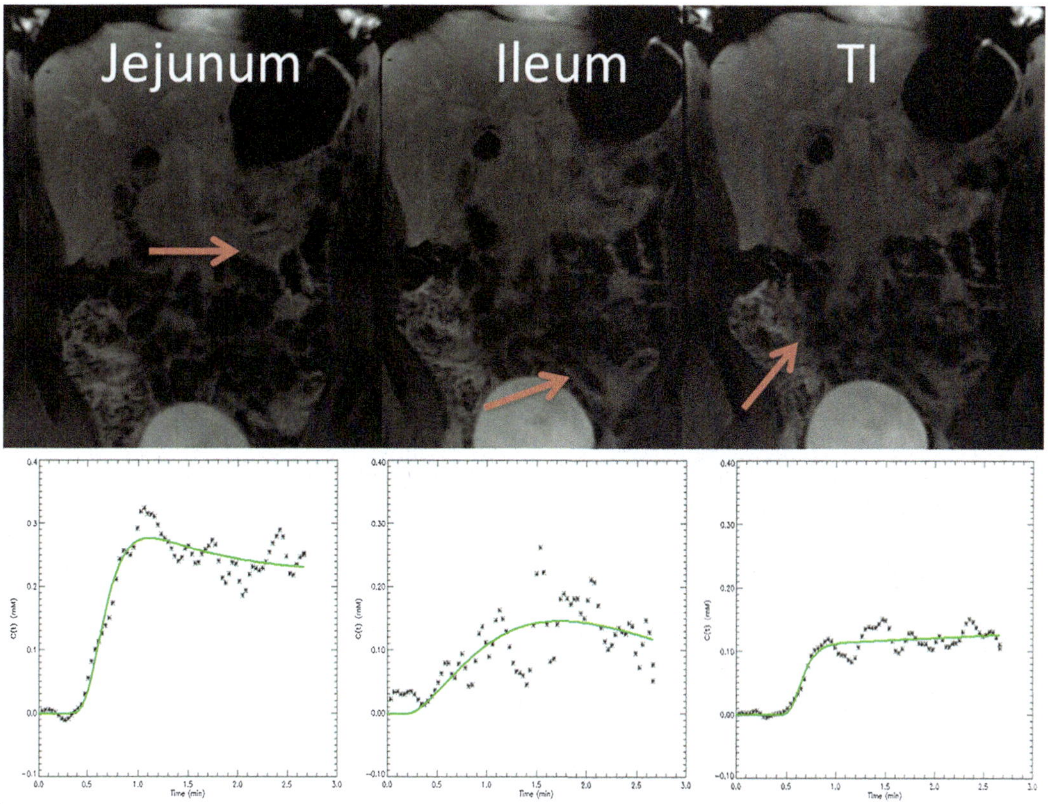

Fig. 9.3 Concentration curves estimating the contrast concentration in various bowel segments in a normal patient showing the normal enhancement pattern. These *curves* are further analyzed to extract quantitative parameter the reflect tissue perfusion

more the restricted diffusion, the lower the ADC value. The ADC value therefore allows for quantitative analysis, a potential strength of DWI. It has long been recognized that certain inflammatory processes may likewise demonstrate restricted diffusion. While this phenomenon is more challenging to explain and is likely multifactorial, it has nevertheless led to an emerging interest in using DWI as a quantifiable indicator of inflammation in the abdomen.

Inflamed bowel segments have been shown to demonstrate restricted diffusion compared to normal bowel [25, 26] (Fig. 9.6). Using DWI and quantitative DCE-MRI parameters, Oto et al. showed that actively inflamed small bowel segments can be differentiated from normal small bowel loops in patients with CD [25]. The combination of DWI and DCE-MRI improved the specificity for detection of active inflammation [25]. DWI was more sensitive than DCE-MRI in that study. Kiryu et al. reported a sensitivity, specificity, and accuracy of 86.0 %, 81.4 %, and 82.4 %, respectively, for DWI in the detection of disease-active segments [27]. In a study [28] of 132 patients including 848 segments of bowel where DWI was compared to standard contrast MR enterography, DWI was found to be accurate in detecting and assessing disease activity and differentiating active from non-active colonic CD. Overall, sensitivity, specificity, and accuracy for detecting active disease were 93.7 %, 98.7 %, and 97.6 %, respectively. The accuracy was higher in colonic disease than in ileal disease. Using the ADC as a quantitative indicator of disease activity, it was found that the ADC was significantly lower in active segments than inactive segments (Fig. 9.7). A threshold ADC value of 1.9×10^{-3} mm²/s was determined based on the

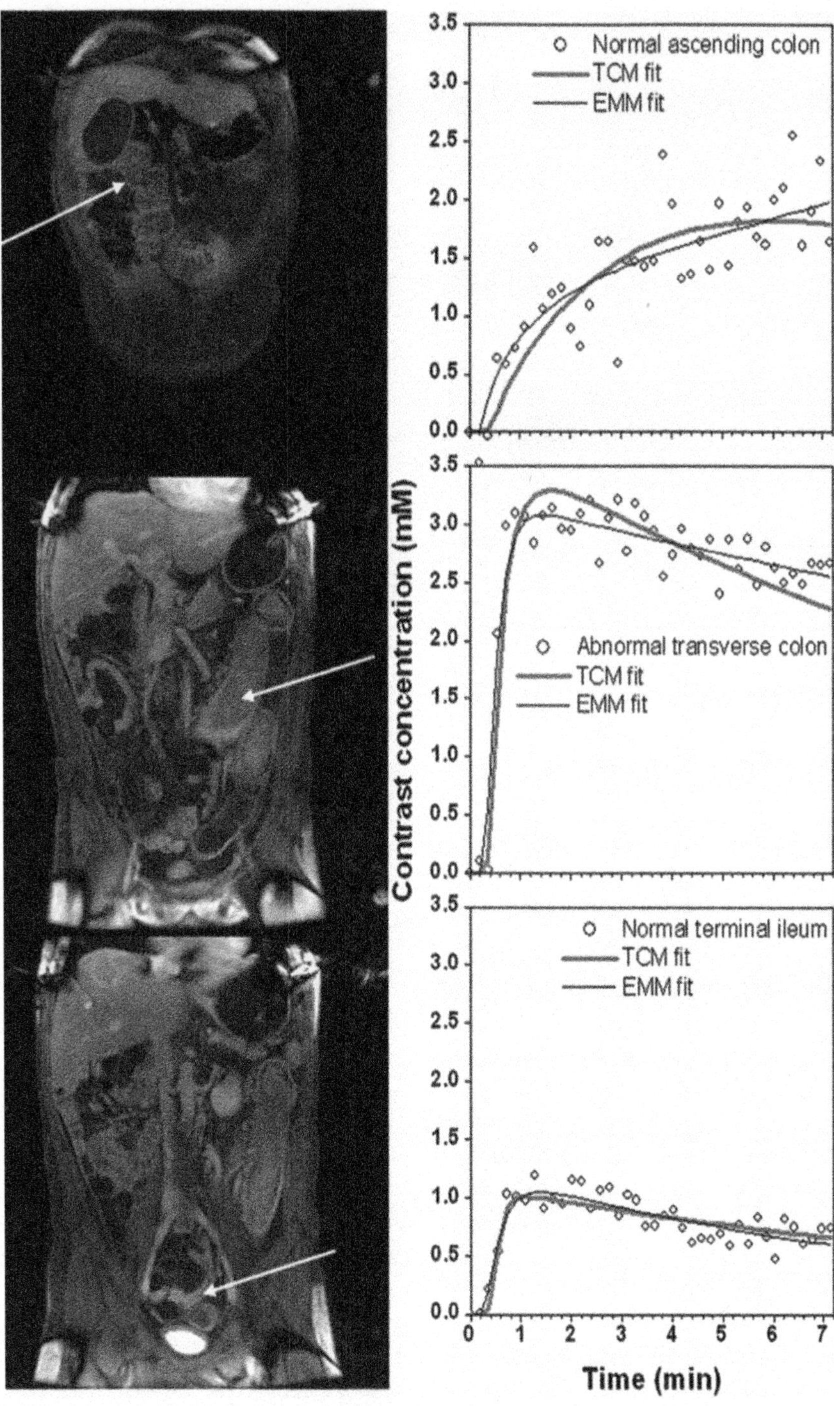

Fig. 9.4 Concentration curves estimating the contrast concentration in abnormal transverse colon (*middle image*) compared to normal ascending colon (*top image*) and normal terminal ileum. The actively inflamed transverse colon demonstrates early hyperenhancement and a degree of washout

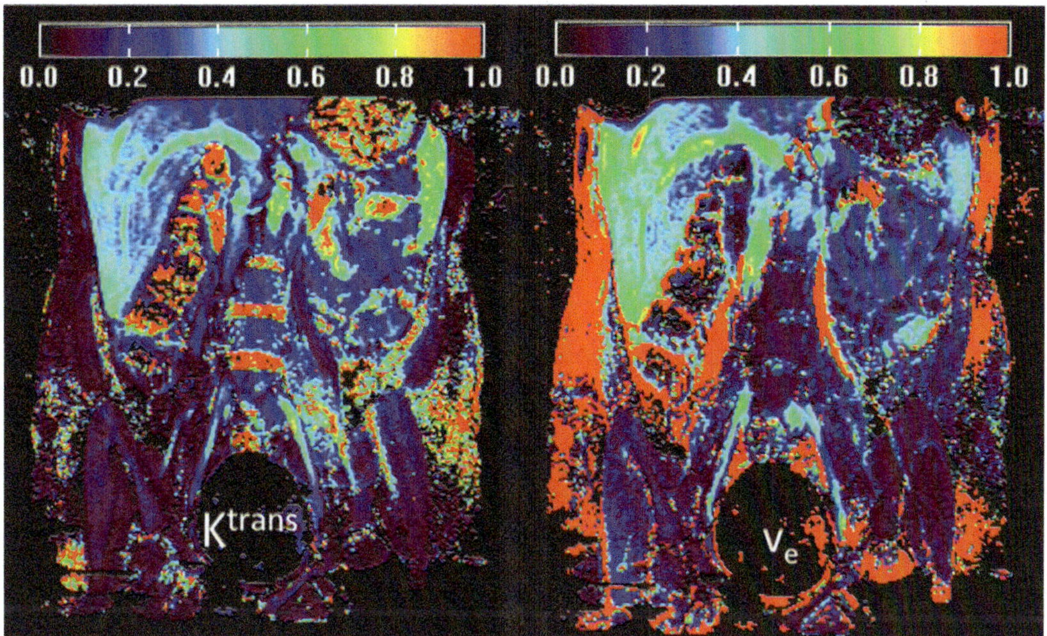

Fig. 9.5 Color maps of two quantitative parameters K^{trans} and V_e obtained from pixel by pixel analysis. These maps, which are commonly employed in other application of the DCE MRI, can be a quick visual to evaluate areas of disease

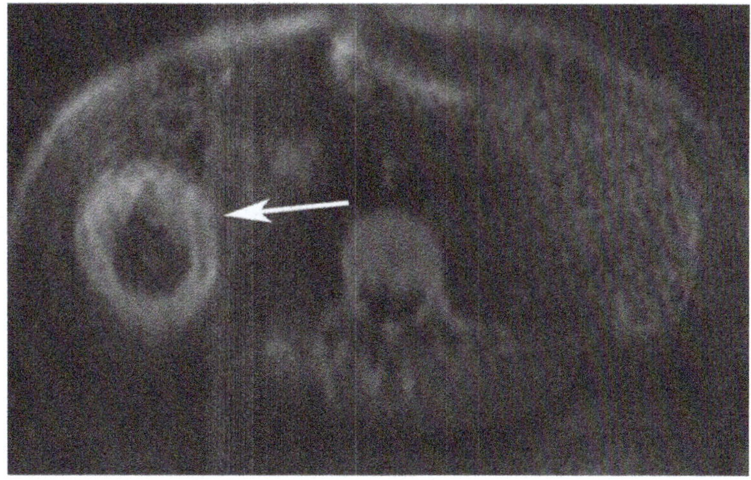

Fig. 9.6 Diffusion weighted imaging demonstrates increased signal in an actively inflamed segment of the ascending colon in the right lower quadrant (*arrow*)

ROC curve which had a sensitivity and specificity of 93.7 % and 96.0 %, respectively, in differentiating active from inactive disease. Based on these results, the authors concluded that a scoring system based on DWI was a reliable tool for assessing inflammation in CD. In another smaller [29] study, DWI was compared to CT enterography demonstrating strong correlation between the two imaging modalities. A study in the pediatric population [30] showed a strong correlation between restricted diffusion and multiple traditional MRI findings of active inflammation including bowel wall thickening, increased arterial phase post-contrast enhancement, striated

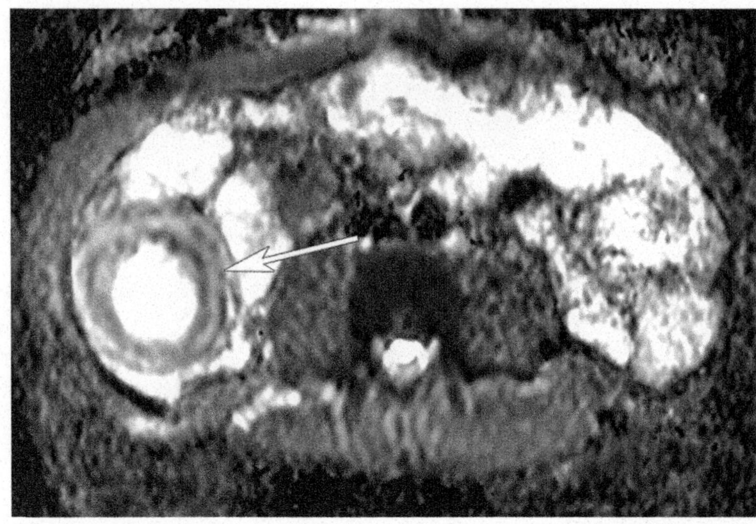

Fig. 9.7 Apparent diffusion coefficient map obtained from analysis of the DWI data which demonstrate low ADC value (*dark signal*) in the wall of an actively inflamed segment of ascending colon in the right lower quadrant (*arrow*)

pattern of arterial phase post-contrast enhancement, increased delayed phase arterial enhancement, and increased adjacent mesenteric inflammatory changes. Another study [31] in the pediatric population has shown that DWI has comparable diagnostic accuracy to contrast enhanced MRI and has the potential to replace the need for contrast. The majority of the studies discussed are limited by the lack of a gold standard such as histopathology; nevertheless, they highlight the potential of DWI in the imaging of CD. In our experience, we are recognizing segments of active disease have greater conspicuity on DWI sequences, which anecdotally increases our sensitivity and confidence in detecting active disease. The future may hold bigger role for DWI in the imaging of CD, particularly given the potential for using the ADC value as quantitative marker of disease activity. One potential role would be in qualitative and quantitative assessment of response to treatment which can be done using the ADC value.

MR Motility Imaging Techniques

MR motility Imaging or cine MR enterography refers to real time images with high temporal resolution (~1 s) obtained by iterative acquisition of ultrafast bSSFP or SSFSE images through a coronal slab of the abdomen to evaluate the small bowel peristalsis. It is used to identify areas of altered motility, specifically focal areas of paralysis or hypomotility. The most direct use of motility imaging is to differentiate areas of functional stenosis from scarring and strictures [23] (Fig. 9.8). In addition, MR motility may complement static images by highlighting areas of subtle disease that may present as area of altered motility. Froehlich et al. [32] detected a larger number of CD-specific findings on cine MR enterography combined with static MR enterography than on static MR enterography alone. They identified segments of altered motility and then evaluated these segments on the static MR enterography to identify corresponding anatomic abnormalities. The CD-specific findings identified included wall thickening, stenosis, wall layering (thickened wall combined with alternating hyperintense and hypointense layers within the wall), ulcers, the comb sign, fistulas, and abscess. They also identified significantly more patients with CD than identified on MR enterography alone. Kitazume et al. described the finding of asymmetric involvement or mesenteric rigidity with antimesenteric flexibility that correlated with longitudinal ulcer in small-bowel CD [33].

The use of motility imaging in clinical practice remains qualitative and largely subjective, however, there is increasing interest in the literature towards more quantitative assessment of motility. Software tools for automated evaluation

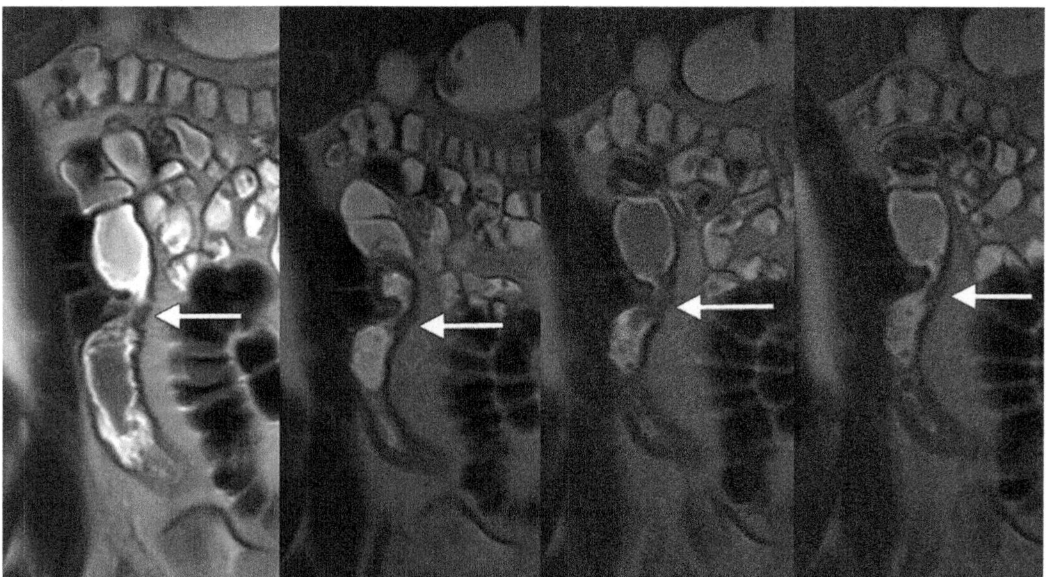

Fig. 9.8 Fixed focal narrowing in the ileum demonstrated on motility imaging (bSSFP cine image). Multiple snapshot images at various time points of the cine image demonstrate the fixed stricture. The bowel loop just proximal to the narrowing is mildly dilated

and quantitative analysis of bowel motility on cine MR enterography techniques have been developed but are not yet commercially available [34–36]. The most commonly reported and perhaps the easiest to conceptualize method to quantify motility is based on tracking the bowel diameter to calculate the number of contraction per minutes, contraction amplitudes, and other variation of contraction assessments [35, 37–41]. Various other methods and parameters have been described in the literature [39, 42–45]. Menys et al. quantified the motility of the terminal ileum using a new parameter, motility index (MI), and showed a significant difference in motility between non-inflamed and inflamed terminal ileum in 28 patients with CD [35]. The MI was negatively correlated with the acute inflammation score that was assigned on biopsy, suggesting a role for quantified motility in assessing disease activity. Similar results were reported by Cullmann et al. with strong correlation between motility changes and histopathologic findings in both active and chronic CD [38]. In a subsequent paper, Menys et al. evaluated changes in motility in and around strictures showing quantifiable differences between prestricture, strictured, and normal bowel [37]. However, in a latter study [39] of motility in 20 healthy volunteers, the authors pointed out the large variation in motility of different segments of small bowel within the same individual and at the same location at different times. On the other hand, global motility quantification was shown to be repeatable in healthy subjects [42] and sensitive to changes induced by medication [42, 44]. These results are useful and relevant in evaluation of CD since it has been shown that global motility is affected in patients with active CD compared to patients with chronic CD and to healthy volunteers even within distant non-affected segments [41]. These global alterations in motility was also shown to correlate with C-reactive protein and calprotectin [46].

There have been two general approaches to acquiring motility imaging with regard to technique. Breath-hold techniques is one approach that avoids the interference from breathing motion when analyzing the motility imaging. However, this allows for only short duration of motility imaging which limits qualitative and quantitative assessment of motility. Alternatively, free breathing techniques allow for longer duration of imaging at the expense of interference from breathing motion. Recently, automated breathing correction have been described [36, 47] and have been shown to be reliable [36].

Magnetization Transfer

Assessing the degree of fibrosis in the affected segments of bowel in CD has major implications on the choice of treatment. While areas of active inflammation may respond to medical therapy, areas of fibrosis usually require surgical intervention. Most of the current imaging techniques provide at best an indirect evaluation of fibrosis with the recognition that there is significant overlap between fibrosis and inflammation on imaging [12, 48]. Magnetization Transfer (MT) is a novel MR technique that promises to directly image and quantify fibrosis differentiating it from edema and inflammation. MT-MRI generates contrast that is primarily determined by the fraction of large macromolecules or immobilized phospholipid cell membranes in tissue, therefore, stiff body substances such as muscle or fibrotic tissue has a high magnetization transfer effect. Adler et al. have shown that MT ratio correlates with tissue collagen in the rat's fibrotic bowel wall injected with peptidoglycan–polysaccharide, but it remained unchanged in the control rats that demonstrated inflammation but no fibrosis [49]. In a subsequent paper, the rats were injected with anti-TNF-alpha after the injection peptidoglycan–polysaccharide which resulted in less intestinal fibrosis and therefore less tissue collagen on histology. MT-MRI measurably demonstrated the decrease in intestinal fibrosis. Pazahr et al. have shown that MT imaging of the small bowel wall is feasible in humans with sufficient image quality and may help with the identification of fibrotic scarring in patients with CD [50]. These early results indicate a potential role for MT in assessing bowel fibrosis. MT-MRI may distinguish between inflammatory changes that can respond to medical management and fibrotic changes that may require surgery or new therapeutic agents. It may also evaluate response to new therapeutic agents targeted at treating fibrotic strictures.

Advances in CT Enterography

With the growing concern about the radiation exposure in younger patients, particularly in patients with CD, there is an ongoing effort to minimize the radiation dose from CT enterography without affecting the diagnostic quality. These dose reduction methods are particularly valuable in patients with CD. The majority of patients with CD are young, increasing the risk of late radiation effects [51]. Additionally, repeated imaging results in a large cumulative radiation dose with some patients receiving five to ten CT scans [52]. Patients with CD also already have background risk of neoplasia and in addition are co-exposed to potentially synergistic agents as part of their medical treatment, which further increases the risk of neoplasia [53].

Standard strategies for minimizing radiation dose have been employed in abdominal imaging [54–57] including use of low tube current, low tube voltage, and automatic tube current modulation. These techniques are limited by their effect on the image quality and noise level. New techniques of iterative reconstruction are allowing for low-dose CTs while maintaining or even improving the image quality.

Iterative reconstruction is a computational technique used to generate images from the raw projection data acquired by the CT scanner. It replaces the currently used conventional technique known as filtered back projection (FBP). Iterative reconstruction techniques generate images with less noise; this translates into the ability to acquire images at lower radiation doses while maintaining a comparable quality and noise level with the conventional methods. The benefits of iterative reconstruction are achieved at the cost of longer computational processing time. True iterative reconstruction methods demand advanced computation hardware and lengthy reconstruction that limits their clinical utility. Hybrid techniques that incorporate both FBP and iterative reconstruction allow more rapid reconstruction which is more practical for clinical applications. Multiple vendor specific variants of these hybrid iterative reconstruction techniques are available commercially.

Using adaptive statistical iterative reconstruction (ASIR), Kambadakone et al. [58] reported a 34 % reduction in radiation dose compared to standard CT without compromise to image quality or noise levels. In fact in this study the image quality was improved and the image noise level was reduced. Kaza et al. [59] compared the standard 120 kVp tube voltage with a low-tube-voltage technique of 80 kVp in which ASIR have been applied. The 80 kVp images were adequately diagnostic with an average dose reduction of 71 %. The image quality was decreased and the noise level was higher on the 80 kVp images, but the accuracy metrics were comparable with the 120 kVp images. Johnson et al. [60] used a low-tube-current of 100 kVp and applied an iterative reconstruction technique known as SAFIRE to achieve a 33 % dose reduction with no loss of image quality or increase in noise. O'Niel et al. [61] were able to reduce the radiation dose to 1.3±0.8 mSv. In the subset of patients with normal or low BMI the mean effective dose was 0.84 mSv. These reduced doses represent more than 70 % dose reduction of the conventional-dose approach used at that institution. To put these values in prospective, the sub-millisievert radiation doses reported here are comparable to radiation doses from standard plain radiographs of the abdomen. In order to achieve this level of dose reduction, the image quality was slightly compromised and a higher noise level was accepted, however, the authors reported that the diagnostic accuracy of the scan was adequate yielding comparable information regarding extent, activity, and complications of CD when compared to conventional-dose technique.

Other noise-reduction techniques have been described that can be applied to CT images without the need for image reconstruction from the raw projection data, as is the case with iterative reconstruction. The advantage of these methods is that they are not tied down to the reconstruction algorithm on the scanner and can be applied using a standard computer at a short processing time. Guimarães et al. [62] applied a novel denoising algorithm (projection-space denoising—PSDN) to CT data obtained at 50 % noise reduction with low-voltage (80 kV) and demonstrated they approached the quality of full-dose exams. It is also possible to combine these various noise-reduction methods to achieve higher quality images at lower doses [55] though the exact combinations and potential compound benefits have yet to be described.

Dual energy CT is perhaps the latest major development in CT scanner technology that is commercially available. Images are acquired simultaneously or near-simultaneously at two energy levels (most commonly 80 and 140 kVp) which can be analyzed to provide information about tissue composition and improve detection of iodine containing substances. The use of dual energy CT in bowel imaging remains relatively uninvestigated. Low kVp images display greater density of contrast agent than standard images [63] and therefore 80 kVp images obtained at dual energy CT may be more helpful for low does enterography protocols [62]. Aside from dose reduction, dual energy CT has the theoretical potential for quantifying the degree of enhancement of the bowel wall. Using dual energy CT, iodine-only images can be obtained that can highlight the degree of mural enhancement. Preliminary studies have used this technique to asses polyp enhancement in phantom model [64] and distinguish mural enhancement from high density intraluminal contrast in animal models [65]. Iodine quantification techniques using dual energy CT have been reported in renal lesions [66] and mediastinal lymph nodes [67]. This suggests a possible role of dual energy CT in quantifying the degree of enhancement as an indicator of inflammation or response to treatment, however, to date there are no studies that have investigated iodine imaging or quantification in CD.

Advances in PET Imaging

While scintigraphy with radiolabeled leukocytes has been considered as an acceptable imaging approach according to the ECCO (European Crohn's and Colitis Organisation) and ESGAR

(European Society of Gastrointestinal and Abdominal Radiology), the potential role of PET-CT is yet to be defined [68]. FDG-PET (Flouro-deoxy-glucose positron emission tomography) is widely used in oncologic imaging where increase in metabolic activity of the tumor leads to increased glucose metabolism which translated into increased FDG update that can be imaged with PET. The increased uptake of FDG in inflammation is recognized as well and is the basis for the use of FDG-PET in imaging of inflammatory bowel disease. The use of PET-CT allows for better localization of the inflamed bowel, which is very important in imaging of CD. The literature supporting the potential role of FDG-PET dates back to the late 1990s [69, 70]. Multiple studies since have demonstrated the ability of PET-CT to identify inflamed small and large bowel [71–75]. In a meta-analysis [76] of seven studies including 219 patients with IBD, the pooled sensitivity was 85 % [95 % confidence interval (CI) 81–88 %], and the pooled specificity was 87 % [95 %CI 84–90 %] for detection of active inflammation. Some of the studies have combined PET with CT enterography showing correlation between area of increased FDG uptake and abnormal segments on CT enterography [77, 78]. Few studies [79, 80] that evaluated the role of PET-CT in delineating the degree of active inflammation versus chronic fibrostenotic strictures found that PET-CT was not reliable in making that distinction. In a small study of seven patients [81], PET was shown to improve therapeutic decisions. In another small study of five patients [82], there was demonstrable decrease in FDG uptake in the affected bowel segments following.

Future developments may focus on new radiopharmaceuticals that can be more specific for inflammation and distinguishing it from normal bowel and from chronic fibrostenotic disease. Technical developments may continue to improve resolution and sensitivity and decrease the radiation dose. Finally, the recent introduction of PET-MR scanners may present an opportunity for a new powerful method of evaluating IBD.

Advances in Ultrasound

Contrast enhanced ultrasound (CEUS) is a relatively new technique for evaluation of bowel wall perfusion in the inflamed bowel segments of patients with CD. Gray scale and color Doppler US are initially performed and an inflamed bowel segment with bowel thickening is selected for further evaluation with CEUS. The segment in question is visualized in real time under US during the IV administration of microbubble contrast agent. The degree and pattern of enhancement of the bowel wall is assessed and has been shown to correlate with disease activity [83, 84]. The enhancement can be further assessed quantitatively using software package installed on the US machine or on separate external workstations. The software can generate brightness-time curve for manually defined regions of interest and different parameters can be calculated from these curves. Most commonly, a threshold brightness value is set to define abnormal versus normal mural enhancement which has been shown to be sensitive for predicting moderate or severe inflammation [85]. Quantitative CEUS is a promising technique to assess disease activity [86, 87] and distinguish inflammation from fibrostenotic lesions [88–90]. The quantitative analysis of enhancement allows for assessment and monitoring of pharmacologic treatment response [91, 92] as well as detection of postoperative recurrence [93].

Another recently described advance in US of CD is US elastography which is a noninvasive method for evaluating tissue stiffness using ultrasound waves. An initial study in CD animal model showed that US elastography can accurately distinguish fibrosis from acutely inflamed bowel [94].

References

1. Sinha R, Rajiah P, Murphy P, Hawker P, Sanders S. Utility of high-resolution MR imaging in demonstrating transmural pathologic changes in Crohn disease. Radiographics. 2009;29(6):1847–67.
2. Sinha R, Murphy P, Sanders S, Ramachandran I, Hawker P, Rawat S, et al. Diagnostic accuracy of

high-resolution MR enterography in Crohn's disease: comparison with surgical and pathological specimen. Clin Radiol. 2013;68(9):917–27.
3. Chang KJ, Kamel IR, Macura KJ, Bluemke DA. 3.0-T MR imaging of the abdomen: comparison with 1.5 T1. Radiographics. 2008;28(7):1983–98.
4. Barth MM, Smith MP, Pedrosa I, Lenkinski RE, Rofsky NM. Body MR imaging at 3.0 T: understanding the opportunities and challenges. Radiographics. 2007;27(5):1445–62.
5. van Gemert-Horsthuis K, Florie J, Hommes DW, Lavini Mphil C, Reitsma JB, van Deventer SJ, et al. Feasibility of evaluating Crohn's disease activity at 3.0 Tesla. J Magn Reson Imaging. 2006;24(2):340–8.
6. Dagia C, Ditchfield M, Kean M, Catto-Smith A. Feasibility of 3-T MRI for the evaluation of Crohn disease in children. Pediatr Radiol. 2010;40(10): 1615–24.
7. Rimola J, Rodriguez S, García-Bosch O, Ordás I, Ayala E, Aceituno M, et al. Magnetic resonance for assessment of disease activity and severity in ileocolonic Crohn's disease. Gut. 2009;58(8):1113–20.
8. Adamek HE, Schantzen W, Rinas U, Goyen M, Ajaj W, Esser C. Ultra-high-field magnetic resonance enterography in the diagnosis of ileitis (neo-)terminalis: a prospective study. J Clin Gastroenterol. 2012;46(4): 311–6.
9. Fiorino G, Bonifacio C, Padrenostro M, Sposta F, Spinelli A, Malesci A, et al. Comparison between 1.5 and 3.0 Tesla magnetic resonance enterography for the assessment of disease activity and complications in ileo-colonic Crohn's disease. Dig Dis Sci. 2013; 58(11):3246–55.
10. Patak MA, von Weymarn C, Froehlich JM. Small bowel MR imaging: 1.5T versus 3T. Magn Reson Imaging Clin N Am. 2007;15(3):383–93.
11. Gonçalves SI, Ziech MLW, Lamerichs R, Stoker J, Nederveen AJ. Optimization of alternating TR-SSFP for fat-suppression in abdominal images at 3T. Magn Reson Med. 2012;67(3):595–600.
12. Zappa M, Stefanescu C, Cazals-Hatem D, Bretagnol F, Deschamps L, Attar A, et al. Which magnetic resonance imaging findings accurately evaluate inflammation in small bowel Crohn's disease? A retrospective comparison with surgical pathologic analysis. Inflamm Bowel Dis. 2011;17(4):984–93.
13. Maccioni F, Bruni A, Viscido A, Colaiacomo MC, Cocco A, Montesani C, et al. MR imaging in patients with Crohn disease: value of T2- versus T1-weighted gadolinium-enhanced MR sequences with use of an oral superparamagnetic contrast agent. Radiology. 2006;238(2):517–30.
14. Low RN, Sebrechts CP, Politoske DA, Bennett MT, Flores S, Snyder RJ, et al. Crohn disease with endoscopic correlation: single-shot fast spin-echo and gadolinium-enhanced fat-suppressed spoiled gradient-echo MR imaging. Radiology. 2002;222(3):652–60.
15. Laghi A, Borrelli O, Paolantonio P, Dito L, de Mesquita MB, Falconieri P, et al. Contrast enhanced magnetic resonance imaging of the terminal ileum in children with Crohn's disease. Gut. 2003;52(3): 393–7.
16. Sempere GAJ, Martinez Sanjuan V, Medina Chulia E, Benages A, Tome Toyosato A, Canelles P, et al. MRI evaluation of inflammatory activity in Crohn's disease. Am J Roentgenol. 2005;184(6):1829–35.
17. Pupillo VA, Di Cesare E, Frieri G, Limbucci N, Tanga M, Masciocchi C. Assessment of inflammatory activity in Crohn's disease by means of dynamic contrast-enhanced MRI. Radiol Med. 2007;112(6):798–809.
18. Del Vescovo R, Sansoni I, Caviglia R, Ribolsi M, Perrone G, Leoncini E, et al. Dynamic contrast enhanced magnetic resonance imaging of the terminal ileum: differentiation of activity of Crohn's disease. Abdom Imaging. 2008;33(4):417–24.
19. Knuesel PR, Kubik RA, Crook DW, Eigenmann F, Froehlich JM. Assessment of dynamic contrast enhancement of the small bowel in active Crohn's disease using 3D MR enterography. Eur J Radiol. 2010; 73(3):607–13.
20. Oto A, Fan X, Mustafi D, Jansen SA, Karczmar GS, Rubin DT, et al. Quantitative analysis of dynamic contrast enhanced MRI for assessment of bowel inflammation in Crohn's disease: pilot study. Acad Radiol. 2009;16(10):1223–30.
21. Horsthuis K, Bipat S, Stokkers PC, Stoker J. Magnetic resonance imaging for evaluation of disease activity in Crohn's disease: a systematic review. Eur Radiol. 2009;19(6):1450–60.
22. Giusti S, Faggioni L, Neri E, Fruzzetti E, Nardini L, Marchi S, et al. Dynamic MRI of the small bowel: usefulness of quantitative contrast-enhancement parameters and time-signal intensity curves for differentiating between active and inactive Crohn's disease. Abdom Imaging. 2010;35(6):646–53.
23. Röttgen R, Grandke T, Grieser C, Lehmkuhl L, Hamm B, Lüdemann L. Measurement of MRI enhancement kinetics for evaluation of inflammatory activity in Crohn's disease. Clin Imaging. 2010;34(1):29–35.
24. Ziech MLW, Lavini C, Caan MWA, Nio CY, Stokkers PCF, Bipat S, et al. Dynamic contrast-enhanced MRI in patients with luminal Crohn's disease. Eur J Radiol. 2012;81(11):3019–27.
25. Oto A, Kayhan A, Williams JTB, Fan X, Yun L, Arkani S, et al. Active Crohn's disease in the small bowel: evaluation by diffusion weighted imaging and quantitative dynamic contrast enhanced MR imaging. J Magn Reson Imaging. 2011;33(3):615–24.
26. Oto A, Zhu F, Kulkarni K, Karczmar GS, Turner JR, Rubin D. Evaluation of diffusion-weighted MR imaging for detection of bowel inflammation in patients with Crohn's disease. Acad Radiol. 2009;16(5): 597–603.
27. Kiryu S, Dodanuki K, Takao H, Watanabe M, Inoue Y, Takazoe M, et al. Free-breathing diffusion-weighted imaging for the assessment of inflammatory activity in Crohn's disease. J Magn Reson Imaging. 2009;29(4):880–6.

28. Hordonneau C, Buisson A, Scanzi J, Goutorbe F, Pereira B, Borderon C, et al. Diffusion-weighted magnetic resonance imaging in ileocolonic Crohn's disease: validation of quantitative index of activity. Am J Gastroenterol. 2014;109(1):89–98.
29. Cakmakci E, Erturk SM, Cakmakci S, Bayram A, Tokgoz S, Caliskan KC, et al. Comparison of the results of computerized tomographic and diffusion-weighted magnetic resonance imaging techniques in inflammatory bowel diseases. Quant Imaging Med Surg. 2013;3(6):327–33.
30. Ream J, Dillman J, Adler J, Khalatbari S, McHugh J, Strouse P, et al. MRI diffusion-weighted imaging (DWI) in pediatric small bowel Crohn disease: correlation with MRI findings of active bowel wall inflammation. Pediatr Radiol. 2013;43(9):1077–85.
31. Neubauer H, Pabst T, Dick A, Machann W, Evangelista L, Wirth C, et al. Small-bowel MRI in children and young adults with Crohn disease: retrospective head-to-head comparison of contrast-enhanced and diffusion-weighted MRI. Pediatr Radiol. 2013;43(1): 103–14.
32. Froehlich JM, Waldherr C, Stoupis C, Erturk SM, Patak MA. MR motility imaging in Crohn's disease improves lesion detection compared with standard MR imaging. Eur Radiol. 2010;20(8):1945–51.
33. Kitazume Y, Satoh S, Hosoi H, Noguchi O, Shibuya H. Cine magnetic resonance imaging evaluation of peristalsis of small bowel with longitudinal ulcer in Crohn disease: preliminary results. J Comput Assist Tomogr. 2007;31(6):876–83.
34. Odille F, Menys A, Ahmed A, Punwani S, Taylor SA, Atkinson D. Quantitative assessment of small bowel motility by nonrigid registration of dynamic MR images. Magn Reson Med. 2012;68(3):783–93.
35. Menys A, Atkinson D, Odille F, Ahmed A, Novelli M, Rodriguez-Justo M, et al. Quantified terminal ileal motility during MR enterography as a potential biomarker of Crohn's disease activity: a preliminary study. Eur Radiol. 2012;22(11):2494–501.
36. Bickelhaupt S, Froehlich JM, Cattin R, Raible S, Bouquet H, Bill U, et al. Software-assisted small bowel motility analysis using free-breathing MRI: feasibility study. J Magn Reson Imaging. 2014;39(1): 17–23.
37. Menys A, Helbren E, Makanyanga J, Emmanuel A, Forbes A, Windsor A, et al. Small bowel strictures in Crohn's disease: a quantitative investigation of intestinal motility using MR enterography. Neurogastroenterol Motil. 2013;25(12):967–e775.
38. Cullmann JL, Bickelhaupt S, Froehlich JM, Szucs-Farkas Z, Tutuian R, Patuto N, et al. MR imaging in Crohn's disease: correlation of MR motility measurement with histopathology in the terminal ileum. Neurogastroenterol Motil. 2013;25(9): 749–e577.
39. Menys A, Plumb A, Atkinson D, Taylor SA. The challenge of segmental small bowel motility quantitation using MR enterography. Br J Radiol. 2014;87(1040): 20140330.
40. Wakamiya M, Furukawa A, Kanasaki S, Murata K. Assessment of small bowel motility function with cine-MRI using balanced steady-state free precession sequence. J Magn Reson Imaging. 2011;33(5): 1235–40.
41. Bickelhaupt S, Froehlich JM, Cattin R, Patuto N, Tutuian R, Wentz KU, et al. Differentiation between active and chronic Crohn's disease using MRI small-bowel motility examinations—initial experience. Clin Radiol. 2013;68(12):1247–53.
42. Menys A, Taylor SA, Emmanuel A, Ahmed A, Plumb AA, Odille F, et al. Global small bowel motility: assessment with dynamic MR imaging. Radiology. 2013;269(2):443–50.
43. Farghal A, Kasmai B, Malcolm PN, Graves MJ, Toms AP. Developing a new measure of small bowel peristalsis with dynamic MR: a proof of concept study. Acta Radiol. 2012;53(6):593–600.
44. van der Paardt MP, Sprengers AMJ, Zijta FM, Lamerichs R, Nederveen AJ, Stoker J. Noninvasive automated motion assessment of intestinal motility by continuously tagged MR imaging. J Magn Reson Imaging. 2014;39(1):9–16.
45. Sprengers AMJ, van der Paardt MP, Zijta FM, Caan MWA, Lamerichs RM, Nederveen AJ, et al. Use of continuously MR tagged imaging for automated motion assessment in the abdomen: a feasibility study. J Magn Reson Imaging. 2012;36(2):492–7.
46. Bickelhaupt S, Pazahr S, Chuck N, Blume I, Froehlich JM, Cattin R, et al. Crohn's disease: small bowel motility impairment correlates with inflammatory-related markers C-reactive protein and calprotectin. Neurogastroenterol Motil. 2013;25(6):467–e363.
47. Hamy V, Menys A, Helbren E, Odille F, Punwani S, Taylor S, et al. Respiratory motion correction in dynamic-MRI: application to small bowel motility quantification during free breathin. Med Image Comput Comput Assist Interv. 2013;16(Pt 2):132–40.
48. Al-Hawary M, Zimmermann EM. A new look at Crohn's disease: novel imaging techniques. Curr Opin Gastroenterol. 2012;28(4):334–40.
49. Adler J, Swanson SD, Schmiedlin-Ren P, Higgins PDR, Golembeski CP, Polydorides AD, et al. Magnetization transfer helps detect intestinal fibrosis in an animal model of Crohn disease. Radiology. 2011;259(1):127–35.
50. Pazahr S, Blume I, Frei P, Chuck N, Nanz D, Rogler G, et al. Magnetization transfer for the assessment of bowel fibrosis in patients with Crohn's disease: initial experience. MAGMA. 2013;26(3):291–301.
51. Palmer L, Herfarth H, Porter CQ, Fordham LA, Sandler RS, Kappelman MD. Diagnostic ionizing radiation exposure in a population-based sample of children with inflammatory bowel diseases. Am J Gastroenterol. 2009;104(11):2816–23.
52. Jaffe TA, Gaca AM, Delaney S, Yoshizumi TT, Toncheva G, Nguyen G, et al. Radiation doses from small-bowel follow-through and abdominopelvic MDCT in Crohn's disease. Am J Roentgenol. 2007; 189(5):1015–22.

53. Desmond AN, O'Regan K, Curran C, McWilliams S, Fitzgerald T, Maher MM, et al. Crohn's disease: factors associated with exposure to high levels of diagnostic radiation. Gut. 2008;57(11):1524–9.
54. McCollough CH, Primak AN, Braun N, Kofler J, Yu L, Christner J. Strategies for reducing radiation dose in CT. Radiol Clin North Am. 2009;47(1):27–40.
55. Del Gaizo AJ, Fletcher JG, Yu L, Paden RG, Spencer GC, Leng S, et al. Reducing radiation dose in CT enterography. Radiographics. 2013;33(4):1109–24.
56. Nakayama Y, Awai K, Funama Y, Hatemura M, Imuta M, Nakaura T, et al. Abdominal CT with low tube voltage: preliminary observations about radiation dose, contrast enhancement, image quality, and noise. Radiology. 2005;237(3):945–51.
57. Funama Y, Awai K, Nakayama Y, Kakei K, Nagasue N, Shimamura M, et al. Radiation dose reduction without degradation of low-contrast detectability at abdominal multisection CT with a low-tube voltage technique: phantom study. Radiology. 2005;237(3): 905–10.
58. Kambadakone AR, Chaudhary NA, Desai GS, Nguyen DD, Kulkarni NM, Sahani DV. Low-dose MDCT and CT enterography of patients with Crohn disease: feasibility of adaptive statistical iterative reconstruction. Am J Roentgenol. 2011;196(6): W743–52.
59. Kaza RK, Platt JF, Al-Hawary MM, Wasnik A, Liu PS, Pandya A. CT enterography at 80 kVp with adaptive statistical iterative reconstruction versus at 120 kVp with standard reconstruction: image quality, diagnostic adequacy, and dose reduction. Am J Roentgenol. 2012;198(5):1084–92.
60. Johnson E, Megibow A, Wehrli N, O'Donnell T, Chandarana H. CT enterography at 100 kVp with iterative reconstruction compared to 120 kVp filtered back projection: evaluation of image quality and radiation dose in the same patients. Abdom Imaging. 2014;39:1255–60.
61. O'Neill S, Mc Laughlin P, Crush L, O'Connor O, Mc Williams S, Craig O, et al. A prospective feasibility study of sub-millisievert abdominopelvic CT using iterative reconstruction in Crohn's disease. Eur Radiol. 2013;23(9):2503–12.
62. Guimarães LS, Fletcher JG, Yu L, Huprich JE, Fidler JL, Manduca A, et al. Feasibility of dose reduction using novel denoising techniques for low kV (80 kV) CT enterography: optimization and validation. Acad Radiol. 2010;17(10):1203–10.
63. Graser A, Johnson TR, Chandarana H, Macari M. Dual energy CT: preliminary observations and potential clinical applications in the abdomen. Eur Radiol. 2009;19(1):13–23.
64. Qu M, Ehman E, Fletcher JG, Huprich JE, Hara AK, Silva AC, et al. Toward biphasic computed tomography (CT) enteric contrast: material classification of luminal bismuth and mural iodine in a small-bowel phantom using dual-energy CT. J Comput Assist Tomogr. 2012;36(5):554–9.
65. Mongan J, Rathnayake S, Fu Y, Wang R, Jones EF, Gao D-W, et al. In vivo differentiation of complementary contrast media at dual-energy CT. Radiology. 2012;265(1):267–72.
66. Mileto A, Marin D, Alfaro-Cordoba M, Ramirez-Giraldo JC, Eusemann CD, Scribano E, et al. Iodine quantification to distinguish clear cell from papillary renal cell carcinoma at dual-energy multidetector CT: a multireader diagnostic performance study. Radiology. 2014;273(3):813–20.
67. Baxa J, Vondráková A, Matoušková T, Růžičková O, Schmidt B, Flohr T, et al. Dual-phase dual-energy CT in patients with lung cancer: assessment of the additional value of iodine quantification in lymph node therapy response. Eur Radiol. 2014;24(8):1981–8.
68. Panes J, Bouhnik Y, Reinisch W, Stoker J, Taylor SA, Baumgart DC, et al. Imaging techniques for assessment of inflammatory bowel disease: joint ECCO and ESGAR evidence-based consensus guidelines. J Crohns Colitis. 2013;7(7):556–85.
69. Bicik I, Bauerfeind P, Breitbach T, von Schulthess GK, Fried M. Inflammatory bowel disease activity measured by positron-emission tomography. Lancet. 1997;350(9073):262.
70. Skehan SJ, Issenman R, Mernagh J, Nahmias C, Jacobson K. 18 F-fluorodeoxyglucose positron tomography in diagnosis of paediatric inflammatory bowel disease. Lancet. 1999;354(9181):836–7.
71. Neurath MF, Vehling D, Schunk K, Holtmann M, Brockmann H, Helisch A, et al. Noninvasive assessment of Crohn's disease activity: a comparison of 18 F-fluorodeoxyglucose positron emission tomography, hydromagnetic resonance imaging, and granulocyte scintigraphy with labeled antibodies. Am J Gastroenterol. 2002;97(8):1978–85.
72. Lemberg DA, Issenman RM, Cawdron R, Green T, Mernagh J, Skehan SJ, et al. Positron emission tomography in the investigation of pediatric inflammatory bowel disease. Inflamm Bowel Dis. 2005;11(8): 733–8.
73. Louis E, Ancion G, Colard A, Spote V, Belaiche J, Hustinx R. Noninvasive assessment of Crohn's disease intestinal lesions with 18 F-FDG PET/CT. J Nucl Med. 2007;48(7):1053–9.
74. Däbritz J, Jasper N, Loeffler M, Weckesser M, Foell D. Noninvasive assessment of pediatric inflammatory bowel disease with 18 F-fluorodeoxyglucose-positron emission tomography and computed tomography. Eur J Gastroenterol Hepatol. 2011;23(1):81–9. doi:10.1097/MEG.0b013e3283410222.
75. Holtmann M, Uenzen M, Helisch A, Dahmen A, Mudter J, Goetz M, et al. 18 F-fluorodeoxyglucose positron-emission tomography (PET) can be used to assess inflammation non-invasively in Crohn's disease. Dig Dis Sci. 2012;57(10):2658–68.
76. Treglia G, Quartuccio N, Sadeghi R, Farchione A, Caldarella C, Bertagna F, et al. Diagnostic performance of fluorine-18-fluorodeoxyglucose positron emission tomography in patients with chronic inflammatory

bowel disease: a systematic review and a meta-analysis. J Crohns Colitis. 2013;7(5):345–54.

77. Groshar D, Bernstine H, Stern D, Sosna J, Eligalashvili M, Gurbuz EG, et al. PET/CT enterography in Crohn disease: correlation of disease activity on CT enterography with 18 F-FDG uptake. J Nucl Med. 2010; 51(7):1009–14.
78. Ahmadi A, Li Q, Muller K, Collins D, Valentine JF, Drane W, et al. Diagnostic value of noninvasive combined fluorine-18 labeled fluoro-2-deoxy-D-glucose positron emission tomography and computed tomography enterography in active Crohn's disease. Inflamm Bowel Dis. 2010;16(6):974–81. doi:10.1002/ibd.21153.
79. Jacene HA, Ginsburg P, Kwon J, Nguyen GC, Montgomery EA, Bayless TM, et al. Prediction of the need for surgical intervention in obstructive Crohn's disease by 18 F-FDG PET/CT. J Nucl Med. 2009;50(11):1751–9.
80. Lenze F, Wessling J, Bremer J, Ullerich H, Spieker T, Weckesser M, et al. Detection and differentiation of inflammatory versus fibromatous Crohn's disease strictures: prospective comparison of 18 F-FDG-PET/CT, MR-enteroclysis, and transabdominal ultrasound versus endoscopic/histologic evaluation. Inflamm Bowel Dis. 2012;18(12):2252–60. doi:10.1002/ibd.22930.
81. Lapp R, Spier B, Perlman S, Jaskowiak C, Reichelderfer M. Clinical utility of positron emission tomography/computed tomography in inflammatory bowel disease. Mol Imaging Biol. 2011;13(3):573–6.
82. Spier B, Perlman S, Jaskowiak C, Reichelderfer M. PET/CT in the evaluation of inflammatory bowel disease: studies in patients before and after treatment. Mol Imaging Biol. 2010;12(1):85–8.
83. Serra C, Menozzi G, Labate AMM, Giangregorio F, Gionchetti P, Beltrami M, et al. Ultrasound assessment of vascularization of the thickened terminal ileum wall in Crohn's disease patients using a low-mechanical index real-time scanning technique with a second generation ultrasound contrast agent. Eur J Radiol. 2007;62(1):114–21.
84. Migaleddu V, Scanu AM, Quaia E, Rocca PC, Dore MP, Scanu D, et al. Contrast-enhanced ultrasonographic evaluation of inflammatory activity in Crohn's disease. Gastroenterology. 2009;137(1):43–52.
85. Ripollés T, Martínez MJ, Paredes JM, Blanc E, Flors L, Delgado F. Crohn disease: correlation of findings at contrast-enhanced US with severity at endoscopy. Radiology. 2009;253(1):241–8.
86. Romanini L, Passamonti M, Navarria M, Lanzarotto F, Villanacci V, Grazioli L, et al. Quantitative analysis of contrast-enhanced ultrasonography of the bowel wall can predict disease activity in inflammatory bowel disease. Eur J Radiol. 2014;83(8):1317–23.
87. De Franco A, Di Veronica A, Armuzzi A, Roberto I, Marzo M, De Pascalis B, et al. Ileal Crohn disease: mural microvascularity quantified with contrast-enhanced US correlates with disease activity. Radiology. 2012;262(2):680–8.
88. Ripollés T, Rausell N, Paredes JM, Grau E, Martínez MJ, Vizuete J. Effectiveness of contrast-enhanced ultrasound for characterisation of intestinal inflammation in Crohn's disease: a comparison with surgical histopathology analysis. J Crohns Colitis. 2013;7(2): 120–8.
89. Quaia E, De Paoli L, Stocca T, Cabibbo B, Casagrande F, Cova MA. The value of small bowel wall contrast enhancement after sulfur hexafluoride-filled microbubble injection to differentiate inflammatory from fibrotic strictures in patients with Crohn's disease. Ultrasound Med Biol. 2012;38(8):1324–32.
90. Nylund K, Jirik R, Mezl M, Leh S, Hausken T, Pfeffer F, et al. Quantitative contrast-enhanced ultrasound comparison between inflammatory and fibrotic lesions in patients with Crohn's disease. Ultrasound Med Biol. 2013;39(7):1197–206.
91. Quaia E, Migaleddu V, Baratella E, Pizzolato R, Rossi A, Grotto M, et al. The diagnostic value of small bowel wall vascularity after sulfur hexafluoride-filled microbubble injection in patients with Crohn's disease. Correlation with the therapeutic effectiveness of specific anti-inflammatory treatment. Eur J Radiol. 2009;69(3):438–44.
92. Quaia E, Cabibbo B, De Paoli L, Toscano W, Poillucci G, Cova M. The value of time-intensity curves obtained after microbubble contrast agent injection to discriminate responders from non-responders to anti-inflammatory medication among patients with Crohn's disease. Eur Radiol. 2013;23(6):1650–9.
93. Paredes JM, Ripollés T, Cortés X, Moreno N, Martínez MJ, Bustamante-Balén M, et al. Contrast-enhanced ultrasonography: usefulness in the assessment of postoperative recurrence of Crohn's disease. J Crohns Colitis. 2013;7(3):192–201.
94. Dillman JR, Stidham RW, Higgins PDR, Moons DS, Johnson LA, Rubin JM. US elastography-derived shear wave velocity helps distinguish acutely inflamed from fibrotic bowel in a Crohn disease animal model. Radiology. 2013;267(3):757–66.

10 Surgery: Small Intestine Terminal Ileum—Resection

S.K. Sharma and J.W. Milsom

Introduction

Patients and medical doctors often perceive Crohn's Disease (CD) surgery as a management "last resort"—i.e., a potentially dangerous outcome only to be contemplated "when all else fails." Terminal Ileal (TI) disease, however, most often coupled with limited disease involving the cecum (ileocecal disease) represents a particular manifestation of CD that solicits a rethinking of this principle. The primary reasons that early surgical therapy should often be considered are: (1) the vast majority of CD patients, regardless of treatment, will require at least one surgical resection during their lifetime, (2) the ultimate development of a short bowel syndrome following CD surgery is extremely unlikely, and (3) surgery achieves quick resolution of symptoms and reduced rates of recurrence with a high safety and low cost profile, especially when compared to a lifetime of immunomodulatory medical therapy [1, 2].

This chapter will examine the key factors that influence surgery for Terminal Ileal Crohn's Disease (TICD), the surgical techniques that are available to the surgeon currently, how to avoid common pitfalls, and sets the stage for a rethinking of our surgical approaches (resection and strictureplasty) that shifts the current mindset of TICD management to an increasingly less invasive, more cost-effective one.

Overview of CD and Surgery

Despite the relatively recent expansion in our knowledge of CD pathophysiology, its definitive cause remains elusive. Population studies and basic science research indicate that CD is likely to be caused by a constellation of familial risk factors, genetic susceptibility loci (as identified by Genome Wide Association Studies [GWAS]), environmental factors including changes to the microbiome, and a dysregulated immunobiological response. CD remains a chronic, relapsing, remitting disease of the alimentary tract with extraintestinal manifestations and to date, no cure.

The symptoms and signs related to TI CD are numerous, invariably including the triad of weight loss, abdominal pain, and diarrhea. Differentiating factors in management relate to formation of strictures (with obstruction), fistulae, abscesses, and bleeding. Surgical intervention, whilst usually inferring resection, should strive to eliminate these problems with an overarching principle of "bowel preservation."

CD patients have lifetime likelihood for surgery of 70–90 % [2, 3]. Fifty percent of CD

S.K. Sharma, MD • J.W. Milsom, MD (✉)
Minimally Invasive New Technologies, Section of Colon and Rectal Surgery, Center for Advanced Digestive Care, Weill Cornell Medical College, New York Presbyterian Hospital, New York, NY 10065, USA
e-mail: sksharma14@gmail.com; mim2035@med.cornell.edu

A. Fichera and M.K. Krane (eds.), *Crohn's Disease: Basic Principles*,
DOI 10.1007/978-3-319-14181-7_10, © Springer International Publishing Switzerland 2015

patients will undergo bowel resection within 10 years of diagnosis [4]. Seventy percent of CD patients undergo a second operation following the first within 10 years [5]. Only 10 % of patients have prolonged clinical remission. Nonetheless, the life expectancy of a CD patient is only minimally reduced compared to the normal population.

Whereas CD can affect any part of the gastrointestinal tract from the mouth to the anus, the TI and cecum are the most commonly affected areas. The disease is limited to the TI in 25 % of CD patients [6]. In the past two decades, there has been a rapid expansion in the use of biological agents to manage CD, despite this, for localized symptomatic ileocecal disease, surgery may be considered a viable first-line alternative to medical therapy [7]. In this context, for unknown reasons, worldwide incidence and rates of IBD are increasing, particularly in developing countries [8, 9].

Terminal Ileum (TI)

The TI is the terminal portion of small intestine and connects to cecum, and is often defined as the small intestine's latter half. In addition to its general absorptive functions, this region specifically acts to resorb vitamin B12 and bile salts. As a consequence, surgery to remove the TI may affect these functions. Most experts in managing patients with CD believe that removal of more than 100 cm of ileum is required before malabsorption of B12 and bile salts begins to occur, however bile salt absorption dysfunction has been reported in as little as 10 cm resection [10].

Diagnosis

The diagnosis of CD is based on specific criteria according to specific guidelines [11]. A spectrum of signs and symptoms will be present on initial patient contact based on the classical triad of abdominal pain, weight loss, and diarrhea, and biopsies should be pursued through endoscopic means to confirm the diagnosis.

A thorough medical history is recommended, followed by a complete physical examination and early involvement of the multidisciplinary team, including the primary care doctor, then gastroenterologist, nutritionist, and surgeon when the disease is considered significant.

Investigations

Relevant investigations will be guided by the initial presentation, but will likely involve blood tests including inflammatory markers (usually CRP, ESR, and the Prometheus testing), stool microscopy, and endoscopic (upper and lower) examination with biopsies. Tuberculosis can be ruled out by appropriate blood or skin testing, and it should be borne in mind, particularly if a patient does not respond well to treatment. Ileal lymphomas may masquerade as a "Crohn's-like" inflammatory mass in the terminal ileum. Histopathological analysis of biopsies from affected segments may reveal architectural abnormalities and inflammation, but most often are not diagnostic for CD. Photodocumentation (particularly via flexible endoscopy) is important, especially for longitudunal disease course and pattern monitoring.

Radiographic imaging studies may be of particular use, especially in cases of suspected obstruction, and plain abdominal radiographs with contrast may reveal the stenotic segment(s). CT and MRI enterography may also be performed to reveal additional information as required. Phenotypical classification of the disease is undertaken according to the Montreal system, denoting the patient age, affected anatomical location (L-category), the stricturing or penetrating nature of the disease (B-category), and extraintestinal manifestations exhibited by the patient [12].

Initial Non-surgical Management of CD

The treatment of Crohn's disease aims to achieve sustained clinical and endoscopic remission (mucosal healing) and to interrupt the progressive destructive disease course that culminates in intestinal failure and associated complications. Lifestyle modifications should be instigated at the earliest possible juncture, in particular tobacco smoking cessation.

Medical Therapy

The medical therapy initiated at the time of diagnosis will depend on the phenotype, disease activity, and comorbidities. Medications likely to be initiated are likely to be the synthetic thiopurines and anti-tumor necrosis factor (TNF) agents. Glucocorticoids are usually reserved for acute small bowel obstruction, and are otherwise avoided in the practice of most gastroenterologists.

During the past three decades, the question of whether IBD medications (particularly biological agents) use has decreased the need for surgery has been seen as controversial. Some studies have reported on a decrease in surgery over time that has been paralleled by an increase in thiopurines and anti-TNF-α medication usage. Concurrently, topical steroid use and oral steroid use has been decreasing. When compared to patients whom had never used medication, only the instigation of azathioprine within the first 3 months of diagnosis reduced risk of surgery. In a separate analysis, the use of long-term oral steroids significantly reduced the need for surgery. In addition, overall no convincing surgery sparing effect of medications was found in a large nationwide cohort study from Denmark [13].

Whereas some groups conclude initiating treatment early reduces rates of surgery, a recent study observed that thiopurine use in CD had doubled in the past 20 years whereas surgery rates fell by one-third. They surmised that thiopurine therapy reduced the risk of surgery; however, early initiation of therapy offered no benefit, so there remains controversy about whether any medication has yet obviated the eventual need for surgical intervention, albeit there may be a postponement [14–18]. Very few data exists comparing medical and surgical treatment for TICD. However, early ileal resection has been shown to result in less future surgeries and less use of medication [19, 20]. When compared to the average lifetime cost of anti-TNF treatment of $24,000–48,000 in the US (wholesale excluding direct and indirect costs) [21], it behoves all surgeons caring for CD patients to partake in an early discussion about when surgical therapy may be appropriate for a patient with TI disease.

Surgical Treatment

Overview

The primary principle of small intestinal CD surgery is to restore function whilst preserving intestinal length. There has been a clear shift over the past several decades away from radical resection, i.e. achieving inflammation-free microscopic margins of resection, to that of minimal surgery intended to remove grossly affected tissue or performing bowel preserving strictureplasty [22]. Resection of grossly diseased segment remains the most common procedure performed in both pediatric and adult populations. Stricturoplasty is an option in select cases, especially in reoperative surgery, as we will discuss later.

Surgical Indications

Failure of Medical Treatment

Symptomatic disease refractory to medical therapy is the most common reason to consider surgical management of TI CD. We use the general principle that "failure of medical management" means:

- No improvement on optimal medical management, or
- Improvement with moderate to severe side-effects of the CD medications, over approximately 6–12 months of consistent treatment
- All of this should be under the guidance of a gastroenterologist who is expert in treatment of CD patients.

Intractable symptoms and manifestations of chronic disease, such as anemia or growth retardation can be included in a constellation of clinical entities that may comprise this group.

Bowel Obstruction

The TI's lumen naturally narrows upon insertion into the cecum, thus inflammatory stricturing at this site may rapidly lead to symptomatic obstruction of varying degrees of severity, culminating in complete blockade, affecting up to 54 % of CD patients [23, 24]. Nearly always, the acute obstructive episode can be managed effectively without surgery, then an elective procedure can be considered.

Fistulae or Abscess

Intraabdominal abscess occurs in 12–28 % of patients with CD. They may be treated medically or with radiologically placed percutaneous drainage catheters. This may provide a temporizing solution for definitive interval surgery. Intermesenteric or intraperitoneal abscess rupture is an indication for emergent surgery after a period of appropriate resuscitation [25].

Fistulae may emanate from the TI to join nearby viscera, including adjacent loops of small or large bowel, bladder, female reproductive organs, retroperitoneal structures including the psoas muscle, or anterolaterally to the skin.

Bowel Perforation

In rare instances, perforation of the bowel can occur, usually within the dilated section of bowel just proximal to a stenotic segment. In these cases, an assessment of patient condition and level of contamination will be mandatory for judgement of stoma formation and interval anastomosis versus a primary procedure, but emergent surgical intervention is mandatory [26].

Ureteral Obstruction

Obstruction of the ureter secondary to CD is another rare, but well-described complication (5–25 % of cases). Inflammation, abscess compression, and secondary fibrosis can all contribute to this presentation. Removal of the offending causative CD issue usually results in resolution of the ureteral obstruction [27].

Major Hemorrhage

Significant acute hemorrhage (urgent need to transfuse two or more units of packed red blood cells) secondary to TICD would be a rare complication and is associated with significant morbidity and some risk of mortality. If the degree of hemorrhage warranted surgical treatment, urgent endoscopy and possibly angiography should be considered to isolate the bleeding location. Pitressin may be infused intravenously or via a mesenteric arterial catheter to control the bleeding in extreme situations [28, 29].

Malignancy

The risk of TICD patients developing a small bowel malignancy is significantly higher than for the general population. One study reported 67 % of CD associated cancers occur in the TI (versus 20–30 % in the general population). The risk of malignancy is increased if a bowel loop bypass has been formed [30].

It is important to remember that combinations of the aforementioned indications may exist and should always be examined for at the time of operation. Imaging studies may falsely underestimate the extent of disease in at least 30 % of cases [31]. In addition, the presence of proximal or distal disease should be examined for (see complications and pitfalls later).

In the vast majority of cases the procedure will be an elective one, however in some, emergent situations may be evident (details on management later).

Pediatric Cases

Pediatric, including adolescent patients (less than 18 years old) account for 25 % of all cases of CD. The rationale for surgery and its consideration do not differ in this group, although consideration to act earlier may be wise, since surgery may offer the quickest means of restoring nutrition and avoiding the immunosuppressive and growth slowing effects of prolonged intractable CD and its medical therapy.

The most common indication for surgery in this age group is also chronic obstruction related to stricturing disease of the TI and cecum. Growth delay is the most common complication found in this age group. Due to their highly specialized nature, pediatric cases are usually managed in tertiary centers. Intraabdominal limited resection surgery for stricturing disease at the terminal ileum (ileocecal valve) is the most common procedure performed. There is a wide range of reported complications (12–77 %) and recurrence rates (16–94 %) in the literature at a median of 1.8 years follow-up [32].

Preoperative Preparation

Anemia and Electrolyte Imbalance

Those patients with preoperative hemoglobin of less than 8 g/dl would benefit from a blood transfusion (aim to bring Hb to above 9). Fluid imbalance and electrolyte abnormalities should be corrected.

Nutritional Support

Malnutrition is commonplace in CD patients and should be assessed for preoperatively. Severe hypoprotinemia (albumin <2.5 g/Dl) is a reliable indicator of poor healing and so primary anastomosis should be avoided and TPN instigated, ideally 5–7 days preoperatively.

Stoma

The vast majority of patients will not require a stoma for isolated ileal disease. However, if any concerns are raised about the possibility of stoma, particularly if the surgery is urgent or emergent, the patient should be marked for stoma preferably in concert with an enterostomal nurse who works closely with the surgical team.

Peri- and Intra-Operative Medications

Intravenous steroids should be given according to the anesthetist protocol during the procedure, but we generally administer IV steroids in the perioperative period to any patient who has been on steroids for any significant interval (longer than 1–2 weeks) within the previous year before operation. Special care should be taken with postoperative steroid regimes in patients on long-term preoperative steroid therapy (see later).

Intravenous prophylactic antibiotics are given 1 h before the procedure and then at intervals during the procedure if more than 2–3 h, then discontinued unless contamination or infection is discovered, then they are continued for up to a week postoperatively. Our hospital protocol is to use cefoxitin 2 g IV (every 2–3 h during operation) as the drug of choice in patients without penicillin allergies, and to use gentamicin 1 mg/kg and clindamycin 600 mg IV (every 6–8 h) in penicillin allergic patients.

Thromboembolic Prophylaxis

CD patients are at a higher risk for thromboembolic complications than the general population. The European Crohn's and Colitis Organization (ECCO) guidelines, in agreement with the American College of Chest Physician guidelines and the Enhanced Recovery After Surgery (ERAS) Society guidelines recommend that IBD patients who undergo abdominal surgery should wear well-fitting compression stockings, receive intermittent pneumatic compression, and receive pharmacological prophylaxis with low-molecular-weight heparin or unfractionated heparin in the perioperative period [33–36].

Immunosuppressive Medication Considerations

A lack of consensus regarding the impact on postoperative outcomes of preoperative IBD medications allows for no clear guidance on when to discontinue treatment preoperatively or reinstate postoperatively.

A prospective study was recently presented at the Digestive Disease Weekly Conference showing that increased serum levels of infliximab 7 days prior to surgery were associated with increased rates of postoperative complications in CD [37]. However, a recent Canadian investigation concluded that a shorter time interval of surgery from last dose was not associated with increased postoperative complications (2 weeks) [37].

Adrenal suppression occurs with prolonged steroid use (more than 7 days). If suppression persists, exogenous steroid dependence ensues, for this reason steroids must *never* be stopped abruptly and should be tapered gradually (the degree of this depends on the clinical case). If stopped too quickly an Addisonian crisis may develop (shock, decreased mental status, etc.). In the immediate postoperative period steroid dosage should be increased accordingly, and maintained at a high level until the patient is stable in their recovery period.

Psychological Support

As part of the multidisciplinary management of CD, patient's psychological needs should always be considered and managed.

Surgical Technique

Open Versus Laparoscopic

Worldwide, open surgery is likely to be the most common technique performed to treat TI CD, but increasingly, particularly in non-emergent cases, laparoscopic methods are preferred by both patients and surgeons. Laparoscopic assisted methods have been used over several decades, and short-term medical advantages have been seen including quicker recovery period, fewer wound complications, and certainly smaller skin incisions, resulting in a better cosmetic result. Overall the benefits appear to be in the early postoperative period, and no clear long-term benefit related to recurrence rates have been seen for laparoscopic assisted surgical interventions. Thus laparoscopic assisted surgery, in centers with surgeons experienced in this method, should be viewed as the optimal approach to surgical treatment of TI disease [38–41], albeit whatever method seems most safe should be the preferred individual patient approach.

Principles and Strategies to Maximize Operative Success

Patient Setup (Including Incisions and/or Cannula Insertions) (See Fig. 10.1)

The patient should be prepared and draped in a modified lithotomy position with adjustable stirrups. This permits access to the perineum if needed, as we favor having the option of on-table endoscopic examination if needed. For open procedures, we prefer the midline laparotomy incision due to its versatility. For laparoscopic cases we place one umbilical port and 2–4 others depending on the exact site of pathology. Generally, we use a 5 mm port in the left lower quadrant, away from the pathology, for insertion of a compressive energy device. Then we insert 3–5 mm ports in each of the other quadrants for the surgeon's second hand and the assistant. Alternatively, a hand-port may be considered at the Pfannenstiel position to aid dissection.

Exploration/Disease Extension

Once access to the abdominal cavity is obtained, a quadrant-by-quadrant inspection of the abdomen and pelvis is undertaken. We usually start in the right upper quadrant and move clockwise to the left upper quadrant, left lower quadrant, right lower quadrant, and finally the pelvis. Next, the entire length of the small intestine is "run,"

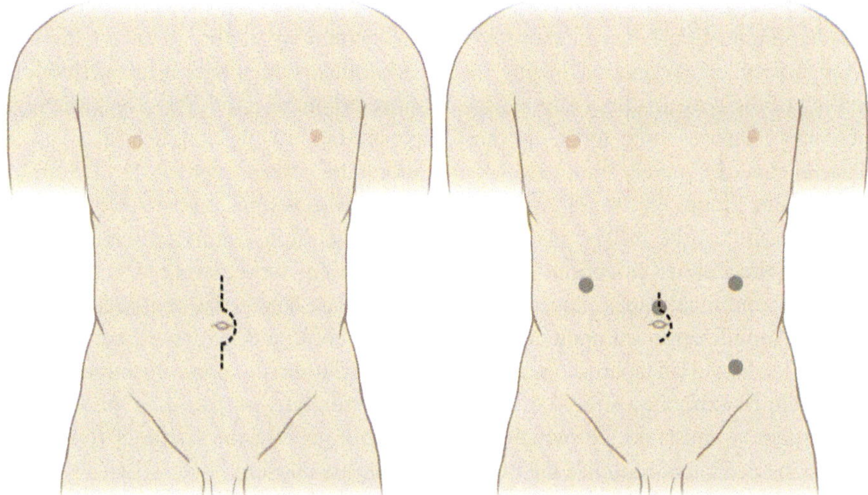

Fig. 10.1 Incisions and port placement for open (*left image*) and laparoscopic (*right image*)

searching for diseased segments, sequelae (such as fistulae and abscesses), fat wrapping, and lymphadenopathy. Photodocumentation of findings should be performed at this time. Disease extension often exceeds that of preoperative investigation, thus the surgeon should anticipate this and, as necessary, seek senior advice. Findings should be accurately documented, photographed, and recorded.

Bowel Preservation

As previously mentioned, there has been a shift in the prevailing attitude to intestinal resection margins from that of radical removal to one of conservation. *Grossly* diseased segments only should be removed and the bowel ends anastomosed should be pliable and free from obvious ulceration, although a few small aphthoid ulcers noted at the anastomotic line should not prompt further resection to "cleaner" margins.

Specific Operative Techniques: Open or Laparoscopic

In this section, we will combine the laparoscopic and open methods in a general description, and point out particular means whereby to utilize laparoscopic methods when relevant. Overall, the principles should be the same!

Resection

The procedure follows three broad steps after thorough exploration: (1) mobilization and resection, (2) anastomosis, and (3) closure. Pitfalls and cautions in each step are highlighted.

Mobilization and Resection

After exploration, the TI should be isolated by tilting the patient with the right side up and moving the proximal small bowel, omentum, and transverse colon away from the disease. We prefer using a compressive energy device such as THUNDERBEAT (Olympus) or Ligasure (Valley Lab), and when laparoscopic methods are used, we generally use the left lower quadrant port (5 mm) for insertion of the energy device to divide mesentery and seal major mesenteric vessels, as well as retroperitoneal or adhesive attachments to the diseased segments.

TICD is frequently associated with matted loops of adjacent small bowel adherent to the diseased TI segment, or with a very dilated small bowel upstream of the disease, filled with intestinal fluid. Matted loops often herald the existence of fistulous communication between those segments. Avoidance of contamination means that gentle handling of the bowel is imperative, especially when using laparoscopic tools, as these 3–5 mm instruments can be very traumatic when grasping a dilated loop of small intestine. Intraluminal contents can be milked proximally and isolated from the planned resection segment, using gently tied umbilical tapes placed at the beginning of the mobilization (in open cases) or after mobilizing the bowel (in laparoscopic cases) through the specimen extraction site.

Next, the surgeon must decide whether to divide the ileocolic pedicle or mobilize the bowel. We usually can isolate the ileocolic pedicle, divide it with the energy device after providing three serial compressions (Fig. 10.2), and proceed with some medial to lateral dissection underneath the terminal ileal and right colon mesentery.

Alternatively, one may go inferior to the TI, mobilize this area, and bring this superiorly away from the retroperitoneum. Usually, the right colon is freed at least up to the hepatic flexure, and in the case of laparoscopy, this mobilization helps to pull the diseased bowel out through the specimen extraction site (periumbilical).

Resection margins should be *minimal*, i.e. avoidance of resecting anything more than gross disease of either side. If only the cecum needs resection on the distal side, this is optimal, since we prefer to avoid laying the new anastomosis anywhere near the duodenum—the more colon resected, the closer the new anastomosis lies to the duodenum. The omentum should be placed over the duodenum to shield it from the new anastomosis (see later). Palpating the bowel along its mesenteric edge assists the surgeon in appreciating diseased and disease free areas. Since we nearly always perform a laparoscopic assisted type of procedure, with the anastomosis done through the specimen extraction site, palpation is invaluable and very feasible whichever method (open or laparoscopic) is chosen.

Once the diseased segment is mobilized, we then draw this upwards through the midline incision (open procedure), or make a 4–7 cm midline incision around the umbilical port and place a wound protective device (e.g., Alexis, Applied Medical, CA, USA—laparoscopic procedure), then draw it outside the abdomen and resect to grossly disease free margins using a GIA-80 mm (Covidien, New Haven, CT, USA), and pass the specimen out of the field (Fig. 10.3). We measure the length of the resected specimen, particularly the length of the small bowel resection, and record this on the operative report. Also the length of the remaining small bowel, if measurable, should be taken and recorded.

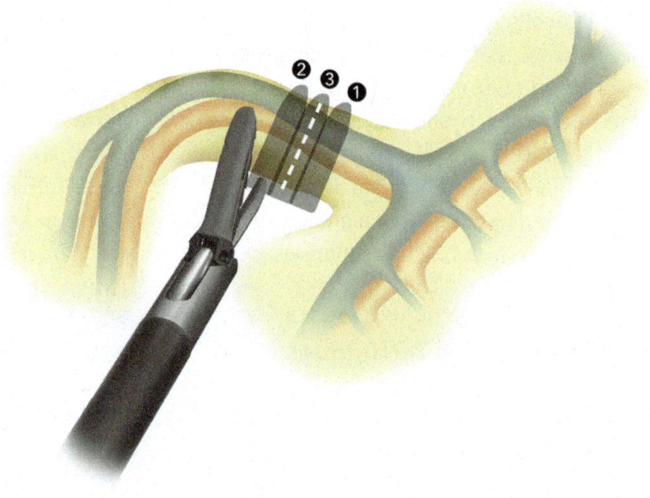

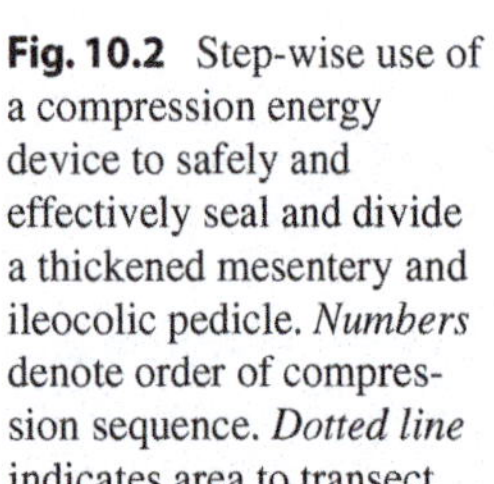

Fig. 10.2 Step-wise use of a compression energy device to safely and effectively seal and divide a thickened mesentery and ileocolic pedicle. *Numbers* denote order of compression sequence. *Dotted line* indicates area to transect

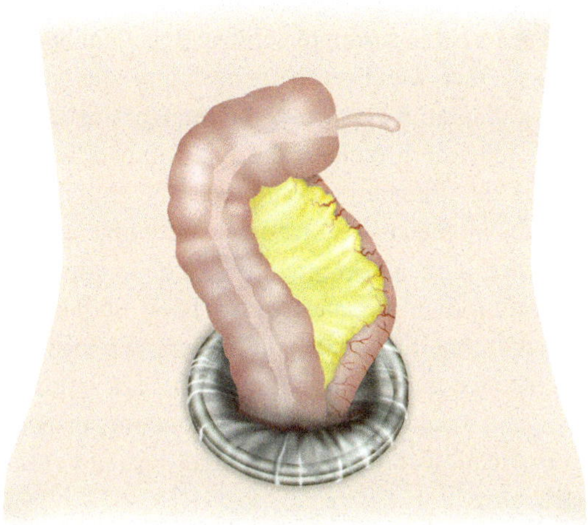

Fig. 10.3 A wound protective device can be used in the umbilical port as the specimen is drawn extracorporeally for resection

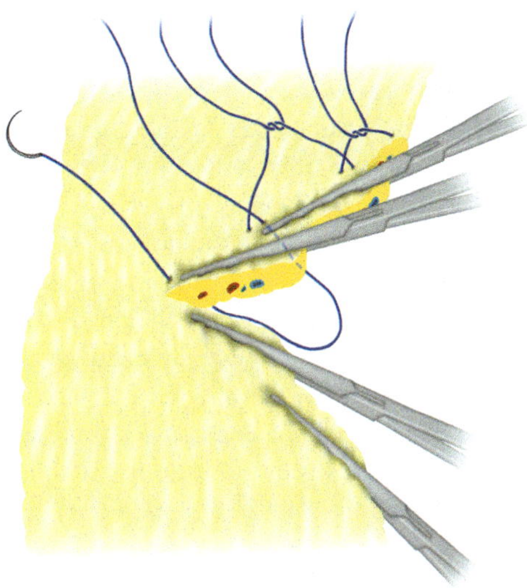

Fig. 10.4 Mesenteric hemorrhage can be minimized during an open operation using overlapping Kocher clamps and 0 or 1-0 horizontal mattress absorbable sutures to control the vascular pedicles and thickened mesentery

Caveats and Pitfalls

1. Be careful to evaluate the true extent of disease, including adherence to significant structures such as the common iliac vessels, gonadal vessels, right ovary and right ureter, at the time of operation. Anticipation avoids structural damage and serious consequences.
2. Be aware that right ureter damage during mobilization is much more likely in CD than other ileal/right colon procedures.
3. Mesenteric hemorrhage during mobilization can occur easily, leading to the dreaded "intramesenteric hematoma." [42] This may be minimized during an open operation using overlapping Kocher clamps and 0 or 1–0 horizontal mattress absorbable sutures to control the vascular pedicles and thickened mesentery (Fig. 10.4). Alternatively, a stepwise use of the compression energy device can safely and effectively seal and divide a thickened mesentery (Fig. 10.2).
4. Stenotic segments other than the surgical can be missed. An inflated Baker tube catheter (Bard medical, Covington Georgia) with its balloon inflated to a 2 cm diameter can be passed intraluminally and passed through the entire length of the small intestine to identify stenotic segments. These may then be either resected or repaired (strictureplasty).

Anastomosis

The core principles of anastomosis should be meticulously adhered to in CD patients, these are: (1) hemostatic control (2) sufficient bowel end blood flow (3) tension free and (4) prevention of bowel torsion.

Anastomotic Segments

The proximal segment of the small bowel anastomotic site should be free of longitudinal ulceration but minor aphthous ulcerations in the lumen of the anastomotic line should not prompt further resection.

The distal large bowel site (rectum, sigmoid, left, and transverse colon) should have been inspected within several months of the operation, and if there is any question the surgeon should be prepared to perform an on-table colonoscopy prior to anastomosis. In our institution we have a colonoscope with CO_2 gas insufflation ready to use during intestinal surgical procedures. The rapid absorption of CO_2 permits the colonoscopy to be performed without concern for prolonged bowel distension since the gas is dissipated within minutes.

Anastomotic Procedure (See Fig. 10.5)

We advocate a stapled functional side-to-side anastomosis, as it is faster, and there are reports that fewer postoperative complications and recurrences have been reported using this method compared to a sutured end-to-side or end-to-end anastomosis (although this is controversial) [43–45]. We use a GIA-80 stapler, and the enterotomy defects can be closed using suturing (3-0 PDS) or stapling techniques (Fig. 10.6). In CD, there seems to be an increased tendency for the enterocolonic staple line to bleed, so we always carefully check it, and oversew the staple line internally (from the luminal side) using a running 3-0 absorbable suture to achieve excellent hemostasis. Once we close the enterotomy site with a linear stapler, we oversew the intersecting staple lines and the crotch of the anastomosis with a series of interrupted sutures. As mentioned above, we then place omentum, if available, over the duodenum and suture it in place, or suture the omentum over the anastomosis itself, in particular shielding it from the duodenum. As a result, if disease recurs, the anastomosis will not immediately be fused to the retroperitoneum, causing complications related to adherence to vital structures.

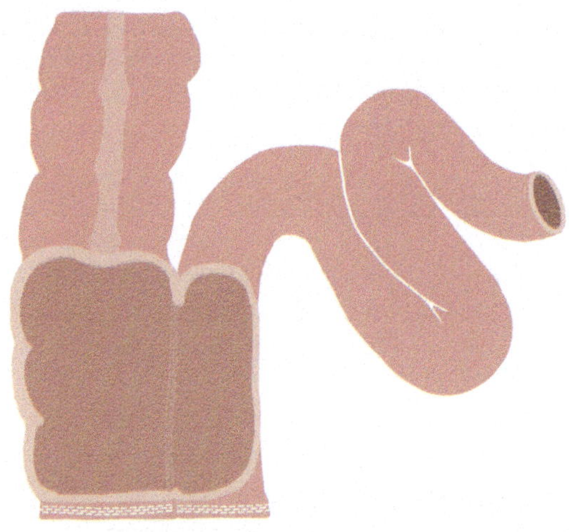

Fig. 10.5 Stapled functional side-to-side anastomosis

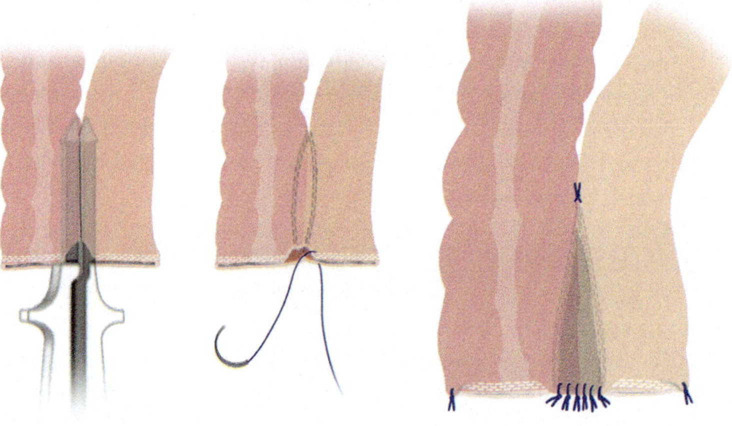

Fig. 10.6 Side-to-side anastomosis: A GIA-80 stapler is used, and the enterotomy defects closed using suturing (3-0 PDS) or stapling techniques. Sutures also be placed at the "trouser crotch" to relieve tension

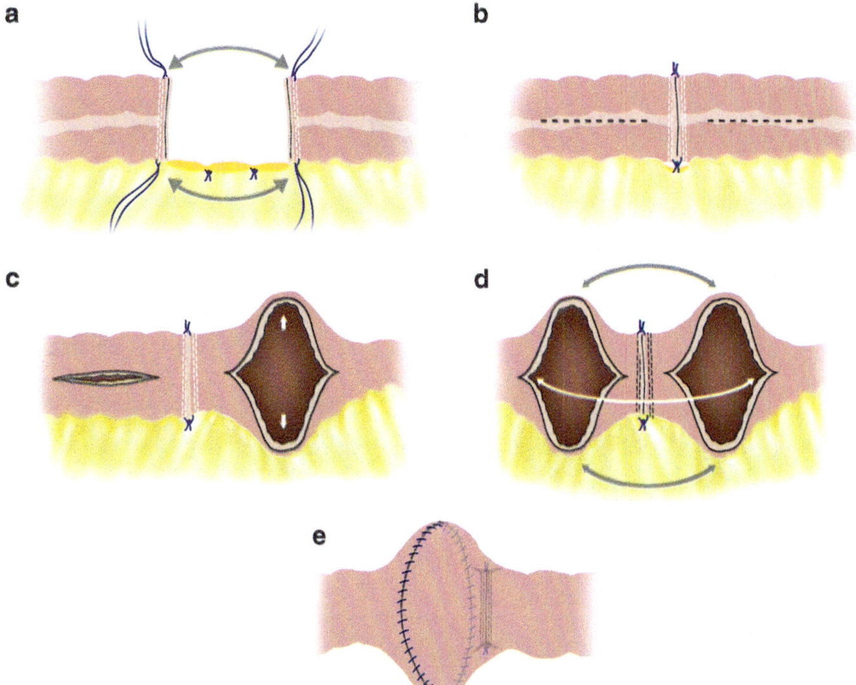

Fig. 10.7 The Kono-S procedure. (**a**) Intestinal segments are divided. Mesentery is preserved. Staple line corners are imbricated and silk sutures are placed and tied. (**b**) The two staple lines are sutured together. (**c**) Longitudunal enterotomies are performed starting no more than 1 cm away from the staple line and extending approximately 7cm. (**d**) The enterotomies are closed transversely with outer layer of 4.0 silk interupted sutures and an inner layer of running 3.0 absorbable suture on the posterior wall. (**e**) Complete anastomosis

Specimen Evaluation and Tissue Procurement

We advocate the evaluation of the specimen prior to operation completion, to ensure complete understanding of the disease process, including the possible presence of a concurrent malignancy. Identification of concerning mucosal changes at this time may be confirmed using frozen section and discussion with a histopathologist. If malignancy is confirmed, an oncologically sound resection should then be performed. If a lymphoma or infectious process is considered, then appropriate touch preps, fresh tissue processing, and cultures may be obtained. Biobanking should also be considered. Also important is the photodocumentation (photo of the gross unopened and opened specimen) at this point, making this a permanent part of the medical record.

Kono-S Anastomotic Procedure (See Fig. 10.7)

A relatively novel anastomotic technique has been developed with the intention of lowering restructuring rates, named the "Kono-S" procedure. The Kono-S is an anti-mesenteric functional end-to-end handsewn anastomosis and in a limited study, 5-year recurrence of CD was less in Kono-S patients than those that had conventional anastomoses [46].

Mesenteric Defect Closure

Closure of the mesenteric defect is not performed if wider than 4-5 fingers. Smaller ones are carefully closed with a 3-0 absorbable running suture.

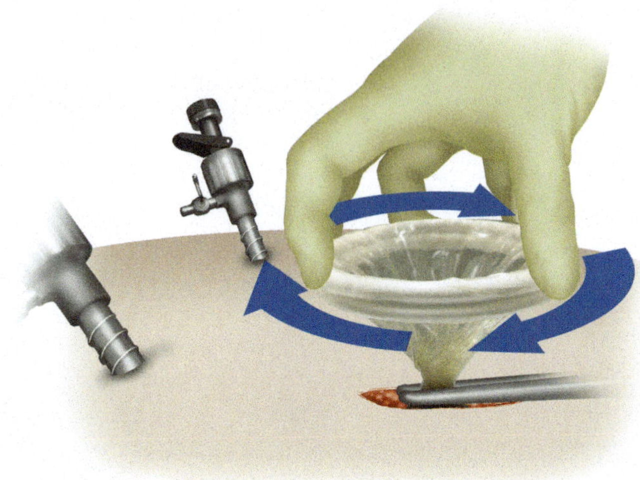

Fig. 10.8 Closure of the umbilical port site by occluding the wound protective device through clockwise rotation and clamping of the retractor neck. This permits a "re-look" after completion of the anastomosis checking for bleeding within the abdominal cavity

Caveats and Pitfalls

1. Avoid placing the anastomosis adjacent to or over the duodenum.
2. Identify and search for stenotic segments upstream.
3. Consider retroperitoneal abscess and treat it.
4. Remove only grossly involved bowel.
5. Have intra-operative endoscopy (with CO_2 insufflation) available.

Final Phase: Closure

Hemostasis should be again evaluated and maintained, looking for intraabdominal clots and at the ileocolic pedicle and mesenteric cut edge. If necessary, we close the umbilical port site by occluding the wound protective device, reinsufflate the abdomen, and relaparoscope the patient to assure hemostasis (Fig. 10.8). Drains may be placed if concurrent septic complications exist, or if a retroperitoneal or pelvic abscess was present. Closed suction drains can be placed into any cavities for up to 2 weeks to allow drainage and irrigation. Laparoscopic and open incisions should be closed according to surgeon training and preference; attention should be paid to the non-traumatic handling of tissues. We will often close the primary skin incision at 2–3 cm intervals but pack the wound with saline soaked gauze for 2–3 days, between the skin sutures, particularly if there is infection or contamination of the surgical site. This seems to lower the incidence of primary wound infection in our experience.

Postoperative Care

The patient is transferred to postoperative nursing unit with routine care instructions. Naso or orogastric tubes are generally removed at the end of the procedure while the patient is still asleep. Antibiotic therapy may need to be continued in the postoperative phase if infectious complications or contamination existed intraoperatively. Glucocorticoid doses may need to be maintained in the immediate postoperative period in those patients with long-standing steroid use. The consequences of an Addisonian crisis may be catastrophic and as such ramping and subsequent tapering regimes of steroids should be clearly prescribed and communicated to the whole team.

Potential Complications

The mortality rate following resection operations for CD approached 2 % in 1980, and likely is below this now, but reports are sparse in the literature [47]. The principal complications are infections (wound and intraabdominal including anastomotic issues), pulmonary problems, adhesive obstruction, and urinary tract infection.

Early Complications

Hemorrhage

Correction of coagulation deficits and hemodynamic maintenance should be first priorities. Use of early endoscopy (colonoscopy) or angiography to identify the bleeding segment may be of use in massive transanal blood loss. Exploration of the abdominal cavity may be the only resort in intraabdominal hemorrhage, and falling blood count in the early postop period should prompt consideration for a rapid return to the operating theater after correction of coagulation deficits.

Sepsis

Abscess formation, wound sepsis, and UTI for the earliest complications of TICD surgery. In such cases, the septic source should be pursued as well as suitable antibiotic regimen instigated. Abscesses can be drained through radiological (CT) guidance or less preferably through operative means.

Late Complications

Fistulae

These are generally either enterocutaneous (EC) or enteroperineal (EP). EC fistulae are commonly associated with technical failure of the anastomosis and are commonly treated conservatively with bowel rest and TPN. Abscesses can be drained percutaneously and through operative approaches. EP fistulae may herald disease recurrence.

Long-Term Complications

Vitamin B12 deficiency may become evident leading to anemia, but this may take 6–12 months or more to become clinically evident. With resection of less than 100 cm, this is extremely unlikely. Cholelithiasis and urolithiasis do occur with increased frequency in the TICD population due to disturbances in the enterohepatic circulation.

Disease recurrence: The reoperation rates for CD recurrence have been reported to be 10–30 % at 5 years, 20–40 % at 10 years, and 40–60 % at 20 years after surgery. The most significant factor affecting postoperative CD recurrence was found to be tobacco smoking. Rutgeerts et al. [48] reported that recurrent lesions were observed endoscopically in the neo-terminal ileum (the proximal site of the ileocolonic anastomosis) within 1 year of resection in 73 % of patients, although only 20 % of the patients had symptoms. Three years after surgery, the endoscopic recurrence rate increased to 85 % and symptomatic recurrence occurred in 34 %. Patients with severe endoscopic lesions within 1 year after resection developed early clinical recurrence. In contrast, patients with no or mild endoscopic lesions had a low frequency of subsequent clinical recurrence. The severity of the endoscopic inflammation in the neo-terminal ileum during the first year after resection was found to be a reliable predictive risk factor for future clinical recurrence. Ileocolonoscopy is the gold standard in the diagnosis of postoperative recurrence by defining the presence and severity of morphologic recurrence and predicting the clinical course. Ileocolonoscopy is recommended within the first year after surgery where treatment decisions may be affected. A recent study from one institution found that recurrence rates following ileocolic CD surgery did not differ between pediatric and adult groups [49].

Special Cases

Bypass and or Proximal Diversion

For certain types of ileocecal CD with associated abscess or phlegmon densely adherent to the retroperitoneum, or during a crisis when the patient undergoes urgent or emergent surgery for obstruction or perforation, bypass or proximal diversion may be used as a surgical solution,

In an investigation by Homan and Dineen [50], CD involving the ileum and cecum was treated with resection in 115 patients, exclusion bypass in 25, and simple bypass in 21. Overall recurrence rates were 25 % for resection, 63 % for exclusion bypass (Eisenhower operation), and 75 % for simple bypass. This difference was accounted for by early recurrence or by persistent disease in the two bypass groups: 21 % for exclusion bypass and 45 % for simple bypass as compared to 3 % for resection.

These results indicate that the recurrence rate following resection is significantly lower than bypass, and continuing disease in the bypassed loop accounts for a high percentage of reoperations in that group. Therefore, as is emphasized repeatedly in this chapter, resection is the surgical treatment of choice for ileocecal CD. Furthermore, there is an increased risk of malignancy in the bypassed segment, with the added concern that this segment cannot be surveyed by conventional means (endoscopic or radiographic).

Stricturoplasty

For TICD, sricuturoplasty may be an option if diffuse disease is encountered at the time of operation or if the risk of short bowel syndrome is significant. Options for stricturoplasty are discussed elsewhere in this book, but broadly are categorized according to the length of the stenotic segment.

Short Strictures (Up to 10 cm) (See Fig. 10.9)

For the management of short strictures, the Heineke–Mikulicz procedure is the most widely used. It is the eponymous description of the longitudinal incision and subsequent transverse closure of the bowel lumen that expands the diameter of the strictured segment.

Long Strictures (Up to 25 cm) (See Fig. 10.10)

For longer strictures we advocate the Finney stricturoplasty, which is essentially a side-to-side handsewn anastomosis.

Strictures longer than 30 cm require resection or utilization of novel procedures, e.g. Michelassi stricturoplasty. The Michelassi stricturoplasty is an isoperistaltic side-to-side anastomosis [51] (see Fig. 10.11).

There are contraindications to stricturoplasty. These are:

1. Excessive tension due to rigid and thickened bowel segments
2. Free perforation of the intestine, particularly with peritonitis
3. Fistula or abscess formation at the intended strictureplasty site
4. Hemorrhagic strictures
5. Multiple strictures within a short segment
6. Malnutrition or hypoalbuminemia (<2.0 g/dL)
7. Suspicion of cancer at the intended strictureplasty site.

Novel Procedures

Over the past several decades, progress in surgical management of intestinal diseases has been significant, but could be summarized as follows:

- Removal of sections of intestine through smaller incisions
- Development of a high definition/magnified view (laparoscopic approach)
- Novel suturing/stapling methods of anastomosing the bowel

While extremely important, these improvements in therapy could be described as mere embellishments of ideas that are really decades old.

In the near future, improved endoscopic capabilities, miniaturization of tools, improved biomaterials, and better external imaging (including image fusion) will provide us with the means to *rethink and improve* our approach to many of the complications of CD that now lead to the surgical interventions that this chapter and many others in this book describe.

There is no reason that new tools and approaches should not emerge in the near future that will permit obstructions to be relieved, abscesses to be drained, bleeding to be stopped, and nutrition to be restored without always applying the age old intestinal surgical principle of "cutting out a piece and sewing it back together."

Fig. 10.9 Heineke–Mikulicz procedure steps. (**a**) Longitudinal incision, at least 1–2 cm beyond the stricture. (**b**) Subsequent transverse closure of the bowel lumen that (**c**) expands the diameter of the strictured segment

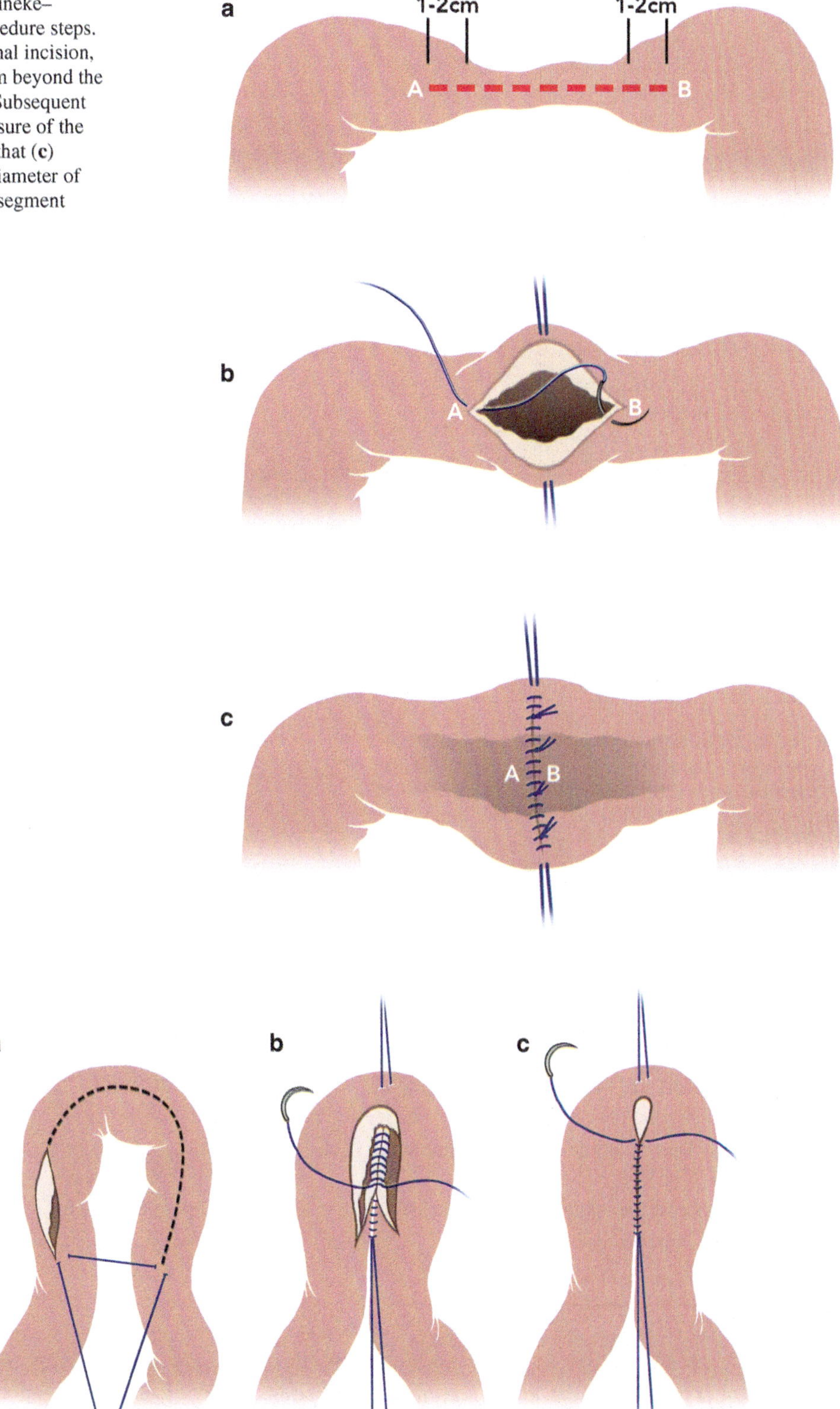

Fig. 10.10 Finney stricturoplasty—a side-to-side hand-sewn anastomosis. (**a**) Continuous incision on the anti-mesenteric side of bowel extending 1–2 cm beyond stricture into "normal" bowel. (**b**) Repair is done by folding the bowel into a "u" shape and closing the posterior side first, using a continuous absorbable suture (*single layer*). (**c**) Final closure of the anterior wall with a continuous suture, single layer

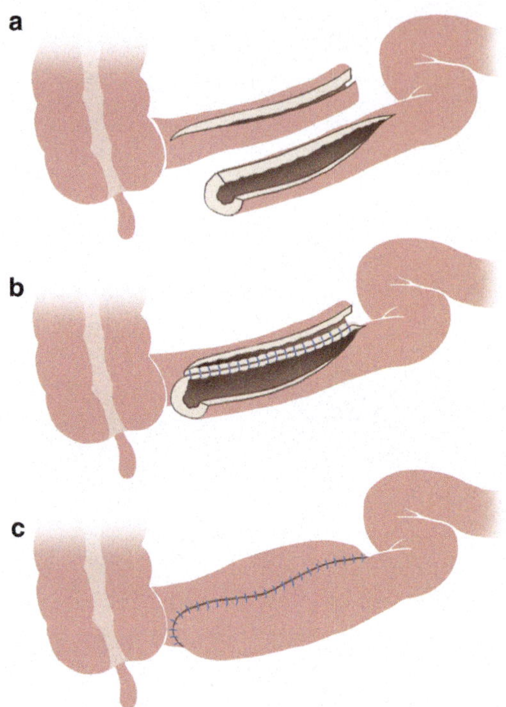

Fig. 10.11 Michelassi stricturoplasty steps—isoperistaltic side-to-side anastomosis. (**a**) Initial opening of the long stricture on its anti-mesenteric side, then dividing of the bowel and a short division of its mesentery in the mid portion. (**b**). Beginning the repair starting with a continuous suture on the posterior side. (**c**) Final closure by running a suture on the anterior side

We believe the luminal channel likely offers us the next platform for dramatically improving outcomes in TI (and other location) CD patients who suffer from the complications of the disease (see Figs. 10.12 and 10.13), but a full discussion of these potentials lies beyond the scope of this chapter. The greatest near-future potential in minimally invasive, bowel sparing management of TICD stricturing may lie in the application of absorbable stents used with better endoscopic tools.

Conclusions

Isolated ileal and ileocecal disease is one of the most common and treatable manifestations of CD. Surgery has a potential curative role, is generally safe with excellent long-term outcomes,

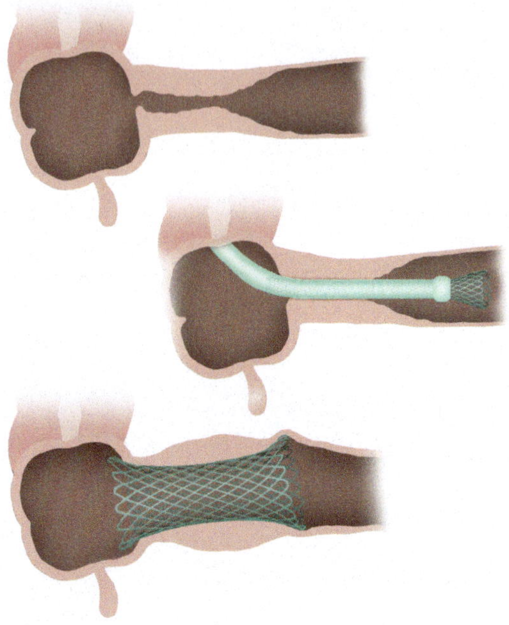

Fig. 10.12 The future: stenosis of the terminal ileum treated through expansion of an intraluminal absorbable stent, with flared ends to prevent migration

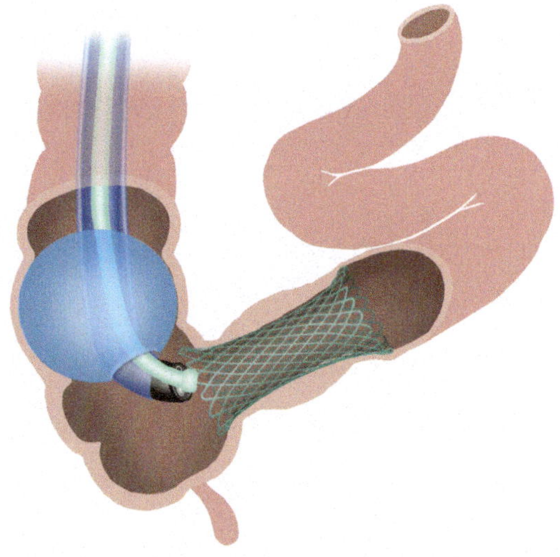

Fig. 10.13 Stent placement can be challenging particularly under current fluoroscopic guidance. This may be improved through use of futuristic endoscopic tools using balloons to stabilize the endoscope tip under development by the authors, stabilizing the endoscope in the cecum, allowing for improved accuracy and safety

and should not be seen as a last resort in TI CD management. The surgeon should become involved in the decision making for CD patients at an early stage through collaborative conferences and clinics with gastroenterology colleagues.

On top of exciting additions to the surgeon's armamentarium are laparoscopic approaches (smaller incisions) and new types of bowel sparing techniques.

Finally, and most intriguing, we believe the stage is now set for a new "endoluminal approach" to treating many of the complications of Crohn's disease, using a combination of better imaging, new biomaterials, and novel biomedical devices that we and others are now developing. Within the next 5 years, we envisage dramatic improvements in the approach to surgical TICD treatment.

References

1. Baumgart DC, Bernstein CN, Abbas Z, Colombel JF, Day AS, D'Haens G, et al. IBD around the world: comparing the epidemiology, diagnosis, and treatment: proceedings of the World Digestive Health Day 2010–Inflammatory Bowel Disease Task Force meeting. Inflamm Bowel Dis. 2011;17(2):639–44.
2. Binder V, Both H, Hansen PK, Hendriksen C, Kreiner S, Torp-Pedersen K. Incidence and prevalence of ulcerative colitis and Crohn's disease in the County of Copenhagen, 1962 to 1978. Gastroenterology. 1982; 83(3):563–8.
3. Peyrin-Biroulet L, Loftus Jr EV, Colombel JF, Sandborn WJ. The natural history of adult Crohn's disease in population-based cohorts. Am J Gastroenterol. 2010;105(2):289–97.
4. Frolkis AD, Lipton DS, Fiest KM, Negron ME, Dykeman J, deBruyn J, et al. Cumulative incidence of second intestinal resection in Crohn's disease: a systematic review and meta-analysis of population-based studies. Am J Gastroenterol. 2014;109(11): 1739–48.
5. De Cruz P, Kamm MA, Prideaux L, Allen PB, Desmond PV. Postoperative recurrent luminal Crohn's disease: a systematic review. Inflamm Bowel Dis. 2012;18(4):758–77.
6. Freeman HJ. Application of the Montreal classification for Crohn's disease to a single clinician database of 1015 patients. Can J Gastroenterol. 2007;21(6): 363–6.
7. Baumgart DC, Sandborn WJ. Inflammatory bowel disease: clinical aspects and established and evolving therapies. Lancet. 2007;369(9573):1641–57.
8. Kaplan GG. IBD: global variations in environmental risk factors for IBD. Nat Rev Gastroenterol Hepatol. 2014;11(12):708–9.
9. Molodecky NA, Soon IS, Rabi DM, Ghali WA, Ferris M, Chernoff G, et al. Increasing incidence and prevalence of the inflammatory bowel diseases with time, based on systematic review. Gastroenterology. 2012;142(1):46–54.e42. quiz e30.
10. Steiner MS, Morton RA. Nutritional and gastrointestinal complications of the use of bowel segments in the lower urinary tract. Urol Clin North Am. 1991; 18(4):743–54.
11. Van Assche G, Dignass A, Panes J, Beaugerie L, Karagiannis J, Allez M, et al. The second European evidence-based Consensus on the diagnosis and management of Crohn's disease: definitions and diagnosis. J Crohns Colitis. 2010;4(1):7–27.
12. Silverberg MS, Satsangi J, Ahmad T, Arnott ID, Bernstein CN, Brant SR, et al. Toward an integrated clinical, molecular and serological classification of inflammatory bowel disease: report of a Working Party of the 2005 Montreal World Congress of Gastroenterology. Can J Gastroenterol. 2005;19(Suppl A):5A–36.
13. Rungoe C, Langholz E, Andersson M, Basit S, Nielsen NM, Wohlfahrt J, et al. Changes in medical treatment and surgery rates in inflammatory bowel disease: a nationwide cohort study 1979–2011. Gut. 2014;63(10):1607–16.
14. Peyrin-Biroulet L, Oussalah A, Williet N, Pillot C, Bresler L, Bigard MA. Impact of azathioprine and tumour necrosis factor antagonists on the need for surgery in newly diagnosed Crohn's disease. Gut. 2011;60(7):930–6.
15. Lakatos PL, Golovics PA, David G, Pandur T, Erdelyi Z, Horvath A, et al. Has there been a change in the natural history of Crohn's disease? Surgical rates and medical management in a population-based inception cohort from Western Hungary between 1977–2009. Am J Gastroenterol. 2012;107(4):579–88.
16. Ramadas AV, Gunesh S, Thomas GA, Williams GT, Hawthorne AB. Natural history of Crohn's disease in a population-based cohort from Cardiff (1986–2003): a study of changes in medical treatment and surgical resection rates. Gut. 2010;59(9):1200–6.
17. Gao X, Yang RP, Chen MH, Xiao YL, He Y, Chen BL, et al. Risk factors for surgery and postoperative recurrence: analysis of a south China cohort with Crohn's disease. Scand J Gastroenterol. 2012;47(10): 1181–91.
18. Bernstein CN, Loftus Jr EV, Ng SC, Lakatos PL, Moum B. Hospitalisations and surgery in Crohn's disease. Gut. 2012;61(4):622–9.
19. Aratari A, Papi C, Leandro G, Viscido A, Capurso L, Caprilli R. Early versus late surgery for ileo-caecal Crohn's disease. Aliment Pharmacol Ther. 2007; 26(10):1303–12.
20. Latella G, Cocco A, Angelucci E, Viscido A, Bacci S, Necozione S, et al. Clinical course of Crohn's disease

first diagnosed at surgery for acute abdomen. Dig Liver Dis. 2009;41(4):269–76.
21. Park KT, Bass D. Inflammatory bowel disease-attributable costs and cost-effective strategies in the United States: a review. Inflamm Bowel Dis. 2011; 17(7):1603–9.
22. Fazio VW, Marchetti F, Church M, Goldblum JR, Lavery C, Hull TL, et al. Effect of resection margins on the recurrence of Crohn's disease in the small bowel. A randomized controlled trial. Ann Surg. 1996;224(4):563–71. discussion 71–3.
23. Farmer RG, Hawk WA, Turnbull Jr RB. Indications for surgery in Crohn's disease: analysis of 500 cases. Gastroenterology. 1976;71(2):245–50.
24. Platell C, Mackay J, Collopy B, Fink R, Ryan P, Woods R. Crohn's disease: a colon and rectal department experience. Aust N Z J Surg. 1995;65(8): 570–5.
25. Nagler SM, Poticha SM. Intraabdominal abscess in regional enteritis. Am J Surg. 1979;137(3):350–4.
26. Greenstein AJ, Mann D, Sachar DB, Aufses Jr AH. Free perforation in Crohn's disease: I. A survey of 99 cases. Am J Gastroenterol. 1985;80(9):682–9.
27. Siminovitch JM, Fazio VW. Ureteral obstruction secondary to Crohn's disease: a need for ureterolysis? Am J Surg. 1980;139(1):95–8.
28. Fazio VW, Zelas P, Weakley FL. Intraoperative angiography and the localization of bleeding from the small intestine. Surg Gynecol Obstet. 1980;151(5): 637–40.
29. Homan WP, Tang CK, Thorbjarnarson B. Acute massive hemorrhage from intestinal Crohn disease. Report of seven cases and review of the literature. Arch Surg. 1976;111(8):901–5.
30. Hawker PC, Gyde SN, Thompson H, Allan RN. Adenocarcinoma of the small intestine complicating Crohn's disease. Gut. 1982;23(3):188–93.
31. Seastedt KP, Trencheva K, Michelassi F, Alsaleh D, Milsom JW, Sonoda T, et al. Accuracy of CT enterography and magnetic resonance enterography imaging to detect lesions preoperatively in patients undergoing surgery for Crohn's disease. Dis Colon Rectum. 2014;57(12):1364–70.
32. Blackburn SC, Wiskin AE, Barnes C, Dick K, Afzal NA, Griffiths DM, et al. Surgery for children with Crohn's disease: indications, complications and outcome. Arch Dis Child. 2014;99(5):420–6.
33. Bernstein CN, Blanchard JF, Houston DS, Wajda A. The incidence of deep venous thrombosis and pulmonary embolism among patients with inflammatory bowel disease: a population-based cohort study. Thromb Haemost. 2001;85(3):430–4.
34. Bernstein CN, Nabalamba A. Hospitalization-based major comorbidity of inflammatory bowel disease in Canada. Can J Gastroenterol. 2007;21(8):507–11.
35. Danese S, Papa A, Saibeni S, Repici A, Malesci A, Vecchi M. Inflammation and coagulation in inflammatory bowel disease: the clot thickens. Am J Gastroenterol. 2007;102(1):174–86.
36. Miehsler W, Reinisch W, Valic E, Osterode W, Tillinger W, Feichtenschlager T, et al. Is inflammatory bowel disease an independent and disease specific risk factor for thromboembolism? Gut. 2004;53(4): 542–8.
37. Waterman M, Xu W, Dinani A, Steinhart AH, Croitoru K, Nguyen GC, et al. Preoperative biological therapy and short-term outcomes of abdominal surgery in patients with inflammatory bowel disease. Gut. 2013; 62(3):387–94.
38. Dasari BV, McKay D, Gardiner K. Laparoscopic versus open surgery for small bowel Crohn's disease. Cochrane Database Syst Rev. 2011;19(1):Cd006956.
39. Eshuis EJ, Slors JF, Stokkers PC, Sprangers MA, Ubbink DT, Cuesta MA, et al. Long-term outcomes following laparoscopically assisted versus open ileocolic resection for Crohn's disease. Br J Surg. 2010; 97(4):563–8.
40. Milsom JW, Hammerhofer KA, Bohm B, Marcello P, Elson P, Fazio VW. Prospective, randomized trial comparing laparoscopic vs. conventional surgery for refractory ileocolic Crohn's disease. Dis Colon Rectum. 2001;44(1):1–8. discussion – 9.
41. Stocchi L, Milsom JW, Fazio VW. Long-term outcomes of laparoscopic versus open ileocolic resection for Crohn's disease: follow-up of a prospective randomized trial. Surgery. 2008;144(4):622–7. discussion 7-8.
42. Fazio VW. Verbal communication. Circa 1990.
43. Ikeuchi H, Kusunoki M, Yamamura T. Long-term results of stapled and hand-sewn anastomoses in patients with Crohn's disease. Dig Surg. 2000; 17(5):493–6.
44. McLeod RS, Wolff BG, Ross S, Parkes R, McKenzie M. Recurrence of Crohn's disease after ileocolic resection is not affected by anastomotic type: results of a multicenter, randomized, controlled trial. Dis Colon Rectum. 2009;52(5):919–27.
45. Zurbuchen U, Kroesen AJ, Knebel P, Betzler MH, Becker H, Bruch HP, et al. Complications after end-to-end vs. side-to-side anastomosis in ileocecal Crohn's disease – early postoperative results from a randomized controlled multi-center trial (ISRCTN-45665492). Langenbeck's Arch Surg. 2013;398(3):467–74.
46. Fichera A, Zoccali M, Kono T. Antimesenteric functional end-to-end handsewn (Kono-S) anastomosis. J Gastrointest Surg. 2012;16(7):1412–6.
47. Lock MR, Farmer RG, Fazio VW, Jagelman DG, Lavery IC, Weakley FL. Recurrence and reoperation for Crohn's disease: the role of disease location in prognosis. N Engl J Med. 1981;304(26):1586–8.
48. Rutgeerts P, Geboes K, Vantrappen G, Beyls J, Kerremans R, Hiele M. Predictability of the postoperative course of Crohn's disease. Gastroenterology. 1990;99(4):956–63.
49. Bobanga ID, Bai S, Swanson MA, Champagne BJ, Reynolds HJ, Delaney CP, et al. Factors influencing disease recurrence after ileocolic resection in adult

and pediatric onset Crohn's disease. Am J Surg. 2014;208(4):591–6.
50. Homan WP, Dineen P. Comparison of the results of resection, bypass, and bypass with exclusion for ileocecal Crohn's disease. Ann Surg. 1978;187(5):530–5.
51. Michelassi F, Taschieri A, Tonelli F, Sasaki I, Poggioli G, Fazio V, et al. An international, multicenter, prospective, observational study of the side-to-side isoperistaltic strictureplasty in Crohn's disease. Dis Colon Rectum. 2007;50(3):277–84.

11 Bowel Sparing Procedures in Crohn's Disease of the Small Intestine

Cheguevara Afaneh and Fabrizio Michelassi

Introduction

Crohn's disease (CD) is a chronic transmural inflammatory disease of the entire gastrointestinal tract. Surgical treatment has a place in the treatment of this condition when complications or failure of medical treatment have occurred. Complications of CD include bowel obstruction, intestinal perforation, abscesses or fistulas, hemorrhage, and malignant transformation. Despite advances in medical therapy, the majority of patients with CD require surgical intervention within 10 years of the initial diagnosis.

Crohn's disease is a recurrent disease. At 5 years after the index operation, the recurrence rate requiring an additional surgical procedure ranges from 16 to 60 % [1, 2], while at 15 years the recurrence rate has been reported as high as 94 % [1]. Thus, preservation of intestinal length and mucosal surface is of utmost importance to avoid the complications of intestinal insufficiency and short bowel syndrome. When the need for surgical treatment is prompted by the presence of a stenosis causing symptomatic obstruction, strictureplasties can be performed to avoid intestinal resections while still addressing the complication at hand.

C. Afaneh, MD • F. Michelassi, MD (✉)
Department of Surgery, New York-Presbyterian Hospital/Weill Cornell Medical Center, New York, NY 10065, USA
e-mail: fam2006@med.cornell.edu

Katariya et al. [3] reported the first series of nine patients undergoing strictureplasties for benign tubercular strictures in the 1970s. Lee et al. [4] adopted this technique in Crohn's strictures of the small bowel. Since then, multiple others have described modifications and adaptations of the original strictureplasties or have contributed additional techniques. This chapter will focus on the use of various strictureplasties in addressing obstructive complications of Crohn's disease.

Indications and Contraindications

Strictureplasties are indicated in patients with strictures of the small bowel. The use of strictureplasties is even more pressing in patients with prior bowel resection of more than 100 cm, existing short bowel syndrome and strictures occurring less than a year from a previous surgery [5]. Strictureplasties have been also performed in the duodenum and at the site of a previous ileocolic anastomotic [6].

In contrast, strictureplasty is not advised in the presence of local sepsis, such as phlegmon or abscess, and generalized peritonitis. Other contraindications to the use of strictureplasty include suspicion of dysplasia or cancer, and an intended strictureplasty at a site next to a diseased segment requiring resection [5, 7]. Although previously viewed as a contraindication, the presence of an enteric fistula surrounded by chronic, as opposed to active, inflammation, is not a contraindication in most cases.

A. Fichera and M.K. Krane (eds.), *Crohn's Disease: Basic Principles*,
DOI 10.1007/978-3-319-14181-7_11, © Springer International Publishing Switzerland 2015

Preoperative Assessment

The extent of disease needs to be investigated preoperatively with the use of radiologic and endoscopic studies. Small bowel disease is best assessed by either computed tomographic scan enterography (CTE) or magnetic resonance enterography (MRE). The use of MRE is preferred based on the increased sensitivity in distinguishing between inflammatory and fibrotic strictures, as the former can be managed medically while the latter is better managed with surgical procedures. The presence of duodenal and colonic disease is better assessed with upper and lower endoscopy. At the time of colonoscopy, the ileocecal valve is intubated and the terminal ileum is assessed.

Patients at increased risk of morbidity should be identified preoperatively with the goal to mitigate the chance of postoperative complications. Several factors have been identified as prognostic for increased morbidity, including preoperative use of corticosteroids, presence of an intra-abdominal abscess, phlegmon and/or a fistula, and malnutrition [8]. Usually corticosteroids cannot be weaned off preoperatively as they are controlling disease symptoms, but abscesses can be drained percutaneously and malnutrition can be addressed with a short course of enteral or parenteral nutrition. Most recently, use of monoclonal anti-tumor necrosis factor (TNF) antibodies has been employed in the treatment of Crohn's disease. Preoperative use of these antibodies has led to an increased risk (approximately 1.5–2 times) of postoperative infectious complications, typically remote from the surgical site [9].

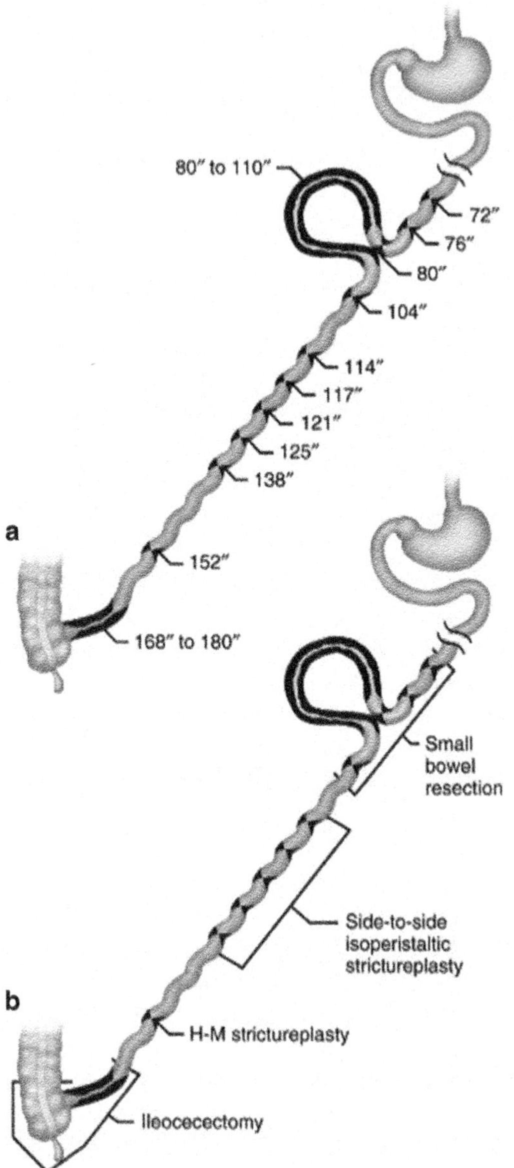

Fig. 11.1 Intraoperative roadmap. (**a**) Design of an intraoperative roadmap and (**b**) surgical plan. This figure was published in *Current Surgical Therapy* John Cameron and Andrew M. Cameron (Ed.) 11th ed., "Stricturoplasty in Crohn's Disease" by Leon Maggiori and Fabrizio Michelassi, p. 118 Copyright Elsevier (2014) Philadelphia, PA

Operative Approach

As with all Crohn's disease patients, the operative approach should always begin with examination of the entire small bowel from the ligament of Treitz to the ileocecal valve. This can be achieved either laparoscopically or via laparotomy. The surgeon should be vigilant in identifying any strictures, phlegmons, abscesses, fistulae, or masses. This portion of the procedure is meant to design a "roadmap" (Fig. 11.1). Once creation of the "roadmap" is complete, the surgeon should develop a surgical strategy based on the number, length, and relative location of all symptomatic Crohn's disease-related complications as previously listed.

Strictureplasty: Types, Techniques, and Technical Considerations

The use of the Heineke–Mikulicz and the Finney strictureplasty in Crohn's stricture was first described more than 30 years ago [4]. Since then modifications of the Heineke–Mikulicz strictureplasties and of the Finney strictureplasty as well as advanced strictureplasty techniques have been proposed [10]. All these techniques can be grouped into various categories: conventional versus non-conventional, short versus long or based on technical difficulty. Yet, the choice of the technique ultimately rests on length, number, and location of strictures. In this section, the major techniques will be presented based on stricture length and modifications of original techniques. At the end, a section will describe choices of strictureplasty based on location in the gastrointestinal tract.

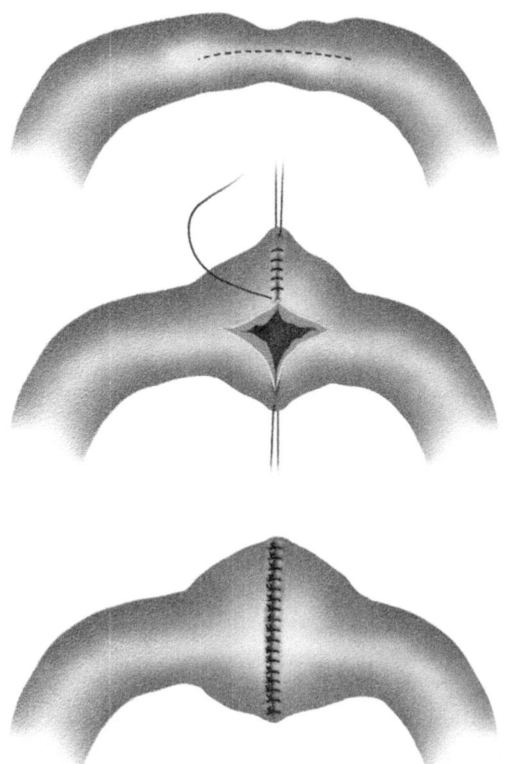

Fig. 11.2 Heineke–Mikulicz Strictureplasty. Heineke–Mikulicz strictureplasty on a short segment stricture. This figure was published in *Current Surgical Therapy* John Cameron and Andrew M. Cameron (Ed.) 11th ed., "Stricturoplasty in Crohn's Disease" by Leon Maggiori and Fabrizio Michelassi, p. 119 Copyright Elsevier (2014) Philadelphia, PA

Strictureplasty Techniques Based on Stricture Length and Modifications

Heineke–Mikulicz Strictureplasty

The Heineke–Mikulicz is the most commonly performed strictureplasty and best used for short (≤7 cm) strictures [5, 10, 11]. A single longitudinal incision is made on the antimesenteric side of the stricture extending approximately 2 cm beyond the thickened segment of bowel, both proximally and distally (Fig. 11.2). The enterotomy is then closed transversely with a single or double layer closure. Our preference is a two-layer closure with a running absorbable 3-0 suture for the inner layer and an interrupted Lembert nonabsorbable 3-0 suture for the outer layer. This strictureplasty enlarges the lumen of the diseased intestine and maintains intestinal transit without creating a blind loop or intestinal stasis.

Judd Strictureplasty

If the strictured segment is complicated by a chronic fistula without a great deal of acute inflammation, a Judd strictureplasty can be performed. After appropriate excision of the fistulous opening and the adjacent inflamed tissue, the stricture is opened longitudinally [10, 11] and the subsequent defect is closed transversally according to the Heineke–Mikulicz strictureplasty technique.

Moskel–Walske–Neumayer Strictureplasty

The Moskel–Walske–Neumayer strictureplasty technique is suitable for short strictures in the setting of dilated proximal bowel [10, 11]. A Y-shaped longitudinal enterotomy is made across the stricture, with the arms of the Y pointing towards the dilated proximal end. The enterotomy is closed in a V-shape, similar to the Heineke–Mikulicz strictureplasty technique. This technique helps mitigate size mismatch between dilated and non-dilated bowel.

Double Heineke–Mikulicz Strictureplasty

The Double Heineke–Mikulicz strictureplasty technique can be used when two short strictures are present in close proximity of each other [5, 10, 11]. A single longitudinal incision is made over the strictured areas including the normal segment of intervening small bowel. An incomplete transverse closure is performed on each strictured segment. This leaves a single longitudinal incision that is closed transversely according to the Heineke–Mikulicz strictureplasty technique.

Finney Strictureplasty

The Finney strictureplasty can be used for strictures longer than 7 cm and shorter than 15 cm [5, 10, 11]. The stricture is folded into a *U* shape (Fig. 11.3). A longitudinal enterotomy is performed midway between the mesenteric and antimesenteric borders so that the two ends of the enterotomy face each other in the two arms of the *U*. The enterotomy is then closed in a running continuous single layer or double layer, as previously described for the Heineke–Mikulicz strictureplasty. This strictureplasty should not be used for strictures longer than 15 cm because the ultimate result is the creation of a large lateral intestinal diverticulum that is susceptible to luminal stasis, bacterial overgrowth, malabsorption, malnutrition, and persistent low grade inflammation [4].

Jaboulay Strictureplasty

The Jaboulay strictureplasty is used for strictures between 10 and 20 cm [10]. The stricture is folded into a *U* shape and two enterotomies are created facing each other to allow for a side-to-side enteroenterostomy performed with a running continuous single layer or double layer, as previously described for the Heineke–Mikulicz strictureplasty. The end result is very similar to the Finney strictureplasty and, like the Finney strictureplasty, as the stricture length increases, so does the chance of developing a lateral diverticulum or blind loop, bacterial overgrowth, malabsorption, malnutrition, and persistent low grade inflammation [4].

Michelassi Strictureplasty

As described by the senior author in 1996, the Michelassi side-to-side isoperistaltic strictureplasty is indicated for long portion of bowel containing multiple short strictures in sequence [11, 12]. This technique has been used on segments of bowel as long as six feet. In this technique,

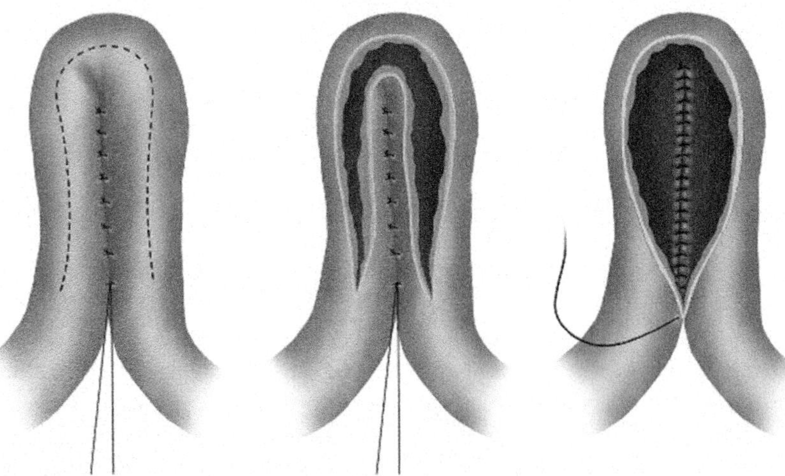

Fig. 11.3 Finney strictureplasty. Finney strictureplasty on a strictured segment of bowel (>7 cm). This figure was published in *Current Surgical Therapy* John Cameron and Andrew M. Cameron (Ed.) 11th ed., "Stricturoplasty in Crohn's Disease" by Leon Maggiori and Fabrizio Michelassi, p. 120 Copyright Elsevier (2014) Philadelphia, PA

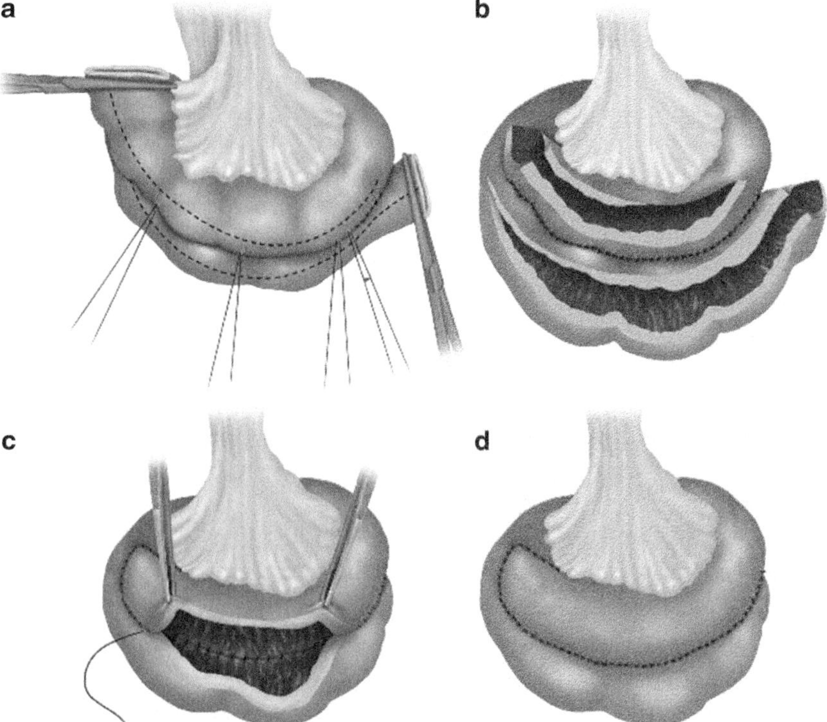

Fig. 11.4 Side-to-side isoperistaltic strictureplasty. The figure demonstrated the Michelassi side-to-side isoperistaltic strictureplasty. (**a**) The two loops of bowel are approximated by a layer of interrupted seromuscular Lembert stitches, with nonabsorbable 3-0 sutures. (**b**) A longitudinal enterotomy is performed on both loops, with ends tapered. (**c**) The outer suture line is reinforced with an internal row of running full-thickness 3-0 absorbable sutures, continued anteriorly as a running Connell suture; this layer is reinforced by an outer layer of interrupted seromuscular Lembert stitches with nonabsorbable 3-0 sutures. (**d**) This figure was published in *Current Surgical Therapy* John Cameron and Andrew M. Cameron (Ed.) 11th ed., Stricturoplasty in Crohn's Disease by Leon Maggiori and Fabrizio Michelassi, p. 120 Copyright Elsevier (2014) Philadelphia, PA

the mesentery of the small bowel loop to undergo the strictureplasty is first divided at its center (Fig. 11.4). The proximal small bowel loop is then moved over the distal one in a side-to-side fashion. The stenotic segments of one loop are placed adjacent to the dilated segments of the other loop. The two loops are then approximated by a layer of interrupted seromuscular Lembert stitches with nonabsorbable 3-0 sutures. A longitudinal enterotomy is performed on both loops, with the intestinal ends tapered to avoid blind ends. Occult malignant disease should be excluded with frozen-section biopsies of suspicious areas of disease, while hemostasis is achieved with suture ligatures or electrocautery. The outer suture line is reinforced with an internal row of running full-thickness 3-0 absorbable sutures, continued anteriorly as a running Connell suture; this layer is reinforced by an outer layer of interrupted seromuscular Lembert stitches with nonabsorbable 3-0 sutures.

The benefits of this technique include relief of intestinal obstruction created by multiple strictures in sequence, avoidance of resecting a long segment of bowel containing normal-absorbing intestine in between strictures, and avoidance of blind and bypassed loops of bowel [10]. This technique may be challenging to perform in the presence of a thickened and shortened mesentery.

Various modifications of the Michelassi strictureplasty have been described. These variations include either incorporation of additional Heineke–Mikulicz strictureplasties at either end of the Michelassi strictureplasty or resection of a segment of bowel prior to moving the proximal small bowel loop over the distal one in a side-to-side fashion if the diseased loop contains a severely diseased segment [5, 10, 11].

Strictureplasty Techniques Based on Location in the Gastrointestinal Tract

Traditionally, strictureplasty techniques have been applied to Crohn's strictures of the jejunum and ileum. With increased experience, these techniques have been exported to other gastrointestinal segments. Heineke–Mikulicz strictureplasties are particularly useful in isolated strictures of the first, second, and third portion of the duodenum. A stricture of the fourth portion of the duodenum is better handled with a Finney strictureplasty involving the first loop of jejunum. Obviously, in the presence of multiple strictures or technical challenge, a gastro-enterostomy still remains a valid option in duodenal disease.

Disease of the terminal ileum is commonly treated with a resection and an ileocolic anastomosis. Yet, recently D'Hoore has trialed the use of the side-to-side isoperistaltic strictureplasty in this location with excellent results (personal communication). Disease of the neo-terminal ileum with a stricture isolated to the ileocolic anastomosis may be treated with a Heineke–Mikulicz strictureplasty.

Crohn's disease of the colon lends itself poorly to be treated with strictureplasty techniques. This is due to the frequently extensive inflammatory nature of colonic Crohn's disease. Only rarely the disease presents itself as an isolated fibrotic stricture located in a segment easily amenable to a strictureplasty. The ascending, transverse, and rectosigmoid colon rather than the flexures and the rectum offer the necessary combination of intestinal wall pliability, lumen size, and mobility to perform a strictureplasty. Yet, even in the most favorable conditions, strictureplasty techniques have resulted in mediocre long-term outcomes [13].

Short-Term Outcomes

The safety and feasibility of strictureplasty for Crohn's disease has been well validated. In a meta-analysis by Yamamoto et al. [8], 1,112 patients who underwent 3,259 strictureplasties were studied. The overall morbidity rate was 13 % and the mortality rate was nil. Only 4 % of patients developed a septic complication, such as anastomotic leak, abscess formation, and fistula. Less than half of these patients required a laparotomy for sepsis. The strictureplasty site was commonly associated with sepsis (78 % of patients). The postoperative hemorrhage rate was 3 %. The authors concluded that strictureplasty techniques were safe.

Strictureplasty has been shown to have favorable outcomes even when compared to small bowel resections for Crohn's disease. In a meta-analysis by Reese et al. [14] 662 patients who underwent strictureplasty or bowel resection were examined. The overall early postoperative complication rate of strictureplasty was 12.7 % compared to 19.1 % in the resection group, septic complications occurred in 8.1 % of strictureplasties, and 11.2 % of intestinal resections, and postoperative hemorrhage rates in 3.0 % vs. 6.7 %, respectively. None of these differences was statistically significant. The authors conclude that strictureplasty is safe and does not confer increased morbidity when compared with resection and anastomosis.

In a meta-analysis by Campbell et al. [5] 1,616 patients who underwent 4,538 strictureplasties were studied and grouped according to conventional (Heineke–Mikulicz or Finney) and non-conventional (Michelassi, modified and others) strictureplasties. The overall morbidity rate was 13 %. The septic complication rate, which also included surgical site infections, was 4.6 % in conventional strictureplasties and 3.8 % in non-conventional strictureplasties. The postoperative hemorrhage rate was 4.6 % in conventional strictureplasties compared to 1.9 % in non-conventional strictureplasties. This meta-analysis proved that non-conventional, advanced strictureplasty techniques do not confer a higher postoperative morbidity risk than conventional, simpler strictureplasty techniques.

The Michelassi side-to-side isoperistaltic strictureplasty has been validated as feasible and safe in several smaller studies. An international multicenter observational study of 184 patients with Crohn's disease who underwent a side-to-side isoperistaltic strictureplasty [15] determined that the overall morbidity rate was low, ranging from 5.7 to 20.8 %. In this series, the length of diseased bowel selected for strictureplasty ranged from 20.8 ± 9.9 cm to 64.3 ± 29.3 cm and synchronous strictureplasties were performed in 41.9–83.3 % of cases.

Long-Term Outcomes

Strictureplasty sites are not immune from disease recurrences. In a meta-analysis by Reese et al. [14] comparing patients undergoing strictureplasty with patients undergoing resections, recurrence in need of surgical treatment occurred in 37.8 % of patients undergoing strictureplasty compared to 31.0 % of those patients undergoing resection. On further analysis, patients undergoing strictureplasty were 8 % more likely to experience surgical recurrence than patients undergoing resection ($P = 0.01$). Yet the site of the recurrence was not specified in this paper.

The site of recurrence was looked at specifically by Tichansky et al. [16]. Although recurrence rates ranged from 23 % for the Finney strictureplasty to 32 % for the Heineke–Mikulicz strictureplasty, when the authors looked at where the recurrence occurred, only in 8 % of cases the recurrence occurred on a previous strictureplasty site, most of the recurrences occurring away from strictureplasty sites.

This observation was confirmed by Fichera et al. who described a series of 78 patients with 134 sites requiring operative intervention (85 requiring resection and 49 amenable to strictureplasty). The authors found significantly fewer recurrences at strictureplasty sites compared to resection sites (45 % vs. 70 %; $P < 0.05$). Similarly, in a meta-analysis by Yamamoto analyzing 1,112 patients who underwent 3,259 strictureplasties, the 5-year site-specific recurrence rate was only 3 % [8].

Experience with recurrences in need of surgery is accumulating slowly after performance of a side-to-side isoperistaltic strictureplasty. One observational study [15] reported a surgical recurrence rate of 7.6 % after a mean follow-up of 35 months. The majority of the recurrences occurred at the inlet and outlet of the side-to-side strictureplasty, leading some authors to advocate performance of a Heineke–Mikulicz strictureplasty at the inlet and outlet, respectively (see under section "Strictureplasty Techniques Based on Stricture Length and Modifications").

Development of small bowel adenocarcinoma has been documented at strictureplasty sites. Surgical biopsies should be obtained at intended sites of strictureplasty if the mucosa appears concerning for a dysplastic or neoplastic transformation. The incidence is fairly low, as Campbell et al. [5] reported rates of 0.34 % in conventional strictureplasties and 0.21 % in non-conventional strictureplasties. Given the rarity of this complications, most surgeons concur that risk of malignant transformation is not sufficient to dissuade performance of a strictureplasty.

Summary

Crohn's disease is a chronic, inflammatory disease of the entire gastrointestinal tract. Surgical indications include obstruction, perforation, hemorrhage, failure to thrive, and failure of medical therapy. Strictureplasty techniques can be employed to relieve strictures causing partial or complete bowel obstruction. The choice of technique depends on the number, length, and location of the stricture(s). Strictureplasty has been shown to be safe and effective, avoids sacrificing absorptive bowel surface, and possibly may have a protective effect against site recurrences. Bowel-sparing techniques are an essential tool in the armamentarium of a surgeon caring for a patient with Crohn's disease.

References

1. Greenstein AH, Sachar DB, Pasternack BS, Janowitz HD. Reoperation and recurrence of Crohn's colitis and ileocolitis crude and cumulative rates. N Engl J Med. 1975;293:685–90.
2. Lennard-Jones JE, Stadler GA. Prognosis after resection of chronic regional ileitis. Gut. 1967;8:332–6.
3. Katariya RN, Sood S, Rao PG, Rao PL. Stricture-plasty for tubercular strictures of the gastro-intestinal tract. Br J Surg. 1977;64:496–8.
4. Lee EC, Papaioannou N. Minimal surgery for chronic obstruction in patients with extensive or universal Crohn's disease. Ann R Coll Surg Engl. 1982; 64:229–33.
5. Campbell L, Ambe R, Weaver J, Marcus SM, Cagir B. Comparison of conventional and nonconventional strictureplasties in Crohn's disease: a systematic review and meta-analysis. Dis Colon Rectum. 2012;55:714–26.
6. Worsey MJ, Hull T, Ryland L, Fazio V. Strictureplasty is an effective option in the operative management of duodenal Crohn's disease. Dis Colon Rectum. 1999; 42:596–600.
7. Milsom JW. Strictureplasty and mechanical dilation in strictured Crohn's disease. In: Michelassi F, Milsom JW, editors. Operative strategies in inflammatory bowel disease. New York: Springer; 1999. p. 259–67.
8. Yamamoto T, Fazio VW, Tekkis PP. Safety and efficacy of strictureplasty for Crohn's disease: a systematic review and meta-analysis. Dis Colon Rectum. 2007;50:1968–86.
9. Kopylov U, Ben-Horin S, Zmora O, Eliakim R, Katz LH. Anti-tumor necrosis factor and postoperative complications in Crohn's disease: systematic review and meta-analysis. Inflamm Bowel Dis. 2012;18: 2404–13.
10. Ambe R, Campbell L, Cagir B. A comprehensive review of strictureplasty techniques in Crohn's disease: types, indications, comparisons, and safety. J Gastrointest Surg. 2012;16:209–17.
11. Maggiori L, Michelassi F. Strictureplasty in Crohn's disease. In: Cameron J, Cameron AM, editors. Current surgical therapy. Philadelphia: Elsevier; 2014. p. 118–22.
12. Michelassi F. Side-to-side isoperistaltic stricture-plasty for multiple Crohn's strictures. Dis Colon Rectum. 1996;39:345–9.
13. Broering DC, Eisenberger CF, Koch A, et al. Strictureplasty for large bowel stenosis in Crohn's disease: quality of life after surgical therapy. Int J Colorectal Dis. 2001;16:81–7.
14. Reese GE, Purkayastha S, Tilney HS, von Roon A, Yamamoto T, Tekkis PP. Strictureplasty vs resection in small bowel Crohn's disease: an evaluation of short-term outcomes and recurrence. Colorectal Dis. 2007;9:686–94.
15. Michelassi F, Taschieri A, Tonelli F, et al. An international, multicenter, prospective, observational study of the side-to-side isoperistaltic strictureplasty in Crohn's disease. Dis Colon Rectum. 2007;50: 277–84.
16. Tichansky D, Cagir B, Yoo E, Marcus S, Fry R. Strictureplasty for Crohn's disease: meta-analysis. Dis Colon Rectum. 2000;43:911–9.

Surgery: Colon

12

Amila Husic and Tonia M. Young-Fadok

Clinical Presentation

Similar to ulcerative colitis, the onset of colonic Crohn's is bimodal, with a first peak occurring in the pediatric and young adult population, and the second amongst patients in the 50–70 age range [1]. A common description is that of anorectal disease preceding that of more proximal disease by several years. Other common presentations include diarrhea which may or may not be bloody, crampy abdominal pain, weight loss, and nutritional deficiencies. Acuity can vary from symptoms evolving over weeks or months, to a patient presenting with a sudden onset of severe, "toxic" colitis.

Colonic Crohn's disease can occur in three main presentations: pancolonic, i.e. involving the entire colon; or segmental with intervening normal mucosa; or the colon may be involved as a "bystander." By definition, the inflammatory process involves all layers of colonic wall, which can lead to perforation, abscess, and/or fistula. The most common site of involvement is the terminal ileum, which can fistulize to colon (most frequently the sigmoid colon) or other pelvic organs such as the bladder or the vaginal cuff. Often, these organs are secondarily involved by the inflammatory process and simple repair at the time of surgery would suffice. In the case of ileosigmoid fistula (Fig. 12.1), colonoscopic examination demonstrating lack of inflammation at the area of fistula confirms that the colon is secondarily involved [2, 3].

Colonic strictures are a common manifestation of Crohn's disease. The treatment may be determined by the length of the stricture and its characteristics, e.g. rigidity secondary to long-standing scarring. Some shorter isolated strictures may be amenable to endoscopy with balloon dilation after biopsy. High grade strictures, long strictures, and active inflammation would be more likely to require segmental resection.

Colon Cancer

Although Crohn's disease does not confer the same increase in colorectal cancer risk compared to ulcerative colitis, there is no doubt that long-standing colitis of any etiology increases the risk of malignancy. A recent Swedish study demonstrated a relative risk of 5.6 in these patients, with higher risk observed in patients with pancolitis [4, 5]. Therefore, current recommendations with regard to screening are similar to those in patients with ulcerative colitis. Surveillance should begin 10 years after onset of the disease symptoms and every 1–2 years thereafter. The areas affected by colitis are most prone to malignant transformation,

A. Husic, MD, FACS
T.M. Young-Fadok, MD, MS, FACS, FASCRS (✉)
Division of Colorectal Surgery, Mayo Clinic
College of Medicine, Phoenix, AZ, USA
e-mail: youngfadok.tonia@mayo.edu

A. Fichera and M.K. Krane (eds.), *Crohn's Disease: Basic Principles*,
DOI 10.1007/978-3-319-14181-7_12, © Springer International Publishing Switzerland 2015

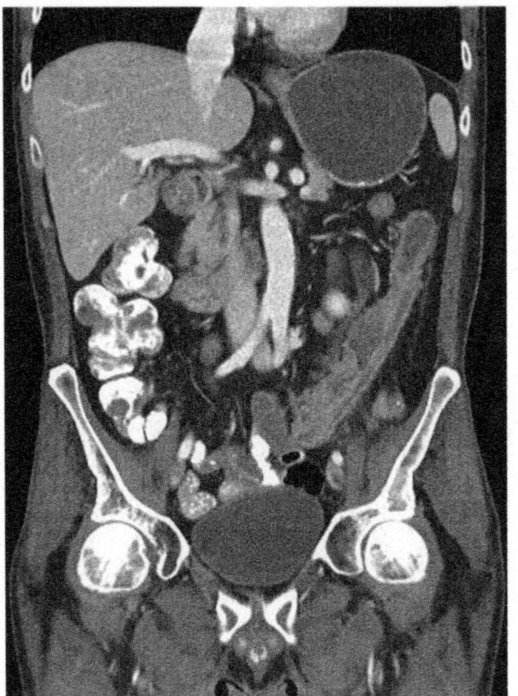

Fig. 12.1 CT scan. Sixty-two-year-old male patient with left-sided Crohn's colitis. Note long abscess cavity lateral to the descending colon

therefore the distribution can affect entire colon. Present recommendations include biopsies of all suspicious lesions, polyps, or masses as well as 2–4 random biopsies every 10 cm.

Finding of high grade dysplasia implies up to a 40 % chance of associated cancer and therefore warrants a total colectomy. Lesions with low grade dysplasia may or may not progress to high grade based on a study demonstrating only 10 % conversion rate at 10 years. Although studies have demonstrated various rates of malignancy at the time of colectomy in patients with low grade dysplasia, a close follow-up is warranted to exclude further progression to malignancy.

Surgical Management

Indications for surgery in a patient with Crohn's colitis can be classified as emergent and elective. Acute perforation with abscess, hemorrhage, obstruction with stricture or fulminant colitis not responsive to medical therapy requires an urgent approach. Most patients, however, proceed to surgery after longstanding and often progressive disease. Chronic anemia, malnutrition, and debilitating diarrhea can all be indications for surgery. In cases of severe anorectal involvement, surgical approaches often involve creation of a stoma, which in many cases is permanent. Therefore, the decision to proceed to surgery in patients with severe associated anorectal disease is often contingent upon the patient's acceptance of permanent colostomy/ileostomy. Establishment of a trusting, long-term relationship between the surgeon and a patient with Crohn's disease is necessary as the decision-making can be complex and involving multiple aspects of patient care. A multidisciplinary approach is often beneficial with a gastroenterologist, primary care physician, and surgeon involved.

Approach

Considering that the majority of Crohn's patients have a relatively low BMI compared to general population, a laparoscopic approach is feasible and should be considered. In addition, these patients are often young and aware of the cosmetic result. This is particularly advocated since there is high likelihood of repeat operative intervention. There is a relatively low rate of conversion to laparotomy, ranging from 7 to 11 % [6, 7]. Even in patients presenting with acute colitis a laparoscopic approach is advisable [8, 9]. Leading to reduced wound infections, intra-abdominal abscesses, and shorter length of hospital stay. In reoperative surgery cases, laparoscopic approach is feasible and does not appear to increase the likelihood of complications [10]. Necessity for further bowel resection and presence of abscess/fistula were found to be risk factors for conversion, as demonstrated in study by Alves et al. [11]. Patients who underwent laparoscopic ileocolic resection had improved outcomes with morbidity for 10 % vs 33 % when compared to the open group, as well as a shorter length of stay 5 vs 7 days [12].

Establishment of initial laparoscopic access can be challenging in reoperative surgery cases.

We have found that a cutdown technique using a supra- or periumbilical incision works well for most cases and provides a satisfactory cosmetic result. The periumbilical incision may be extended as needed and allow for exteriorization of small bowel and mobilized segments of colon.

Placement of accessory ports is influenced based on the location of the involved segment. For proctocolectomy, we have found that port distribution in a "diamond" pattern is most versatile, with the Hasson port located supraumbilically, and three 5 mm working ports: suprapubic, LLQ, and RUQ. Occasionally, a fifth port can be placed in LUQ to assist in mobilization of omentum and transverse mesocolon, although this is frequently not necessary in a patient with little intra-abdominal fat. Since many of these operations will include a creation of ileostomy or colostomy, the planned ostomy site can be used to guide placement of lateral ports, to avoid unnecessary incisions. Some centers also employ a hand-assist port, which is most commonly introduced via Pfannenstiel incision. It has been our practice to perform the mobilization laparoscopically, and then perform an extracorporeal anastomosis through a periumbilical incision, which is also used as the specimen extraction site. In thin patients, with a relatively favorable anatomy and no history of previous surgery, a single port approach can be considered [13].

When anastomosing two segments, it is important to examine the intestinal lumen for ulcerations or other signs of mucosal disease. The use of a stapler vs handsewn technique is often a matter of personal preference of the surgeon. A systematic review assessing the anastomotic leak rate in Crohn's patients undergoing ileocolic resection found a higher leak rate in patients undergoing handsewn end-to-end anastomosis, compared to other configurations [14]. Due to the larger caliber of colon compared to small bowel, however, stapled side-to-side anastomosis allows for easier construction of the anastomosis. Handsewn anastomosis may be considered in general when dealing with a significant discrepancy in thickness of bowel wall as a consequence of prolonged obstructive symptoms.

Postoperative Care

Increasing implementation of ERAS protocols has led to faster patient recovery and shorter length of stay. Numerous studies have documented the benefit of this approach in both adult and pediatric patients [15, 16]. Frequently, these patients have a high narcotic tolerance due to chronic abdominal pain, therefore a dedicated pain service is often helpful in transitioning the patient to oral therapy. It is important to note that medical therapies for Crohn's disease should generally be discontinued in the perioperative period, except for corticosteroid therapy which needs a gradual taper.

Segmental Resection

The distribution of colonic Crohn's disease is highly variable with approximately a third of the patients presenting with right-sided disease, and remainder with left-sided disease (Fig. 12.2) or pancolitis. Of particular importance in surgical planning is the extent and degree of anorectal involvement since that can limit potential reconstructive options. For isolated segmental disease, a local resection of that portion of bowel is a reasonable alternative to more aggressive approaches. This option is commonly utilized in an elective setting, where the extent of disease is known and documented, for example an existing stenosis or a fistula. Primary anastomosis is often possible, except in cases of anorectal involvement or gross contamination (Fig. 12.3). Since this approach involves a creation of an anastomosis, the patient's nutritional and medication-related factors need to be optimized. In particular, if the patient is receiving concomitant treatment with biologic agents, the patient should ideally be outside the therapeutic window. For infliximab this period is 6–8 weeks, adalimumab 2 weeks, and cimzia 4 weeks. The decision to proceed is contingent on patient's understanding of risks associated, in particular the risk of anastomotic leak and recurrent disease.

Unlike ulcerative colitis for which total proctocolectomy is curative, Crohn's disease can often

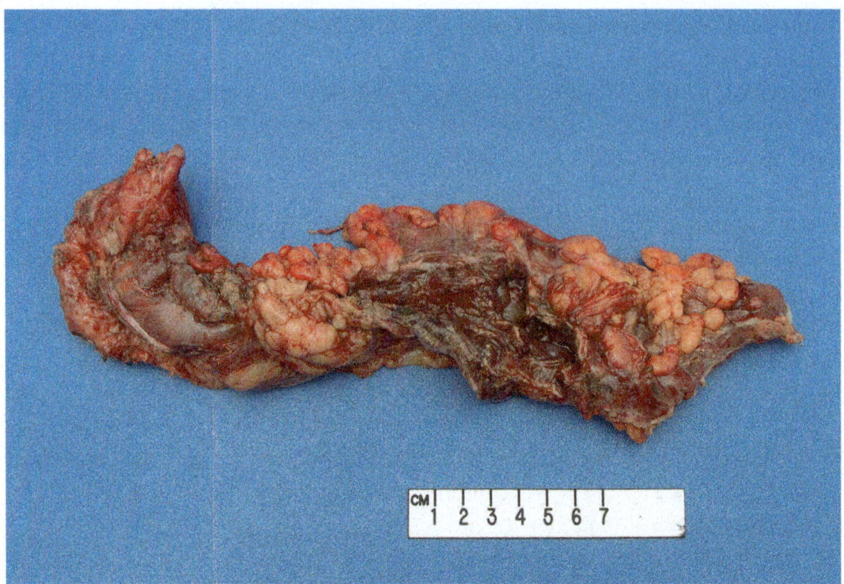

Fig. 12.2 Operative specimen following left colectomy, Hartmann procedure, and mucus fistula

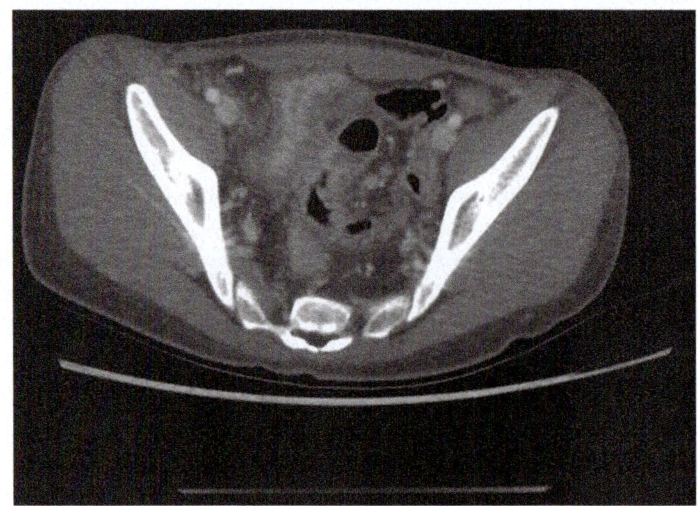

Fig. 12.3 CT scan. Eighteen-year-old male with ileocecal disease plus ileosigmoid fistula and active localized sigmoid Crohn's colitis. Patient underwent ileocecectomy and segmental resection of the distal sigmoid laparoscopically

recur after surgical resection. Risks of recurrence have been estimated in the literature in the order of 40 %, as reported in the study by Fichera et al. [7]. This study also found shorter time for disease recurrence in patients who underwent segmental colectomy as well as higher likelihood of requiring long-term medications. Patients with isolated distal disease were more likely to ultimately require a stoma, warranting that a more extensive resection should be considered at the time of initial operation.

The advantages of segmental resection are reflected in improving the patient's functional outcome, namely decrease in frequency of bowel movements, as well as avoidance of stoma. In one study, 86 % of patients remained stoma free long-term after segmental resection [17]. Similarly, a retrospective analysis by Martel demonstrated no difference in postoperative complications with respect to segmental colectomy vs more extensive approach [18]. Another study found the risk of having a stoma after initial segmental colonic resection to be 44 %, after a mean follow-up of 8.3 years [19]. A large retrospective analysis of 833 patients with Crohn's disease analyzed the risks factors for postoperative disease recurrence. Perianal disease, ileorectal anastomosis, and segmental resection were found to be independent risk factors [20].

Surgical experience involving strictureplasty is limited in colonic Crohn's disease likely because the colon does not actively participate in digestion and absorption of nutrients and therefore preserving a few inches is of questionable clinical benefit.

Total Colectomy with Ileorectal Anastomosis

Ileorectal anastomosis is an option in patients with pancolitis who have relative rectal sparing. This procedure can often be safely performed as a single stage. When presentation of colonic Crohn's is complicated by toxic colitis or an abscess, strong consideration should be given to performing the procedure in two stages, particularly in a severely immunosuppressed and/or nutritionally depleted patient. Patient selection is important with regard to age and sphincter function. Poor sphincter control can lead to incontinence and inferior functional outcome. Thorough evaluation should include obtaining details of any history of perianal surgery, rectal prolapse, obstetric history, or any other trauma to the perineum that might affect sphincter muscles and their nerve supply. The patient should be questioned on frequency of "accidents" and undergo anal manometry or ultrasound evaluation if there is a high clinical suspicion for sphincter injury. Preoperative counseling is important, as some patients will be better served with permanent ileostomy, even if the rectum is left in place. Despite the success of initial surgery, many patients will develop further problems over time. A study by Elton et al. demonstrated that approximately half of the patients who undergo ileorectal anastomosis would ultimately require a permanent ileostomy [21]. The most common complications were development of strictures and fistulas. Overall functional outcome in most patients included 3–5 bowel movements per day [21]. In general, this procedure is most appropriate for younger patients with good sphincter function and relative rectal sparing who wish to avoid a permanent ileostomy.

Another study by Cattan et al. retrospectively examined rate of recurrence after ileorectal anastomosis in 118 patients. Despite disease recurrence rate of 83 % at 10 years, 63 % of patients retained a functioning ileorectal anastomosis [22]. Extraintestinal manifestations and previous ileal disease were associated with a higher risk of recurrence.

A recent retrospective review by Riordan similarly found a 5- and 10-year rate of functional ileorectal anastomosis of 87 % and 72 %, respectively [23]. Their reported leak rate was 7.4 %.

The construction of ileorectal anastomosis can be performed end-to-end, end-to-side, or side-to-side using a stapler or a handsewn technique. We prefer the straight laparoscopic approach using the EEA stapler for a side-to-end anastomosis with the terminal ileum. Consideration should be given to a diverting ileostomy, especially in patients with nutritional or immunologic deficiencies.

Subtotal Colectomy with End Ileostomy

Subtotal colectomy with end ileostomy is most suitable for patients with extensive colonic disease with rectal sparing who are not candidates for ileorectal anastomosis. Patient preference plays a role in selection as well as any risk factors with regard to incontinence. Regardless of patient's ultimate desire for GI continuity, this procedure is often indicated as the first stage in dealing with acute presentation of severe colonic Crohn's disease, where construction of an anastomosis would be inadvisable. This approach is also advocated in patients with short duration acute colitis, since on initial presentation it may be difficult to differentiate between ulcerative colitis and Crohn's disease in a patient with limited prior history and evaluation. Completion proctectomy or ileorectal anastomosis may be performed at a later date if indicated.

At the time of colectomy, the rectal stump is divided just above the level of the sacral promontory. Care should be taken during division of sigmoid mesentery to preserve the superior rectal pedicle. Some authors advocate leaving a long sigmoid stump as a mucus fistula which can be used to decompress, irrigate, and evaluate the remaining rectum [24, 25]. While this is an option, we have found that leaving a large-caliber transanal drain for 48 h accomplishes the same goal, with minimal patient discomfort and therefore avoids the need for a mucus fistula.

The fate of the defunctioned rectal stump was investigated in a study by Guillem et al. where they reviewed 47 cases of excluded rectal segment. Perianal disease at initial presentation was predictive of a need for proctectomy, while terminal ileal disease and inflammatory changes in the rectum did not carry a significant risk. The disease recurrence in the remnant was noted to be 70 % at 5 years, requiring completion proctectomy in half of the patients [26].

The authors concluded that the patients with perianal disease undergoing colectomy for Crohn's colitis should probably be candidates for proctocolectomy or early completion proctectomy.

It is important to note the importance of surveillance proctoscopy in patients with rectal remnant. Although the exact rate of colorectal malignancy is unknown, several cases have been described in the literature [27].

At increased risk are patients with longstanding active anorectal Crohn's fistulas in which both squamous cell and adenocarcinomas have been reported and conferred a poor prognosis [28].

Proctocolectomy with End Ileostomy

For a patient with pancolitis and severe perianal disease, proctocolectomy is the procedure of choice. In this scenario, patients are left with a permanent end ileostomy. The advantages of this approach in patients with Crohn's disease isolated to the colon are minimizing the risks of recurrent disease and the need for further operative intervention. Disadvantages include the extensive initial operation, which includes pelvic dissection. In both men and women, there are associated risks, primarily with sexual dysfunction due to the potential injury to hypogastric nerves and nervi erigentes [29].

There are several options for addressing the anal sphincter during proctectomy. In patients with severe perianal disease, a complete anoperineal resection might be the most appropriate. This can, however, lead to wound complications and pelvic sepsis in over 20 % of patients. Yamamoto et al. demonstrated that factors conferring significantly greater risk of perineal sinus were younger age, rectal involvement, perianal sepsis, high fistulas, extrasphincteric excision, and fecal contamination at operation [30].

An intersphincteric approach can be used as an alternative, where the external sphincter muscle and part of the mesorectum are left in place. Some authors advocate a completely transperineal approach with complete proctectomy performed in prone position [31].

In select patients, a low Hartmann procedure can be offered, where the rectum is stapled off at the level of the pelvic floor. This option might help younger patients with decision-making to undergo surgery since their anal sphincter will be preserved for potential future restorative procedure. The risks are persistent fistulizing perianal disease, in particular a development of a chronic presacral sinus, presumably resulting from staple line breakdown.

Proctocolectomy with Ileal Pouch Anal Anastomosis

While restorative proctocolectomy with creation of ileal pouch is generally an option in patients with ulcerative colitis, this procedure has not been accepted as a treatment plan in patients with colonic Crohn's disease [32].

The concern is a high risk of disease occurrence in the pouch as well as the need for extensive surgery and small bowel resection should the pouch require removal. Several studies have challenged this notion, often in cases where Crohn's disease was diagnosed after creation of ileal pouch.

Initial study published on the subject was by a French group in 1996 where out of 31 patients, 6 (19 %) experienced Crohn's related complications necessitating further surgery [33]. Long-term follow-up of this cohort found a pouch excision rate of 10 % [34]. A more recent study from Cleveland clinic incorporated three groups of patients who underwent IPAA with Crohn's colitis—those where surgery was performed intentionally, those where Crohn's was diagnosed on final pathology, and those with delayed diagnosis. The 10-year pouch retention rate was 71 % and was lower in patients who had delayed diagnosis. Patients with a pouch reported good quality of life scores with respect to continence and number of daily bowel movements (7 on average) [35].

In contrast to the studies above, researchers from Lahey Clinic reported a complication rate of 93 % with 29 % eventual rate of pouch loss or diversion. The most common complications were development of perineal abscess/fistula, pouchitis, and pouch-anal stricture. The authors found no preoperative clinical, endoscopic, and pathologic risk factors that were predictive of pouch failure [36].

Similarly, a British study examined a subset of patients who underwent IPAA and had 57.5 % pouch failure rate when diagnosed with Crohn's disease or indeterminate colitis favoring Crohn's, while patients with UC were found to have pouch failure of 11.5 %, while no differences were observed with regard to bowel function and incontinence [37].

Considering these findings, a few surgeons have offered ileal pouch anal anastomosis in highly select patients with isolated colonic Crohn's disease. In these patients, affected segments should be confined to colon, with no perianal or small bowel involvement. While the creation of an ileal pouch in a patient with Crohn's disease is controversial, there is no doubt that these patients require extensive counseling and long-term medical therapy for Crohn's disease. In the US the controversy persists and this is not considered an option in a patient with known Crohn's colitis.

References

1. Johnston RD, Logan RF. What is the peak age for onset of IBD? Inflamm Bowel Dis. 2008;14 (Suppl 2):S4–5
2. Block GE, Schraut WH. The operative treatment of Crohn's enteritis complicated by ileosigmoid fistula. Ann Surg. 1982;196(3):356–60.
3. Heimann T, Greenstein AJ, Aufses Jr AH. Surgical management of ileosigmoid fistula in Crohn's disease. Am J Gastroenterol. 1979;72(1):21–4.
4. Laukoetter MG, et al. Intestinal cancer risk in Crohn's disease: a meta-analysis. J Gastrointest Surg. 2011; 15(4):576–83.
5. Canavan C, Abrams KR, Mayberry J. Meta-analysis: colorectal and small bowel cancer risk in patients with Crohn's disease. Aliment Pharmacol Ther. 2006;23(8): 1097–104.
6. Umanskiy K, et al. Laparoscopic colectomy for Crohn's colitis. A large prospective comparative study. J Gastrointest Surg. 2010;14(4):658–63.
7. Fichera A, et al. Long-term outcome of surgically treated Crohn's colitis: a prospective study. Dis Colon Rectum. 2005;48(5):963–9.
8. da Luz Moreira A, et al. Laparoscopic surgery for patients with Crohn's colitis: a case-matched study. J Gastrointest Surg. 2007;11(11):1529–33.
9. Messenger DE, et al. Subtotal colectomy in severe ulcerative and Crohn's colitis: what benefit does the laparoscopic approach confer? Dis Colon Rectum. 2014;57(12):1349–57.
10. Tavernier M, Lebreton G, Alves A. Laparoscopic surgery for complex Crohn's disease. J Visc Surg. 2013;150(6):389–93.
11. Alves A, et al. Factors that predict conversion in 69 consecutive patients undergoing laparoscopic ileocecal resection for Crohn's disease: a prospective study. Dis Colon Rectum. 2005;48(12):2302–8.
12. Rosman AS, Melis M, Fichera A. Metaanalysis of trials comparing laparoscopic and open surgery for Crohn's disease. Surg Endosc. 2005;19(12):1549–55.
13. Champagne BJ, et al. Single-incision versus standard multiport laparoscopic colectomy: a multicenter, case-controlled comparison. Ann Surg. 2012;255(1): 66–9.
14. Choy PY, et al. Stapled versus handsewn methods for ileocolic anastomoses. Cochrane Database Syst Rev. 2011;9:CD004320.
15. Fierens J, et al. Enhanced recovery after surgery (ERAS) protocol: prospective study of outcome in colorectal surgery. Acta Chir Belg. 2012;112(5): 355–8.

16. Lassen K, et al. Consensus review of optimal perioperative care in colorectal surgery: Enhanced Recovery After Surgery (ERAS) Group recommendations. Arch Surg. 2009;144(10):961–9.
17. Prabhakar LP, et al. Avoiding a stoma: role for segmental or abdominal colectomy in Crohn's colitis. Dis Colon Rectum. 1997;40(1):71–8.
18. Martel P, et al. Crohn's colitis: experience with segmental resections; results in a series of 84 patients. J Am Coll Surg. 2002;194(4):448–53.
19. Polle SW, et al. Recurrence after segmental resection for colonic Crohn's disease. Br J Surg. 2005;92(9): 1143–9.
20. Bernell O, Lapidus A, Hellers G. Recurrence after colectomy in Crohn's colitis. Dis Colon Rectum. 2001;44(5):647–54. discussion 654.
21. Elton C, et al. Mortality, morbidity and functional outcome after ileorectal anastomosis. Br J Surg. 2003;90(1):59–65.
22. Cattan P, et al. Fate of the rectum in patients undergoing total colectomy for Crohn's disease. Br J Surg. 2002;89(4):454–9.
23. O'Riordan JM, et al. Long-term outcome of colectomy and ileorectal anastomosis for Crohn's colitis. Dis Colon Rectum. 2011;54(11):1347–54.
24. Ng RL, et al. Subcutaneous rectal stump closure after emergency subtotal colectomy. Br J Surg. 1992; 79(7):701–3.
25. Grieco MB, et al. Toxic megacolon complicating Crohn's colitis. Ann Surg. 1980;191(1):75–80.
26. Guillem JG, et al. Factors predictive of persistent or recurrent Crohn's disease in excluded rectal segments. Dis Colon Rectum. 1992;35(8):768–72.
27. Cirincione E, Gorfine SR, Bauer JJ. Is Hartmann's procedure safe in Crohn's disease? Report of three cases. Dis Colon Rectum. 2000;43(4):544–7.
28. Church JM, et al. The relationship between fistulas in Crohn's disease and associated carcinoma. Report of four cases and review of the literature. Dis Colon Rectum. 1985;28(5):361–6.
29. Yamamoto T, Watanabe T. Surgery for luminal Crohn's disease. World J Gastroenterol. 2014;20(1): 78–90.
30. Yamamoto T, et al. Persistent perineal sinus after proctocolectomy for Crohn's disease. Dis Colon Rectum. 1999;42(1):96–101.
31. Gardenbroek TJ, et al. Surgery for Crohn's disease: new developments. Dig Surg. 2012;29(4):275–80.
32. Hyman NH, et al. Consequences of ileal pouch-anal anastomosis for Crohn's colitis. Dis Colon Rectum. 1991;34(8):653–7.
33. Panis Y, et al. Ileal pouch/anal anastomosis for Crohn's disease. Lancet. 1996;347(9005):854–7.
34. Regimbeau JM, et al. Long-term results of ileal pouch-anal anastomosis for colorectal Crohn's disease. Dis Colon Rectum. 2001;44(6):769–78.
35. Nisar PJ, et al. Factors associated with ileoanal pouch failure in patients developing early or late pouch-related fistula. Dis Colon Rectum. 2011;54(4): 446–53.
36. Braveman JM, et al. The fate of the ileal pouch in patients developing Crohn's disease. Dis Colon Rectum. 2004;47(10):1613–9.
37. Tekkis PP, et al. Long-term outcomes of restorative proctocolectomy for Crohn's disease and indeterminate colitis. Colorectal Dis. 2005;7(3):218–23.

13 Surgery: Perineum

Patricia L. Roberts

Introduction

While Crohn's disease was initially described as terminal ileitis in 1932 [1], there were a number of reports of anal fistulizing disease which was most likely a manifestation of anal Crohn's disease in the nineteenth and early twentieth century. Colles described fistulizing rectal and perianal disease in children in 1829 [2] and Gabriel described anal fistulas and giant cells in 30 patients in the absence of tuberculosis [3]. Penner and Crohn subsequently recognized anal lesions in 20 out of 110 patients with Crohn's disease in 1938 [4]. Perianal disease is now recognized as a distinct phenotype of Crohn's and the susceptibility locus on chromosome five has been identified.

The exact incidence of patients with Crohn's disease who have perianal manifestations ranges from 14 to 38 % [5–8]. The range is due in part to the definition of perianal disease and how diligently perianal disease was sought after and diagnosed. Studies that include skin tags and hemorrhoids have a higher incidence of perianal disease, while studies which include abscess, fistula, and fissure only have a lower incidence of perianal disease.

Patients with colonic Crohn's disease are more likely to have perianal disease; the likelihood is higher, the more distal the intestinal disease is. Crohn's disease involving the anus only is rare and a small minority of patients present with anal disease only [8]. Manifestations of perianal Crohn's disease include anal fissures, anal ulcerations, anorectal abscess or fistulas including rectovaginal fistulas, anal stricture, and perianal skin tags disease. While these lesions are not pathognomonic of Crohn's, the diagnosis should be suspected in patients who have multiple anal lesions, lateral fissures, deep ulcerations, a stricture at the anorectal ring, and multiple fistulas.

Examination and Diagnosis

The initial patient history should focus on the extent of Crohn's, prior medical treatments, and prior resections. A history of prior anal surgery or obstetric trauma should be noted.

Initial assessment consists of visual inspection and palpation of the perianal skin and anal canal. Large anal tags may overly fissures and anal ulcerations; retraction of the buttocks is necessary to note these findings. The presence of prior scarring is noted as well as the external opening

P. L. Roberts, MD (✉)
Department of Colon and Rectal Surgery, Division of Surgery, Lahey Hospital and Medical Center, 41 Mall Road, Burlington, MA 01805, USA

Tufts University School of Medicine, Boston, MA, USA
e-mail: patricia.l.roberts@lahey.org

A. Fichera and M.K. Krane (eds.), *Crohn's Disease: Basic Principles*,
DOI 10.1007/978-3-319-14181-7_13, © Springer International Publishing Switzerland 2015

of any fistula tracts. If an external opening is noted, one should attempt to palpate a tract. A palpable tract generally notes a more superficial fistula and is helpful in facilitating the identification of the internal opening. Digital rectal examination combined with anoscopy is performed to identify the tone of the sphincter, identify an internal opening or secondary tract, note the presence of associated sepsis or abscess and note a stricture of the anorectal ring. A flexible sigmoidoscopy or colonoscopy is helpful to assess the degree of rectal inflammation and assess the distensibility of the rectum.

Patients with active proctitis and associated anorectal sepsis may be too tender to examine in the office, and examination under anesthesia (EUA) is indicated. EUA also permits use of various probes to assess fistula tracts and potential injection of hydrogen peroxide or methylene blue to identify the internal opening. Gentle probing, palpation of the tract with the educated index finger, and application of Goodsall's rule are helpful to identify the internal opening of fistula tracts. Goodsall's rule states if the anus is divided by a line drawn transversely through the anus, a fistula with an anterior external opening will follow a radial course to the anal canal and a fistula with a posterior external opening will curve posteriorly to enter the crypt in the midline [9]. The accuracy of Goodsall's rule has been reexamined. In a study of 110 male and 72 female patients, of whom 63 had Crohn's disease, anterior fistulas were more frequent in women and in patients with Crohn's disease [10]. Posterior fistulas were more common in men and in patients without Crohn's disease. Goodsall's rule was more accurate for posterior than anterior fistulas and was not affected by the presence of inflammatory bowel disease [10, 11].

Imaging and Other Considerations

Imaging is not necessary in the majority of patients with Crohn's disease but is a useful adjunct in patients with complex or multiple fistulas and patients with recurrent anal fistulas (Figs. 13.1, 13.2, and 13.3). The history and physical examination and overall assessment of the patient should include a review or prior imaging and endoscopic examinations.

Fistulography

Fistulography entails cannulating the external opening of a fistula, injecting contrast material and obtaining images. Although fistulography has fallen somewhat out of vogue particularly with the use of MRI, I still find fistulography valuable in selected cases, particularly those patients who have long pararectal tracts. In these patients,

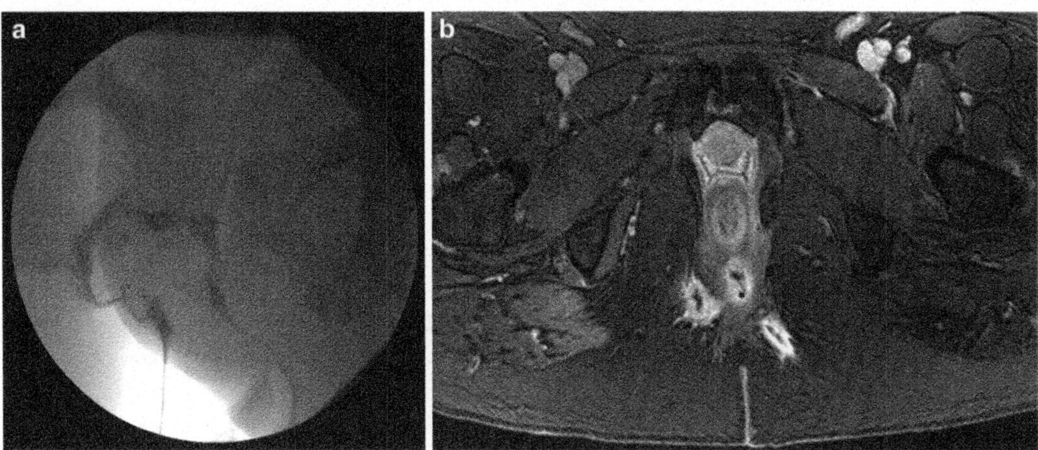

Fig. 13.1 Two images of a patient with a transphincteric fistula shown on sinogram (fistulogram) (**a**) and on MRI (**b**)

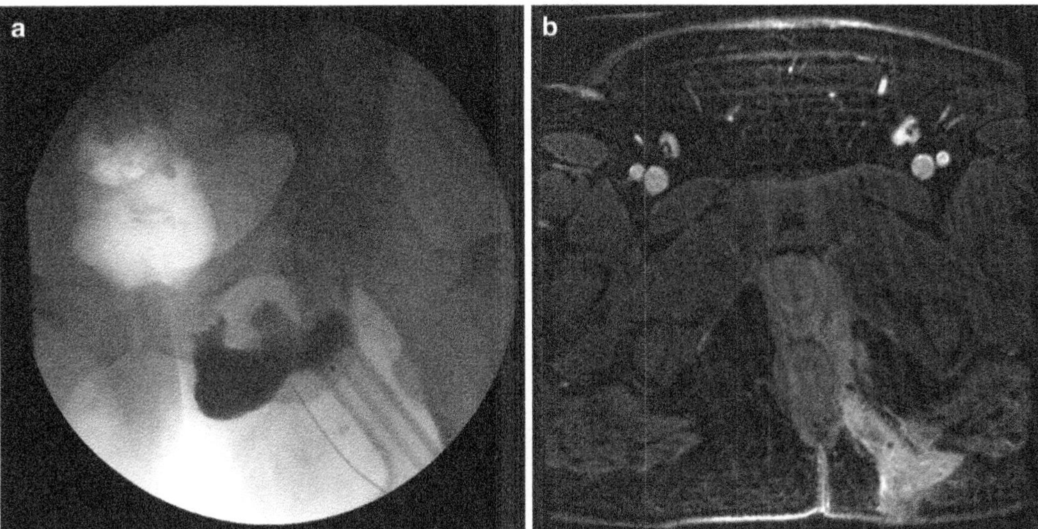

Fig. 13.2 Two images of a patient with a complex suprasphincteric fistula shown on fistulogram (**a**) and MRI (**b**) MRI can distinguish between fibrosis and infection and assess complex tracts

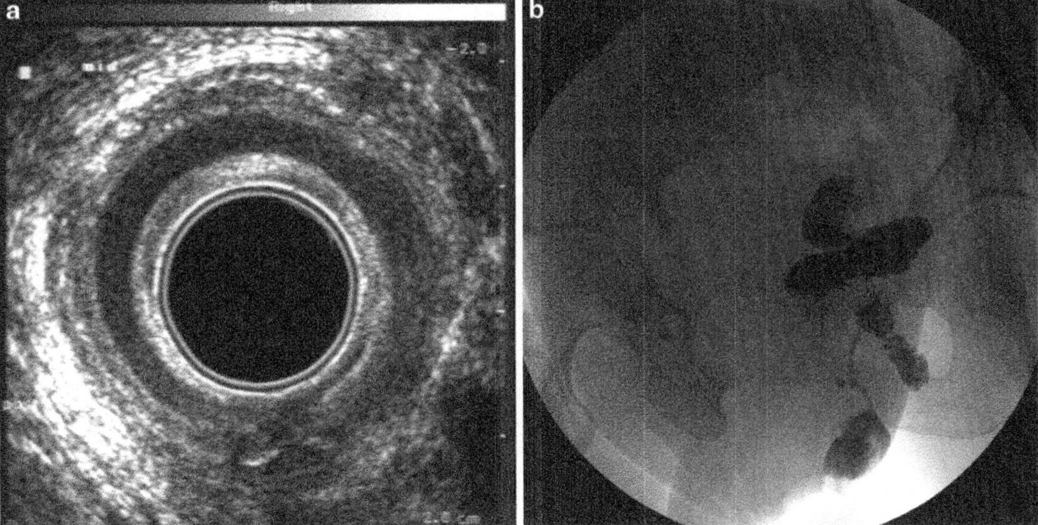

Fig. 13.3 This patient had a complex intersphincteric fistula with a secondary track and large cavity demonstrated on fistulogram (**b**) and ultrasound (**a**)

fistulography is a straightforward examination to look for communication with remote organs such as small bowel or sigmoid colon.

Endoanal Ultrasound

Although ultrasound is not needed in the majority of patients with anorectal abscess and fistula, it is useful in selected patients with Crohn's disease particularly those with complex fistulas including horseshoe fistulas, high tracts, multiple fistulas, and secondary tracts. Accuracy rates of 80–89 % have been reported [12–16]. Three dimensional ultrasound techniques combined with hydrogen peroxide injection have been reported with concordance rates of 90 % (comparable to the accuracy of MRI) [17, 18]. Ultrasound remains operator dependent with excellent results from selected centers.

Magnetic Resonance Imaging

Magnetic resonance imaging (MRI) has the ability to distinguish anal sepsis and granulation tissue from anal sphincter musculature and is useful to delineate additional or more complex disease in patients with Crohn's. In some studies, additional or more complex disease was noted in 40 % of patients which altered the operative plan [19, 20].

MRI has been reported to have accuracy rates as high as 90 % for delineating fistula tracts and the relationship to the sphincter and identifying the internal opening [17, 18]. While imaging is not necessary for the majority of patients, it is helpful in patients with complex disease and those with recurrent disease. The findings of MRI must then be correlated with the intraoperative findings; at times, the sophistication of imaging exceeds our ability to delineate the tracts intraoperatively.

Clinical Course and Approach to Treatment

The clinical course of perianal Crohn's disease is variable but in general, patients have a more disabling clinical course with the development of more extra-intestinal manifestations and less response to steroids. Close collaboration with the surgeon, primary care physician, and gastroenterologist is essential for optimal outcomes. The goals of treatment include maintaining continence and avoiding a stoma if possible, improving the quality of life, limiting the risk of recurrent disease, timing surgical interventions, and optimizing medical therapy.

A number of classification systems have been devised for assessment of perianal Crohn's disease. Hughes proposed the Cardiff classification system in which each major manifestation of perianal Crohn's disease is graded on a 2 point scale [21]. The American Gastroenterological Association technical review in 2003 [6] proposed an empiric approach, including physical exam and endoscopic examination with classification of fistulas as simple or complex. A perianal Crohn's disease activity index was described by Irvine in 1995 to evaluate five categories of morbidity in patients with perianal Crohn's including presence of fistula discharge and pain, restriction of daily activity, restriction of sexual activity, type of perianal disease, and degree of induration [22]. No classification system is widely used or accepted but collectively they provide a framework to categorize perianal disease.

Treatment of anal Crohn's disease involves coordination of medical and surgical therapy. Drugs with efficacy for treating perianal Crohn's disease include antibiotics (especially metronidazole and ciprofloxacin), immunosuppressives (azathioprine and 6-mercaptopurine), calcineurin inhibitors (cyclosporine and tacrolimus), and biological agents (infliximab, adalimumab, and certolizumab). Please refer to Chap. 4 for specific details.

The use of antibiotics has been a mainstay in the treatment of fistulas and anorectal abscesses associated with perianal Crohn's disease. Despite the widespread use, there are very few controlled trials in the literature and the existing trials have a small sample size. Clinical response generally occurs after 6–8 weeks, fistula drainage decreases but does not cease and drainage and symptoms recur with discontinuation of the antibiotic. In a recent trial to evaluate the results of ciprofloxacin and metronidazole in the treatment of perianal Crohn's disease, remission and response seemed to occur more commonly after ciprofloxacin [23]. Once again, the sample size was small (25 patients). A limiting factor with antibiotic therapy has been the development of adverse events with long-term therapy including sensory neuropathy with the use of metronidazole and the risk of tendon rupture with ciprofloxacin. To avoid the adverse events with systemic therapy, metronidazole 10 % ointment has also been evaluated in a randomized controlled trial [24]. In this trial, 74 patients with anal fistula were randomized to application of placebo ointment or metronidazole 10 % ointment three times a day. A significant difference was not noted but patient in the metronidazole arm had reduction in discharge and perianal pain.

The use of anti-TNF alpha agents has substantially changed the approach to management of patients with Crohn's disease and in particular those with fistulizing disease. The initial data on efficacy was published in 1999 with 94 patients with fistulizing Crohn's disease randomized to infliximab or placebo at 0, 2, and 6 weeks [25]. 55 % of patients randomized to the 5 mg/kg dose of infliximab had fistula closure compared to 13 % of patients randomized to placebo. Subsequently the ACCENT II trial demonstrated superiority of infliximab over placebo for long-term healing [26]. A more recent study showed that combination therapy of adalimumab and ciprofloxacin resulted in a higher fistula closure rate and resulted in better quality of life than adalimumab alone [27].

Perirectal Abscess

Abscesses are common in patients with Crohn's disease occurring in 23–62 % of patients and are a common indication for anal surgery. They may present in any of the perirectal spaces—intersphincteric, perianal, ischiorectal, and supralevator. Patients may also present with a postanal space abscess with poorly characterized rectal pain and no external signs of sepsis. The presentation of patients with perirectal abscess and Crohn's disease is similar to patients without Crohn's presenting with anal pain, fever, and a lump or swelling on examination. Any patient with unexplained rectal pain should be considered to have an abscess until proven otherwise. While ischiorectal and perianal abscesses are common, patients with Crohn's disease are more likely to have more complex abscesses.

The diagnosis of an abscess is usually straightforward on history and physical examination. EUA is performed if the patient is too tender to examination in the office. Simple abscesses can be drained under local anesthesia in the office setting. The majority of patients including those with more complex abscesses, recurrent abscesses, and abscesses associated with other perianal manifestations of Crohn's disease are generally best drained in the operating room where a thorough examination can be performed. Endorectal ultrasound, CT scan, or MRI is generally not needed but may be useful adjuncts to diagnosis selective abscesses, particularly those in the supralevator space [28]. A deep perianal abscess also known as a postanal space abscess may be difficult to diagnose. Patients often complain of perianal pain and have no external signs of sepsis. Digital rectal examination reveals a tender boggy feel of the anal canal posteriorly. The deep postanal space is bounded superiorly by the levator ani, inferiorly by the anococcygeal ligament, medially by the anal sphincter/rectal wall.

Once an abscess is diagnosed, incision and drainage is performed. Drainage is performed as close to the anal canal as possible with care to avoid sphincter damage and to have any resultant fistula have a shorter tract. We have also used mushroom catheters for patients with deep abscesses, complex abscesses, and large cavities and in a cohort of 38 patients have found a slight benefit in patients who underwent catheter drainage in terms of a lower risk or recurrent abscess and a lower risk of proctectomy [29].

Some patients may not have a discrete collection of pus, but rather inflammatory induration. These patients are challenging to treat and may require long-term antibiotic therapy. Our preference is to not use antibiotics in the majority of patients with simple abscesses and to reserve use of antibiotics to patients with multiple abscesses, cellulitis, and other manifestations of anal Crohn's.

Fistula-in-Ano

The majority of patients with an anorectal abscess and Crohn's will develop an anal fistula and approximately 25 % of patients with Crohn's disease will develop a perianal fistula during the course of their disease [30]. Patients with Crohn's disease develop anal fistulas for two reasons: one mechanism (which can also occur in patients who do not have Crohn's) is a consequence of anorectal abscess where the origin of the abscess is the anal glands at the base of the crypts. The other cause of fistula is ulceration or anal fistulas which burrow and result in the formation of fistulas.

The Parks classification system is the most commonly used system to describe anal fistulas [31]. Based on the relationship to the anal sphincter, fistulas are classified as superficial, intersphincteric, transphincteric, extrasphincteric, and suprasphincteric. The system applies to fistulas around the anal canal but does not include fistulas to other organs such as rectovaginal and rectourethral fistulas. The American Gastroenterological Association technical review panel has suggested that fistulas should be classified as simple or complex [6]. Simple fistulas traverse only a small portion of the anal sphincter and do not involve other organs. Complex fistulas involve a substantial part of the anal sphincter and may involve other organs. This system may be more useful in approaching Crohn's fistulas. Some investigators have considered all Crohn's fistulas to be complex.

The approach to perianal fistulas depends on the degree of complexity of the fistula, the presence or absence of involvement of the rectum and colon with active Crohn's disease and inflammation, the presence of other anal manifestations of Crohn's disease, and whether the patient has had additional surgery/bowel resection. Flexible sigmoidoscopy or colonoscopy is helpful to assess the extent of disease and in particular note the degree of rectal inflammation. Healing rates are substantially lower for anorectal procedures in patients with active proctitis [30]. Evaluation of the fistulas involves EUA with inspection and palpation of the tracts and gentle probing. This may be combined with injection of dilute hydrogen peroxide to delineate the internal opening and identify any other unsuspected tracts. For patients with multiple fistula tracts, complex high fistulas, and multiple previous procedures with significant scarring, other imaging may be helpful prior to exam under anesthesia. CT, fistulography, MRI, and endorectal ultrasound have all been used.

Treatment

In approaching the surgical management of anal fistulas in association with Crohn's disease the main options include no surgical intervention, placement of draining setons, and all other options including fistulotomy, endorectal sliding flap, fibrin glue, collagen fistula plug, and LIFT procedure. In determining the best treatment option, one needs to consider the extent of anorectal disease and complexity of the fistula, the status of the anal sphincter and continence, the associated intestinal Crohn's disease, especially proctitis, bowel function, and prior anorectal and abdominal operations.

The treatment of anal fistulas in patients with Crohn's disease is aimed at reducing symptoms and in selected cases, healing or curing the fistula. A small number of patients with anal fistulas and associated Crohn's disease have asymptomatic fistulas. These fistulas require no surgical intervention and may remain asymptomatic for long periods of time. Surgical intervention for such patients is not indicated as it subjects the patient to the potential morbidity of surgery without a clear benefit [32–34].

Fistulotomy

A number of publications and the Practice Parameters of the American Society of Colon and Rectal Surgeons for perianal abscess and fistula-in-ano state that fistulotomy is safe and effective for superficial fistulas with no associated incontinence [6, 35]. Fistulotomy must be considered with caution in patients with Crohn's disease given the relapsing nature of the disease and the potential need for multiple bowel resections or other anorectal procedures and should only be used for the most superficial fistulas (involving internal sphincter). Healing rates after simple fistulotomy have been reported in 56–100 % of patients with mild incontinence rates of 6–12 % [35–39].

Setons

A noncutting seton is one of the most common treatments of anal fistula associated with Crohn's disease. A seton helps to prevent abscess formation, keeps the tract open while facilitating drainage and improving symptoms. Multiple setons can be used for patient with multiple tracts (so-called watering can perineum). Setons may also be used as a bridge to other treatments including biologics.

Setons are well tolerated and patients report good quality of life with setons in place. They may remain in place for many years). Removal of setons results in recurrent anorectal abscess/fistula in up to 80 % of patients [12–14, 40, 41]. My clinical impression is that with time, setons appear to become more superficial suggesting that they gradually cut through the tissue and result in more superficial fistula.

Endorectal Sliding Flap

Endorectal sliding flaps have been used in a variety of clinical settings where simply laying open the fistula tract is not an option. Complex fistulas including those involving a substantial portion of the external sphincter, transphincteric, suprasphincteric, extrasphincteric, and rectovaginal and rectourethral fistulas in addition to anterior fistulas in women are fistulas which may be treated with endorectal advancement flap. The perianal skin may also be used as an anocutaneous advancement flaps. In patients with Crohn's disease relative contraindications include the presence of undrained sepsis and the presence of active disease, especially Crohn's proctitis. Flaps generally cannot be performed with an underlying anorectal stricture which precludes the ability to raise the flap and work intrarectally.

Endorectal sliding (advancement flaps) involves mobilizing a well-vascularized flap of tissue around the internal opening which may consist of mucosa, submucosa, or circular muscle and then advancing the flap to cover over the site of the sutured internal opening. Mucosal flaps may not have adequate vascularity and thicker flaps which include the wall of the rectum (and the internal sphincter) may have a high rate of associated incontinence. The use of fibrin glue as an adjunct has not improved the success rate of flaps.

There are small series of endorectal advancement flaps in patients with Crohn's disease. Soltani and Kaiser [42] performed a systematic review of endorectal advancement flaps for cryptoglandular and Crohn's fistula-in-ano. Over a 30-year period there were 35 studies of 2,065 patients and 1,654 patients underwent advancement flaps for cryptoglandular or Crohn's disease. The quality of the studies was limited with a number of methodological and design flaws. The weighted success for fistula healing was 64 % for patients with Crohn's disease (compared to 80.8 % in patients with cryptoglandular fistulas and the associated incontinence was 13.2 % in cryptoglandular patients versus 9.4 % in patients with Crohn's disease [42].

In patients with Crohn's disease, ongoing proctitis is a relative contradiction to endorectal advancement flap. It is also important to note that if a flap fails, generally the patient is initially more symptomatic—presumably because the internal opening from the failed flap is larger than the initial internal opening associated with the fistula [43].

Fibrin Glue

Fibrin glue may be used as autologous fibrin glue or commercially available fibrin glue. The latter is generally used and entails two syringes of fibrinogen and thrombin injected together into the tract to essentially "caulk" the fistula. The thrombin is activated to form a clot which seals the fistula tract. While the early reports from one group showed healing of 68–85 % of patients with anal fistulas in 1 year, these results have been difficult to replicate particularly in patients with Crohn's disease [44, 45]. An open label randomized controlled trial looked at 77 patients with Crohn's disease and anal fistulas. Half of the patients had complex fistulas [46]. Patients were randomized to either fibrin glue or to removal of the seton with observation. The end point of the trial was clinical remission which was defined as the absence of drainage, perianal pain, or abscess. Remission was observed in 38 % of patients in the fibrin glue arm and only 16 % of patients in the removal of the seton and observation arm showing a clear advantage for fibrin glue. A retrospective review of the use of fibrin glue for complex fistulas had similar results with healing in 31 % of patients with Crohn's disease [47]. Most fistulas were noted to have initial healing but "recrudescence" occurred within 3 months.

Despite these results, fibrin glue has had some appeal as it is simple to perform with minimal morbidity. If the procedure fails, patients have a persistent symptomatic fistula and may require a return trip to the operating room for replacement of the seton.

Fistula Plug

The bioprosthetic fistula plug has been used both to close the primary internal opening of a fistula and to serve as a matrix for obliteration of the fistula tract. The plug essentially acts as a collagen scaffold upon which the patient's cells grow, incorporate, and heal the tract over a 3-month time period. Initial results were promising with fistula closure rates of 83 % for all types of complex fistulas at a median of 12 months and a closure rate of 80 % in patients with Crohn's disease [48, 49].

Subsequent studies have failed to replicate these results. Two systematic reviews have examined the results of anal fistula plug in an extremely heterogeneous group of patients [50, 51]. Garg et al. reviewed 317 patients in 12 studies who underwent placement of an anal fistula plug. Patients with rectovaginal fistulas were excluded. The follow-up ranged from 3.5 to 12 months. The success rate in patients with Crohn's disease ranged from 29 to 86 %. For all patients, the rate of abscess formation or local sepsis was 4–19 % and the plug extrusion rate was 4–41 %. An additional review looked at 530 patients in 20 studies [51]. Rectovaginal, anovaginal, rectourethral, and ileoanal pouch fistulas were excluded in addition to studies with a mean or median follow-up of 3 months or less. There were 488 non-Crohn's patients and 42 Crohn's patients. The pooled proportion of patients achieving fistula closure was similar in the non-Crohn's patients (0.54, 95 % CI 0.50–0.59) to the proportion in the Crohn's patients (0.55, 95 % CI 0.39–0.70). The overall plug extrusion rate was 8.7 %. The authors concluded that the anal fistula plug has not been adequately evaluated in patients with Crohn's disease.

Although anal fistula plug is associated with low morbidity and warrants consideration in selected patient with anal fistulas and Crohn's disease, the cost of the plug combined with the additional treatments needed if plug failure, extrusion or local abscess or sepsis ensue should be considered when considering this treatment.

LIFT Procedure

The ligation of the intersphincteric fistula tract (LIFT) procedure was first introduced by Rojanasakul et al. [52]. The procedure involves ligation of the fistula tract in the groove between the internal and external sphincter, does not involve cutting of the sphincter and thus, continence should be preserved. Some surgeons feel that placement of a seton 8–12 weeks prior to performing the LIFT procedure is helpful to eliminate sepsis in the area and allow for the tract to mature [53]. Active sepsis and active inflammatory bowel disease (especially proctitis) are relative contraindications to the procedure. The procedure involves a curvilinear skin incision over the intersphincteric groove, dissection of the fistula tract, ligation and division of the fistula tract, and closure of the wound.

One prospective series has evaluated the 2 and 12-month outcomes of 15 patients with Crohn's disease who underwent the LIFT procedure for transphincteric fistulas [54]. Fistula healing and two validated quality of life indices were assessed. Ultimately, nine patients healed after the LIFT procedure and six failed. If the LIFT procedure failed, the ensuing intersphincteric fistula was easier to treat. Of interest, 20 % of patients developed additional new fistulas which were most likely a manifestation on ongoing perianal Crohn's disease and not complications of the LIFT procedure.

Failures of the LIFT procedure in combined series generally result in persistence of the internal opening with drainage and failure of wound healing of the intersphincteric incision [55]. One would anticipate that poor wound healing (at the LIFT site) and persistence of the internal opening might be higher in patients with Crohn's disease.

Fecal Diversion

For patients with unrelenting symptoms from perianal disease, fecal diversion may be performed. Diversion generally is performed with a laparoscopic loop ileostomy and may be done as a temporary measure. Risk factors for the need for diversion include Crohn's colitis, anal stricture, and multiple complex fistulas ("watering can perineum"). Diversion results in improvement of symptoms in over 80 % of patients, and while it is theoretically temporary, less than 50 % of patients ultimately have the stoma reversed. Nevertheless, it results in improvement in quality of life for the majority of patients and may help patients adapt to a stoma. Active rectal disease is a predictor of failure.

Proctectomy

Ultimately, proctectomy is required in 5–31 % of patients. The risk of requiring proctectomy is higher in patients with complex fistulas, associated rectovaginal fistulas, deep ulceration, and supralevator abscesses. Although proctectomy may be done by an intersphincteric approach, minimizing the size of the perineal excision, wound healing is slow and may be associated with perineal sinus formation and a non-healing wound in 25–50 % of patients.

Rectovaginal Fistula

Rectovaginal fistulas occur in up to 10 % of women with Crohn's disease and have varying symptoms [56]. The majority of the fistulas are low fistulas; symptoms are worse the higher the fistula. The treatment is aimed at decreasing fistula drainage to a minimal level that is acceptable or if possible, to cure the fistula [6]. The ultimate cure rate of patients with rectovaginal fistula and Crohn's remains lower than those patients with fistulas of obstetric origin; a number of operations may be needed to achieve cure of the fistulas. Patients with Crohn's and rectovaginal fistulas therefore needed to be informed of the challenges of treating such fistulas, the need for fecal diversion, and the multitude of operations which may be needed. Ultimate healing rates of under 50 % are common.

One of the largest series of Crohn's related rectovaginal fistulas reviewed 65 women with a median follow-up of 44.6 months [57]. Ultimately 30 patients (46.2 %) had successful healing. Repair methods included advancement flap ($n=47$), episioproctotomy ($n=8$), coloanal anastomosis ($n=7$), and fibrin glue or plug ($n=3$). Of the 28 women who were sexually active (43.1 %), nine had dyspareunia. The nine women with dyspareunia all had unhealed fistulas. Immunomodulators were associated with successful healing and smoking and steroids were associated with failure of the repair.

Treatment options for rectovaginal fistula are dependent on the state of the rectum, with active proctitis a contraindication to a local repair and the presence of an anorectal stricture making certain repairs such as an endorectal advancement flap challenging. Some surgeons have advocated vaginal advancement flaps instead of endorectal advancement flaps, but a recent systematic review of 11 studies of 219 patients revealed no difference in outcome of rectal or vaginal advancement flaps [58]. Most repairs are performed with fecal diversion. If a fistula recurs after repair, it is generally much larger and more symptomatic initially, an important point to emphasize in the preoperative discussion with the patient.

A number of medical therapies have been used to treat rectovaginal fistulas often combined with surgical intervention. In uncontrolled series, 6-mercaptopurine, infliximab, cyclosporine, and tacrolimus have all been used to treat rectovaginal fistulas. The results of treatment of rectovaginal fistulas are worse than results for perinal fistulas. In the Accent 2 trial, a subgroup of patients with Crohn's and rectovaginal fistulas was examined [59]. In this study, 25 of 138 women (18.1 %) had a rectovaginal fistula. Infliximab was better than placebo but the results were poorer than perianal fistulas.

Anal Skin Tags

Perianal skin tags are quite common and occur in up to 70 % of patients with anal Crohn's disease. They are typically described as waxy tags or so-called elephant ears and may have a violaceous hue.

Tags are believed to results from recurrent fissures or fistulas associated with lymphatic obstruction [60, 61]. They are typically soft and nontender. Pain associated with tags suggests an underlying abscess or a fissure or anal ulceration associated with the tag.

Despite patient's complaints of the appearance of the tag and difficulty with anal hygiene, excision is rarely indicated and can be associated with poor healing.

Hemorrhoids

Hemorrhoids have an estimated incidence of 24 % in the general population and an estimated 7 % incidence in patients with Crohn's disease [62]. The classical teaching has been to avoid hemorrhoid surgery in patients with Crohn's disease because of the concern of poor wound healing noted in prior studies. In 1977, Jeffrey and colleagues reported 62 patients with inflammatory bowel disease who underwent hemorrhoidectomy [63]. There were 20 patients with Crohn's disease and ultimately six required proctectomy.

More recent studies of properly selected patients have been associated with good outcomes. Patients with Crohn's disease and hemorrhoids may have exacerbation of hemorrhoidal symptoms from active disease particularly ongoing diarrhea. Initial medical treatment is aimed at regulating bowel movements; as patients with Crohn's disease rarely have constipation, the initial medical treatment is aimed at controlling loose bowel in addition to topical ointments and Sitz baths. Surgery or hemorrhoid banding may be considered selectively. Wolkomir and Luchtefeld reported a series of 17 patients with successful healing in 88 % of Crohn's patients who underwent hemorrhoid surgery [64]. A series of 13 patients with Crohn's disease who underwent Doppler artery ligation had no complications and a success rate of 77 % at 13 months [65]. An additional series of patients with anal disease and Crohn's disease was associated with a 41 % complication rate in 11 patients who underwent an open hemorrhoidectomy, 3 who underwent a closed hemorrhoidectomy, 1 patient who underwent a PPH, and 2 patients who had rubber band ligation [66]. Given the prevalence of hemorrhoids in the general population and the paucity of data of hemorrhoid surgery in patients with Crohn's disease in addition to concerns of poor healing, stricture and potentially even the need for proctectomy, hemorrhoidectomy is rarely indicated and should be approached with caution in patients with Crohn's disease.

Fissures

Anal fissures are common in patients with Crohn's disease. The most common location (similar to garden variety fissures) is the posterior midline followed by the anterior midline [67]. However, up to 20 % of patients with Crohn's disease and an anal fissure may have a lateral location and many fissures are asymptomatic. A fissure in a lateral location may be the first sign of Crohn's disease. The etiology of Crohn's fissures is probably twofold either due to ischemia similar to the etiology of idiopathic fissures or secondary to ongoing inflammatory disease and associated ulcerations in the anorectum. An abscess or fistula may also develop in approximately one quarter of patients with Crohn's disease and an anal fissure [68]. Fissures may, on occasion, be painless.

Medical management is the first step in treatment including Sitz baths and topical preparations. Patients with Crohn's disease rarely have constipation and thus the fiber preparations utilized in idiopathic fissures are not necessary. The majority of anal fissures in patients with Crohn's disease heal with medical management [69]. There is limited data on the use of nitrates and the use of botulinum toxin for anal fissure. Older studies have suggested a success rate of up to 88 % of sphincterotomy in selected patients without active disease [68]. With more recent concerns of a higher than previously anticipated risk of incontinence after sphincterotomy, this procedure is uncommonly performed now for anal fissures and associated Crohn's disease. A recent review of 14 patients with Crohn's disease and associated anal fissure noted a 57 % complication rate in eight patients who underwent injection of botulinum toxin with or without fissurectomy and six patients who underwent lateral internal sphincterotomy [66].

Strictures

Anal and low rectal strictures are common and have been reported in up to 10 % of patients [70]. These strictures are easily diagnosed on digital, anoscopic, or proctoscopic examination. If the patient is asymptomatic, no treatment is warranted. Some degree of stricture may actually improve bowel function in a patient with diarrhea and Crohn's.

These strictures are usually a manifestation of ongoing active Crohn's disease, with either active proctitis or ongoing sepsis from anorectal disease. Symptomatic fibrotic strictures can be treated by dilatation which, depending on the site, can either be finer dilatation or dilatation with a balloon. A small number of patients will require diversion and/or proctectomy for symptomatic strictures. Strictures may also be associated with anal cancer particularly in patients with longstanding disease and appropriate biopsies and assessment in addition to dilatation should be performed in such patients.

A recent series looked at the natural history of 102 patients with Crohn's disease and anorectal stricture particularly examining the role of biologics [71]. There were 37 men and 65 women with a mean duration of Crohn's disease of 8.9 years. Female gender and introduction or optimization of TNF alpha antagonist treatment decreased the risk of an unfavorable outcome. Two patients developed anal adenocarcinoma and ultimately over a median follow-up of 2.8 years 52 of the 88 patients (59 %) had healing of the stricture.

Neoplasia and Anal Crohn's

Patients with Crohn's disease have not only an increased risk for colorectal cancer but also an increased risk for the development of squamous cell carcinoma and adenocarcinoma of the anus, particularly in longstanding fistula tracts. Risk factors include longstanding duration of disease and active anorectal disease. Detection can be difficult; my practice is to biopsy, curette, and excise the external opening of fistulas of all patients with a long duration of disease. One study suggested a distinct MRI appearance of perineal carcinoma in Crohn's disease [72]. The MRI of six patients with cancer (four mucinous adenocarcinoma and two squamous carcinoma) was compared with 18 patients with Crohn's disease and perianal fistulas. An irregular internal wall and delayed enhancing tissue was seen only in the patients with cancer. Patients with mucinous adenocarcinoma also had a pattern of lobulated fluid filled cavies with delayed internal tissue enhancement.

Conclusion

Perianal Crohn's disease is challenging to treat for both the patient and the physician. Optimal treatment depends on close collaboration of the primary care physician, the gastroenterologist, and the surgeon.

References

1. Crohn BB, Ginzberg L, Oppenheimer GD. Regional ileitis: a pathologic and clinical entity. JAMA. 1932; 99:32.
2. Colles A. Practical observations upon certain diseases of intestines, colon and rectum. Dublin Hosp Rep. 1830;5:131.
3. Gabriel WB. Results of an experimental and histological investigation into seventy-five cases of rectal fistulae. Proc R Soc Med. 1921;14:156–61.
4. Penner A, Crohn BB. Perianal fistulae as a complication of regional ileitis. Ann Surg. 1938;108(5):867–73.
5. Hellers G, Bergstrand O, Ewerth S, Holmstrom B. Occurrence and outcome after primary treatment of anal fistulae in Crohn's disease. Gut. 1980;21(6): 525–7.
6. Sandborn WJ, Fazio VW, Feagan BG, Hanauer SB. American Gastroenterological Association Clinical Practice Committee. AGA technical review on perianal Crohn's disease. Gastroenterology. 2003;125(5): 1508–30.
7. Schwartz DA, Loftus Jr EV, Tremaine WJ, et al. The natural history of fistulizing Crohn's disease in

Olmsted County, Minnesota. Gastroenterology. 2002; 122(4):875–80.
8. Willliams DR, Coller JA, Corman ML, Nugent FW, Veidenheimer MC. Anal complications in Crohn's disease. Dis Colon Rectum. 1981;24(1):22–4.
9. Goodsall DH, Miles WE. Anorectal fistula. Dis Colon Rectum. 1982;25:262–78.
10. Corremans G, Docks S, Wyndacle J, et al. Do anal fistulas in Crohn's disease behave differently and defy Goodsall's rule more frequently than fistulas that are cryptoglandular in origin? Am J Gastroenterol. 2003;98:2732–5.
11. Cirocco WC, Reilly JC. Challenging the predictive accuracy of Goodsall's rule for anal fistulas. Dis Colon Rectum. 1992;35:537–42.
12. Buchanan GN, Halligan S, Bartram CI, William AB, Tarroni D, Cohen CR. Clinical examination, endosonography and MR imaging in preoperative assessment of fistula-in-ano: comparison with outcome based reference standard. Radiology. 2004;233: 674–81.
13. Buchanan GN, Bartram CI, Williams AB, Halligan S, Cohen CR. Value of hydrogen peroxide enhancement of three-dimensional endoanal ultrasound in fistula-in-ano. Dis Colon Rectum. 2004;48:141–7.
14. Buchanan GN, Owen HA, Torkington J, Lunniss PJ, Nicholls RJ, Cohen CR. Long-term outcome following loose-seton technique for external sphincter preservation in complex anal fistula. Br J Surg. 2004;91(4):476–80.
15. Toyonaga T, Matsushima M, Tanaka Y, et al. Microbiological analysis and endoanal ultrasonography for diagnosis of anal fistula in acute anorectal sepsis. Int J Colorectal Dis. 2007;22:209–13.
16. Toyonaga T, Tanaka Y, Song JF, et al. Comparison of accuracy of physical examination and endoanal ultrasonography for preoperative assessment in patients with acute and chronic anal fistula. Tech Coloproctol. 2008;12:217–23.
17. West RL, Zimmerman DD, Dwarkasing S, et al. Prospective comparison of hydrogen peroxide-enhanced three-dimensional endoanal ultrasonography and endoanal magnetic resonance imaging of perianal fistulas. Dis Colon Rectum. 2003;46: 1407–15.
18. West RL, Dwarkasing S, Felt-Bersma RJ, et al. Hydrogen peroxide-enhanced three-dimensional endoanal ultrasonography and endoanal magnetic resonance imaging in evaluating perianal fistulas: agreement and patient preference. Eur J Gastroenterol Hepatol. 2004;15:1319–24.
19. Beets-Tan RG, Beets GI, van der Hoop AG, et al. Preoperative MR imaging of anal fistulas: does it really help the surgeon? Radiology. 2001;218(1): 75–84.
20. Buchanan GN, Halligan S, Williams AB, et al. Magnetic resonance imaging for primary fistula in ano. Br J Surg. 2003;90(7):877–81.
21. Hughes LE. Clinical classification of perianal Crohn's diseases. Dis Colon Rectum. 1992;35:928–32.
22. Irvine EJ. Usual therapy improves perianal Crohn's disease as measured by a new disease activity index. McMaster IBD Study Group. J Clin Gastroenterol. 1995;20:27–32.
23. Thia KT, Mahadevan U, Feagan BG, et al. Ciprofloxacin or metronidazole for the treatment of perianal fistulas in patients with Crohn's disease: a randomized, double-blind, placebo-controlled pilot study. Inflamm Bowel Dis. 2009;15:17–24.
24. Maedal U, Ng SC, Durdey P, et al. Randomized clinical trial of metronidazole ointment versus placebo in perianal Crohn's disease. Br J Surg. 2010;97:1340–7.
25. Present DH, Rutgeerts P, Targan S, et al. Infliximab for the treatment of fistulas in patients with Crohn's disease. N Engl J Med. 1999;340:1398–405.
26. Sands BE, Anderson FH, Bernstein CN, et al. Infliximab maintenance therapy for fistulizing Crohn's disease. N Engl J Med. 2004;350:876–85.
27. Dewint P, Hansen B, Verhey E. Adalimumab combined with ciprofloxacin is superior to adalimumab monotherapy in perianal fistula closure in Crohn's disease: a randomized double-blind, placebo controlled trial (ADAFI). Gut. 2014;63:292–9.
28. Caliste X, Nazir S, Goode T, et al. Sensitivity of computer tomography in detection of perirectal abscess. Am Surg. 2011;77(2):166–8.
29. Pritchard TJ, Schoetz Jr DJ, Roberts PL, Murray JJ, et al. Perirectal abscess in Crohn's disease. Drainage and outcome. Dis Colon Rectum. 1990;33(11):922–7.
30. Wise PE, Schwartz DA. Management of perianal Crohn's disease. Clin Gastroenterol Hepatol. 2006; 4(4):426–30.
31. Parks AG, Gordon PH, Hardcastle JD. A classification of fistula-in-ano. Br J Surg. 1976;63(1):1–12.
32. Solomon MJ. Fistulae and abscesses in symptomatic perianal Crohn's disease. Int J Colorectal Dis. 1996;11:222–6.
33. Mardini HE, Schwarts DA. Treatment of perianal fistula and abscess: Crohn's and non-Crohn's. Curr Treat Options Gastroenterol. 2007;10:211–20.
34. Steele SR, Kumar R, Feingold DL, Rafferty JL, Buie WD. Practice parameters for the management of perianal abscess and fistula-in-ano. Dis Colon Rectum. 2011;54:1465–74.
35. Sangwan YP, Schoetz Jr DJ, Murray JJ, et al. Perianal Crohn's disease: results of local surgical treatment. Dis Colon Rectum. 1996;39:529–53.
36. Davies M, Harris D, Lohana P, et al. The surgical management of fistula-in-ano in a specialist colorectal unit. Int J Colorectal Dis. 2008;23:833–8.
37. Williams JG, MacLeod CA, Rothenberger DA, Goldberg SM. Seton treatment of high anal fistulae. Br J Surg. 1991;78:1159–61.
38. Williamson PR, Hellinger MD, Larah SW, Ferrara A. Twenty year review of the surgical management of perianal Crohn's disease. Dis Colon Rectum. 1995; 38:389–92.
39. Pescatori M, Interisano A, Basso L. Management of perianal Crohn's disease: results of a multicenter trial in Italy. Dis Colon Rectum. 1994;38:121–4.

40. Faucheron JL, Saint-Marc O, Guibert L, Parc R. Long-term seton drainage for high anal fistulas in Crohn's disease-a sphincter salving operation? Dis Colon Rectum. 1996;39(2):208–11.
41. Eitan A, Koliada M, Bickel A. The use of the loose seton technique of a definitive treatment for recurrent and persistent high transphincteric anal fistulas: a long-term outcome. J Gastrointest Surg. 2009;13(6): 1116–9.
42. Soltani A, Kaiser AM. Endorectal advancement flap for cryptoglandular or Crohn's fistula-in-ano. Dis Colon Rectum. 2010;53(4):486–95.
43. Poritz L. How should complex perianal Crohn's disease be treated in the Remicade era. J Gastrointest Surg. 2006;10(5):633–4.
44. Cintron JR, Park JJ, Orsay CP, Peal RK, Nelson RL, Abcarian H. Repair of fistulas-in-ano using autologous fibrin tissue adhesive. Dis Colon Rectum. 1999;42(5):607–13.
45. Cintron JR, Park JJ, Orsay CP, et al. Repair of fistulas-in-ano using fibrin adhesive: long-term follow-up. Dis Colon Rectum. 2000;43(7):944–9. discussion 949–50.
46. Grimaud JC, Munoz-Bongrand N, Siproudhis L, et al. Groupe d'Etude Therapeutique des Affections Inflammatoires du Tube Digestif. Fibrin glue is effective healing perianal fistulas in patients with Crohn's disease. Gastroenterology. 2010;138(7):2275–81.
47. Loungnarath R, Dietz DW, Mutch MG, Birnbaum EH, Kodner IJ, Fleshman JW. Fibrin glue treatment of complex anal fistulas has low success rate. Dis Colon Rectum. 2004;47(4):432–6.
48. O'Connor L, Champagne BJ, Ferguson MA, Orangio GR, Schertzer ME, Armstrong DN. Efficacy of anal fistula plug in closure of Crohn's anorectal fistulas. Dis Colon Rectum. 2006;49:1569–73.
49. Champagne BJ, O'Connor LM, Ferguson M, Orangiio GR, Schertzer ME, Armstrong DN. Efficacy of anal fistula plug in closure of cryptoglandular fistulas: long-term follow-up. Dis Colon Rectum. 2006;49:1817–21.
50. Garg P, Song J, Bhatia A, Kalia H, Menon GR. The efficacy of anal fistulas plus in fistula-in-ano: a systematic review. Colorectal Dis. 2010;12910:965–70.
51. O'Riordan JM, Datta I, Johnstron C, Baxter NN. A systematic review of the anal fistula plus for patients with Crohn's and non-Crohn's related fistula-in-ano. Dis Colon Rectum. 2012;55(3):351–8.
52. Rojanasakul A, Pattanaarun J, Sahakitrungruang C, Tantiphlachiva K. Total anal sphincter saving technique for fistula-in-ano; the ligation of intersphincteric fistula tract. J Med Assoc Thai. 2007;90:581–6.
53. Moloo H, Bleier JIS, Goldberg SM. Ligation of the intersphincteric fistula tract (LIFT). In Wexner SD, Fleshman JW, editors. Colon and rectal surgery anorectal operations – master techniques in general surgery. Philadelphia, PA: Wolters Kluwer Health Lippincott, Williams & Wilkins; 2012. p. 79–84.
54. Gingold DS, Murrell ZA, Fleshner PR. A prospective evaluation of the ligation of the intersphincteric tract procedure for complex anal fistula in patients with Crohn disease. Ann Surg. 2013;00:1–5.
55. Tan KK, Tan IJ, Lim FS, Koh DC, Tsang CB. The anatomy of failures following the ligation of the intersphincteric tract technique for anal fistula: a review of 93 patients over 4 years. Dis Colon Rectum. 2011;54(11):1368–72.
56. Radcliffe AG, Ritchie JK, Hawley PR, Lennard-Jones JE, Northover JM. Anovaginal and rectovaginal fistulas in Crohn's disease. Dis Colon Rectum. 1988;31:94–9.
57. El-Gazzaz G, Hull T, Mignanelli E, Hammel J, Gurland B, Zutshi M. Analysis of function and predictors of failure in women undergoing repair of Crohn's related rectovaginal fistula. J Gastrointest Surg. 2010;14(5):824–9.
58. Ruffolo C, Scarpa M, Bassi N, Angriman I. A systematic review on advancement flaps for rectovaginal fistula in Crohn's disease: transrectal v. transvaginal approach. Colorectal Dis. 2010;12:1183–91.
59. Sands B, Van Deventer S, Bernstein C, et al. Long term treatment of fistulizing Crohn's disease: response to infliximab in the ACCENT II trial through 54 weeks (Abs). Gastroenterology. 2001;122:A81.
60. Ingle SB, Loftus Jr EV. The natural history of perianal Crohn's disease. Dig Liver Dis. 2007;39(100):963–9.
61. Singh B, Mortensen NJ, Jewell DP, George B. Perianal Crohn's disease. Br J Surg. 2004;91(7):801–14.
62. Lewis RT, Maron DJ. Anorectal Crohn's disease. Surg Clin North Am. 2010;90:83–97.
63. Jeffrey PJ, Parks AG, Ritchie JK. Treatment of haemorrhoids in patients with inflammatory bowel disease. Lancet. 1977;1:1084–5.
64. Wolkomir AF, Luchtefeld MA. Surgery for symptomatic hemorrhoids and anal fissures in Crohn's disease. Dis Colon Rectum. 1993;36(6):545–7.
65. Karin E, Avital S, Dotan I, Skornick Y, Greenberg R. Doppler-guided haemorrhoidal artery ligation in patients with Crohn's disease. Colorectal Dis. 2012;14(1):111–4.
66. D'Ugo S, Franceschilli L, Cadeddu F, Leccesi L, et al. Medical and surgical treatment of haemorrhoids and anal fissure in Crohn's disease: a critical appraisal. BMC Gastroenterol. 2013;13:47.
67. Sweeney JL, Ritchie JK, Nicholls R. Anal fissure in Crohn's disease. Br J Surg. 1988;75:56–67.
68. Fleshner PR, Schoetz Jr DJ, Roberts PL, et al. Anal fissure in Crohn's disease: a plea for aggressive management. Dis Colon Rectum. 1995;38:1137–43.
69. Steele SR. Operative management of Crohn's disease of the colon including anorectal disease. Surg Clin North Am. 2007;87(3):611–31.
70. Keighley MR, Allan RN. Current status and influence of operation on perianal Crohn's disease. Int J Colorectal Dis. 1986;1(2):104–7.
71. Brouchard C, Siproudhis L, Wallenhorst T, et al. Anorectal stricture in 102 patients with Crohn's disease: natural history in the era of biologics. Aliment Pharmacol Ther. 2014;40(7):796–803.
72. Lad SV, Haider MA, Brown CJ, Mcleod RS. MRI appearance of perianal carcinoma in Crohn's disease. J Magn Reson Imaging. 2007;26(6):1659–62.

14 Perineal Reconstruction in Crohn's Disease

Essie Kueberuwa and Larry J. Gottlieb

Introduction

It is estimated that approximately 14 % of patients with Crohn's disease will ultimately require proctectomy for failure of both medical and local surgical therapy [1]. Unfortunately, proctectomy for Crohn's disease is associated with a high risk for perineal wound complications [2]. The presence of transphincteric and supralevator fistulas can cause a stiff, fibrotic, and inflamed field in which tension free, re-approximation of the native tissues post excision is challenging. When present, concomitant perianal sepsis secondary to abscesses, undrained fistulas, or sinus tracts can further increase the risk of infection related wound complications. In the setting of Crohn's disease with complex perianal fistulization, wide excision of perianal skin is necessitated [3] and primary edge-to-edge closure can be extremely difficult, if not impossible.

E. Kueberuwa, MD
Section of Plastic and Reconstructive Surgery, Department of Surgery, University of Chicago, 5841 S. Maryland Avenue, MC 6035, Chicago, IL, USA
e-mail: Essie.Kueberuwa@uchospitals.edu

L.J. Gottlieb, MD, FACS (✉)
Department of Surgery, Section of Plastic and Reconstructive Surgery, University of Chicago, 5841 S. Maryland Avenue, MC 6035, Chicago, IL, USA
e-mail: lgottlie@surgery.bsd.uchicago.edu

Rectal and anal fistulization can also occur to adjacent structures such as vagina, urethra, or bladder. On occasions, Crohn's disease can be complicated by malignancy, further increasing the size of the extirpated specimen resulting in massive defects. Patient factors such as immunosuppression, steroid dependence, and compromised nutritional status further increase the risk of wound dehiscence and other wound healing complications.

Patient Selection

The goal of perineal reconstruction is reliable wound closure with healthy, well-vascularized tissue, sealing of the pelvic floor, obliteration of pelvic or perineal dead space, and skin closure without tension. Whether treating a persistent perineal wound or prophylactically trying to prevent one, reliable wound closure can only be accomplished after sepsis has been cleared and infected, diseased, and scarred tissue is adequately debrided. The best method of closure is patient specific and is a factor of the size and location of the defect, planned future treatments, donor site availability, and patient/surgeon preference. When it is anticipated that pelvic tissues and/or perineal skin will not be able to be primary approximated at the time of proctocolectomy, pre-operative consultation and coordination with a reconstructive plastic surgeon should be considered to discuss timing and manner of wound closure. If indeed the wound is

A. Fichera and M.K. Krane (eds.), *Crohn's Disease: Basic Principles*,
DOI 10.1007/978-3-319-14181-7_14, © Springer International Publishing Switzerland 2015

amenable to acute closure, then considerations of reconstruction or sealing of the pelvic floor as well as options of providing flap closure to fill perineal "dead" space and, if needed, to add skin to facilitate perineal skin closure should be discussed. This prophylactic reconstructive surgery at the time of extirpation will optimize the likelihood of successful healing.

In cases where the defect is not amenable to primary approximation of immediately local tissue, reconstruction generally requires transfer of local, regional, or distant tissue in the form of a well-vascularized flap into the defect. When flap closure is performed at the time of proctectomy, flap choice is frequently predicated on and limited to what flaps are available depending on patient positioning as well as previous scars and stoma. Procedures are usually performed under general anesthesia (with or without epidural supplementation), with sequential compression boots, subcutaneous heparin prophylaxis, antibiotic prophylaxis, and pressure point padding.

Consultation with a reconstructive plastic surgeon post procedure should be considered in patients with persistent perineal wounds, and in patients who did not heal a wound that was intentionally left open or subsequently broke down after primary repair.

Primary Closure

When surgical proctectomy was first introduced, primary closure of the perineal wound was advocated. However, because of the high incidence of severe wound complications, this practice was abandoned and perineal wounds were left open for packing with intended healing by secondary intention [2]. Healing by secondary intent has its own limitations due to prolonged convalescence, and in fact may be painful, and puts patients at high risk for the development of chronic, persistent perineal sinus development. Despite this, the practice remained popular until the 1960s when perineal wound closure with closed suction drainage was proposed by Burge and Tompkin [4]. Numerous studies subsequently evaluated the outcomes of primary closure of the perineal wound versus closure by secondary intent, with the conclusion that primary closure is superior [5–9]. Thus the current standard for closure when attempting to directly reapproximate local tissues is to do so primarily with the utilization of closed suction drainage. This method has been demonstrated to facilitate more rapid healing, decreased cost, improved quality of life, and less need for prolonged nursing/wound care [10]. Primary perineal wound closure is usually performed in a layered fashion using absorbable sutures. The goal is to reapproximate tissue without undue tension and distortion of adjacent anatomical structures. Even in the best hands, primary closure of the perineum following proctectomy has a high incidence of complications. Wound infection rates are reported at 11–16 % [11] and delayed healing is a frequent issue. In instances where the levator muscles are divided laterally along pelvic bones and there is a large potential perineal dead space, the patient is at risk for a perineal hernia. Whenever possible, it is imperative to identify patients at risk for tenuous or challenging perineal wound closures pre-operatively and in an attempt to mitigate perineal wound complications, alternative methods other than direct primary local tissue re-approximation should be considered. Delayed wound closure or healing by secondary intention should be considered in wounds that are severely contaminated from multiple abscesses, sinuses, and fistulae where infection is unable to be cleared by surgical extirpation/debridement (Fig. 14.1).

Negative Pressure Wound Therapy

The utilization of a negative pressure wound therapy (NPWT) device for large perineal defects secondary to Necrotizing Fasciitis and Fournier's Gangrene is well described [12]. Its utilization in combination with an omental flap in abdominal perineal resection has been described in case studies and small series in the literature [13]. NPWT devices using sponge or gauze are frequently more comfortable and better tolerated than traditional packing and topical dressing changes. In the non-infected patient, it is typically changed 2–3 times per week by a wound care specialist rather than multiple times per day for traditional

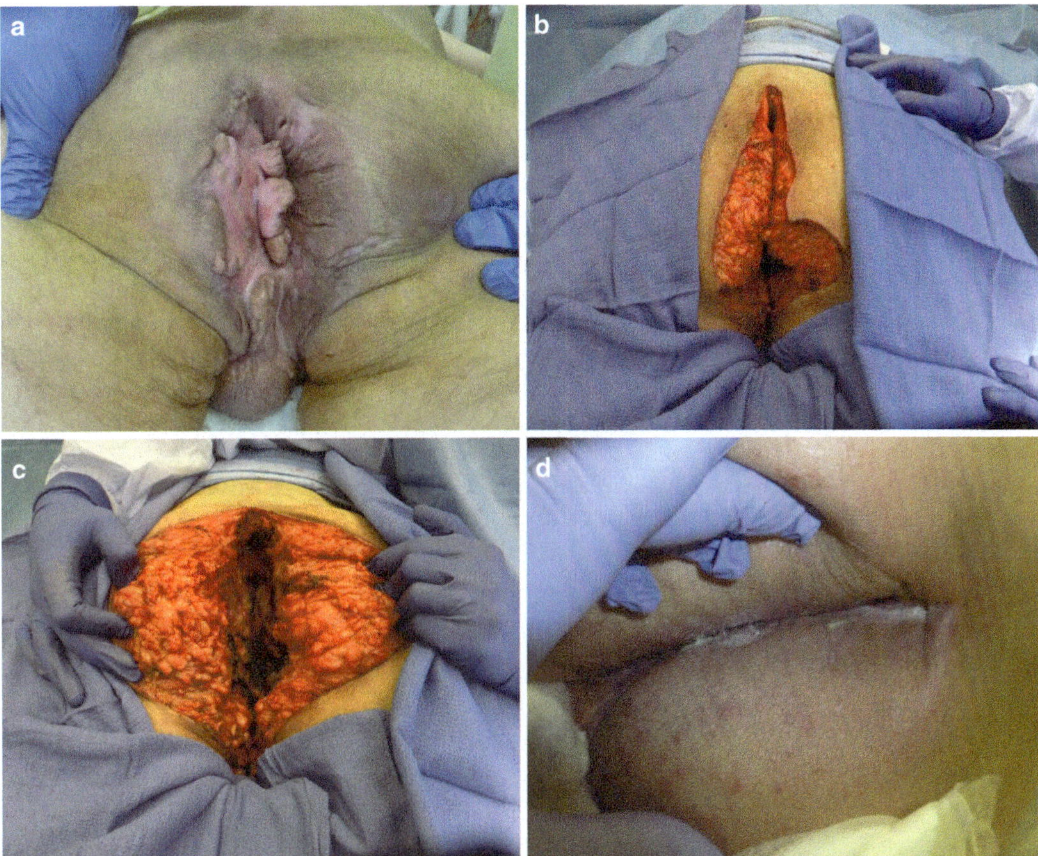

Fig. 14.1 (**a**) 40-year-old male with severe perineal Crohn's disease. (**b**) Extent of skin excision (**c**) Extirpation including resection of coccyx unable to clear infection. Wound left open to be treated with topical antimicrobial and subsequently an NPWT devise. (**d**) Wound almost totally closed at 6 months post-op

dressings. This device theoretically decreases the time of wound healing by assisting collapse of the potential space, increasing angiogenesis and revascularization and promoting the deposition of granulation tissue [12]. The downside of NPWT devices is that it is frequently difficult to obtain a negative pressure seal in the perineum especially in an ambulatory patient and the patients are tethered to the device for many weeks or months.

Perineal Reconstruction

The leading causes of perineal wound healing issues in Crohn's patients are inadequate debridement of infected tissue, failure to obliterate perineal dead space, and tension on the perineal skin closure. In patients where perineal tissue cannot be primarily re-approximated then this space should be filled with well-vascularized tissue. Muscle, de-epithelialized myocutaneous, adipose/fascial and omental flaps have all been used successfully to fill perineal dead space and seal the pelvic floor to minimize wound healing issues and avoid perineal herniation. When there is a cutaneous deficit, skin should be transferred to allow for perineal skin closure without tension. The skin may be transferred independently based on the plethora of axial or perforating vessels from the pudendal vascular system in the region. Alternatively skin may be transferred as part of a more distant myocutaneous flap, or as a chimeric flap [14, 15]. If the extirpation includes a portion of or all of the vagina and or vulva, then skin may be required for vaginal/vulva reconstruction as well.

The use of myocutaneous flap transfer has been shown to reduce pelvic wound complications after abdominal perineal resections [16, 17]. Hurst et al. demonstrated that immediate primary closure using flaps as an adjunct in Crohn's patients can augment perineal wound healing and avoid the morbidity associated with an open wound [2]. There are a variety of local, regional, and distant flap options which can be advanced, transposed, or rotated on their vascular pedicle, into the defect. The vascular leash of most of the major regional muscle, musculocutaneous, fasciocutaneous, and perforator flaps is along a circumference of a 20 cm diameter circle over the perineum (Fig. 14.2). When choosing one flap or another, consideration is given to the volume of tissue needed, the size of the skin paddle required, availability of donor site and intraoperative positioning, as well as surgeon and patient preferences. Ultimately the reconstructive method of choice should be the most reliable technique that addresses the patients' individual needs and optimizes the likelihood of successful perineal wound healing with minimal morbidity.

Muscle Flaps

The four most common regional muscles used for filling dead space in the perineum are the Rectus Abdominis, Gracilis, Vastus Lateralis, and Inferior Gluteal muscles.

Rectus Abdominis Muscle Flap

The rectus abdominis muscle (RAM) is transferred to the perineum based on its inferior vascular pedicle, the deep inferior epigastric artery, and vein. It is easily harvested in the supine position

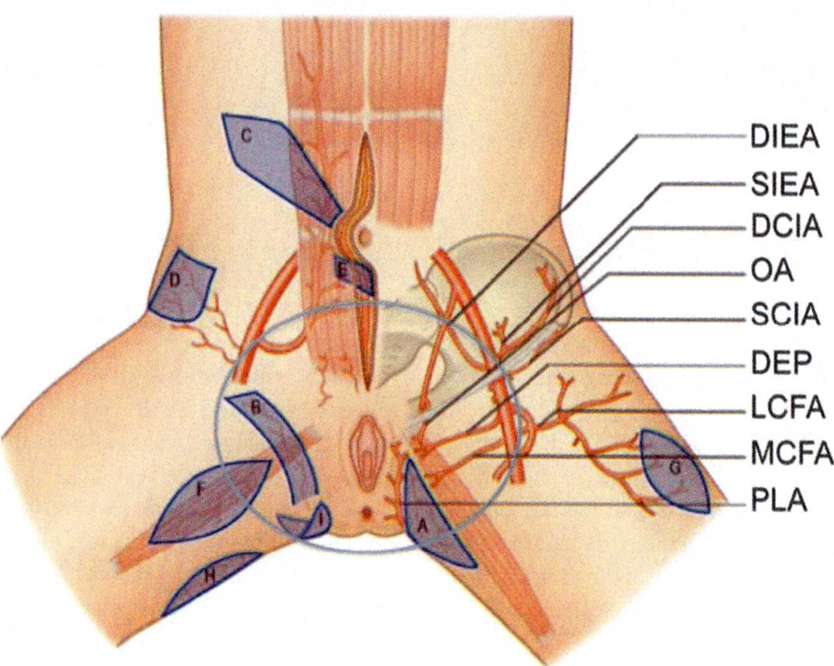

Fig. 14.2 The pivot points of most loco-regional flaps used for perineal reconstruction are located along the circumference of a 20 cm diameter circle centered over the perineum. (**a**) V-Y advancement flap, from medial thigh or inferior gluteal area. (**b**) Pudendal thigh flap. (**c**) Oblique rectus abdominis myocutaneous (*ORAM*) or deep inferior epigastric artery perforator (*DIEP*) flap. (**d**) Superficial inferior epigastric artery (*SIEA*) flap or extended superficial circumflex iliac artery (*SCIA*) flap (**e**) Rectus abdominis musculoperitoneal (*RAMP*) flap (**f**) Gracilis myocutaneous flap, shown with vertical skin paddle (**g**) Anterolateral thigh (*ALT*) flap (**h**) Gluteal thigh flap (**i**) Gluteal fold flap *DCIA* deep circumflex iliac artery, *OA* anterior branch of obturator artery, *DEPA* deep external pudendal artery, *LCFA* lateral circumflex femoral artery, *MCFA* medial circumflex femoral artery, *PLA* posterior labial artery (branch of pudendal artery)

and can be taken with or without a skin paddle. The RAM or myocutaneous flap has become the workhorse flap for perineal reconstruction. As a muscle only flap, it is an excellent option to interpose healthy tissue between resected and repaired rectal-vaginal fistulae. With the addition of a portion of the posterior rectus sheath and peritoneum (RAMP), this musculoperitoneal flap has been used to patch small defects in the vagina without the bulk of a myocutaneous flap [18]. A single RAM flap may not have enough volume to fill the dead space of large pelvic wounds and the addition of another flap or including the overlying fat is frequently required to completely fill this space. The vertical orientation of the skin paddle of a rectus abdominis myocutaneous flap (VRAM) is generally used when more volume is required and a relatively small amount of skin is required to reconstruct the posterior wall of the vagina and/or to minimize tension on the perineal suture line. If a large amount of skin is required for perineal and/or vaginal reconstruction, then an oblique orientation of the rectus abdominis muscle (ORAM) is preferred (Fig. 14.3). Advantages of the ORAM include a longer skin paddle with increased reach and arc of rotation. The donor site is usually more easily closed with this orientation and only a limited amount of rectus fascia needs to be included in the harvest of this flap. If the clitoris requires resection (usually for cancer), a sensory innervated flap can be fashioned on the 8th intercostal nerve, with neurorrhaphy to the clitoral nerve [19] or to the pudendal nerve [20].

The conventional description of the rectus abdominis flap delivers it into the pelvis via a transpelvic route [16, 21]. Ho et al. [22] described a more direct prepelvic version with the VRAM flap entering through an anterior perforation in the perineal membrane and so shortening the course and enhancing the reach of the flap. The flap is equally applicable in the case of large pure perineal defects without pelvic wounds by tunneling via extrapelvic approach through a prepubic subcutaneous route.

Previous transverse abdominal incisions that transected both recti and the presence of bilateral ostomies generally render this work horse flap unavailable for use.

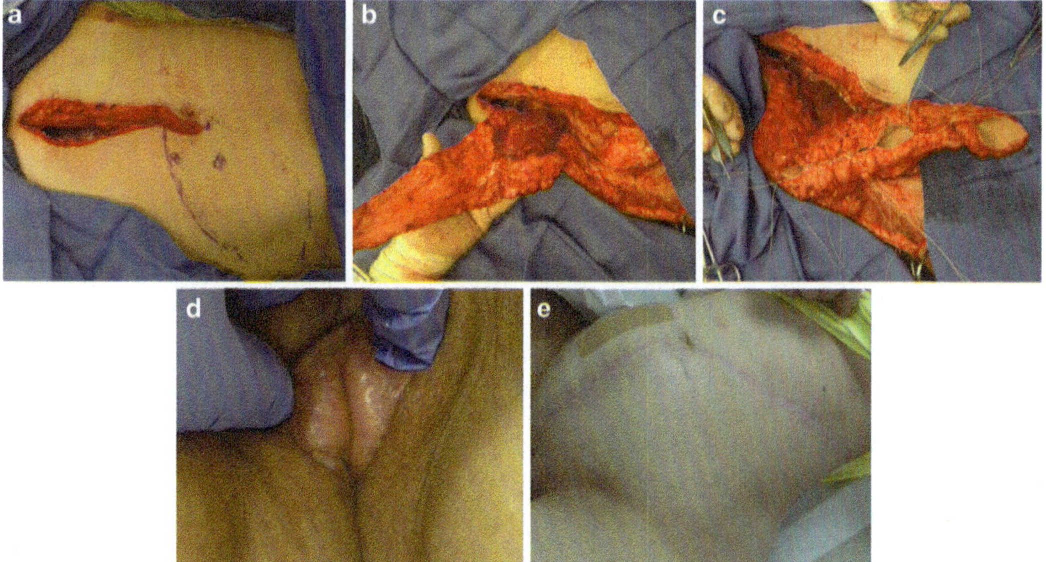

Fig. 14.3 (**a**) Lower midline abdominal incision with intraoperative design of a left oblique rectus abdominis myocutaneous (*ORAM*) flap for a 45-year-old woman undergoing pelvic exenteration. The skin island can extend from the umbilicus to the mid-axillary line. (**b**) Flap elevated. Note rectus muscle attachment to inferior portion of flap (**c**) Skin flap being "tubed" to construct a vagina which will subsequently passed transpelvically (**d**) 4-month follow-up demonstrating introitus of vagina reconstructed with ORAM. (**e**) Abdominal scar at 4 months post-op

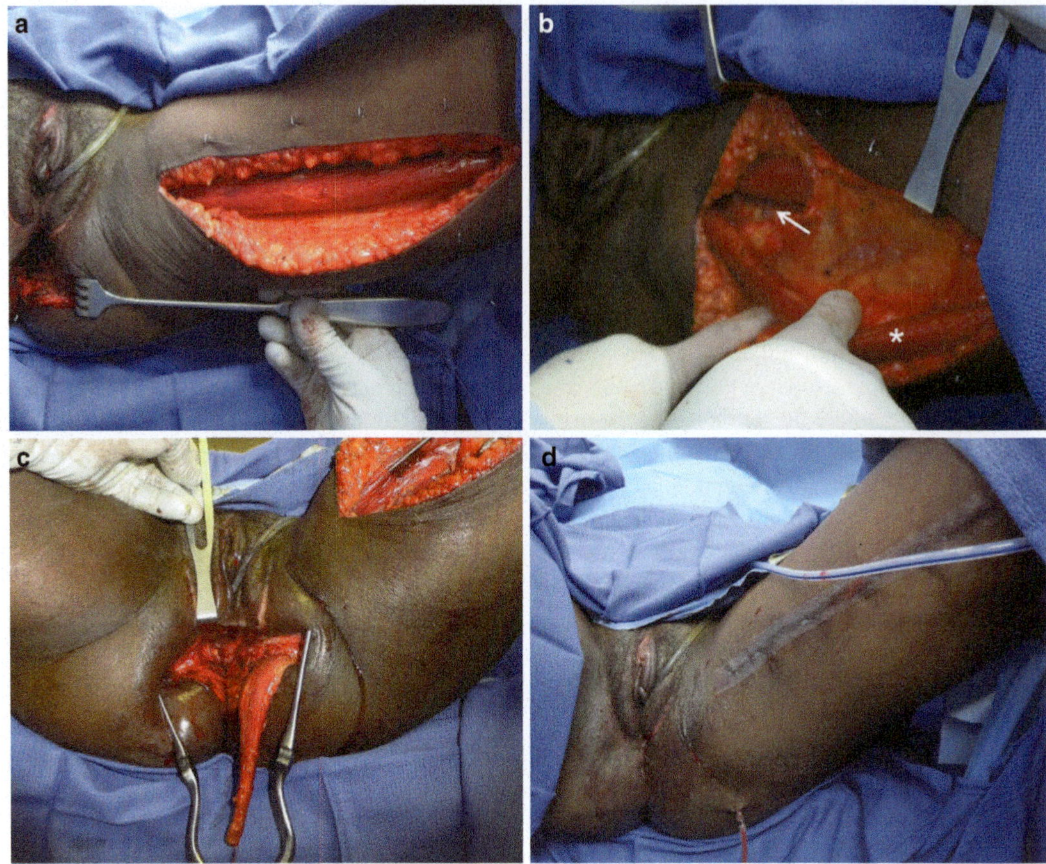

Fig. 14.4 (**a**) Gracilis muscle visible after incision in medial thigh skin in patient with a relatively shallow perineal defect. (**b**) Dominant pedicle (*arrow*) of gracilis muscle (*asterisk*) as it course beneath adductor longus muscle (**c**) after distal end is divided and then passed under subcutaneous tunnel (note relatively small volume of muscle available for perineal fill) (**d**) After muscle placed in perineal wound and incisions closed

Gracilis Flap

The gracilis muscle and myocutaneous flaps have been used for vaginal, vulva, and perineal reconstruction since their original description by McGraw in the mid-1970s [23]. The gracilis muscle is a superficial muscle located in the medial thigh, and functions as a thigh adductor and knee flexor but whose absence is inconsequential to the patient. Its dominant blood supply, the medial circumflex femoral artery, which is a branch off the profunda femora, enters the muscle approximately 10 cm below the pubic symphysis. This flap is straightforward to dissect in lithotomy with minimal donor site morbidity. Although the vascularity of the muscle is reliable and this flap has been used extensively to reconstruct perineal wounds [23, 24], the volume or bulk of muscle tissue available to fill large defects is quite limited [25]. The limitation of the longitudinally oriented Gracilis myocutaneous flap is that skin paddle overlying the distal 1/3 of the muscle is often unreliable. Thus in our practice, we have reserved the gracilis muscle flap for relatively shallow perineal wounds, or to interpose between repaired distal fistulae (Fig. 14.4). One study compared the outcome of 133 cancer patients who had undergone abdomino-perineal resection or pelvic exenteration closed with either VRAM or gracilis flaps. This study found that the gracilis flap group had a significantly greater incidence of major complications [26] (42 % versus 15 %) than the VRAM flap group. They also had significantly

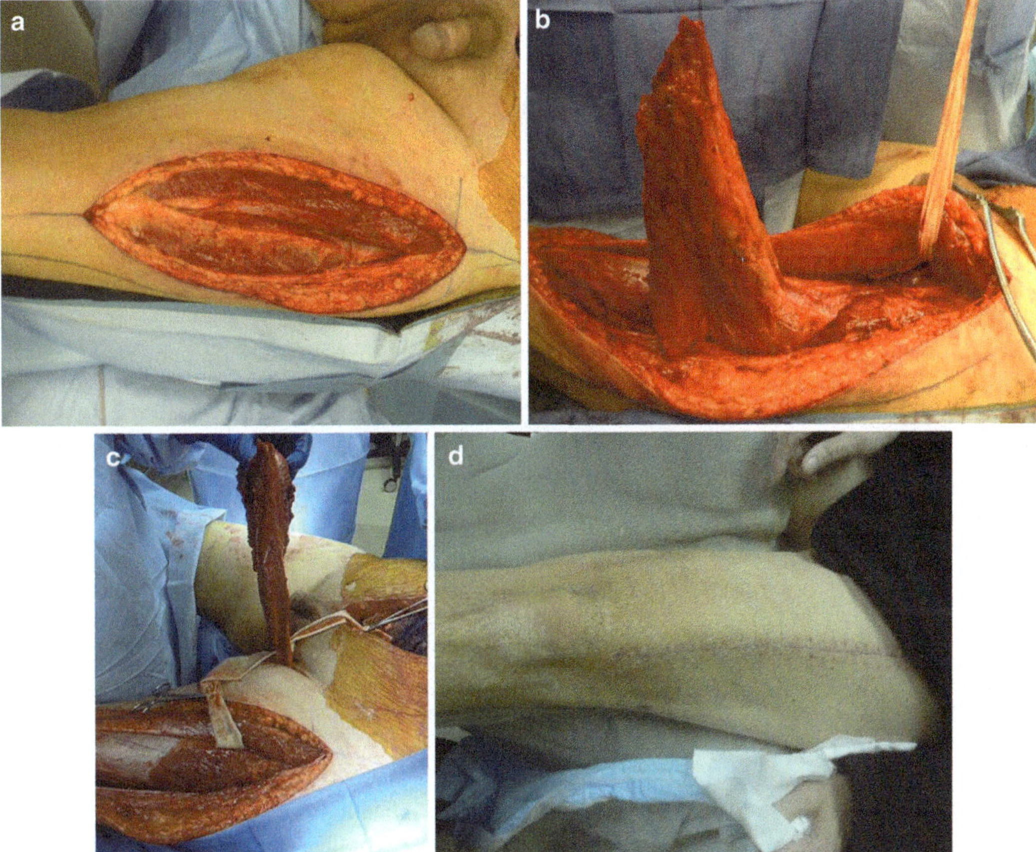

Fig. 14.5 (**a**) Thigh incision demonstrating the underlying musculature (**b**) Vastus lateralis muscle being elevated (**c**) After the flap is passed medially under rectus femoris and sartorius muscles (it will subsequently be passed into the perineal space) (**d**). Resulting scar on thigh

higher rates of donor-site cellulitis: 26 % (gracilis group) versus 6 % (VRAM group) and recipient-site complications, including recipient site cellulitis (21 % versus 4 %), pelvic abscess (32 % versus 6 %), and major wound dehiscence (21 % versus 5 %). The group concluded that in their patient population, the VRAM was superior to gracilis flaps in perineal cancer reconstruction.

Anterior Lateral Thigh Flap

The anterior lateral thigh (ALT) flap can be used as a regional pedicled flap based off the lateral circumflex femoral artery (LCFA), which is a branch of the profunda femoris. It is versatile and may be designed as a fasciocutaneous flap, a muscle (Vastus Lateralis) flap, a musculocutaneous flap, or a chimeric flap. In order to comfortably transpose this flap into the perineum and extend its reach without tension, the flap is passed beneath rectus femoris and sartorius muscles thus transposing the pivot point of the vascular pedicle medial to the sartorius muscle (Fig. 14.5). The advantage of this flap is the potential for bulk and volume and a reliable skin paddle, however the donor site is quite visible on the anterior thigh. If a skin graft is required for closure, it can lead to an unsightly scar.

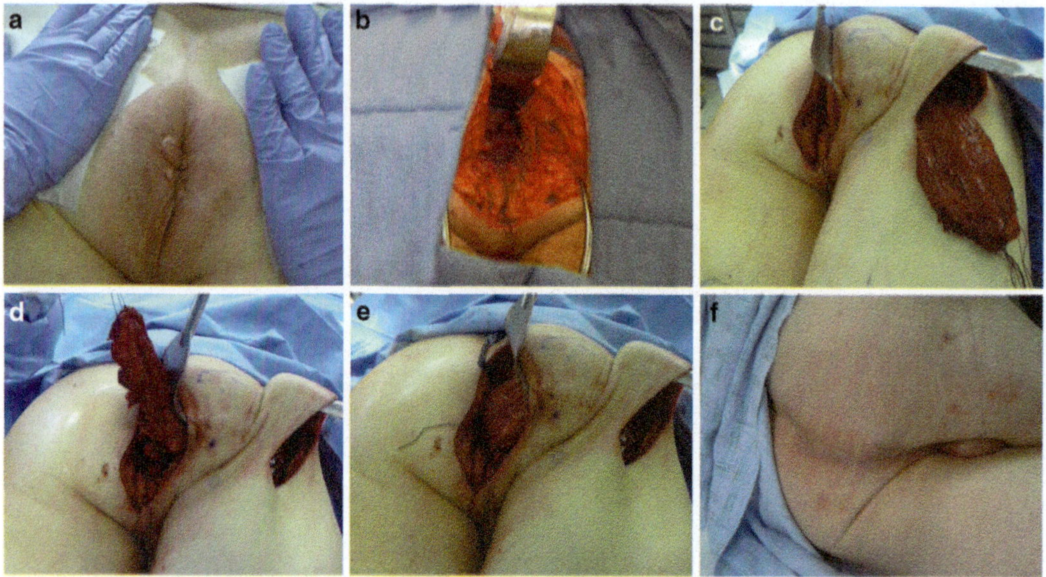

Fig. 14.6 (**a**) 62-year-old male with severe chronic Crohn's proctitis with a diffusely infiltrating rectal cancer. (**b**) Extirpative defect with large perineal dead space (**c**) Inferior gluteal muscle harvested through a counter-incision in lateral gluteal crease (laid on the skin to demonstrate amount of muscle harvested.) (**d**) Inferior gluteal muscle passed through subcutaneous tunnel pivoting on the inferior gluteal neurovascular bundle. (**e**) Muscle inset to fill perineal space. (**f**) Skin closed primarily shown here at 5 weeks post-op

Inferior Gluteal Muscle Flap

The inferior gluteal muscle is a large muscle that acts as an adductor and external rotator of the limb. It attaches to the lateral border of the sacrum and inserts into the iliotibial band of the fascia lata, the deeper fibers of the lower portion of the muscle insert into the gluteal tuberosity between the vastus lateralis and adductor magnus. It is supplied by the inferior gluteal artery which exits the greater sciatic foramen emerging between the piriformis and coccygeus approximately 5 cm above the ischial tuberosity. It may be transferred as a muscle flap, a myocutaneous compound flap or as a myocutaneous chimeric flap. When the perineal defect is relatively shallow, the medial aspect of the muscle is elevated through the perineal wound and the overlying skin island is usually designed as a V-Y and advanced medially with the muscle [27]. If the perineal defect is more extensive, it is usually best to elevate the muscle without overlying skin and transposing it to fill perineal dead space (Fig. 14.6). This flap can be elevated with the patient either in a jack-knife or lithotomy position. The medial aspect is approached through the perineal wound and lateral extent of the muscle may be accessed through a counter-incision in the lateral portion of the inferior gluteal crease. If additional skin is required to accomplish perineal wound closure without tension, the overlying skin can be rotated or advanced medially. Alternatively, a gluteal thigh flap may be elevated in combination with the inferior gluteal muscle flap based on the descending branch of the inferior gluteal artery which allows independent placement of the skin [15]. Harvest of the inferior gluteal muscle may cause a contour deformity of the inferior lateral buttock but is well tolerated even in ambulatory patients.

Cutaneous/Fasciocutaneous Flaps

Skin can be included in all the muscle flaps described above. In addition, skin flaps may be used independently of the muscles as perforator flaps, as V-Y advancement, transposition, rotation,

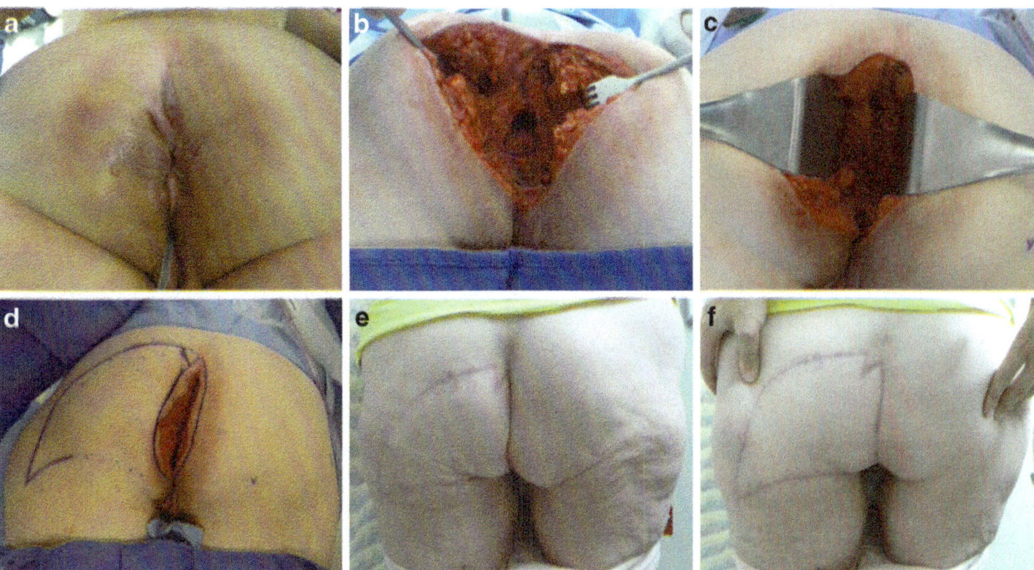

Fig. 14.7 (**a**) 61-year-old female with a 30-year history of Crohn's disease complicated by adenocarcinoma of rectum. (**b**) Extirpative defect (**c**) The levator aponeurosis and pelvic musculature was able to be closed to seal the pelvic floor. (**d**) The potential perineal space was obliterated by securing the medial edge of each gluteal muscle together as well as Scarpa's fascia. Although the debrided skin edges could be brought together, it was felt that there would be too much tension with sitting and normal activity. Therefore, a large crescent V-Y advancement flap was designed. (**e**) Note the buttock symmetry at 4 months follow-up (**d**) with cheeks spread

and propeller flaps. These terms describe methods of elevating local skin and subcutaneous tissue directly adjacent to the perineal defect, and moving them short distances, whilst attached to their original blood supply. Local cutaneous/fasciocutaneous flaps are muscle sparing and generally less morbid than the muscle flaps previously described.

V-Y Advancement Flaps

Transferring skin in a V-Y fashion allows skin closure without tension. Skin, fascia, and subcutaneous tissue can be recruited from the medial thigh and inferior gluteal area, and advanced toward the midline in a V-Y fashion. When these flaps are designed on the medial aspect of the thigh, the blood supply is from perforator vessels from the pudendal, medial circumflex femoral, or obturator vessels. The skin overlying the gluteal muscles may be advanced in a V-Y fashion based on perforating vessels from the superior and/or inferior gluteal arteries and veins (Fig. 14.7). These flaps have the potential to provide high volume, well-vascularized and sensate skin, with acceptable scars, minimal morbidity, and high reliability.

Gluteal Thigh Flap

The skin island of the gluteal thigh flap is centered over a point midway between greater trochanter and ischial tuberosity, perpendicular to gluteal crease. The flap can be designed to extend down to within 8 cm of the popliteal fossa. The pedicle of the gluteal thigh flap, the descending branch of the inferior gluteal artery can be separated from beneath the gluteal muscle and dissected to its take-off from the inferior gluteal artery as it emerges from underneath the piriformis muscle, allowing independent placement of the muscle in the cavity and the thigh skin paddle on the surface. This technique allows for independent movement of the inferior gluteal muscle or independent movement of the posterior thigh skin or two separate tissue transfers as a chimeric flap based on a single pedicle (Fig. 14.8).

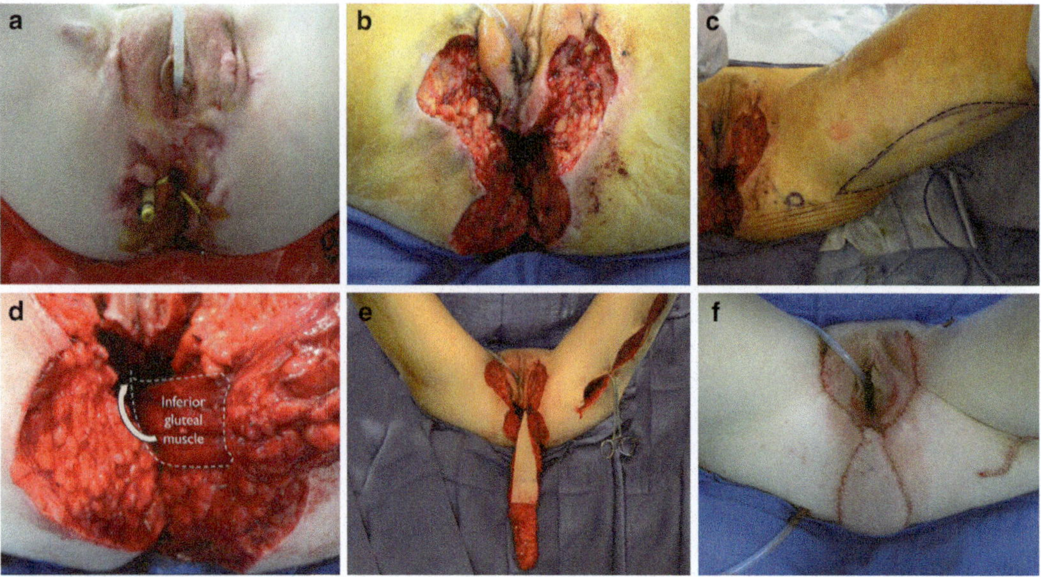

Fig. 14.8 (**a**) Severe perianal and perineal Crohn's disease in a 26-year-old woman with multiple fistulae, sinuses, and abscesses. After proctectomy and excision of all involved soft tissue (**b**), an inferior gluteal artery chimera flap was designed (**c**) with inferior gluteal muscle and a posterior thigh flap both based on separate branches of the left inferior gluteal artery (**d**). Muscle flap transposed into pelvic defect (**e**). Posterior thigh skin paddle passed under skin bridge and de-epithelialized distally to provide more bulk for obliterating defect (**f**). Final inset of posterior thigh flap with closure of groin wounds

Gluteal Fold Flap

A fasciocutaneous flap can be designed from skin overlying the infragluteal fold. This flap is based off perforators from the internal pudendal artery. Shahzad et al. [28] report the use of a gluteal fold flap in perineal reconstruction for Crohn's disease. It can be harvested with the patient in lithotomy or jack-knife positions. The donor site is generally well concealed causing minimal buttock asymmetry, especially when bilateral flaps are harvested. The flap width is limited to about 8 cm, and length limited to 15 cm. This fasciocutaneous flap can be de-epithelialized to fill perineal dead space or used to resurface perianal skin loss (Fig. 14.9). Patients are allowed to ambulate early postoperatively but advised to not sit on the donor site for a number of weeks postoperatively.

Pudendal Artery Flaps

The pudendal artery (PA) originates from the internal iliac artery in the pelvis, emerging deep to ischial tuberosity in the trajectory of the ischiorectal fossa. A number of perforators (3–5) branch off the PA and nourish perineal skin directly. This rich and interconnecting blood supply allows for the design of freestyle pedicled perforator flaps, random or axial pattern flaps which are thin and pliable with inconspicuous donor scars.

Martius Flap

The Martius flap, originally described by Henrique Martius for repair of urethrovaginal fistula in 1928, is a pedicled flap containing the labia majora fat pad with or without the overlying skin and underlying bulbocavernosus muscle in females. It may be harvested from either labia majora and is based on the perineal branch of the pudendal artery. It is a small flap usually utilized to augment the repair of rectal-vaginal fistulae. It is transposed through a subcutaneous tunnel to overlie the rectal closure and separate the rectal and vaginal walls with healthy, well-vascularized tissue (Fig. 14.10).

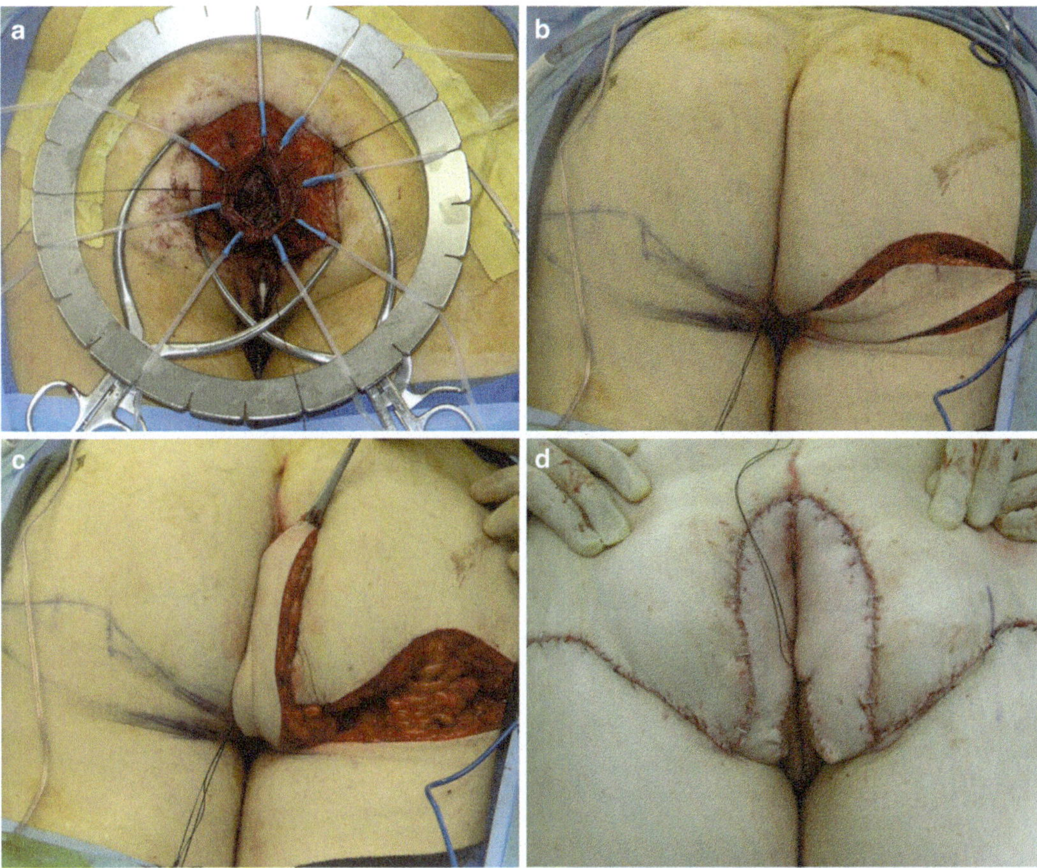

Fig. 14.9 (**a**) Circumferential perianal skin excision. (**b**) Right gluteal fold flap elevated (**c**) Right gluteal fold flap transposed to close right side of wound. (**d**) Bilateral gluteal fold flaps inset

Omentum

A pedicled greater omentum flap, when available, can be used to help obliterate dead space in the pelvis and/or help seal the pelvic floor. It has the advantage of being harvested through a laparotomy incision without creating additional surgical scars. The flap can be based off either the right or left gastroepiploic vessels, with the right side usually providing the dominant blood supply. The flap is elevated by dissecting the omentum off the transverse mesocolon and dividing the branches of the gastroepiploic vessels going to the greater curve of the stomach. It can be elongated by dividing some of the vascular arcades to comfortably reach the perineum (Fig. 14.11). This flap is often unavailable in many Crohn's patients due to multiple abdominal surgeries, and extensive intraabdominal scarring and adhesions. It also cannot provide any skin for a perineal defect, and may lack sufficient volume to truly fill all pelvic and perineal dead space following an extensive proctocolectomy. It is best used in conjunction with muscle and cutaneous flaps for perineal reconstructions with large soft tissue and skin defects.

Acellular Dermal Matrix

Acellular dermal matrix is a biological prosthetic implant, which is used to augment structural support during reconstructive procedures. Its uses are well documented in breast and abdominal

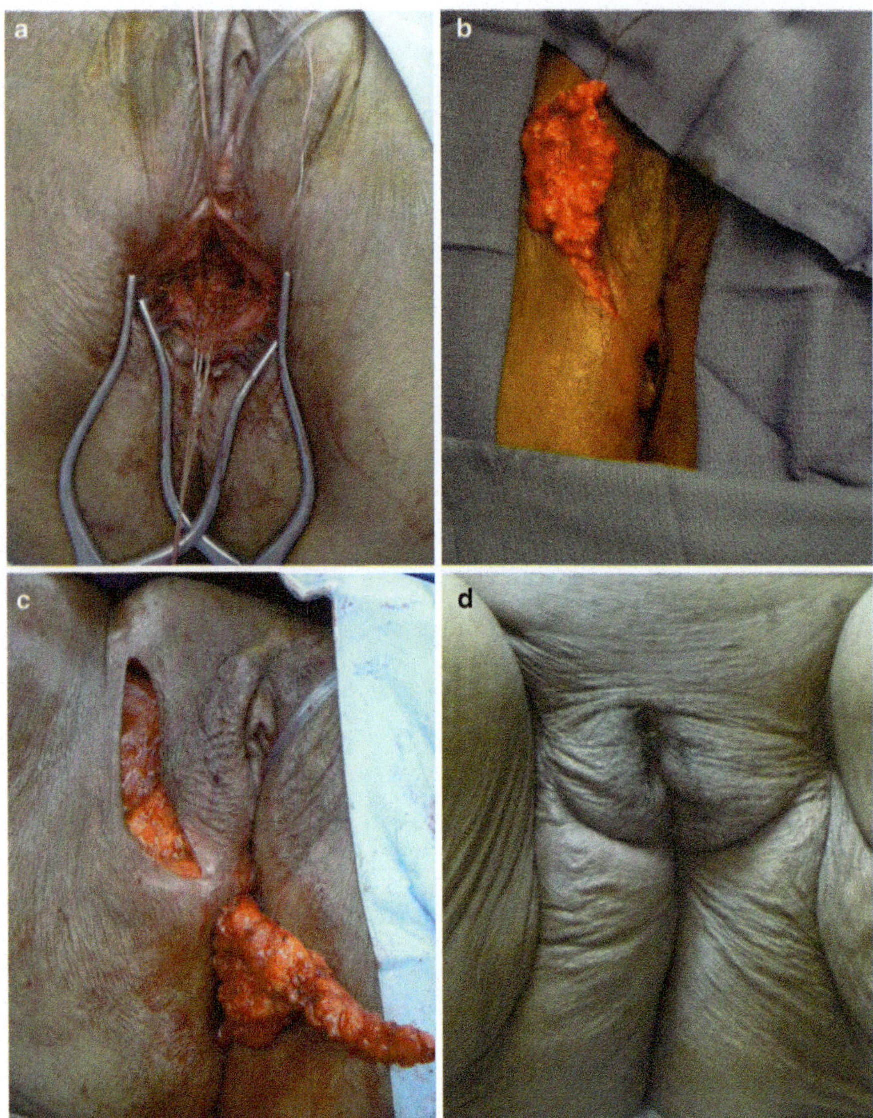

Fig. 14.10 (**a**) Rectal-vaginal fistula divided and repaired (**b**) Martius adipose flap elevated (**c**) Martius adipose flap transposed under skin bridge (to be placed between rectal and vaginal repair) (**d**) Incisions healed 3 months post-op

wall reconstruction, and there are a number of studies describing its use in pelvic reconstruction to restore support for intraabdominal organs following larger exenterative procedures [29]. The purpose of prosthetic placement is to reinforce pelvic floor reconstructions and minimize risk of perineal hernias. When used in conjunction with vascularized soft tissue flaps, the literature to date suggests it may lower perineal hernia incidence and increase healing rates without increased rates of infection [30].

Summary

Perineal reconstruction in Crohn's disease is best addressed with a multidisciplinary approach. The individual patient's specific needs must be assessed on a case-by-case basis. Attention must be given to previous surgeries, scars, donor site availabilities, and future therapeutic plans. Consideration must also be given to the size and location of the defect on the perineum, as well as

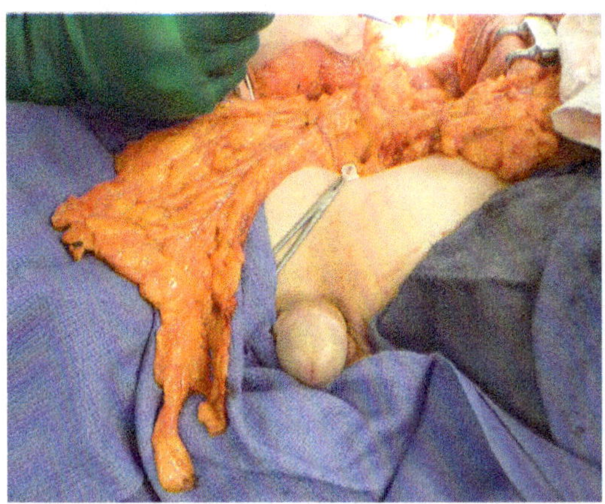

Fig. 14.11 Omental flap based on right gastroepiploic vessels laid on top of skin to demonstrate volume of tissue potentially available to fill pelvic and perineal wounds

patient characteristics which directly affect the likelihood of healing, such as nutritional status, the presence of perineal sepsis, immunosuppression, and steroid dependence. The reconstructive option of choice should afford the patient the best likelihood of successful healing, using safest and least morbid technique. If perineal closure cannot be achieved with edge-to-edge opposition of viable wound edges in a tension free manner, transfer of local and regional flaps should be considered. Pure perineal skin defects are best addressed with local fasciocutaneous tissue flaps based off the internal pudendal, inferior gluteal, and medial thigh systems. In larger defects such as proctectomy with or without visceral fistula resection, Crohn's disease complicated by cancer or massive perianal skin excisions, goals include sealing the pelvic floor thereby preventing the prolapse of intraabdominal contents into the perineal space, filling perineal dead space by the transposition of bulky vascularized tissue to potentiate wound healing and tension free closure of perineal skin.

References

1. Fields S, Rosainz L, Korelitz BI, Panagopoulos G, Schneider J. Rectal strictures in Crohn's disease and coexisting perirectal complications. Inflamm Bowel Dis. 2008;14:29–31.
2. Hurst RD, Gottlieb LJ, Cruciiti P, Melis M, Rubin M, Michelassi F. Primary closure of complicated perineal wounds with myocutaneous and fasciocutaneous flaps after proctectomy for Crohn's disease. Surgery. 2001;130:767–72.
3. Broader JH, Masselink BA, Oates GD, Alexander-Williams J. Management of the pelvic space after proctectomy. Br J Surg. 1974;61:94–7.
4. Burge H, Tompkin AM. The perineal wound after excision of the rectum. Postgrad Med J. 1960;36:519.
5. Elliot MS, Todd IP. Primary suture of the perineal wound using constant suction and irrigation, following rectal excision for inflammatory bowel disease. Ann R Coll Surg Engl. 1985;67:6–7.
6. McLeod R, Cohen Z, Langer B, Taylor B. Primary perineal wound closure following excision of the rectum. Can J Surg. 1983;26:122–4.
7. Marks CG, Ritchie JK, Todd IP, Wadsworth J. Primary suture of the perineal wound following rectal excision for inflammatory bowel disease. Br J Surg. 1978;65: 560–4.
8. Warshaw AL, Ottinger LW, Bartlett MK. Primary perineal closure after proctocolectomy for inflammatory bowel disease. Prevention of the persistent perineal sinus. Am J Surg. 1977;133:414–9.
9. Delalande JP, Hay JM, Fingerhut A, Kohlmann G, Paquet JC. Perineal wound management after abdominoperineal rectal excision for carcinoma with unsatisfactory hemostasis or gross septic contamination: primary closure vs. packing. A multicenter, controlled trial. French Association for Surgical Research. Dis Colon Rectum. 1994;37:890–6.
10. Irvin TT, Goligher JC. A controlled clinical trial of three different methods of perineal wound management following excision of the rectum. Br J Surg. 1975;62:287–91.
11. El-Gazzaz G, Kiran RP, Lavery I. Wound complications in rectal cancer patients undergoing primary closure of the perineal wound after abdominoperineal resection. Dis Colon Rectum. 2009;52:1962–6.
12. Kumar S, O'Donnell M, Khan K, Dunne P, Carey D, Lee J. Successful treatment of perineal necrotising fasciitis and associated pubic bone osteomyelitis with the vacuum assisted closure system. World J Surg Oncol. 2008;6:67–71.
13. Cresti S, Ouaïssi M, Sielezneff I, Chaix JB, Pirro N, Berthet B, Consentino B, Sastre B. Advantage of vacuum assisted closure on healing of wound associated with omentoplasty after abdominoperineal excision: a case report. World J Surg Oncol. 2008;6:136.
14. Windhofer C, Michlits W, Heuberger A, Papp C. Perineal reconstruction after rectal and anal disease using the local fascio-cutaneous-infragluteal flap: a new and reliable technique. Surgery. 2011;149:284–90.
15. Agarwal JP, Agarwal BS, Adler N, Gottlieb LJ. Intrinsic chimera flaps: a review. Ann Plast Surg. 2009;4:462–7.
16. Chessin DB, Hartley J, Cohen AM, et al. Rectus flap reconstruction decreases perineal wound complications after pelvic chemoradiation and surgery: a cohort study. Ann Surg Oncol. 2005;12:104–10.
17. Butler CE, Rodriguez-Bigas MA. Pelvic reconstruction after abdominoperineal resection: is it worthwhile. Ann Surg Oncol. 2005;12:91–4.

18. Höckel M. The transversus and rectus abdominis musculoperitoneal (TRAMP) composite flap for vulvovaginal reconstruction. Plast Reconstr Surg. 1996;97:455–9.
19. Gottlieb LJ, Alizadeh K. Restoration of erogenous sensation to the neo vagina neurosensory rectus abdominus myocutaneous flap. Published Abstract. American Society for Reconstructive Microsurgery Annual Meeting. Hawaii; 1999.
20. Di Benedetto G, Siquini W, Bertani A, Grassetti L. Vulvo-perineal reconstruction with a reverse sensitive rectus abdominis salvage flap in a multi recurrent anal carcinoma. J Plast Reconstr Aesthet Surg. 2010;63(2): e127–9.
21. Petrie N, Branagan G, McGuiness C, et al. Reconstruction of the perineum following anorectal cancer excision. Int J Colorectal Dis. 2009;24:97–104.
22. Ho K, Warrier S, Solomon MJ, et al. A prepelvic tunnel for the rectus abdominis myocutaneous flap in perineal reconstruction. J Plast Reconstr Aesthet Surg. 2006;59:1415–9.
23. McCraw JB, Massey FM, Shanklin KD, et al. Vaginal reconstruction with gracilis myocutaneous flaps. Plast Reconstr Surg. 1976;58:176–83.
24. Lee YT, Lee JM. Gracilis myocutaneous flap for the coverage of an extensive scrotoperineal defect and protection of the ruptured urethra and testes. Yonsei Med J. 1990;31:187–90.
25. Shibata D, Hyland W, Busse P, Kim HK, Sentovich SM, Steele Jr G, Bleday R. Immediate reconstruction of the perineal wound with gracilis muscle flaps following abdominoperineal resection and intraoperative radiation therapy for recurrent carcinoma of the rectum. Ann Surg Oncol. 1999; 6:33–7.
26. Nelson RA, Butler CE. Surgical outcomes of VRAM versus thigh flaps for immediate reconstruction of pelvic and perineal cancer resection defects. Plast Reconstr Surg. 2009;123:175–83.
27. Di Mauro D, D'Hoore A, Penninckx F. V-Y bilateral gluteus maximus myocutaneous advancement flap in the reconstruction of large perineal defects after resection of pelvic malignancies. Colorectal Dis. 2008;11:508–12.
28. Shahzad F, Wong KY, Di Candia M, Menon M, Malata CM. Gluteal fold flap in perineal reconstruction for Crohn's disease-associated fistulae. J Plast Reconstr Aesthet Surg. 2014;67(11):1587–90.
29. Said H, Bevers M, Butler C. Reconstruction of the pelvic floor and perineum with human acellular dermal matrix and thigh flaps following pelvic exenteration. Gynecol Oncol. 2007;107:578–82.
30. Wille-Jorgensen P, Pilsgaard B, Moller P. Reconstruction of the pelvic floor with a biological mesh after abdominoperineal excision for rectal cancer. Int J Colorectal Dis. 2009;24:323–5.

15 Surgery: Surgical Quality

Amy L. Halverson

Preoperative Optimization

Nearly half of the patients diagnosed with Crohn's disease will eventually require surgery. Efforts to optimize outcomes of surgery for Crohn's disease patients should start in the preoperative period. The goal of medical therapy is to optimize the quality of life for individuals with Crohn's disease. A shared understanding between the gastroenterologist, surgeon, and patient regarding the limitations of medical therapy and criteria for transitioning to surgical therapy will help to facilitate optimal patient care. The ideal timing of surgery involves consideration of the patient's quality of life, ability to maintain adequate nutrition, and response to pharmacologic therapy. Prolonged attempts at medical treatment without adequate clinical response or aggressive medical therapy in the setting of stricturing disease should be recognized and avoided. Perioperative management should include coordination of care between surgeon, gastroenterologist as well as radiologists, primary care physicians, psychologists, and enterostomal therapists [1].

A.L. Halverson, MD, FACS, FASCRS (✉)
Department of Surgery, Section of Colon and Rectal Surgery, Northwestern University Feinberg School of Medicine, 676 North St. Claire, Suite 650, Chicago, IL 60611, USA
e-mail: Ahalverson@nmff.org

In preparing patients for surgery, one should recognize factors that may contribute to postoperative morbidity. These may include malnutrition, preoperative steroid use, older age, smoking, and other medical comorbidities. Poor nutrition in individuals with Crohn's disease may result from decreased nutrient absorption, systemic inflammation, and anorexia. Indicators of poor nutrition include weight loss >10 % within the past 3–6 months, basic metabolic index < 18.5 kg/m^2, and serum albumin < 3.0 g/dL [2]. Several studies have reported increased rates of anastomotic leaks with an albumin below 3.5 g/dL. Makela and colleagues compared 44 patients with anastomotic leaks to matched controls and found that hypoalbuminemia and weight loss greater than 5 kg were significantly associated with leaks [3, 4]. Options to reduce the effect of under-nutrition on outcome may include utilizing a temporary stoma or providing parenteral nutrition prior to surgery. Several groups that advocate for preoperative nutritional supplementation have reported relatively low complication rates in patients who received preoperative parenteral nutrition [5–8].

Given that many patients are on immunosuppressive therapy prior to surgery, numerous studies evaluating the effect of preoperative glucocorticoids and more recently anti-tumor necrosis factor on postoperative morbidity have conflicting reports. Some studies have shown an association between postoperative complications and preoperative steroid use [7–13] while others have not [14, 15]. Similarly, several studies have reported

A. Fichera and M.K. Krane (eds.), *Crohn's Disease: Basic Principles*,
DOI 10.1007/978-3-319-14181-7_15, © Springer International Publishing Switzerland 2015

increased postoperative morbidity in patients treated with anti-tumor necrosis factor therapy at the time of surgery [16] and others have not observed such a relationship [15, 17–19].

Often patients with Crohn's disease may present with multiple risk factors, which have an additive effect on postoperative morbidity. Yamamoto and colleagues reviewed 566 bowel resections for Crohn's disease. They identified preoperative albumin less than 3.0 g/dL, preoperative steroid use, the presence of an abscess and the presence of a fistula at the time of surgery to be associated with postoperative complications [9]. Patients with zero, one, or two risk factors had a postoperative septic complication rate of 5 %, 16 %, and 14 %, respectively. Patients with three risk factors had a complication rate of 29 % and with all four risk factors the complication rate was 50 %. Alves and colleagues studied 161 patients undergoing ileocolic resection for Crohn's disease [8]. Identified risk factors for postoperative infectious complications included hypoproteinemia (protein serum level less than 60 g/L), intra-abdominal abscess identified at the time of surgery, preoperative steroid use more than 3 months, and multiple acute episodes of Crohn's disease prior to surgery. Patients with zero or one risk factor did not experience a postoperative infections complication. The infection rates in patients with two and three risk factors were 16 and 26 %. Two patients with all four risk factors developed infections complications.

The preoperative discussion with the patient is important for shared decision making and patient satisfaction. Having patients with increased knowledge and confidence who are more actively involved in the care process may lead to improved outcomes and decreased costs [20]. A preoperative discussion should cover the potential risks, benefits, and alternatives to surgery. It may address modifiable and nonmodifiable operative risk factors. Decision support tools such as the NSQIP universal surgical risk calculator may facilitate the discussion. The surgical risk calculator utilizes 21 preoperative factors (demographics, comorbidities, procedure) to estimate the risk of perioperative morbidity. Risk factors that may be especially applicable to individuals with Crohn's disease include chronic steroid use, whether the patient is a current smoker and whether the procedure is an emergency case [21].

Smoking is a modifiable risk factor that should be included in the preoperative discussion with patients who smoke. Smoking within 1 year of surgery increases postoperative complications [22]. Smoking cessation prior to surgery results in reduced vasoconstriction, reduced risk of venous thromboembolism, and improved wound healing [23–25]. While quitting smoking is a challenge for most patients, there are interventions that can help patients quit. Evidence shows that patients are more likely to quit smoking when advised by a health care professional and brief interventions of just a few minutes may increase rates of cessation [26]. The American College of Surgeons has produced a patient education resource that may be accessed at https://www.facs.org/~/media/files/education/patient%20ed/quitsmoking.ashx.

Perioperative Processes to Minimize Postoperative Morbidity

Risk assessment and adherence to evidence-based practices may reduce common postoperative complications. As surgical site infection (SSI) is one of the most common complications following bowel surgery, investigators have placed much effort in identifying methods to reduce surgical site infection. Common practices to reduce the rate of SSI that are well supported in the literature and in professional society include the appropriate timing and dosing of preoperative antibiotics and the use of antiseptic skin preparation. Other practices that are supported by weaker evidence or are inconsistently supported but that appeal to conventional wisdom include maintaining intraoperative normothermia, appropriate glycemic control, the use of uncontaminated instruments for abdominal wound closure, and selective wound closure in the setting of intraoperative contamination. The effectiveness of preoperative administration of intravenous antibiotics is supported by high quality evidence. A recent Cochrane review reported a risk reduction in postoperative wound infection when prophylactic antibiotics were used compared to placebo/no treatment 39–13 %, risk ratio 0.34, 95 % confidence interval 0.28–0.41) [27]. The antibiotics should be administered prior to skin incision and discontinued 24 h after surgery in clean-contaminated cases [28]. Antibiotics should cover bowel flora. Commonly used regimens include cefazolin and metronidazole or a second generation cephalosporin. Despite the broad acceptance of preoperative intravenous antibiotics the effectiveness of this practice may be lessened by variable adherence to recommended guidelines. A preoperative checklist may improve compliance with preoperative antibiotic administration. Awad and colleagues reported an increase in the number of patients who received prophylactic antibiotics within 60 min of incision from 84 to 96 % after implementation of a medical team training program. Similarly, Paull and colleagues reported a significant increase in on-time antibiotics from 92 to 97 %, ($p=0.01$) after implementation of preoperative briefings [29].

The role of oral preoperative antibiotics preparation has been controversial. More recently, several studies support the use of oral antibiotics. In a retrospective study using Veterans Affairs Surgical Quality Improvement Program, Cannon and colleagues found that among 9,940 patients who underwent colorectal resections, those who had no bowel preparation or mechanical preparation only had a SSI rate of 18.1 and 20 %, whereas those who received oral antibiotics or oral antibiotics with mechanical bowel preparation had SSI rates of 8.3 and 9.2 %. The use of oral antibiotics alone was associated with a 67 % decrease in SSI (OR = 0.33, 95 % CI 0.21–0.50) [30]. Additionally, a study from the Michigan State Surgical Quality Collaborative compared 370 matched pairs of patients undergoing bowel surgery. The authors reported an SSI rate of 4.5 % among patients receiving mechanical bowel preparation and oral nonabsorbable antibiotics compared to an SSI rate of 9.6 % in those receiving mechanical bowel preparation without oral antibiotics ($p=0.001$) [31]. In a systematic review and meta-analysis Bellows and colleagues reinforced the benefits of oral preoperative antibiotics. Among 2,669 patients in 16 randomized controlled trials, patients randomized to oral antibiotics had a lower infectious complication rate compared to those without oral antibiotics, relative risk 0.57 (95 % CI, 0.43–0.76) [32].

Controversy also exists as to the optimal formulation for antiseptic skin preparation. Lee and colleagues performed a systematic review that included nine randomized controlled trials with a total of 3,614 patients. The authors found a significantly lower rate of SSI with chlorhexidine antisepsis compared to iodine based skin preparations, adjusted risk ratio 0.64 [95 % confidence interval, 0.51–0.08] [33]. In a prospective randomized trial in patients undergoing bowel resection, Dovovich and colleagues also reported significantly decreased rates of SSI with chlorhexidine compared to iodine based skin preparation formulations (9.5 vs. 16.1 %, relative risk 0.59; 95 % confidence interval, 0.41–0.85) [34]. In contrast, a study from the Washington State Surgical Care and Outcomes Program compared SSI in a cohort of 7,669 clean-contaminated surgical cases and found that risk-adjusted rates of SSI were not significantly different between the different skin preparations [35]. The overall SSI rate was 4.6 %. The risk-adjusted rates were 0.85 ($p=0.28$ for chlorhexidine, 1.10 ($p=0.06$) for chlorhexidine in isopropyl alcohol, 0.98 ($p=0.96$) for povidone-iodine and 0.93 ($p=0.51$) for iodine-povacrylex in isopropyl alcohol.

Cima and colleagues from the Mayo clinic elegantly demonstrated how implementation of a bundle of processes can effectively reduce surgical site infections [36]. Their multidisciplinary team developed a protocol with process steps that spanned the preoperative and postoperative care periods. The key components of this protocol included preoperative showering on the night before and the day of surgery and adherence to preoperative antibiotic administration guidelines and chlorhexidine skin prep. Prior to skin closure, the operating team changed gloves and switched to uncontaminated instruments for the fascia closure. Pre and postoperatively patients were instructed on hand hygiene and wound care, including recognizing and reporting signs and symptoms of wound infections. The implementation of the SSI rate reduction bundle resulted in an overall SSI rate reduction from 9.8 to 4.0 %, $p<0.05$. Superficial SSU decreased from 4.9 to 1.5 %, $p<0.05$. The authors emphasize the importance of standardized processes that minimize variance among providers as well as patient and staff education to insure compliance with protocols.

Patients with Crohn's disease are at increased risk for venous thromboembolic (VTE) events [37, 38]. Postoperative VTE events occur in approximately 2.5 % of patients with inflammatory bowel disease undergoing abdominal surgery. This rate is more than twice the rate of 1 % seen in non-inflammatory bowel disease patients [39, 40]. This increased risk is multifactorial and includes disease-related factors such as anemia, hypoalbuminemia, and malnutrition [39]. Genetic and acquired factors such as smoking and steroid and oral contraceptive use also play a role. In the disease process, inflammatory mediators activate proteases originating from the coagulation and fibrinolysis system. The increased thrombosis persists even when patients are in remission [41]. The American Gastroenterological Association and the Canadian Association for Gastroenterology recommend chemoprophylaxis for all inpatients with inflammatory bowel disease, even if their reason for admission is not related to their inflammatory bowel disease [42].

The American College of Chest Physicians guidelines recommends that individuals undergoing abdominal surgery who are at increased risk for VTE events receive mechanical prophylaxis and chemoprophylaxis with low molecular weight heparin or low-dose unfractionated heparin [43]. These recommendations utilize two different risk assessment models. In each model, major abdominal surgery is considered to be of increased risk. The Patient Safety in Surgery Study model assigns increased risk for albumin <3.5 g/dL. The Caprini model assigns additional risk to individuals with a history of inflammatory bowel disease [44]. These recommendations do not specify the timing of initiation of prophylaxis. The ASCRS practice parameters describe the typical dose of unfractionated heparin as 5,000 units administered within 2 h prior to surgery [45]. The colorectal surgeons at our institution routinely administer 5,000 units of unfractionated heparin just prior to induction of anesthesia. The decision between postoperative prophylaxis with low-dose unfractionated heparin or low molecular weight heparin is based on several factors. Advantages of low molecular weight heparin include once-daily dosing and a lower risk of heparin-induced thrombocytopenia, 2.7 % versus 0 % in a prospective randomized study by Warkentin and colleagues [46]. Patients with renal insufficiency should receive low-dose unfractionated heparin. Also, there remains some controversy on the safety of LMWH in patients with an epidural catheter. Currently, there are no guidelines that recommend prolonged anticoagulation in IBD patients. However, Gross and colleagues performed a retrospective study of 45,964 patients with IBD and colorectal cancer using the American College of Surgeons National Surgical Quality Improvement Program who underwent abdominal surgery [47]. Patients with inflammatory bowel disease had a higher rate of VTE at 30-day post surgery compared to cancer patients (2.7 vs. 2.1 %, $p<0.001$). The authors argue that IBD patients should receive VTE prophylaxis for 4 weeks post discharge.

Until recently, concerns about perioperative adrenal insufficiency and resulting hemodynamic instability in patients taking corticosteroids led physicians to routinely administer perioperative high-dose corticosteroids to patients receiving steroids. This practice is not supported by current literature. In 2008 Marik and colleagues performed a meta-analysis that included two randomized controlled studies of stress dose steroids versus placebo and several cohort studies of patients undergoing surgery without stress dose steroids. No clinical difference was observed between patients receiving high-dose steroids and those receiving the equivalent of their daily dose of steroids [48]. Zaghayan and colleagues recently performed a randomized, noninferiority trial in 92 steroid treated inflammatory bowel disease patients undergoing colorectal surgery. Patients were randomly assigned to receive hydrocortisone 100 mg three times daily followed by taper or hydrocortisone equivalent to one third of their usual daily dose three times daily followed by taper. The primary endpoint, absence of hypotension on postoperative day 1, was observed in 95 % of the patients receiving high-dose steroids and 96 % of patients on low-dose steroids, 95 % confidence interval −0.08 to 0.09, $p=0.007$ [49].

Standardized perioperative care protocols have resulted in decreased complications, earlier hospital discharges, and overall improved outcomes. Key components common to various enhanced recovery include patient education to gain buy-in and mange patient's expectations. After surgery there is early initiation of oral intake and minimization of opiate analgesics, limited intravenous fluids and early removal of urinary catheters and early ambulation. Some protocols attempt to minimize preoperative physiologic stress by withholding bowel preparation, allowing preoperative oral fluids and the use of oral carbohydrate supplements. The concept of enhanced recovery was introduced by Kehlet in the late 1990s [50]. This group reported that enhanced recovery could be safely applied to patients undergoing open surgery for Crohn's disease [51]. In 2007 Maessen and colleagues published a multicenter European study that included five sites [52]. The study included patients undergoing elective, open colorectal resections above the peritoneal resection. The authors reported a median length of stay of 5 days. The readmission rate was 14 percent. This report emphasized the need for patient and care team education and care coordination. Factors highly associated with early discharge included the hospital's experience with the enhanced recovery protocol. They found that in hospitals with less experience executing the protocol, only half of the patients who met criteria for discharge on postoperative day 2–3 were actually discharged. This delay in discharge was attributed to patient expectations and care team compliance with the protocol.

The advantages of enhanced recovery seen following open surgery have persisted in minimally invasive surgery. The impact of enhanced recovery in minimally invasive surgery was reported by Lovely and colleagues from the Mayo clinic [53]. The authors compared an enhanced recovery program to a preexisting fast-track pathway. The main differences between the two protocols were elimination of intravenous patient controlled analgesia, avoidance of fluid overload, and more specific ambulation goals in the enhanced recovery group. The enhanced recovery program further reduced length of stay, and decreased overall hospital costs and was associated with similar complication and readmission rates. Another study by Spinelli and colleagues reported the results of implementation of an enhanced recovery program specifically in patients undergoing laparoscopic ileocolic resection for Crohn's disease [54]. It is notable that studies of enhanced recovery have been limited to patients undergoing elective surgery. Contraindications include emergent procedures, ASA 4 or higher, patients with severe malnutrition and limited mobility.

Postoperative hospital readmission is currently an area of focus in assessing quality of surgical care. Intestinal surgery is associated with readmission rates of 10–15 % for elective surgery and up to 21 % for urgent or emergent surgery [55]. Readmission rates following surgery for Crohn's disease are similar to those reported for other indications for surgical resection [56]. Aside from postoperative complications, Frolkis and colleagues identified emergent admission at the time of surgery and the presence of a stoma to be risk factors for 90-day postoperative readmission. Common causes for readmission after intestinal surgery include ileus, obstruction, dehydration or electrolyte disturbances, and surgical site infection. In addition to avoiding postoperative complications, Halverson and colleagues identified processes measures that may potentially reduce postoperative readmissions [55]. These emphasize the importance of identifying and mitigating risk factors for readmission. This includes evaluating the patient for comorbidities, patient education regarding the anticipated operative and perioperative care plan and communication with the patient's primary care physician. Patients who are anticipated to have a stoma created at the time of surgery should undergo preoperative counseling and stoma site selection. This group endorsed the implementation of a standardized perioperative care protocol. Postoperative processes included thorough evaluation of the patient's discharged needs. The patient should receive discharge instructions detailing how to manage medications, wound care instructions, stoma care in applicable, and dietary and activity restrictions. Patients should also be educated on signs and symptoms of common postoperative complications and when to call or go to an emergency department.

Patients with new ileostomies are especially at risk for readmission for dehydration. Nagle and colleagues successfully addressed this problem by implementing a care pathway for individuals with new ileostomies [57]. The fundamental components of this pathway include preoperative education about ileostomy, standardized patient education materials, and a strong emphasis on patients becoming self-sufficient with stoma care, including strict tracking of stoma output. Their program involved engaging and educating a multidisciplinary team of nurses, patient care technicians, enterostomal therapists, and home care providers.

Summary

Providing quality surgical care requires that surgeons incorporate practices that are supported by the best available evidence. Processes important to the surgical care of patients with Crohn's disease are summarized in Table 15.1. Our practices need to be continuously re-evaluated as new evidence is presented and our understanding of how patient characteristics, disease processes, and therapeutic interventions affect outcomes evolves. One must recognize that optimal care requires communication and the coordinated efforts of individuals from multiple disciplines. Central to providing optimal, patient-centered care is consistently informing patients of their treatment options and providing education that supports patients playing an active role in their care.

Table 15.1 Optimization of surgical care

Optimization of surgical care
Preoperative
Nutrition assessment
Smoking cessation
Address existing abdominal infection
Patient counseling and education
Patient counseling and stoma site marking when applicable
Perioperative
Oral nonabsorbable antibiotics
Preoperative briefing/checklist
Intravenous prophylactic antibiotics
Venous thromboembolism prophylaxis
Administer corticosteroids equivalent to patient's usual daily steroid dose
Standardized perioperative care protocol
Patient education regarding stoma care when applicable
Postoperative
Written discharge instructions
Educate patients and caretakers regarding care of the incision as well as identifying and reporting signs and symptoms of postoperative complications

References

1. Spinelli A, Allocca M, Jovani M, Danese S. Review article: optimal preparation for surgery in Crohn's disease. Aliment Pharmacol Ther. 2014;40(9):1009–22.
2. Lochs H, Dejong C, Hammarqvist F, Hebuterne X, Leon-Sanz M, Schutz T, et al. ESPEN guidelines on enteral nutrition: gastroenterology. Clin Nutr. 2006;25(2):260–74.
3. Makela JT, Kiviniemi H, Laitinen S. Risk factors for anastomotic leakage after left-sided colorectal resection with rectal anastomosis. Dis Colon Rectum. 2003;46(5):653–60.
4. Suding P, Jensen E, Abramson MA, Itani K, Wilson SE. Definitive risk factors for anastomotic leaks in elective open colorectal resection. Arch Surg. 2008;143(9):907–11. Discussion 11–2.
5. Smedh K, Andersson M, Johansson H, Hagberg T. Preoperative management is more important than choice of sutured or stapled anastomosis in Crohn's disease. Eur J Surg. 2002;168(3):154–7.
6. Jacobson S. Early postoperative complications in patients with Crohn's disease given and not given preoperative total parenteral nutrition. Scand J Gastroenterol. 2012;47(2):170–7.
7. Zerbib P, Koriche D, Truant S, Bouras AF, Vernier-Massouille G, Seguy D, et al. Pre-operative management is associated with low rate of post-operative morbidity in penetrating Crohn's disease. Aliment Pharmacol Ther. 2010;32(3):459–65.
8. Alves A, Panis Y, Bouhnik Y, Pocard M, Vicaut E, Valleur P. Risk factors for intra-abdominal septic complications after a first ileocecal resection for Crohn's disease: a multivariate analysis in 161 consecutive patients. Dis Colon Rectum. 2007;50(3):331–6.
9. Yamamoto T, Allan RN, Keighley MR. Risk factors for intra-abdominal sepsis after surgery in Crohn's disease. Dis Colon Rectum. 2000;43(8):1141–5.
10. Post S, Betzler M, von Ditfurth B, Schurmann G, Kuppers P, Herfarth C. Risks of intestinal anastomoses in Crohn's disease. Ann Surg. 1991;213(1):37–42.

11. Aberra FN, Lewis JD, Hass D, Rombeau JL, Osborne B, Lichtenstein GR. Corticosteroids and immunomodulators: postoperative infectious complication risk in inflammatory bowel disease patients. Gastroenterology. 2003;125(2):320–7.
12. Subramanian V, Saxena S, Kang JY, Pollok RC. Preoperative steroid use and risk of postoperative complications in patients with inflammatory bowel disease undergoing abdominal surgery. Am J Gastroenterol. 2008;103(9):2373–81.
13. Tzivanakis A, Singh JC, Guy RJ, Travis SP, Mortensen NJ, George BD. Influence of risk factors on the safety of ileocolic anastomosis in Crohn's disease surgery. Dis Colon Rectum. 2012;55(5):558–62.
14. Bruewer M, Utech M, Rijcken EJ, Anthoni C, Laukoetter MG, Kersting S, et al. Preoperative steroid administration: effect on morbidity among patients undergoing intestinal bowel resection for Crohns disease. World J Surg. 2003;27(12):1306–10.
15. Canedo J, Lee SH, Pinto R, Murad-Regadas S, Rosen L, Wexner SD. Surgical resection in Crohn's disease: is immunosuppressive medication associated with higher postoperative infection rates? Colo Dis. 2011;13(11):1294–8.
16. Appau KA, Fazio VW, Shen B, Church JM, Lashner B, Remzi F, et al. Use of infliximab within 3 months of ileocolonic resection is associated with adverse postoperative outcomes in Crohn's patients. J Gastrointest Surg. 2008;12(10):1738–44.
17. Mascarenhas C, Nunoo R, Asgeirsson T, Rivera R, Kim D, Hoedema R, et al. Outcomes of ileocolic resection and right hemicolectomies for Crohn's patients in comparison with non-Crohn's patients and the impact of perioperative immunosuppressive therapy with biologics and steroids on inpatient complications. Am J Surg. 2012;203(3):375–8. Discussion 8.
18. Colombel JF, Loftus Jr EV, Tremaine WJ, Pemberton JH, Wolff BG, Young-Fadok T, et al. Early postoperative complications are not increased in patients with Crohn's disease treated perioperatively with infliximab or immunosuppressive therapy. Am J Gastroenterol. 2004;99(5):878–83.
19. Marchal L, D'Haens G, Van Assche G, Vermeire S, Noman M, Ferrante M, et al. The risk of post-operative complications associated with infliximab therapy for Crohn's disease: a controlled cohort study. Aliment Pharmacol Ther. 2004;19(7):749–54.
20. Hibbard JH, Greene J, Overton V. Patients with lower activation associated with higher costs; delivery systems should know their patient's scores. Health Aff. 2013;32(2):216–22.
21. Bilimoria KY, Liu Y, Paruch JL, Zhou L, Kmiecik TE, Ko CY, et al. Development and evaluation of the universal ACS NSQIP surgical risk calculator: a decision aid and informed consent tool for patients and surgeons. J Am Coll Surg. 2013;217(5):833–42e1–3.
22. Kamath AS, Vaughan Sarrazin M, Vander Weg MW, Cai X, Cullen J, Katz DA. Hospital costs associated with smoking in veterans undergoing general surgery. J Am Coll Surg. 2012;214(6):901–8e1.
23. Lindstrom D, Sadr Azodi O, Wladis A, Tonnesen H, Linder S, Nasell H, et al. Effects of a perioperative smoking cessation intervention on postoperative complications: a randomized trial. Ann Surg. 2008;248(5):739–45.
24. Moller AM, Villebro N, Pedersen T, Tonnesen H. Effect of preoperative smoking intervention on postoperative complications: a randomised clinical trial. Lancet. 2002;359(9301):114–7.
25. Sorensen LT. Wound healing and infection in surgery. The clinical impact of smoking and smoking cessation: a systematic review and meta-analysis. Arch Surg. 2012;147(4):373–83.
26. A clinical practice guideline for treating tobacco use and dependence: a US Public Health Service report. The tobacco use and dependence clinical practice guideline panel, staff, and consortium representatives. JAMA. 2000;283(24):3244–54.
27. Nelson RL, Gladman E, Barbateskovic M. Antimicrobial prophylaxis for colorectal surgery. Cochrane Database Syst Rev. 2014;5, CD001181.
28. Bratzler DW, Houck PM, Surgical Infection Prevention Guidelines Writers Workgroup, American Academy of Orthopaedic Surgeons, American Association of Critical Care Nurses, American Association of Nurse Anesthetists, et al. Antimicrobial prophylaxis for surgery: an advisory statement from the National Surgical Infection Prevention Project. Clin Infect Dis. 2004;38(12):1706–15.
29. Paull DE, Mazzia LM, Wood SD, Theis MS, Robinson LD, Carney B, et al. Briefing guide study: preoperative briefing and postoperative debriefing checklists in the veterans health administration medical team training program. Am J Surg. 2010;200(5):620–3.
30. Cannon JA, Altom LK, Deierhoi RJ, Morris M, Richman JS, Vick CC, et al. Preoperative oral antibiotics reduce surgical site infection following elective colorectal resections. Dis Colon Rectum. 2012; 55(11):1160–6.
31. Englesbe MJ, Brooks L, Kubus J, Luchtefeld M, Lynch J, Senagore A, et al. A statewide assessment of surgical site infection following colectomy: the role of oral antibiotics. Ann Surg. 2010;252(3):514–9. Discussion 9–20.
32. Bellows CF, Mills KT, Kelly TN, Gagliardi G. Combination of oral non-absorbable and intravenous antibiotics versus intravenous antibiotics alone in the prevention of surgical site infections after colorectal surgery: a meta-analysis of randomized controlled trials. Tech Coloproctol. 2011;15(4):385–95.
33. Lee I, Agarwal RK, Lee BY, Fishman NO, Umscheid CA. Systematic review and cost analysis comparing use of chlorhexidine with use of iodine for preoperative skin antisepsis to prevent surgical site infection. Infect Control Hosp Epidemiol. 2010;31(12): 1219–29.
34. Darouiche RO, Wall Jr MJ, Itani KM, Otterson MF, Webb AL, Carrick MM, et al. Chlorhexidine-alcohol versus povidone-iodine for surgical-site antisepsis. N Engl J Med. 2010;362(1):18–26.

35. Hakkarainen TW, Dellinger EP, Evans HL, Farjah F, Farrokhi E, Steele SR, et al. Comparative effectiveness of skin antiseptic agents in reducing surgical site infections: a report from the Washington state surgical care and outcomes assessment program. J Am Coll Surg. 2014;218(3):336–44.
36. Cima R, Dankbar E, Lovely J, Pendlimari R, Aronhalt K, Nehring S, et al. Colorectal surgery surgical site infection reduction program: a national surgical quality improvement program–driven multidisciplinary single-institution experience. J Am Coll Surg. 2013;216(1):23–33.
37. Bernstein CN, Blanchard JF, Houston DS, Wajda A. The incidence of deep venous thrombosis and pulmonary embolism among patients with inflammatory bowel disease: a population-based cohort study. Thromb Haemost. 2001;85(3):430–4.
38. Miehsler W, Reinisch W, Valic E, Osterode W, Tillinger W, Feichtenschlager T, et al. Is inflammatory bowel disease an independent and disease specific risk factor for thromboembolism? Gut. 2004;53(4): 542–8.
39. Wallaert JB, De Martino RR, Marsicovetere PS, Goodney PP, Finlayson SR, Murray JJ, et al. Venous thromboembolism after surgery for inflammatory bowel disease: are there modifiable risk factors? Data from ACS NSQIP. Dis Colon Rectum. 2012;55(11): 1138–44.
40. Merrill A, Millham F. Increased risk of postoperative deep vein thrombosis and pulmonary embolism in patients with inflammatory bowel disease: a study of National Surgical Quality Improvement Program patients. Arch Surg. 2012;147(2):120–4.
41. Owczarek D, Cibor D, Glowacki MK, Rodacki T, Mach T. Inflammatory bowel disease: epidemiology, pathology and risk factors for hypercoagulability. World J Gastroenterol. 2014;20(1):53–63.
42. Nguyen GC, Bernstein CN, Bitton A, Chan AK, Griffiths AM, Leontiadis GI, et al. Consensus statements on the risk, prevention, and treatment of venous thromboembolism in inflammatory bowel disease: Canadian Association of Gastroenterology. Gastroenterology. 2014;146(3):835–48e6.
43. Kearon C, Akl EA, Comerota AJ, Prandoni P, Bounameaux H, Goldhaber SZ, et al. Antithrombotic therapy for VTE disease: antithrombotic therapy and prevention of thrombosis, 9th ed: American college of chest physicians evidence-based clinical practice guidelines. Chest. 2012;141(2 Suppl):e419S–94.
44. Bahl V, Hu HM, Henke PK, Wakefield TW, Campbell Jr DA, Caprini JA. A validation study of a retrospective venous thromboembolism risk scoring method. Ann Surg. 2010;251(2):344–50.
45. Stahl TJ, Gregorcyk SG, Hyman NH, Buie WD. Standards practice task force of the American Society of C, Rectal S. Practice parameters for the prevention of venous thrombosis. Dis Colon Rectum. 2006;49(10):1477–83.
46. Warkentin TE, Levine MN, Hirsh J, Horsewood P, Roberts RS, Gent M, et al. Heparin-induced thrombocytopenia in patients treated with low-molecular-weight heparin or unfractionated heparin. N Engl J Med. 1995;332(20):1330–5.
47. Gross ME, Vogler SA, Mone MC, Sheng X, Sklow B. The importance of extended postoperative venous thromboembolism prophylaxis in IBD: a National Surgical Quality Improvement Program analysis. Dis Colon Rectum. 2014;57(4):482–9.
48. Marik PE, Varon J. Requirement of perioperative stress doses of corticosteroids: a systematic review of the literature. Arch Surg. 2008;143(12):1222–6.
49. Zaghiyan K, Melmed GY, Berel D, Ovsepyan G, Murrell Z, Fleshner P. A prospective, randomized, noninferiority trial of steroid dosing after major colorectal surgery. Ann Surg. 2014;259(1):32–7.
50. Kehlet H. Multimodal approach to control postoperative pathophysiology and rehabilitation. Br J Anaesth. 1997;78(5):606–17.
51. Andersen J, Kehlet H. Fast track open ileo-colic resections for Crohn's disease. Color Dis. 2005; 7(4):394–7.
52. Maessen J, Dejong CH, Hausel J, Nygren J, Lassen K, Andersen J, et al. A protocol is not enough to implement an enhanced recovery programme for colorectal resection. Br J Surg. 2007;94(2):224–31.
53. Lovely JK, Maxson PM, Jacob AK, Cima RR, Horlocker TT, Hebl JR, et al. Case-matched series of enhanced versus standard recovery pathway in minimally invasive colorectal surgery. Br J Surg. 2012;99(1):120–6.
54. Spinelli A, Bazzi P, Sacchi M, Danese S, Fiorino G, Malesci A, et al. Short-term outcomes of laparoscopy combined with enhanced recovery pathway after ileocecal resection for Crohn's disease: a case-matched analysis. J Gastrointest Surg. 2013;17(1):126–32; discussion 32.
55. Halverson AL, Sellers MM, Bilimoria KY, Hawn MT, Williams MV, McLeod RS, et al. Identification of process measures to reduce postoperative readmission. J Gastrointest Surg. 2014;18(8):1407–15.
56. Frolkis A, Kaplan GG, Patel AB, Faris P, Quan H, Jette N, et al. Postoperative complications and emergent readmission in children and adults with inflammatory bowel disease who undergo intestinal resection: a population-based study. Inflamm Bowel Dis. 2014;20(8):1316–23.
57. Nagle D, Pare T, Keenan E, Marcet K, Tizio S, Poylin V. Ileostomy pathway virtually eliminates readmissions for dehydration in new ostomates. Dis Colon Rectum. 2012;55(12):1266–72.

Recurrent CD: Medical Prophylaxis 16

Britt Christensen and David T. Rubin

Abbreviations

CD	Crohn's disease
FC	Fecal calprotectin
IMM	Immunomodulator

Introduction

Following surgical resection in Crohn's disease (CD), post-operative recurrence remains a significant problem. Endoscopic recurrence rates at or proximal to the surgical anastomosis are reported to be between 70 and 90 % within 1 year [1, 2]. In addition, up to 50 % of patients will require a repeat operation for recurrence within 5 years and up to 70 % will require repeat surgery within 20 years [3–6]. Prevention of this post-operative recurrence is essential to prevent both disease relapse and a second negative outcome such as surgery [7]. However optimal monitoring and medical management of patients with CD after surgery is still controversial.

B. Christensen, BSc, MBBS, MPH • D.T. Rubin, MD (✉)
Section of Gastroenterology, Hepatology and Nutrition, The University of Chicago Medicine, 5841 S. Maryland Avenue, MC4076, Room M410, Chicago, IL 60637, USA
e-mail: britt.christensen@uchospitals.edu; drubin@medicine.bsd.uchicago.edu

Relapse Rates and Predictors of Relapse

Clinical relapse rates at 1 year are estimated to be between 10 and 38 % [8]. However clinical relapse is much less frequent than endoscopic recurrence with studies suggesting an endoscopic recurrence rate as high as 90 % in those not receiving medical prophylaxis 1 year after surgery [1, 2]. Endoscopic findings that indicate recurrence include small aphthous ulcers, deep linear ulcers, mucosal inflammation, fistulae, and strictures [9]. These varying degrees of endoscopic disease activity may be seen within 3 months of surgery in more than 70 % of patients [2]. The most common site of recurrence is the surgical anastomosis, especially the proximal side of the anastomosis [1]. The cause of recurrence at this location is believed to be due to luminal contents, specifically intestinal flora [10].

The most consistently recognized risk factors for recurrence include smoking cigarettes, perforating type disease, perianal fistula, prior CD surgery, and ileocolonic disease compared with colonic and small intestinal disease patterns [11–15]. Shorter disease duration till first operation, and younger age at first operation are also likely risk factors [11]. It is unclear if having clear margins at the time of surgery, having a smaller length of resection or if the types of anastomosis are associated with improved outcomes [12, 14–16].

A. Fichera and M.K. Krane (eds.), *Crohn's Disease: Basic Principles*,
DOI 10.1007/978-3-319-14181-7_16, © Springer International Publishing Switzerland 2015

Bacteria and gut contents play a significant role in post-operative recurrence. If a patient is diverted proximal to the anastomosis, a sustained remission at the anastomosis is achieved without medical therapy [17]. In a study by D'Haens et al. of patients with an ileal resection and primary anastomosis but with proximal diversion of luminal contents by a diverting ileostomy, no recurrence was noted by endoscopy [17]. However following reinfusion of ileostomy contents into the diverted distal ileum, there was histologic evidence of inflammation within 1 week, thus demonstrating the critical role of luminal contents in reactivation of CD [17].

Assessing Post-Operative Recurrence Risk

Patients with any of the risk factors mentioned have a high likelihood of recurrence and are the patient subgroup in which prophylactic medical therapy should be strongly considered. The assessment of post-operative risk recurrence should occur pre-operatively. All available options should be discussed with the patient. In addition open communication between the GI physicians and the surgical teams needs to occur with clarification of the type, extent and severity of disease, and discussion regarding plans for immune suppression. Due to the high recurrence rates seen it is worthwhile being proactive and to institute preventative strategies in high-risk patient groups. Post-operative ileocecectomy should be seen as the ideal opportunity for prevention of symptomatic disease and complications from the disease.

Assessment of Recurrence

Clinical symptoms should not be relied upon to assess for post-operative recurrence. Inflammation is often present in asymptomatic patients and there is poor correlation between clinical and endoscopic findings in the post-operative setting [18, 19]. The most commonly used endoscopic scoring system to assess disease recurrence after ileal or ileocolonic resection in CD is the Rutgeerts' score (Fig. 16.1) [1]. This score looks at the presence and severity of recurrence in the

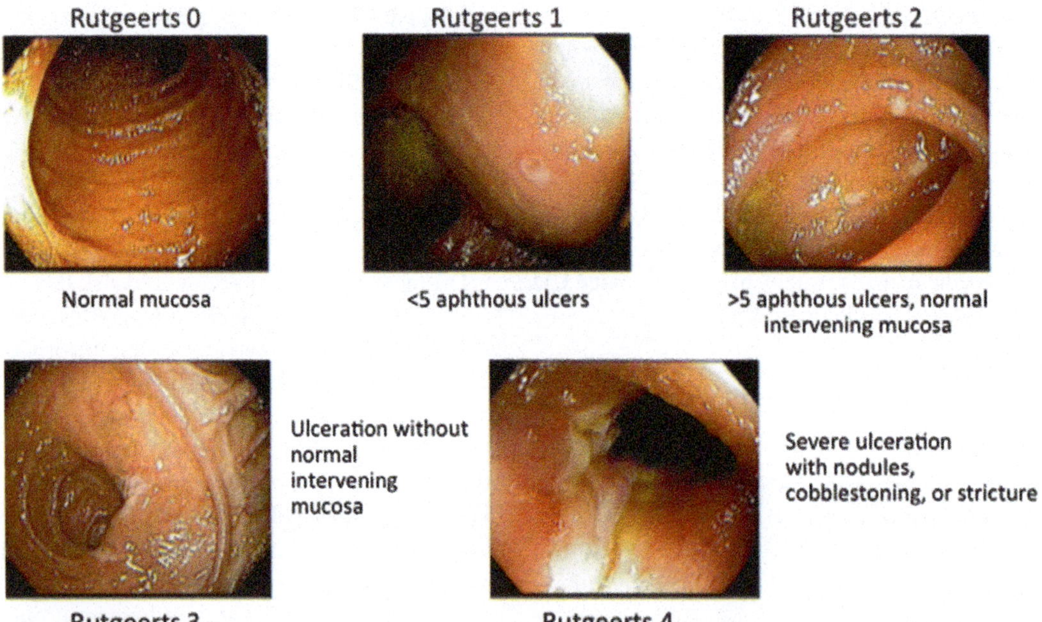

Fig. 16.1 Rutgeerts' score for post-operative endoscopic recurrence

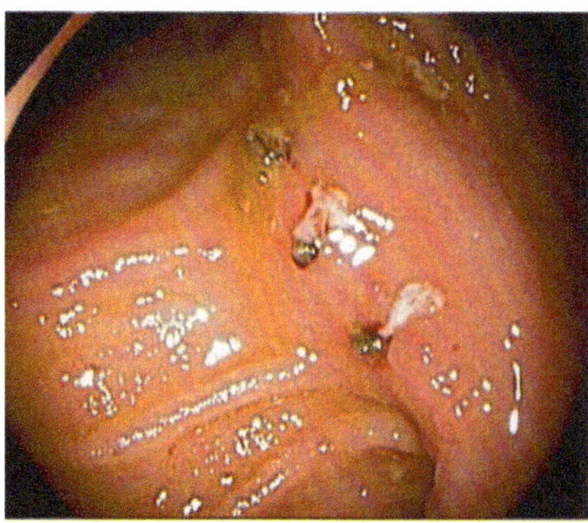

Fig. 16.2 Suture related trauma at the post-operative anastomosis

neoterminal ileum and at the ileocolonic anastomosis. When utilizing this scoring system it is important to acknowledge that ulcers at the anastomosis may not always be related to disease recurrence. It is quite common to have suture related trauma (Fig. 16.2) or marginal ulceration/ischemia at this location and such ulcers should be excluded from the scoring system. Rutgeerts' score is used to determine initiation of medical therapy as it has been found to correlate with the prognosis of clinical disease recurrence with those having a score of i-0 or i-1 having less than 5 % chance of clinical recurrence within 3 years. This is in comparison with i-2, i-3, and i-4, which correlate with a clinical recurrence risk of 14 %, 40 %, and 90 %, respectively [1, 20]. Due to the fact that endoscopic recurrence precedes clinical recurrence and that most recurrence occurs within the first year [20] it is recommended that an ileocolonoscopy be performed within 6–12 months of surgery.

Fecal Calprotectin for Assessing Post-Operative Recurrence

As endoscopy is an invasive test that potentiates a risk to the patient, there has been interest in the use of surrogate markers to monitor for disease recurrence in the post-operative setting. The most promising is that of fecal calprotectin (FC). FC levels correlate well with endoscopic recurrence as measured by the Rutgeerts' score [21, 22]. Sorrentino et al. measured FC in 25 patients every 2 months following surgery and found that FC corresponds to endoscopic recurrence [22]. Additionally, patients that received anti-TNF therapy to treat this recurrence and had endoscopic improvement also had improvement of their FC [22]. Another study by Wright et al. of 136 patients who had a calprotectin measured pre-operatively and at 6 months post-operatively found that a cutoff of 100 μg/g FC could be used to monitor for disease recurrence with a sensitivity of 0.89 and a negative predictive value of 91 %, concluding that the use of fecal calprotectin to monitor patients in the post-operative setting may allow for 41 % of patients to avoid colonoscopy [23]. This has also been demonstrated by Lobaton et al. who found that the medium FC for those with i0–i1 disease was 98 μg/g versus 234.5 μg/g in those with i2–i4 disease [24]. Finally in a study by Yamamoto and Kotze, a cutoff value of 170 μg/g for FC had a sensitivity of 0.83 and a specificity of 0.93 to predict clinical recurrence [25]. Although at this stage it is premature to rely on FC alone to monitor for disease recurrence, growing evidence suggests it will play an increasing role in the future, with colonoscopy reserved for patients with an elevated FC.

Symptoms After Crohn's Surgery Are Not Always Inflammatory

It is important to note that patients may have diarrhea or pain following their operation that may not be due to CD recurrence (Table 16.1). Therefore before treating symptomatic disease recurrence in the post-operative setting, objective markers of disease activity should be sought. Ideally this is with endoscopy, although FC may be a viable substitute. As clinical symptoms and endoscopic activity poorly correlate, treatment should be based on endoscopic activity or a surrogate marker, not on clinical symptoms in order to prevent both over- and under-treatment of the patient.

Table 16.1 Symptoms, etiology, and treatment of problems post CD surgery

Symptoms	Cause	Treatments
Post-operative pain	Mucosal pain/healing	Limited analgesia, regional anesthesia when possible
Diarrhea	Post-resection "diarrhesis" (rapid transit due to absence of obstruction and muscular hypertrophy)	Anti-diarrheals
Diarrhea	Bile salts	Bile acid sequestrant
Abdominal pain ± bloating, nausea, vomiting, and constipation	Narcotic bowel	NO narcotics!
Bloating, diarrhea	Bacterial overgrowth	Antibiotics

Medical Prophylaxis Options

A resection often clears all disease in a patient with CD and provides an ideal opportunity to prevent further symptomatic disease. The risks of medical over-treatment need to be acknowledged, however, under-treatment in the post-operative setting will lead to disease recurrence in the majority of patients. In the current era of treatment for IBD, our aims include the prevention of progressive disease, disability, and future surgical intervention. Therefore prophylactic therapy should be considered in most patients.

Minimal Benefit: Probiotics/5-ASA Medications/Corticosteroids

As antibiotics prevent recurrent disease it has been hypothesized that changing the microbiotica may have benefits in preventing recurrence. However studies have failed to demonstrate any benefit in the post-operative setting with the use of probiotics [26, 27]. 5-ASA medications are also appealing due to their minimal side effect profile and low cost, however results are inconsistent and their effect on clinical and endoscopic outcomes is mild at best [28–30]. Corticosteroids (both systemic and budesonide) have shown little benefit in preventing post-operative recurrence [31, 32].

Moderate Benefit: Antibiotics/Immunomodulators

Due to the evidence that suggests that bacteria are in part responsible for recurrence of CD following resection there have been a number of studies looking at the role of antibiotics to prevent recurrence. Nitroimidazole antibiotics (metronidazole and ornidazole) are the most commonly studied medication. Rutgeerts et al. demonstrated that recurrence, defined as i2 or greater, was decreased at 3 months from 75 % in the placebo group to 52 % ($p=0.09$) in those taking metronidazole and severe recurrence decreased from 43 to 13 % ($p=0.02$). Clinical recurrence was also decreased at 12 months (25 % versus 4 %, $p=0.044$) [33]. In addition metronidazole seems to have a beneficial effect when added to azathioprine as combination therapy at preventing post-operative recurrence with rates of endoscopic recurrence at 12 months of 44 % in the combination therapy group compared to 69 % in those on monotherapy with azathioprine ($p=0.048$) [34]. Patients were also more likely to have no lesions seen at 12 months (22 % no lesions in combination group versus 3.5 % no lesions seen in the azathioprine monotherapy group, $p=0.03$). We therefore recommend that if patients can tolerate it that most be placed on 3 months of metronidazole in the post-operative setting. The dose should not be higher than 1 g/day to minimize the risk of neuropathy.

Immunomodulator (IMM) monotherapy also seems to have a modest effect on reducing post-operative recurrence. A meta-analysis of 433 patients who were placed on immunomodulators versus placebo found that thiopurines were more effective than placebo at preventing severe endoscopic recurrence at 1 year (i2–4) (mean diff 15 %, 1.8–29 %, $p=0.026$, NNT=7) but were not more effective at preventing very severe (i3–4) recurrence [35]. In regard to clinical relapse, thiopurines were more effective than placebo in preventing clinical relapse at 1 year (mean difference 8 %, CI 95 %: 1–15 %, $p=0.021$, NNT=13) and 2 years (mean difference 13 %, CI 95 %: 2–24 %, $p=0.018$, NNT=8) [35].

High Benefit: Biological Therapy

Biological therapies have been found to have the greatest impact in decreasing post-operative recurrence in CD. An initial study by Regueiro et al. demonstrated that anti-TNF therapy could decrease endoscopic recurrence from 84.6 % in the placebo arm to 9.1 % in those receiving infliximab at 1 year (endoscopic recurrence i2–4) [36]. In the second year of follow-up, patients were offered open access infliximab and it was found that remission was maintained over the 2-year period in those who continued on infliximab. In addition, anti-TNF naïve patients who developed endoscopic CD recurrence 1 year after their respective surgery had endoscopic improvement but not cure with infliximab and those who stopped their infliximab at 1 year in the setting of no recurrence developed endoscopic recurrence at 2 years [36, 37]. This demonstrates the need for early and prolonged treatment in such high-risk patients.

Adalimumab also appears to be effective in the post-operative setting. A study of 51 patients by Savarino et al. demonstrated that recurrence of CD was only 6.3 % at 2 years in patients treated with adalimumab post-operatively compared to 64.7 % in patients treated with azathioprine alone and 83.3 % in patients treated with mesalamine alone [7]. Preliminary data from the POCER study has also shown benefit with adalimumab therapy demonstrating that at 6 months 94 % of high-risk patients treated with post-operative adalimumab remain in endoscopic remission (i0–i1) versus 62 % treated with a thiopurine ($p=0.02$) [38].

There is currently no data in the post-operative setting for cetolizumab pegol, natalizumab, or vedolizumab.

A Proposed Monitoring and Treatment Algorithm for Post-Operative CD

Treatment in the post-operative should be individualized for each patient. The benefits of early assessment and titration of medical therapy based on disease recurrence are evident in the preliminary results from the POCER study [39]. This study found that at risk patients treated immediately after surgery followed by colonoscopy performed at 6 months and treatment step-up if recurrence occurred had significantly better outcomes compared to patients treated immediately after surgery with optimal drug therapy but followed without early colonoscopy assessment (Fig. 16.3).

Low risk patients are those that have long-standing CD (>10 years) who are undergoing their first surgical resection for a short (<10 cm), fibrostenotic lesion. These patients progress slowly, so no chronic therapy is required initially. In high-risk patients including those who smoke, have penetrating disease or perianal disease, or have a history of previous resection, initiating or continuing anti-TNF therapy with IMM immediately in the post-operative setting should be considered. Moderate risk patients are those who do not fit into the aforementioned categories and in these patients we treat with an IMM monotherapy in the post-operative period.

In regard to monitoring patients in the post-operative setting, there is currently no standardized approach. As calprotectin levels remain high for the first 2 months and then lower in those patients who do not have CD recurrence it is our practice to measure FC in patients at 3 months post surgery. As FC<100 mg/kg has a high specificity

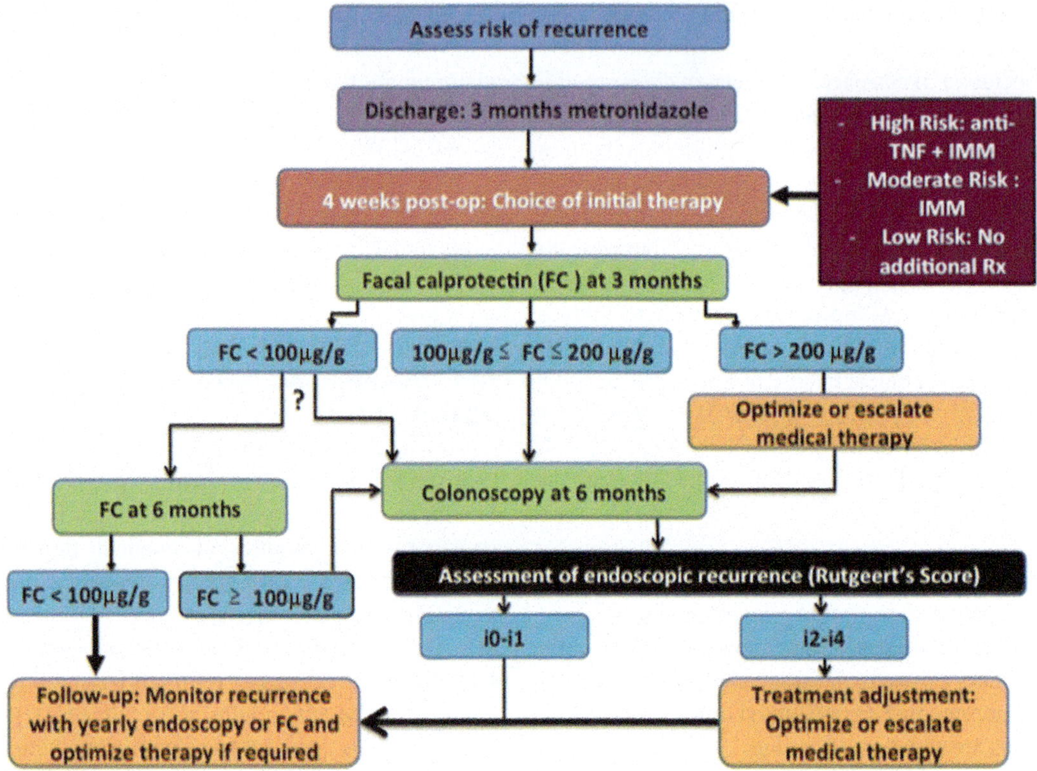

Fig. 16.3 An updated algorithm for predicting and preventing recurrence of post-operative CD

for lack of mucosal lesions, in patients who have an FC<100 mg/kg we continue to monitor and either repeat an FC or perform a colonoscopy at 6 months. If the FC is still below 100 mg/kg or the colonoscopy shows i0–i1 disease at 6 months, we continue the patients' current medical regime.

Evidence suggests that patients with a calprotectin higher than 100 mg/kg should have a colonoscopy at 6 months [23]. However we risk-stratify these patients depending on the level of their calprotectin. In the study by Sorrentino et al. [22], patients who had no post-operative recurrence had FC levels below 200 mg/kg. Therefore if patients have an FC level higher than 200 mg/kg, we optimize or escalate their medical therapy at 3 months with a view to then perform a colonoscopy at 6 months. In patients who have an FC of between 100 and 200 mg/kg we continue their current medical therapy and perform a colonoscopy at 6 months.

At colonoscopy, in patients with i0–i1 disease, current medical therapy may be continued and in patients with i2 or greater recurrence, then initiation, optimization, or escalation of therapy should occur. This can be in the form of commencing IMM or anti-TNF therapy and optimizing dosage of current IMM or anti-TNF therapy. To confirm that IMMs are not under-dosed, the metabolic profile should be assessed with dose increase if required or if shunting is present considering the use of allopurinol. In regard to therapeutic monitoring of anti-TNF therapies, depending on the anti-TNF level and the presence or not of antibodies, options include increasing the dose, decreasing the dosing interval, switching therapy to another drug within the same class or switching therapy to a drug outside the class, or adding a drug to the ongoing treatment regimen. The choice of which strategy to employ is based on careful assessment of the patient by history, examination, and increasingly therapeutic drug monitoring.

Once a patient has had their medical therapy optimized and their post-operative recurrence is stable we review them on a 6–12 monthly basis utilizing a 12 monthly objective marker of recurrence being either that of FC or colonoscopy. If objective evidence of recurrence occurs, then we recommend further optimizing therapy using the techniques discussed.

Conclusion

Surgical resection is an appropriate treatment option in many patients with CD and should be embraced. However, post-operative recurrence of CD is very common. The post-operative setting should be viewed as an ideal opportunity to prevent recurrence of symptomatic disease. It is therefore imperative to understand the patient's risk of recurrence, weigh the risks and benefits of long-term treatment based on this risk and be proactive in preventing recurrence. Antibiotics, immunomodulators, and anti-TNF therapies have all been shown to have efficacy in the post-operative setting. However, there is also increasing evidence for an approach that includes assessment with a 3-month FC and a 6-month colonoscopy to further risk-stratify patients. Although the optimal approach to monitoring and therapy is still unknown, an individualized approach based on a patients' risk profile is most appropriate. We propose an updated algorithm approach to risk stratification and prevention.

References

1. Rutgeerts P, Geboes K, Vantrappen G, Beyls J, Kerremans R, Hiele M. Predictability of the postoperative course of Crohn's disease. Gastroenterology. 1990;99:956–63.
2. Olaison G, Smedh K, Sjodahl R. Natural course of Crohn's disease after ileocolic resection: endoscopically visualised ileal ulcers preceding symptoms. Gut. 1992;33:331–5.
3. Michelassi F, Balestracci T, Chappell R, Block GE. Primary and recurrent Crohn's disease. Experience with 1379 patients. Ann Surg. 1991;214:230–8. discussion 8–40.
4. Terdiman JP. Prevention of postoperative recurrence in Crohn's disease. Clin Gastroenterol Hepatol. 2008;6:616–20.
5. Sachar DB. Patterns of postoperative recurrence in Crohn's disease. Scand J Gastroenterol Suppl. 1990;172:35–8.
6. Sachar DB. The problem of postoperative recurrence of Crohn's disease. Med Clin North Am. 1990;74: 183–8.
7. Savarino E, Bodini G, Dulbecco P, Assandri L, Bruzzone L, Mazza F, et al. Adalimumab is more effective than azathioprine and mesalamine at preventing postoperative recurrence of Crohn's disease: a randomized controlled trial. Am J Gastroenterol. 2013;108:1731–42.
8. Renna S, Camma C, Modesto I, Cabibbo G, Scimeca D, Civitavecchia G, et al. Meta-analysis of the placebo rates of clinical relapse and severe endoscopic recurrence in postoperative Crohn's disease. Gastroenterology. 2008;135:1500–9.
9. Cho SM, Cho SW, Regueiro M. Postoperative management of Crohn disease. Med Clin North Am. 2010;94:179–88.
10. Cameron JL, Hamilton SR, Coleman J, Sitzmann JV, Bayless TM. Patterns of ileal recurrence in Crohn's disease. A prospective randomized study. Ann Surg. 1992;215:546–51. discussion 51-2.
11. Whelan G, Farmer RG, Fazio VW, Goormastic M. Recurrence after surgery in Crohn's disease. Relationship to location of disease (clinical pattern) and surgical indication. Gastroenterology. 1985;88: 1826–33.
12. Bernell O, Lapidus A, Hellers G. Risk factors for surgery and recurrence in 907 patients with primary ileocaecal Crohn's disease. Br J Surg. 2000;87: 1697–701.
13. D'Haens GR, Gasparaitis AE, Hanauer SB. Duration of recurrent ileitis after ileocolonic resection correlates with presurgical extent of Crohn's disease. Gut. 1995;36:715–7.
14. Greenstein AJ, Lachman P, Sachar DB, Springhorn J, Heimann T, Janowitz HD, et al. Perforating and nonperforating indications for repeated operations in Crohn's disease: evidence for two clinical forms. Gut. 1988;29:588–92.
15. Bernell O, Lapidus A, Hellers G. Risk factors for surgery and postoperative recurrence in Crohn's disease. Ann Surg. 2000;231:38–45.
16. Lautenbach E, Berlin JA, Lichtenstein GR. Risk factors for early postoperative recurrence of Crohn's disease. Gastroenterology. 1998;115:259–67.
17. D'Haens GR, Geboes K, Peeters M, Baert F, Penninckx F, Rutgeerts P. Early lesions of recurrent Crohn's disease caused by infusion of intestinal contents in excluded ileum. Gastroenterology. 1998; 114:262–7.
18. McLeod RS, Wolff BG, Steinhart AH, Carryer PW, O'Rourke K, Andrews DF, et al. Prophylactic mesalamine treatment decreases postoperative recurrence of Crohn's disease. Gastroenterology. 1995;109: 404–13.

19. Calabrese E, Petruzziello C, Onali S, Condino G, Zorzi F, Pallone F, et al. Severity of postoperative recurrence in Crohn's disease: correlation between endoscopic and sonographic findings. Inflamm Bowel Dis. 2009;15:1635–42.
20. Rutgeerts P, Geboes K, Vantrappen G, Kerremans R, Coenegrachts JL, Coremans G. Natural history of recurrent Crohn's disease at the ileocolonic anastomosis after curative surgery. Gut. 1984;25: 665–72.
21. Sorrentino D, Paviotti A, Terrosu G, Avellini C, Geraci M, Zarifi D. Low-dose maintenance therapy with infliximab prevents postsurgical recurrence of Crohn's disease. Clin Gastroenterol Hepatol. 2010;8:591–9 e1; quiz e78–9.
22. Sorrentino D, Terrosu G, Paviotti A, Geraci M, Avellini C, Zoli G, et al. Early diagnosis and treatment of postoperative endoscopic recurrence of Crohn's disease: partial benefit by infliximab—a pilot study. Dig Dis Sci. 2012;57:1341–8.
23. Wright E, De Cruz P, Kamm M, Hamilton A, Hamilton K, Ritchie K, et al. Feacal calprotectin is superior to feacal lactoferrin and S100A12 as a surrogate marker for post-operative Crohn's disease endoscopic recurrence. Prospective longitudinal endoscopic validation. Results from the POCER study. Gastroenterology. 2014;146:S-174.
24. Lobaton T, Lopez-Garcia A, Rodriguez-Moranta F, Ruiz A, Rodriguez L, Guardiola J. A new rapid test for fecal calprotectin predicts endoscopic remission and postoperative recurrence in Crohn's disease. J Crohns Colitis. 2013;7:e641–51.
25. Yamamoto T, Kotze PG. Is fecal calprotectin useful for monitoring endoscopic disease activity in patients with postoperative Crohn's disease? J Crohns Colitis. 2013;7:e712.
26. Prantera C, Scribano ML, Falasco G, Andreoli A, Luzi C. Ineffectiveness of probiotics in preventing recurrence after curative resection for Crohn's disease: a randomised controlled trial with Lactobacillus GG. Gut. 2002;51:405–9.
27. Chermesh I, Tamir A, Reshef R, Chowers Y, Suissa A, Katz D, et al. Failure of Synbiotic 2000 to prevent postoperative recurrence of Crohn's disease. Dig Dis Sci. 2007;52:385–9.
28. Cottone M, Camma C. Mesalamine and relapse prevention in Crohn's disease. Gastroenterology. 2000; 119:597.
29. Caprilli R, Cottone M, Tonelli F, Sturniolo G, Castiglione F, Annese V, et al. Two mesalazine regimens in the prevention of the post-operative recurrence of Crohn's disease: a pragmatic, double-blind, randomized controlled trial. Aliment Pharmacol Ther. 2003; 17:517–23.
30. Sutherland LR, Martin F, Bailey RJ, Fedorak RN, Poleski M, Dallaire C, et al. A randomized, placebo-controlled, double-blind trial of mesalamine in the maintenance of remission of Crohn's disease. The Canadian Mesalamine for Remission of Crohn's Disease Study Group. Gastroenterology. 1997;112: 1069–77.
31. Steinhart AH, Ewe K, Griffiths AM, Modigliani R, Thomsen OO. Corticosteroids for maintenance of remission in Crohn's disease. Cochrane Database Syst Rev. 2003:CD000301.
32. Hellers G, Cortot A, Jewell D, Leijonmarck CE, Lofberg R, Malchow H, et al. Oral budesonide for prevention of postsurgical recurrence in Crohn's disease. The IOIBD Budesonide Study Group. Gastroenterology. 1999;116:294–300.
33. Rutgeerts P, Van Assche G, Vermeire S, D'Haens G, Baert F, Noman M, et al. Ornidazole for prophylaxis of postoperative Crohn's disease recurrence: a randomized, double-blind, placebo-controlled trial. Gastroenterology. 2005;128:856–61.
34. D'Haens GR, Vermeire S, Van Assche G, Noman M, Aerden I, Van Olmen G, et al. Therapy of metronidazole with azathioprine to prevent postoperative recurrence of Crohn's disease: a controlled randomized trial. Gastroenterology. 2008;135:1123–9.
35. Peyrin-Biroulet L, Deltenre P, Ardizzone S, D'Haens G, Hanauer SB, Herfarth H, et al. Azathioprine and 6-mercaptopurine for the prevention of postoperative recurrence in Crohn's disease: a meta-analysis. Am J Gastroenterol. 2009;104:2089–96.
36. Regueiro M, Schraut W, Baidoo L, Kip KE, Sepulveda AR, Pesci M, et al. Infliximab prevents Crohn's disease recurrence after ileal resection. Gastroenterology. 2009;136:441–50. quiz 716.
37. Regueiro M, Kip KE, Baidoo L, Swoger JM, Schraut W. Postoperative therapy with infliximab prevents long-term Crohn's disease recurrence. Clin Gastroenterol Hepatol. 2014;12:1494–502.
38. De Cruz P, Kamm MA, Hamilton AL, Ritchie KJ, Gorelik A, Liew D, et al. 1161 adalimumab prevents post-operative Crohn's disease recurrence, and is superior to thiopurines: early results from the POCER study. Gastroenterology. 2012;142:S-212.
39. De Cruz P, Kamm MA, Hamilton AL, Ritchie KJ, Krejany S, Gorelik A, et al. 925j optimising post-operative Crohn's disease management: best drug therapy alone versus colonoscopic monitoring with treatment step-up. The POCER study. Gastroenterology. 2013;144:S-164.

Recurrent CD: Surgical Prophylaxis—Kono-S Anastomosis

17

Toru Kono and Alessandro Fichera

Introduction

Since the first publication in 1932 by Burrill Crohn and his colleagues at the Mount Sinai Hospital in New York, the number of patients worldwide with Crohn's disease (CD) has been continuously increasing [1]. Today, there are more than one million CD patients around the world, with a recent significant increase in Asia and South America. In Japan, the prevalence of CD has increased dramatically in the 1990s; and the nationwide population of CD patients is currently approaching 40,000 patients. Researchers have reported that 70 % of CD patients undergo enterectomy or other surgical interventions within 10 years of diagnosis, with high postoperative rates of anastomotic recurrence and stenosis necessitating repeat surgery [2]. In patients treated with surgical anastomosis, CD recurrence was diagnosed endoscopically in 70–90 % within 1 year, and 20–30 % of surgical patients required a second surgery within 5 years [2]. Despite recent advances in pharmacotherapy [3, 4], there are currently no drugs that can either alleviate fixed stenotic lesions or significantly improve the natural history of CD [5–9]. While strictureplasty has been reported to relieve obstruction due to stenotic lesions [10], no surgical strategies have been developed to prevent postoperative anastomotic recurrences [11, 12].

In September 2003, Kono and his colleagues at the Asahikawa Medical University Hospital, Hokkaido, Japan, started to use their unique surgical technique for preventing anastomotic strictures (Kono-S anastomosis) in patients with CD [13, 14]. Since then, their approach has been adopted at several other medical institutions in Japan. In May 2010, this novel anastomotic procedure was introduced at the University of Chicago Hospital, and subsequently the University of Washington Medical Center, and the Weill Cornell Medical Center [15]. More than 400 CD patients around the world have been treated using this technique. With a mean follow-up of 5 years, none have required reoperative surgery for anastomotic recurrence as of September 2013. There is also a low incidence of endoscopically detected CD recurrence at the anastomotic site. A prospective, randomized, multicenter study led by the Weill Cornell Medical Center researchers in collaboration with the University of Washington Medical Center is currently underway [12]. This chapter will outline the standard Kono-S anastomosis

T. Kono, MD, PhD, FACS (✉)
Advanced Surgery Center, Department of Surgery, Sapporo Higashi Tokushukai Hospital, 3-1, N-33, E-14, Higahi-ku, Sapporo, Hokkaido 0650033, Japan
e-mail: kono@toru-kono.com

A. Fichera, MD, FACS, FASCRS
Division of General Surgery, Department of Surgery, University of Washington Medical Center, 1959 NE Pacific Street, Box 356410, Room BB-414, Seattle, WA 98195, USA
e-mail: afichera@uw.edu

A. Fichera and M.K. Krane (eds.), *Crohn's Disease: Basic Principles*,
DOI 10.1007/978-3-319-14181-7_17, © Springer International Publishing Switzerland 2015

procedure, adopted at the First International Consensus Conference on Kono-S Anastomosis held in September 2011 in Kyoto, Japan [16]. This chapter will also describe the fundamental differences between the Kono-S and the stapled functional end-to-end anastomosis and other anastomotic techniques.

Kono-S Anastomosis Procedure

The Kono-S anastomosis technique is illustrated here using the example of an ileal stenosis, one of the most common types of CD lesion.

Confirmation of the Lesion

Surgical success hinges on detailed preoperative evaluation of the lesions and other parts of the intestinal tract, which may be often compromised by adhesions, multiple disease foci, and other causes. Whether using the open or laparoscopic approach, the surgeon must carefully trace and examine the patient's small bowel starting from the ligament of Treitz. Surgical lysis of adhesions may be necessary for mobilization of the gastrointestinal tract. The surgeon determines the length of the small intestine as well as the extent of the disease, using sterile tape measure or other appropriate tools. Before making the final decision on the surgical procedure intraoperatively, the surgeon may need to endoscopically evaluate the identified lesions and the future remnant tract segments to ensure that no active lesions were missed in the preoperative assessment (Fig. 17.1).

Determination of the Location and the Resection Margin

Attention must be paid to exclude ulcers and other active lesions from the anastomotic site. Although the presence of inactive lesions may be permitted, ideally the surgeon should select an area completely free of disease, keeping in mind at the same time that the bowel must be spared to the maximum extent possible. A 2-cm margin from the edge of macroscopically visible diseased bowel is recommended proximally and distally [17].

Division of the Mesentery for Maximum Preservation of Vascularization and Innervation

CD is a chronic and repeated transmural inflammatory process that also damages the intrinsic intestinal nervous system. The submucosal plexus is particularly susceptible to damage due to its location and morphology. Regeneration of nerve fibers takes much longer (years) than mucosal healing (weeks). Therefore, even after mucosal healing has completely occurred, neuronal regeneration is incomplete. In fact in CD, regional total intestinal and mucosal-submucosal blood flow was reduced to half that of healthy individuals, probably due to reduced levels of the potent vasodilator calcitonin gene-related peptide (CGRP) in the submucosal plexus [18–20]. Poor mucosal blood flow contributes to intestinal ulceration in various clinical conditions including perforation, fistula formation, and excess fibrosis which causes intestinal stenosis.

In peripheral nerve regeneration, it is difficult for nerves to regenerate across large gaps due to the inability to sustain nerve regeneration for long periods of time. Therefore, after reviewing the conventional method of dividing the mesentery where lymphovascular vessels and nerves branch into the intestinal wall, we decided to adopt a new approach.

Usually, a fan-shaped portion of the mesentery spanning the proximal and distal resection margins is removed in order to remove lymph nodes. However, such a procedure likely delays postoperative neural regeneration, because the nerves are severed relatively proximally. The nerves should be divided as close to the intestinal wall as possible to allow for early neural regeneration at the anastomotic site, which will contribute to maintaining its blood supply (Fig. 17.2). Postoperative decreases in intestinal blood flow may be involved in anastomotic recurrence [20].

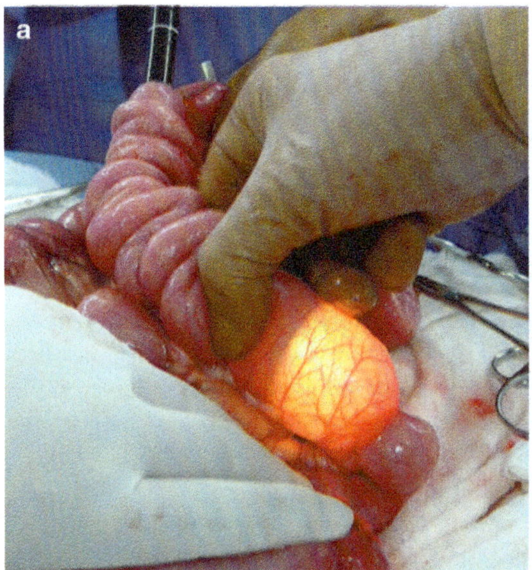

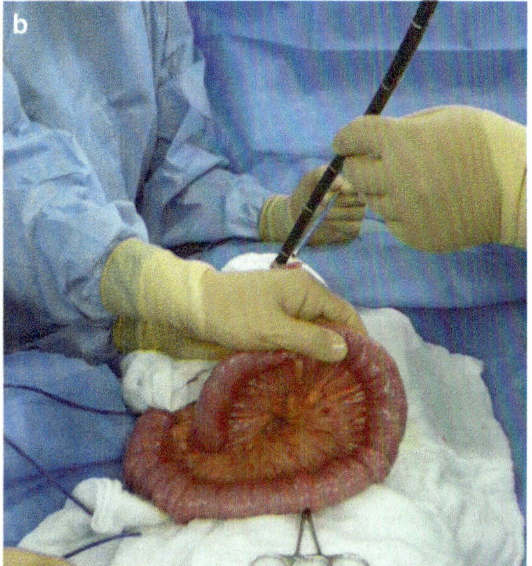

Fig. 17.1 Intraoperative endoscopy. The whole bowel is inspected carefully for diseased segments using an endoscope via an enterotomy placed at a stenosis site. Intraoperative endoscopy is performed by a gastroenterologist in specific cases when unexpected incidental surgical findings are noted upon exploration

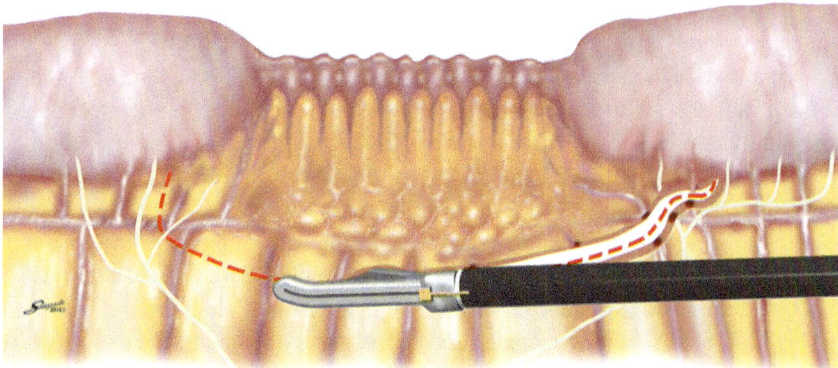

Fig. 17.2 Mesentery is divided using a tissue sealing device close to the intestinal wall to preserve vascularization and innervation

Retaining as much of the mesentery as possible is critical for optimizing blood supply to the anastomosis.

Wherever possible, the use of a tissue sealing device is recommended. Since mesenteric nerves and vessels are to be severed close to the intestinal wall, suture ligature should be avoided to prevent surgical site infection. Hemostasis should be carefully performed in patients with mesenteric inflammation and hypertrophy, which may cause unexpected bleeding. The surgeon must take special care to leave intact the mesentery in the vicinity of the resection margins to the greatest extent possible for optimal postoperative reinnervation and revascularization of the anastomosis.

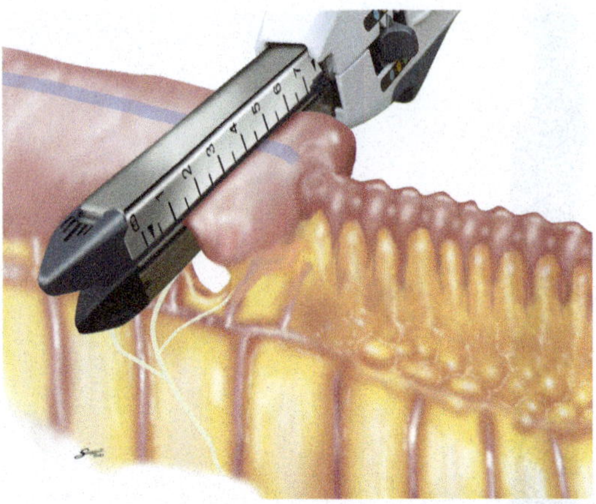

Fig. 17.3 Before dividing the bowel, a longitudinal line is drawn at the antimesenteric side. Bowel is divided transversely placing the linear stapler perpendicular to the intestinal lumen and the mesentery is located in the middle of the staple lines

Use of Automatic Staplers and Creation of a Reinforced Structure: Creation of the Supporting Column

According to conventional anastomotic procedures, the bowel is divided with the long axis of the automatic cutting stapler parallel to the mesenteric plane. In our procedure, however, the two-row or three-row automatic stapler is positioned perpendicular to the mesentery and the longitudinal axis of the intestine so that the mesenteric plane will fall at the midpoint of the transverse staple line (Fig. 17.3a). Three-row staplers are preferable to two-row staplers with respect to the mechanical rigidity of the structure that will be created using the stapled ends. At this point, the surgeon may use a surgical skin marker to draw a longitudinal line of approximately 10 cm along the antimesenteric wall of both sides of the segment to be resected. These lines will serve as a useful indicator for the location and orientation of stapling (Fig. 17.3). Experimental data suggest that the surgeon should wait for a minimum of 2 min so that intestinal tissue can be evenly compressed for secure staple closure (Fig. 17.3) [21]. It is advisable to wait one more minute after firing the device especially in presence of edematous tissue.

Automatic stapling may result in less effective closure at the corners (Fig. 17.4). Consequently, the surgeon is advised to imbricate and reinforce the corners of the staple lines with absorbable sutures (Fig. 17.4). The sutures used to reinforce the proximal and distal ends are tied together to approximate the corresponding corners of the stumps (Fig. 17.5). Then, the two staple lines are sewn together with 3-0 or 4-0 absorbable sutures in order to construct a "supporting column", a structure that helps prevent mechanical deformation of the anastomosis (Fig. 17.5). The supporting column will be located just behind the posterior wall of the anastomosis. The supporting column provides a rigid mechanical support that will prevent mechanical deformation and functional constriction of the lumen of the anastomosis.

Construction of the Anastomosis

An incision is made along the longitudinal line marked on the antimesenteric wall, starting at a position between 5 and 10 mm from the edge of the supporting column (Fig. 17.6a). If the incision starts within 5 mm of the supporting column, it will render the anastomotic procedure technically difficult, and increase the risk of an insufficient blood supply. In contrast, if the opening starts more than 10 mm away from the supporting column, the mechanical reinforcement of the supporting column may be compromised. With the first assistant holding the incision open with forceps, the surgeon extends the longitudinal opening until a transverse lumen of 7–8 cm is created (Fig. 17.6b). Since CD intestinal tracts may vary significantly in elasticity, the size of the opening must be accurately measured. The desired diameters for the anastomosis are 7 and 8 cm for the small and large intestines, respectively.

Either a Gambee or Albert suture pattern can be used for closing the posterior wall. If the wall thickness of the two ends differs considerably, the Gambee technique is preferable. The proximal side of the distal lumen and the distal side of the proximal lumen are approximated by passing long sutures on non-detachable needles from the inside to the outside of one

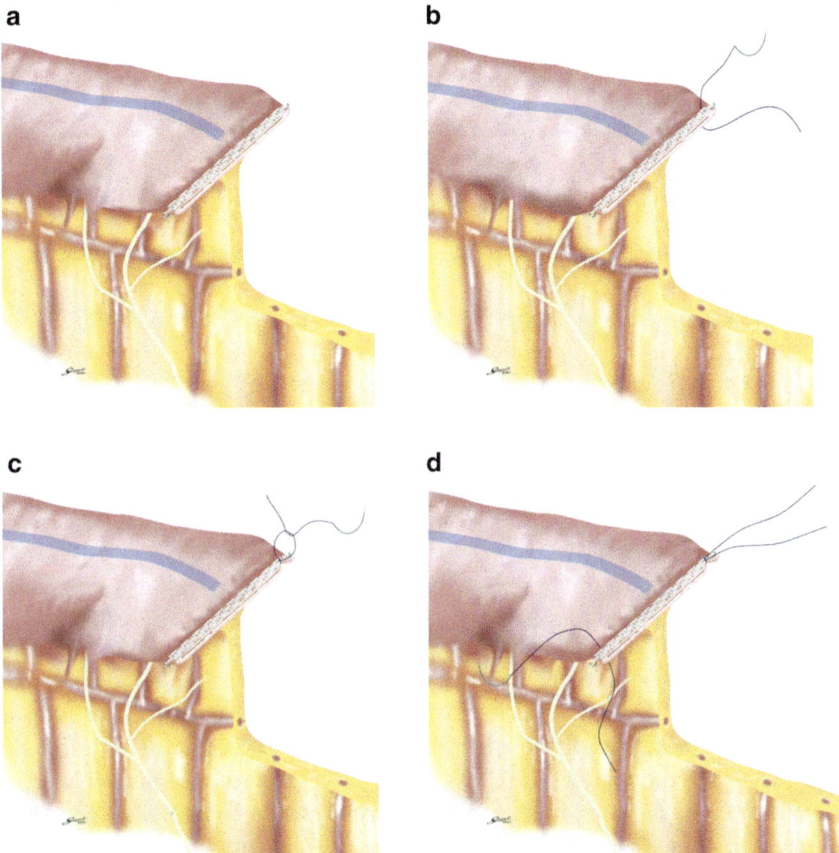

Fig. 17.4 (**a**) Intestinal segment divided by linear stapler. The corners of the staple line are at risk of leaks and bleeding. (**b**), (**c**) Both corners of the staple lines are reinforced and imbricated. (**d**) The sutures are tied together to construct the "supporting column"

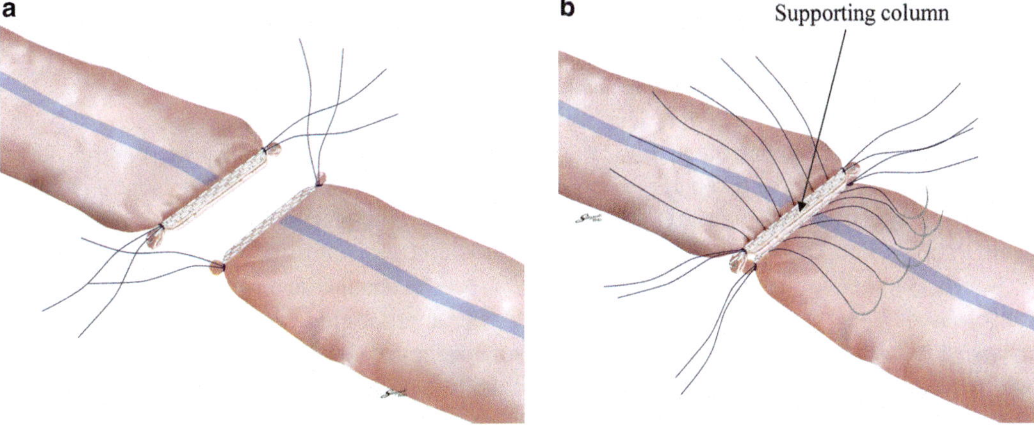

Fig. 17.5 (**a**) The suture threads used to reinforce the proximal and distal ends are tied together in order to create a "supporting column". Adjustments are made to compensate for differences in stump size. (**b**) The staple lines are securely sewn together using interrupted stitches. The "supporting column", helps preventing distortion due to relapse at the anastomotic site

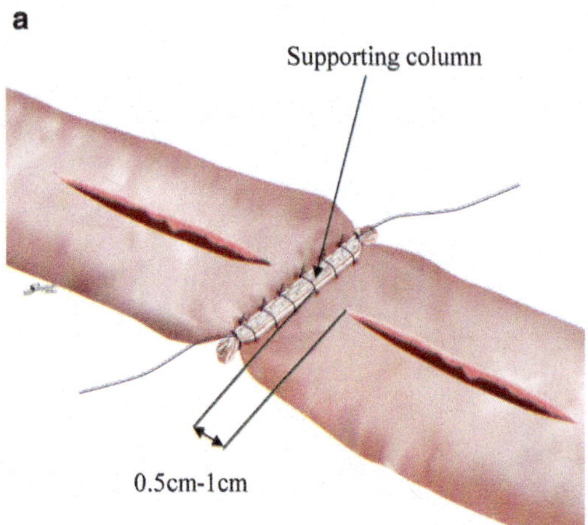

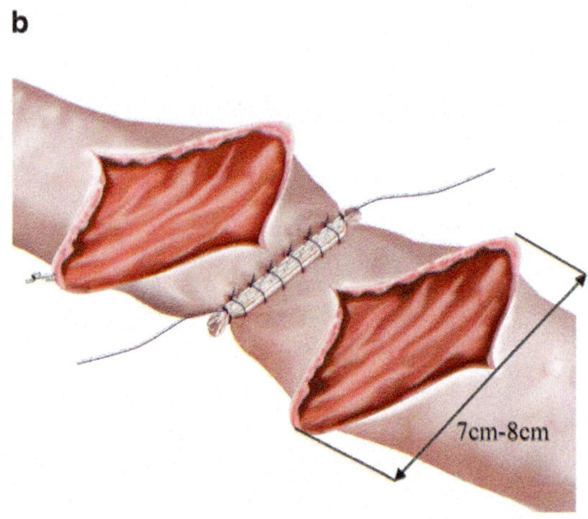

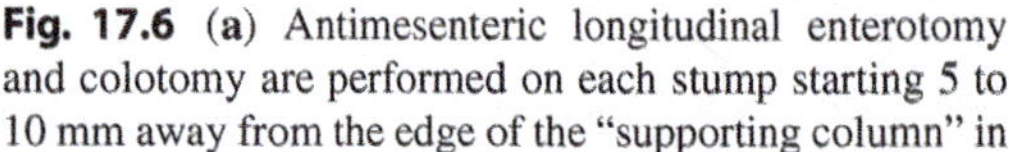

Fig. 17.6 (**a**) Antimesenteric longitudinal enterotomy and colotomy are performed on each stump starting 5 to 10 mm away from the edge of the "supporting column" in order to obtain the optimal effect of the "supporting column" on the anastomosis. (**b**) Enterotomy and colotomy are extended to allow a transverse lumen of 7 cm to 8 cm

opening and from the outside to the inside of the other at the points most distal to the long axis of the intestine (Fig. 17.7a). Next, a short suture with a removable needle is used to join the midpoints of the anastomotic edges using the Gambee technique (Fig. 17.7a). Separate long sutures on non-detachable needles are used to close the posterior wall, starting from the center, i.e., proximal to the long axis (Fig. 17.7b). These sutures are tied to the pre-existing long sutures with non-detachable needles, which are to be used for subsequent closure of the anterior wall. The supporting column will be located immediately behind the posterior wall of the anastomosis. The surgeon is advised to keep at least a 7-mm stitch distance for continuous sutures to ensure sufficient blood flow to the anastomosis. Care must be taken not to pull too hard on stretchable sutures when tying them, to avoid limiting blood flow.

Either Gambee or layer-to-layer suturing can be used. The suture-carrying needles that remained from the suturing of the posterior wall are passed through the edge of the stoma from the inside to the outside. On the side closer to the surgeon, the needle is passed through the colon (distal end), whereas the needle is passed through the ileum (proximal end) on the side further from the surgeon. The surgeon sutures the proximal half of the anastomotic edges and ties the suture (Fig. 17.7c). Another short suture with a detachable needle is placed and tied at the center of the anastomosis. The long suture with the non-detachable needle is left in place. Next, the surgeon closes the distal half of the stomal rim and ties this suture to the pre-existing suture (Fig. 17.7c). With this technique, the mesenteric attachment, a frequent site of pathological changes, ends up aligned with the midpoint of the supporting column (Fig. 17.7d).

Closure of the Mesenteric Defect and Covering the Anastomotic Structure

The surgeon may close the mesenteric defect when appropriate. Since both ends of the supporting column extend beyond the edges of the anastomosed intestinal tract, the anastomotic structure should be covered by omentum or other appropriate fatty tissue to prevent intestinal adhesions. In order to relieve the anastomotic structure of excess mechanical tension, the surgeon may fix the anastomosis to the omentum or other fatty tissue placed over the anterior wall with a few stitches. In this case, stitches should be made along the short axis of the intestinal tract to prevent interference with intestinal blood flow.

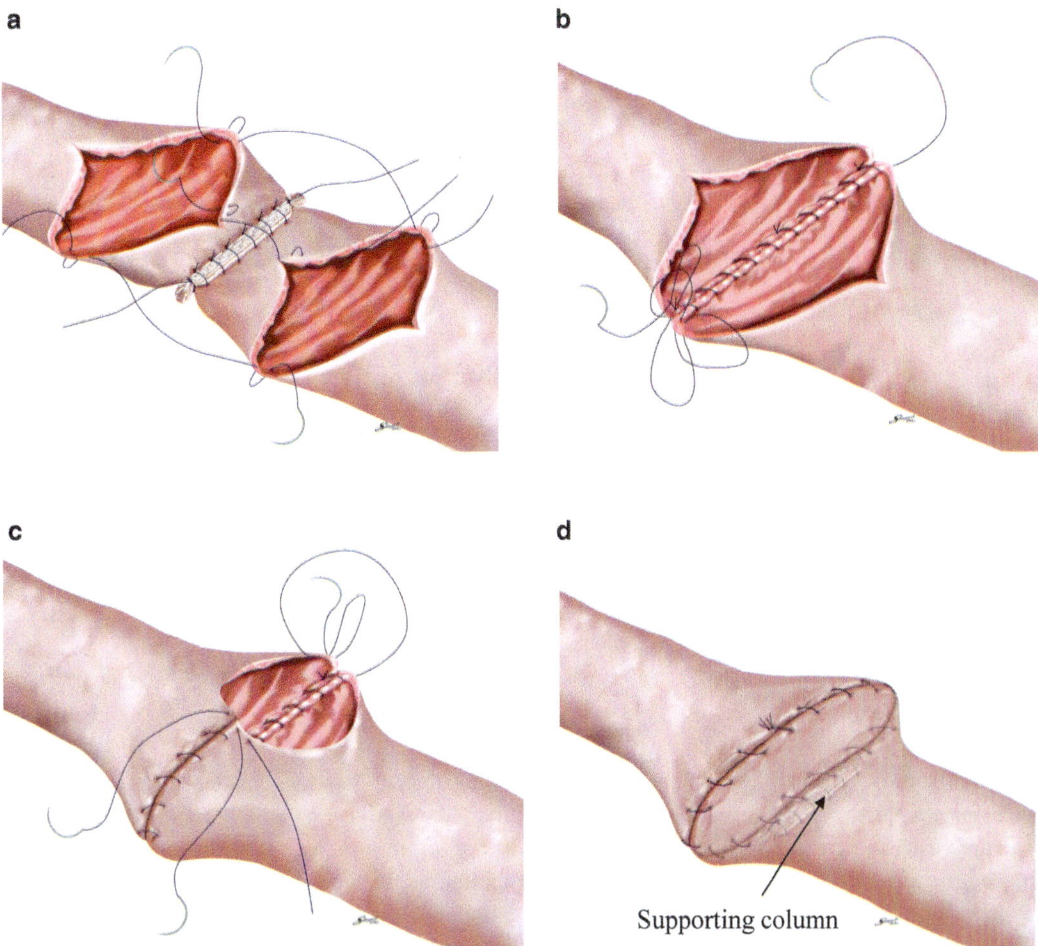

Fig. 17.7 Closure of the anastomotic stoma and completion of the Kono-S anastomosis. (**a**) Posterior wall stitches. Two Gambee sutures are started the first at the points most distal to the long axis of the intestine and the second at the center of the posterior edge. (**b**) Posterior wall closure. Another non-detachable suture goes to close the pre-existing suture at the point most distal to the long axis, which is to be used for subsequent closure of the posterior wall. (**c**) Anterior wall closure. The posterior wall sutures are used to close the anterior wall. The surgeon sutures the proximal half of the anterior wall and ties another short suture with a detachable needle is placed at the center of the anastomosis. Next, the surgeon closes the distal half of the anterior wall and ties this suture to the pre-existing suture. (**d**) Completion of the Kono-S anastomosis. The arrow indicates the supporting column that is closely located at the posterior wall

Potential Application

In order to form a wide anastomosis, the Kono-S technique requires healthy intestinal segments for at least 10 cm both proximal and distal to the area to be resected. Consequently, this technique requires careful preoperative surgical planning and intraoperative decision-making, especially when it is used to treat terminal ileal stenosis requiring preservation of the ileocecal valve, rectal stenosis, or multiple short skipped strictures. With this technique, the anastomosis is handsewn. Sewing by hand renders this technique technically difficult to perform using a totally laparoscopic approach.

One major advantage is that the supporting column can help reduce mechanical tension on the anastomotic site. Therefore, the Kono-S technique is also suitable for ileorectal anastomoses or any types of anastomoses that are likely to suffer from undue tension. In addition, this approach is effective for anastomosing segments

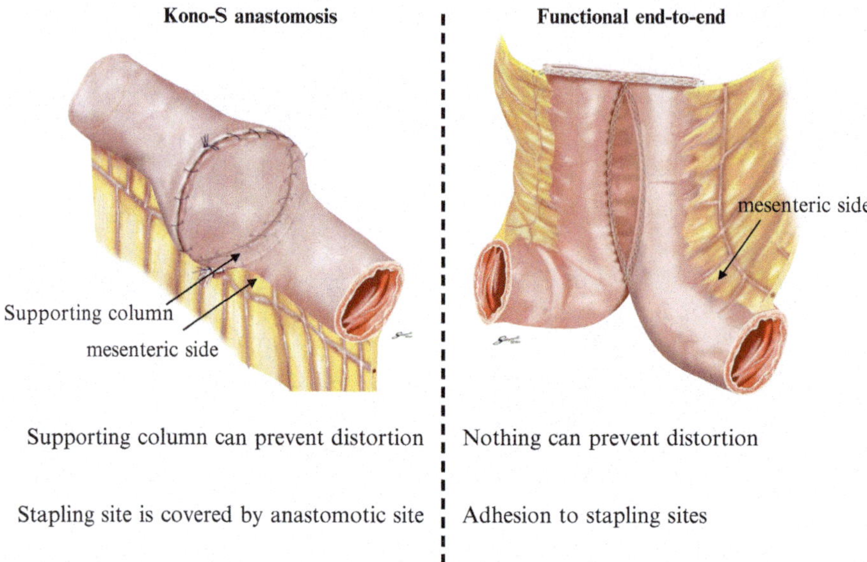

Fig. 17.8 Comparison of the advantages and disadvantages of handsewn and stapled functional end-to-end anastomoses

of significantly different calibers, because incisions are made along the long axis of the intestinal tract so that similar lumen sizes can be created irrespective of diameter.

Effects of Surgical Prophylaxis According to the Type of Surgery

Anastomotic Configurations

Recent meta-analyses of surgical outcomes by the type of anastomosis revealed that end-to-end anastomosis was not associated with significant differences in perianastomotic recurrence or reoperation compared to side-to-side, side-to-end, and end-to-side configurations, but they were associated with increased anastomotic leak rates [22, 23]. In addition, the end-to-end configuration provides smaller lumens than the side-to-side configuration, which is more likely to interrupt the blood supply to the anastomotic site as a result of suturing of the mesenteric aspect of the intestinal tract, a common site of pathological changes [17, 22–24]. Consequently, the side-to-side anastomosis is considered more effective than the end-to-end configuration and is used more often in clinical practice. The Kono-S technique, a type of side-to-side anastomosis, appeared therefore to be superior to the end-to-end anastomotic approach. The differences between Kono-S and other types of anastomotic techniques are summarized in Fig. 17.8.

Handsewn Versus Stapled Anastomoses

Intestinal anastomosis can be performed in a handsewn or stapled fashion. With the recent increase in the use of laparoscopic techniques, the side-to-side stapled anastomosis has become increasingly popular [23, 25–27]. However, stapled anastomoses have several disadvantages compared to handsewn anastomosis in CD. First, once the handsewn segments are completely healed, the anastomotic site recovers elasticity and becomes capable of expanding or shrinking in response to changes in intraluminal pressure more effectively than stapled bowels [28].

Second, stapled lines are more likely to undergo eversion and subsequent adhesion formation. Since CD is associated with a high incidence of flare-ups and recurrences in the perianastomotic region, stapling is associated with a higher probability of adhesion formation between the anastomosis and other parts of the intestine. Clinicians often encounter cases where anastomotic deformation caused by adhesions interferes with the use of endoscopy. Stapled anastomoses often result in complex strictures, for which endoscopic balloon dilatation, the only realistic alternative to intestinal surgery, is technically challenging [29, 30]. In addition, techniques involving stapling, which provide uniform lumen sizes, are less flexible; have higher incidences of anastomotic bleeding and overactive inflammatory responses have been reported [26, 28, 31]. These disadvantages warn against the indiscriminate use of stapling techniques. The authors strongly recommend using handsewn techniques for intestinal anastomosis in patients with CD.

Laparoscopic Versus Open Surgery

Laparoscopy-assisted surgery has been increasingly used in CD. Its short-term safety has been established, and the advantages reported in the literature include better cosmetic outcomes, earlier postoperative recovery, less pain, and shorter hospital stay [32–37]. However, CD is among the most challenging diseases to treat laparoscopically, particularly when the patients have multiple diseased segments or intraabdominal abscesses [38]. Long-term results of laparoscopic and conventional surgeries for CD in the Netherlands and the USA have been reported [25, 39]. These studies suggested that laparoscopic surgery is not superior in terms of reoperation rates.

Conclusion

Our antimesenteric functional end-to-end handsewn (Kono-S) anastomosis technique reduces the incidence of deformation and stenosis of the anastomotic site. This technique helps preserve the blood supply to the surgical site and promote neural regeneration. It reduces anastomotic recurrences and facilitates endoscopic evaluation. The Kono-S procedure has the potential to become the standard of care for CD in the future.

References

1. Crohn BB, Ginzburg L, Oppenheimer GD. Landmark article Oct 15, 1932. Regional ileitis. A pathological and clinical entity. By Burril B. Crohn, Leon Ginzburg, and Gordon D. Oppenheimer. JAMA. 1984;251(1):73–9. PMID: 6361290.
2. Fichera A, Michelassi F. Surgical treatment of Crohn's disease. J Gastrointest Surg. 2007;11(6):791–803. PMID: 17562122.
3. Regueiro M, Kip KE, Baidoo L, Swoger JM, Schraut W. Postoperative therapy with infliximab prevents long-term Crohn's disease recurrence. Clin Gastroenterol Hepatol. 2014;12:1494–502. PMID: 24440221.
4. van Lent AU, D'Haens GR. Management of postoperative recurrence of Crohn's disease. Dig Dis. 2013;31(2):222–8. PMID: 24030230.
5. Limketkai BN, Bayless TM. Editorial: can stenosis in ileal Crohn's disease be prevented by current therapy? Am J Gastroenterol. 2013;108(11):1755–6. PMID: 24192948.
6. Cosnes J, Bourrier A, Laharie D, Nahon S, Bouhnik Y, Carbonnel F, et al. Early administration of azathioprine vs conventional management of Crohn's disease: a randomized controlled trial. Gastroenterology. 2013;145(4):758–65.e2. quiz e14–5. PMID: 23644079.
7. Cosnes J, Nion-Larmurier I, Beaugerie L, Afchain P, Tiret E, Gendre JP. Impact of the increasing use of immunosuppressants in Crohn's disease on the need for intestinal surgery. Gut. 2005;54(2):237–41. PMCID: 1774826.
8. Lazarev M, Ullman T, Schraut WH, Kip KE, Saul M, Regueiro M. Small bowel resection rates in Crohn's disease and the indication for surgery over time: experience from a large tertiary care center. Inflamm Bowel Dis. 2010;16(5):830–5. PMID: 19798731.
9. Vuitton L, Koch S, Peyrin-Biroulet L. Preventing postoperative recurrence in Crohn's disease: what does the future hold? Drugs. 2013;73(16):1749–59. PMID: 24132799.
10. Yamamoto T, Fazio VW, Tekkis PP. Safety and efficacy of strictureplasty for Crohn's disease: a systematic review and meta-analysis. Dis Colon Rectum. 2007;50(11):1968–86. PMID: 17762967.
11. Yamamoto T, Watanabe T. Surgery for luminal Crohn's disease. World J Gastroenterol. 2014;20(1): 78–90. PMCID: 3886035.
12. Michelassi F. Crohn's recurrence after intestinal resection and anastomosis. Dig Dis Sci. 2014;59(7):1352–3. PMID: 24671451.

13. Kono T, Ashida T, Ebisawa Y, Chisato N, Okamoto K, Katsuno H, et al. A new antimesenteric functional end-to-end handsewn anastomosis: surgical prevention of anastomotic recurrence in Crohn's disease. Dis Colon Rectum. 2011;54(5):586–92. PMID: 21471760.
14. Kono T, Ebisawa Y, Chisato N, Okamoto K, Maemoto A, Ashida T, et al. A new combined stapled and handsewn side-to-side anastomosis after resection for Crohn's disease. Gastroenterology. 2010;138:S691.
15. Fichera A, Zoccali M, Kono T. Antimesenteric functional end-to-end handsewn (Kono-S) anastomosis. J Gastrointest Surg. 2012;16(7):1412–6. PMID: 22580840.
16. Kono T, Fichera A. Kono-S anastomosis for Crohn's disease: narrative. Colorectal Dis. 2014;16:833. PMID: 25040294.
17. Fazio VW, Marchetti F, Church M, Goldblum JR, Lavery C, Hull TL, et al. Effect of resection margins on the recurrence of Crohn's disease in the small bowel. A randomized controlled trial. Ann Surg. 1996; 224(4):563–71. discussion 71–3. PMID: 8857860.
18. Hulten L, Lindhagen J, Lundgren O, Fasth S, Ahren C. Regional intestinal blood flow in ulcerative colitis and Crohn's disease. Gastroenterology. 1977;72(3): 388–96. PMID: 832785.
19. Kono T, Omiya Y, Hira Y, Kaneko A, Chiba S, Suzuki T, et al. Daikenchuto (TU-100) ameliorates colon microvascular dysfunction via endogenous adrenomedullin in Crohn's disease rat model. J Gastroenterol. 2011;46(10):1187–96. PMID: 21808981.
20. Carr ND, Pullan BR, Schofield PF. Microvascular studies in non-specific inflammatory bowel disease. Gut. 1986;27(5):542–9. PMID: 3699563.
21. Nakayama S, Hasegawa S, Nagayama S, Kato S, Hida K, Tanaka E, et al. The importance of precompression time for secure stapling with a linear stapler. Surg Endosc. 2011;25(7):2382–6. PMID: 21184102.
22. Simillis C, Purkayastha S, Yamamoto T, Strong SA, Darzi AW, Tekkis PP. A meta-analysis comparing conventional end-to-end anastomosis vs. other anastomotic configurations after resection in Crohn's disease. Dis Colon Rectum. 2007;50(10):1674–87. PMID: 17682822.
23. He X, Chen Z, Huang J, Lian L, Rouniyar S, Wu X, et al. Stapled side-to-side anastomosis might be better than handsewn end-to-end anastomosis in ileocolic resection for Crohn's disease: a meta-analysis. Dig Dis Sci. 2014;59(7):1544–51. PMID: 24500450.
24. Regueiro M. Management and prevention of postoperative Crohn's disease. Inflamm Bowel Dis. 2009;15(10):1583–90. PMID: 19322907.
25. Eshuis EJ, Polle SW, Slors JF, Hommes DW, Sprangers MA, Gouma DJ, et al. Long-term surgical recurrence, morbidity, quality of life, and body image of laparoscopic-assisted vs. open ileocolic resection for Crohn's disease: a comparative study. Dis Colon Rectum. 2008;51(6):858–67. PMID: 18266036.
26. Resegotti A, Astegiano M, Farina EC, Ciccone G, Avagnina G, Giustetto A, et al. Side-to-side stapled anastomosis strongly reduces anastomotic leak rates in Crohn's disease surgery. Dis Colon Rectum. 2005;48(3):464–8. PMID: 15719193.
27. Sica GS, Iaculli E, Benavoli D, Biancone L, Calabrese E, Onali S, et al. Laparoscopic versus open ileocolonic resection in Crohn's disease: short- and long-term results from a prospective longitudinal study. J Gastrointest Surg. 2008;12(6):1094–102. PMID: 18027061.
28. Dziki AJ, Duncan MD, Harmon JW, Saini N, Malthaner RA, Trad KS, et al. Advantages of handsewn over stapled bowel anastomosis. Dis Colon Rectum. 1991;34(6):442–8. PMID: 1953849.
29. Hassan C, Zullo A, De Francesco V, Ierardi E, Giustini M, Pitidis A, et al. Systematic review: endoscopic dilatation in Crohn's disease. Aliment Pharmacol Ther. 2007;26(11–12):1457–64. PMID: 17903236.
30. Atreja A, Aggarwal A, Dwivedi S, Rieder F, Lopez R, Lashner BA, et al. Safety and efficacy of endoscopic dilation for primary and anastomotic Crohn's disease strictures. J Crohns Colitis. 2014;8(5):392–400. PMID: 24189349.
31. Galandiuk S. Stapled and hand-sewn anastomoses in Crohn's disease. Dig Surg. 1998;15(6):655. PMID: 9890783.
32. Maartense S, Dunker MS, Slors JF, Cuesta MA, Pierik EG, Gouma DJ, et al. Laparoscopic-assisted versus open ileocolic resection for Crohn's disease: a randomized trial. Ann Surg. 2006;243(2):143–9. discussion 50–3. PMID: 16432345.
33. Milsom JW. Laparoscopic surgery in the treatment of Crohn's disease. Surg Clin North Am. 2005;85(1):25–34. PMID: 15619526.
34. Milsom JW, Hammerhofer KA, Bohm B, Marcello P, Elson P, Fazio VW. Prospective, randomized trial comparing laparoscopic vs. conventional surgery for refractory ileocolic Crohn's disease. Dis Colon Rectum. 2001;44(1):1–8. discussion 9. PMID: 11805557.
35. Nguyen SQ, Teitelbaum E, Sabnis AA, Bonaccorso A, Tabrizian P, Salky B. Laparoscopic resection for Crohn's disease: an experience with 335 cases. Surg Endosc. 2009;23:2380–4. PMID: 19263141.
36. Roses RE, Rombeau JL. Recent trends in the surgical management of inflammatory bowel disease. World J Gastroenterol. 2008;14(3):408–12. PMID: 18200663.
37. Tan JJ, Tjandra JJ. Laparoscopic surgery for Crohn's disease: a meta-analysis. Dis Colon Rectum. 2007;50(5):576–85. PMID: 17380366.
38. Fichera A. Laparoscopic treatment of Crohn's disease. World J Surg. 2011;35(7):1500–4. PMID: 21384239.
39. Stocchi L, Milsom JW, Fazio VW. Long-term outcomes of laparoscopic versus open ileocolic resection for Crohn's disease: follow-up of a prospective randomized trial. Surgery. 2008;144(4):622–7. discussion 7–8. PMID: 18847647.

18 Recurrent Crohn's Disease: Surgical Treatment

Roger D. Hurst

The nature of Crohn's disease is such that it is a recurring disorder for which there is no cure. After effective surgical resection, long-term recurrence is the typical clinical course. Between 50 and 70 % of patients undergoing surgical treatment of their disease will ultimately require further surgical intervention [1–3]. As such, many of the surgical procedures undertaken for the management of Crohn's disease are performed in patients who have already had prior surgical treatment. Surgical strategies and approaches for recurrent Crohn's disease for the most part mirror the surgical treatment of primary Crohn's disease. There are, however, nuances that the surgeon should consider when re-operating on patients with Crohn's disease. The purpose of this section is to review these issues.

Indications for Surgery

Indications for surgical treatment of recurrent Crohn's disease are essentially the same as for primary Crohn's disease with failure of medical management with intractability, intestinal obstruction, fistula, abscess, perforation, and hemorrhage being the most common. Other indications include growth retardation in children and risk of malignancy in patients with difficult to assess colonic strictures or dysplasia [4].

Management Strategies

Because eventual recurrence of disease is so common, the approach to Crohn's disease should be seen as a continuum, rather than a series of episodic, independent surgical interventions. As such, planning for a second or subsequent surgical intervention should begin with the initial operation. It cannot be emphasized enough that the surgical strategies for the management of Crohn's disease should always be conducted in a manner that anticipates recurrence of disease and the need for future surgeries. As an example, patients with a pattern of disease that puts them at long-term risk for a stoma should have their surgical incisions placed so as to preserve potential future stoma sites even if there is no consideration for a stoma at the current operation.

Clear documentation is an important aspect of the long-term surgical management of Crohn's disease. To assist any future operative management, at the time of the initial surgery the accessible portions of the GI tract should be evaluated with its condition and length fully documented in the operative report. Additionally, if at all possible, it is best to avoid unorthodox procedures or procedures that result in unusual or confusing anatomy. If an unusual anatomic rearrangement

R.D. Hurst, MD, FRCS(Ed), FACS (✉)
University of Chicago Pritzker School of Medicine, Chicago, IL, USA
e-mail: rhurst@surgery.bsd.uchicago.edu

A. Fichera and M.K. Krane (eds.), *Crohn's Disease: Basic Principles*,
DOI 10.1007/978-3-319-14181-7_18, © Springer International Publishing Switzerland 2015

is necessary, then a clear and unambiguous description of the anatomy should be made in the operative report. All patients should be given ready access if not copies of their operative and pathology reports so that they can be easily conveyed and reviewed for those caring for the patient in the future. Conversely when contemplating surgery for recurrent Crohn's disease it is critically important to review all previous operative reports in order to have the best understanding of the patient's anatomy. Special attention should be given to the overall anatomy of the gastrointestinal tract, and areas that have been bypassed, diverted, or excluded should be noted. Specific locations of previous anastomoses and strictureplasties should also be noted. Any potential alterations in the vascular anatomy of the GI tract should also be considered. For instance, when anticipating surgery on the left colon it is important to know if the collaterals through the inferior mesenteric vessels and the marginal artery of Drummond may have been disrupted by prior surgery.

Because surgical interventions can be separated by many years and in some cases decades, institutional policies for routine destruction of medical records after a certain period of time can be an obstacle to optimal management of patients with Crohn's disease. It is yet to be seen if the widespread application of the electronic medical record will result in a more universal adoption of long-term archiving of records rather than an all too common practice of destroying records once minimal statutory requirements for preservation have been met.

Preoperative Evaluation

The preoperative workup for patients with recurrent disease should include a thorough evaluation of the gastrointestinal tract with imaging studies and endoscopic examinations. This is of particular importance for patients with recurrent disease as intraoperative assessment may be limited by the presence of significant intra-abdominal adhesions. All patients with recurrent disease should undergo either a small bowel follow-through, a CT enterography, or MRI enterography with dedicated protocol. These studies should be scrutinized for evidence of multifocal disease with skip lesions. Areas of disease and presences of complications such as stricture, fistula, or abscess should also be noted. Small bowel imaging should also be studied to assess the overall anatomy of the intestine with special attention to post-surgical alterations and length of disease and length of remaining normal small intestine. Preoperative colonoscopy should be performed to assess the colon for the presence and extent of disease, to assess the terminal ileum or neoterminal ileum, and to evaluate the patency of any ileocolonic anastomoses.

Typically, but certainly not always, the recurrent disease develops in the same location as the initial primary disease. Stricturing disease tends to recur as stricturing disease and penetrating or fistulous disease tends to recur as fistulous disease, but again this is far from universal. Additionally there is often a correlation between length of involved intestine with primary disease and the length of intestine involved with recurrent disease with patients experiencing short segment primary disease being more likely to have short segment recurrence while patients with long segment primary disease are more likely to have recurrent disease over a long segment [5]. The complications of Crohn's disease occur with both primary and recurrent disease with a couple of interesting exceptions. Curiously ileo-vesical fistula is an occasionally seen complication of primary disease but is quite rare as a manifestation of recurrent disease. Ileo-vesical fistulas are seen much less commonly in patients who have undergone prior intestinal resection for Crohn's disease and it is not entirely clear why this would be the case [6, 7]. On the other hand, ileoduodenal fistulas, infrequent complications of Crohn's disease under any circumstances, are seen more often after prior resection. This is likely due to the fact that after an ileocolonic resection, the removal of the descending colon results in the positioning of the neo-terminal ileum to rest directly on top of the duodenum.

Surgical Techniques

As previously indicated, surgery for recurrent disease for the most part mirrors the surgery for primary disease. Areas of disease should be resected to grossly normal margins, and standard anastomotic techniques and appropriate use of abdominal wall stomas apply. However, special consideration and discussion of strictureplasty, laparoscopy, and lysis of adhesions as part of the management of recurrent disease is in order.

Strictureplasty

In an attempt to avoid the debilitating consequences of the short gut syndrome intestinal strictureplasties are utilized to avoid resection and preserve absorptive capacity. For patients with recurrent Crohn's disease such techniques are often an imperative. Strictureplasty techniques include the Heineke–Mikulicz, the Finney, and the Michelassi strictureplasty with the Heineke–Mikulicz being the most common technique employed [8].

Recurrent disease frequently occurs at the location of a previous anastomosis and in some cases can result in focal stricture formation. For these patients the feasibility of strictureplasty at a previous anastomotic site comes into question. A limited number of studies have reported on both the long-term and short-term outcomes of intestinal strictureplasty at a previous anastomotic site [9–11]. These reports suggest that strictureplasty of a previous ileocolonic anastomosis has similar results when compared to re-resection and anastomosis. Thus strictureplasty for recurrent disease resulting in focal stricture at a previous anastomosis is an acceptable option in selected cases. These reports, however, do not provide details regarding the specific techniques of the original anastomosis and it is not clear if all types of anastomoses are equally appropriate for a subsequent strictureplasty. It would seem, however, that an end-to-end anastomosis would be the most amenable to strictureplasty, while the appropriateness of strictureplasty in side-to-side anastomosis is less clear. The available published literature on strictureplasty of a previous anastomosis is for the most part limited to strictureplasty of ileocolonic anastomoses, but it would seem reasonable to conclude that the technique can also be applied to recurrent disease at a previous small bowel to small bowel anastomosis. No matter what the configuration or the location of the previous anastomosis it is important to emphasize that strictureplasty of a previous anastomosis should only be performed for short segment stricturing disease without any associated fistulas or abscesses. Additionally the ideal strictureplasty technique for this type of recurrent disease would be the Heineke–Mikulicz strictureplasty.

There is no published experience of strictureplasty for recurrent disease at a previous strictureplasty site, i.e., there is no published experience for strictureplasty of a previous strictureplasty. This may be the case because strictureplasty is so effective at preventing recurrence at the strictureplasty site itself as only 10 % of patients undergoing strictureplasty require reoperation at the previous strictureplasty site [12]. Focal strictures at a previous strictureplasty site are so unusual that the possibility of malignancy must be seriously considered and adequate assessment of the tissue with biopsy should be undertaken before considering leaving the tissue in situ [13]. From a technical standpoint it would be possible to perform an extension of either a previous Heineke–Mikulicz or a Finney strictureplasty that would allow for reestablishment of patency of the intestinal lumen.

Laparoscopic Surgery

Laparoscopic resection has become the standard for management of primary stricturing Crohn's disease of the terminal ileum. When compared to standard open surgery, laparoscopic resection for Crohn's disease is associated with shorter hospital stays and faster recovery times. Additionally laparoscopic resection decreases the adhesion formation and thus facilitates future surgical interventions. Multiple centers have reported on the value of laparoscopic surgery for primary

Crohn's disease [14–17]. Published data regarding the use of laparoscopic techniques for recurrent disease, on the other hand, is limited, but available data seems to indicate that laparoscopic surgery for recurrent Crohn's disease has an acceptable safety profile [18, 19]. Reported conversion rates for laparoscopic resection or recurrent disease range from between 6 and 30 % depending upon the series [18, 20]. Laparoscopic surgery for recurrent Crohn's disease is associated with longer operative times when compared to primary laparoscopic resection [18, 19, 21]. The currently available published experience with laparoscopic resection for recurrent Crohn's disease suggests that this is an approach that is not often utilized. Major centers that have reported on their experience indicate that laparoscopic surgery for recurrent disease is performed at an average of only two to three cases a year even at recognized IBD centers [20, 21]. This would suggest that the published experience is colored by highly selected application of this technique in patients with recurrent Crohn's disease.

The primary impediment to laparoscopic surgery for patients with recurrent Crohn's disease is the presence of adhesions; either inflammatory from the recurrent Crohn's disease or postoperative from the previous surgery. Therefore patient selection based upon the likelihood of significant adhesive disease would seem important. One rarely considered benefit from laparoscopic surgery for Crohn's disease is a lower risk for postoperative adhesions which in turn facilitates the subsequent operation for recurrent disease, be it either open or laparoscopic.

Management of Adhesions

Most patients with recurrent Crohn's disease will have intra-abdominal adhesions that will impact on the planned surgical treatment of the recurrent disease. These adhesions can either be inflammatory from the Crohn's disease itself or they can be of the typical post-surgical variety. For all cases of surgical management of recurrent intra-abdominal Crohn's disease significant adhesion formation must be anticipated and appropriate strategies employed.

At the time of laparotomy or laparoscopy for Crohn's disease it is preferable to perform an inspection and evaluation of the entire small intestine. Such an evaluation may be inhibited by the presence of adhesions and the surgeon must weigh the benefit of a detailed intraoperative evaluation against the risk of extensive adhesiolysis and the potential for injury to normal structures. This decision is based upon a variety of factors including the patient's condition, symptoms, reliability of preoperative imaging studies and endoscopic exams, and the extent and density of the adhesions. For instance, in a case where preoperative studies demonstrate focal recurrence of the ileum but a normal appearing proximal small bowel with no evidence of skip lesions and at the time of surgery the patient is found to have severe dense adhesions involving the jejunum, an argument can be made to limit the adhesiolysis to what is necessary to perform the required resection or strictureplasty, while leaving severe jejunal adhesions intact to avoid injury to what is most likely otherwise normal small intestine. Conversely if the jejunal adhesions are light and are easily separated without risk of injury, or if preoperative studies do not provide adequate confidence that the jejunum is free of significant Crohn's disease, then the advantage would be to separate the adhered loops of bowel and perform a full examination.

As with any redo operation, surgery for recurrent Crohn's disease requires special attention regarding operative technique [22, 23]. Care must be undertaken when first entering the peritoneal cavity so as not to injure intestine that may be adherent to the anterior abdominal wall. At times it may be necessary to extend the incision into a previously un-incised area in order to safely enter the abdomen. In these cases when incising the fascia it is best to avoid electrocautery, but instead to use the knife to slowly divide the fascia with multiple shallow strokes of the blade. This technique provides better control of the depth of incision and lessens the likelihood of injury to the underlying intestine.

As a general strategy easily separate adhesions should be divided before attacking the more difficult or dense adhesions. This approach often allows for better exposure of the more difficult adhesions and can provide differing avenues to better define planes surrounding the more severe adhesions. Also as a general rule it is best to stay within the natural surgical planes whenever possible. The old adage of "it's better to leave fascia on the bowel than leave bowel on the fascia" may be true, but it is even better to stay in the correct plane for a clean dissection. Adequate visualization is key to the safe management of intra-abdominal adhesions and dividing tissue without clear visualization of the surgical plane is to be avoided. Minimizing blood loss that may obscure the visibility of the point of dissection is critical. This can best be accomplished by staying within the natural surgical planes to avoid injury to small blood vessels. When necessary, judicious use of electrocautery can be employed. For difficult cases it is ideal to have an experienced first assistant who can appropriately adjust the lighting and provide exposure through effective retraction, and who is skilled at using the suction device to keep the point of dissection clear of blood and fluids.

Oftentimes with even a small amount of blood loss, the tissues can become stained with blood making it difficult to discern the correct surgical plane or path. Under these circumstances simply washing the area with a stream of irrigation can improve the contrast between the planes and allow for safe dissection. A technique that is often useful to facilitate dissection of difficult adhesions is that of hydrodissection [24]. With this technique saline is gently injected into the surgical planes (Fig. 18.1). This provides an effect that is essentially an artificially induced edema of the adhesions and it separates adhered structures so that the plane of dissection can be more easily seen. This technique is useful in exposing surgical planes in mild or moderately dense adhesions but unfortunately it is not effective for the most severe adhesions where structures are fused together and the planes are obliterated by fibrosis.

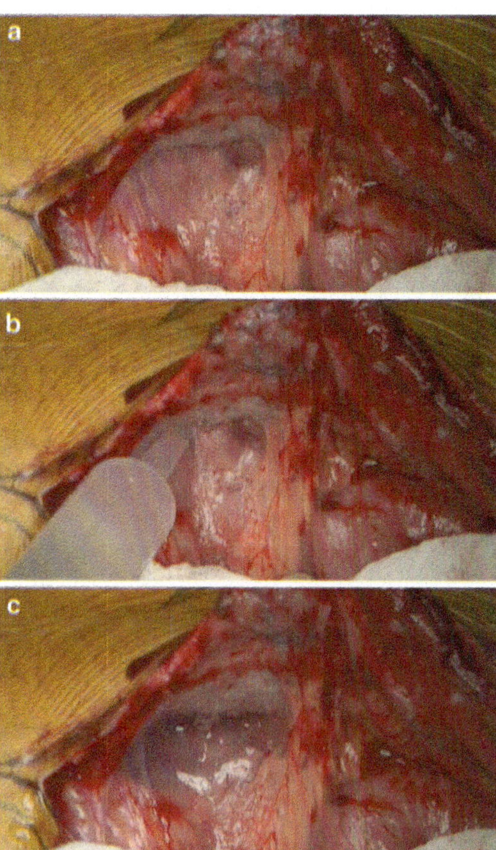

Fig. 18.1 Severe postoperative adhesions in a patient with recurrent Crohn's disease (**a**). Hydrodissection (**b**) is utilized to separate the small bowel from the abdominal wall (**c**) and thus facilitate the lysis of adhesions. (Reprinted with permission from the University of Chicago Colorectal Surgery Archives)

Perioperative Morbidity

Available data comparing the risk for postoperative complications for patients undergoing resection for primary Crohn's disease versus those undergoing resection for recurrent disease is somewhat limited. Most studies regarding the surgical outcomes for patients with Crohn's disease combine data for primary and recurrent disease cases. Heimann et al. looking at 74 patients undergoing resection for recurrent disease found that on average patients with recurrent disease required shorter resections (60 cm vs. 46 cm), and were more likely to require an ileostomy [25]. These patients also had an increased risk for requiring a blood transfusion, however, overall outcomes were similar between patients undergoing surgery for primary disease and those undergoing surgery for recurrent disease. Brouquet et al. reported a case control study comparing ileocolonic resection for recurrent Crohn's disease (54 patients) versus primary ileocecal resection for Crohn's disease (57 patients) [26]. They reported a significant increased risk for postoperative complications in the recurrent group primarily from an increase in the risk for intra-abdominal abscess. Other studies that have compared the morbidity associated with recurrent versus primary Crohn's disease are limited to laparoscopic surgery and these studies have not shown a significant difference in the risk for perioperative complications [18, 19, 21]. Overall it appears that the risk for perioperative complications for patients undergoing surgery for recurrent disease is similar to those undergoing surgery for primary disease.

Summary

A large number of operations performed for Crohn's disease are undertaken in patients for recurrent disease. This poses special challenges that must be considered in the overall management of patients with Crohn's disease and the recurrent nature of Crohn's disease must always be kept in mind from the outset of surgical treatment.

References

1. Greenstein AJ, Sachar DB, Pasternack BS, Janowitz HD. Reoperation and recurrence in Crohn's colitis and ileocolitis crude and cumulative rates. N Engl J Med. 1975;293:685–90.
2. Mekhjian HS, Switz DM, Watts HD, Deren JJ, Katon RM, Beman FM. National cooperative Crohn's disease study: factors determining recurrence of Crohn's disease after surgery. Gastroenterology. 1979;77: 907–13.
3. Whelan G, Farmer RG, Fazio VW, Goormastic M. Recurrence after surgery in Crohn's disease. Relationship to location of disease (clinical pattern) and surgical indication. Gastroenterology. 1985;88: 1826–33.
4. Michelassi F. Indications for surgical treatment in ulcerative colitis and Crohn's disease. In: Michelassi F, Milsom JW, editors. Operative strategies in inflammatory bowel disease. New York: Springer; 1999. p. 150–3.
5. D'haens G, Baert F, Gasparaitis A, Hanauer S. Length and type of recurrent ileitis after ileal resection correlate with presurgical features in Crohn's disease. Inflamm Bowel Dis. 1997;3:249–53.
6. Hurst RD, Molinari M, Chung TP, Rubin M, Michelassi F. Prospective study of the features, indications, and surgical treatment in 513 consecutive patients affected by Crohn's disease. Surgery. 1997;122:661–7. discussion 7–8.
7. Schraut WH, Chapman C, Abraham VS. Operative treatment of Crohn's ileocolitis complicated by ileosigmoid and ileovesical fistulae. Ann Surg. 1988; 207:48–51.
8. Ambe R, Campbell L, Cagir B. A comprehensive review of strictureplasty techniques in Crohn's disease: types, indications, comparisons, and safety. J Gastrointest Surg. 2012;16:209–17.
9. Sharif H, Alexander-Williams J. Strictureplasty for ileo-colic anastomotic strictures in Crohn's disease. Int J Colorectal Dis. 1991;6:214–6.
10. Tjandra JJ, Fazio VW. Strictureplasty for ileocolic anastomotic strictures in Crohn's disease. Dis Colon Rectum. 1993;36:1099–103. discussion 103–4.
11. Yamamoto T, Keighley MR. Long-term results of strictureplasty for ileocolonic anastomotic recurrence in Crohn's disease. J Gastrointest Surg. 1999;3: 555–60.
12. Yamamoto T, Fazio VW, Tekkis PP. Safety and efficacy of strictureplasty for Crohn's disease: a systematic review and meta-analysis. Dis Colon Rectum. 2007;50:1968–86.
13. Michelassi F, Sultan S. Surgical treatment of complex small bowel Crohn disease. Ann Surg. 2014;260: 230–5.
14. Dasari BV, McKay D, Gardiner K. Laparoscopic versus open surgery for small bowel Crohn's disease. Cochrane Database Syst Rev. 2011;(1):CD006956.
15. Maartense S, Dunker MS, Slors JF, et al. Laparoscopic-assisted versus open ileocolic resection for Crohn's disease: a randomized trial. Ann Surg. 2006;243:143–9. discussion 50–3.
16. Milsom JW, Hammerhofer KA, Böhm B, Marcello P, Elson P, Fazio VW. Prospective, randomized trial comparing laparoscopic vs. conventional surgery for refractory ileocolic Crohn's disease. Dis Colon Rectum. 2001;44:1–8. Discussion -9.
17. Nguyen SQ, Teitelbaum E, Sabnis AA, Bonaccorso A, Tabrizian P, Salky B. Laparoscopic resection for Crohn's disease: an experience with 335 cases. Surg Endosc. 2009;23:2380–4.
18. Chaudhary B, Glancy D, Dixon AR. Laparoscopic surgery for recurrent ileocolic Crohn's disease is as

safe and effective as primary resection. Colorectal Dis. 2011;13:1413–6.
19. Hasegawa H, Watanabe M, Nishibori H, Okabayashi K, Hibi T, Kitajima M. Laparoscopic surgery for recurrent Crohn's disease. Br J Surg. 2003;90: 970–3.
20. Brouquet A, Bretagnol F, Soprani A, Valleur P, Bouhnik Y, Panis Y. A laparoscopic approach to iterative ileocolonic resection for the recurrence of Crohn's disease. Surg Endosc. 2010;24:879–87.
21. Holubar SD, Dozois EJ, Privitera A, et al. Laparoscopic surgery for recurrent ileocolic Crohn's disease. Inflamm Bowel Dis. 2010;16:1382–6.
22. Coleman MG, McLain AD, Moran BJ. Impact of previous surgery on time taken for incision and division of adhesions during laparotomy. Dis Colon Rectum. 2000;43:1297–9.
23. Jobanputra S, Wexner SD. Systematic guide to complex cases from adhesive disease. Colorectal Dis. 2007;9 Suppl 2:54–9.
24. Bokey EL, Keating JP, Zelas P. Hydrodissection: an easy way to dissect anatomical planes and complex adhesions. Aust N Z J Surg. 1997;67:643–4.
25. Heimann TM, Greenstein AJ, Lewis B, Kaufman D, Heimann DM, Aufses AH. Comparison of primary and reoperative surgery in patients with Crohn's disease. Ann Surg. 1998;227:492–5.
26. Brouquet A, Blanc B, Bretagnol F, Valleur P, Bouhnik Y, Panis Y. Surgery for intestinal Crohn's disease recurrence. Surgery. 2010;148:936–46.

19 Extraintestinal Manifestations of Crohn's Disease

Kara De Felice and Laura E. Raffals

Musculoskeletal Manifestations

Musculoskeletal manifestations in CD patients are common (Table 19.1). In population-based European inflammatory bowel disease (IBD) cohorts, the prevalence of any musculoskeletal symptom was 36 % in Crohn's disease.

Sacroiliitis and Ankylosing Spondylitis

Axial arthropathies are common in CD (5–22 %) patients. Axial arthropathies are independent of CD activity and sometimes can present prior to the diagnosis of CD. Patients can be asymptomatic or have lower back pain and morning stiffness. Patients with sacroiliitis are frequently asymptomatic, even when inflammation is detected on plain film or MRI in the sacroiliac joints. A small percentage of these patients do progress to ankylosing spondylitis which results in inflammation of vertebral joints and ligaments (Fig. 19.1). The HLA-B27 genotype appears to increase the risk of progression to ankylosing spondylitis in these patients. There is a strong link between CD and ankylosing spondylitis. Up to 10 % of patients with IBD have ankylosing spondylitis. Interestingly, up to 70 % of patients with ankylosing spondylitis will have clinically asymptomatic ileitis on colonoscopy. Of these patients, 5–10 % are eventually diagnosed with IBD (whether UC or CD). The genetic link, HLA B27, is thought to play a major role. Moreover, there is a threefold increase risk of first degree relatives of patients with ankylosing spondylitis developing IBD [1].

The gold standard for diagnosing axial arthropathies is MRI, since it detects lesions that may not be apparent on plain film. The disease course of axial arthropathies, especially ankylosing spondylitis, is progressive despite the underlying CD activity. Treatment involves aggressive physical therapy, pain management, and anti-inflammatory agents such as nonsteroidal anti-inflammatory drugs (NSAIDs). Anti-TNFα agents (infliximab, adalimumab, etanercept, and golimumab) are indicated in patients who do not respond to conservative treatment. Caution is advised in using NSAIDs since they can exacerbate underlying CD.

Peripheral Arthritis

Type I arthropathy is an oligoarticular arthritis, involving less than five joints. Patients present

K. De Felice, MD
Mayo Clinic Hospital-Rochester Methodist Campus, Rochester, MN, USA

L.E. Raffals, MD (✉)
Department of Gastroenterology and Hepatology, May Clinic, Rochester, MN, USA
e-mail: Raffals.Laura@mayo.edu

A. Fichera and M.K. Krane (eds.), *Crohn's Disease: Basic Principles*,
DOI 10.1007/978-3-319-14181-7_19, © Springer International Publishing Switzerland 2015

Table 19.1 Musculoskeletal manifestations of CD

Spondyloarthropathy	Metabolic bone disease
Axial skeleton	Osteopenia and osteoporosis
Sacroiliitis	Osteomalacia
Ankylosing spondylitis	Osteonecrosis
Peripheral	
Type 1: oligoarticular	
Type 2: polyarticular	

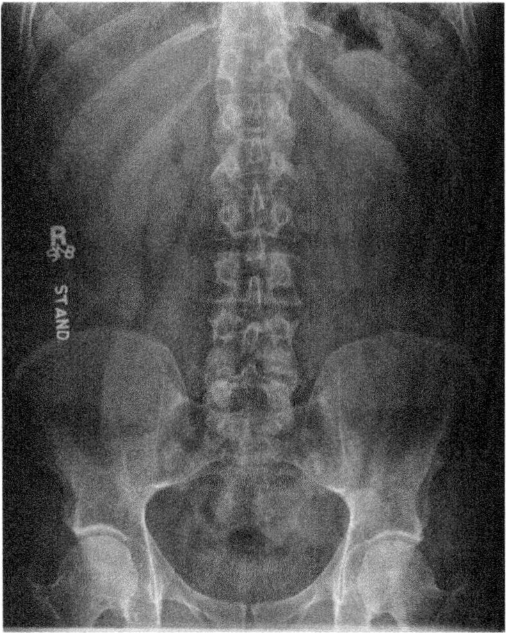

Fig. 19.1 Sacroiliitis with signs of spondyloarthropathy in the lower thoracic and lumbar spine

with swollen, tender joints with limited movement. Plain films usually do not reveal joint destruction and this arthropathy is not associated with long-term sequelae. The peripheral arthritis parallels the underlying CD activity, and therefore medical or surgical treatment of the luminal CD results in improvement of the peripheral arthritis. It is most common in those patients with colonic CD involvement.

Type II arthropathy is a chronic, symmetric polyarthritis that mimics rheumatoid arthritis although the rheumatoid factor is negative in these patients. Type II arthropathy is independent of underlying CD; therefore, this arthropathy can be active even in the setting of quiescent CD. Treatment consists of physical activity, pain management, anti-inflammatory agents, sulfasalazine, and oral or intra-articular corticosteroids. Methotrexate and anti-TNFα agents have also been used successfully in refractory cases [2].

Osteopenia and Osteoporosis

A decrease in bone mineral density is common in CD patients. The prevalence of osteoporosis in all patients with IBD is roughly 15 %. The cause of bone loss is multifactorial and could be a result of circulating cytokines increasing bone resorption, malabsorption of calcium and vitamin D, use of corticosteroids, cigarette smoking, and low level of physical activity.

The American Gastroenterological Association (AGA) guidelines recommend dual energy X-ray absorptiometry (DXA) screening in IBD patients with one or more risk factors: postmenopausal, history of vertebral fractures, chronic systemic corticosteroid use, male >50 years of age, or hypogonadism. If the initial DXA is normal, the AGA recommends repeat testing in 2–3 years [3].

Treatment for osteopenia includes regular weight-bearing exercise, minimizing corticosteroid use, smoking cessation, and calcium (1,500 mg daily) and vitamin D (400–800 IU daily) supplementation. Patients with osteoporosis should be referred to an endocrinologist and are often treated with bisphosphonates, calcitonin, or recombinant parathyroid hormone.

Ocular Manifestations

Eye manifestations occur in 2–5 % of CD patients and should prompt a rapid referral to an ophthalmologist to accurately diagnose and treat the underlying ocular disease (Table 19.2).

Anterior Uveitis

Anterior uveitis (including iritis) presents as acute or chronic changes in vision, photophobia, redness

Table 19.2 Ocular manifestations in CD

Inflammatory	Steroid-induced
Anterior uveitis	Glaucoma
Scleritis	Cataracts
Episcleritis	
Retinitis	

of the eye, and ocular pain. The acute form of anterior uveitis is associated with HLA B27 in 50 % of patients. In these patients who are HLA B27 positive, the uveitis may not parallel CD activity. The chronic form of anterior uveitis is not associated with HLA B27 and often improves with treatment of the underlying CD [4].

CD patients with changes in vision should be seen by ophthalmology promptly to undergo a slit-lamp exam. Leukocytes are seen in the aqueous humor of the anterior chamber on slit-lamp examination. Treatment should be instituted to prevent complications and permanent vision loss. Treatment with topical or systemic steroids, immunomodulator therapy, and anti-TNFα agents has been successful.

Scleritis and Episcleritis

Patients with episcleritis or scleritis present with acute hyperemia and burning of the eye. Vision is usually intact in patients suffering from episcleritis. Scleritis is a more severe condition and may impair vision. Prompt evaluation by an ophthalmologist should be done to accurately diagnose the underlying eye disease and institute appropriate therapy, preventing long-term vision loss. Episcleritis and scleritis generally present before or during flares of CD, and improve with treatment of the underlying CD and topical steroids and/or oral steroids.

Dermatologic Manifestations

Numerous skin disorders have been associated with CD (Table 19.3). The two most common skin disorders are erythema nodosum (EN) and pyoderma gangrenosum (PG).

Table 19.3 Dermatologic manifestations of CD

Common	Rare
Pyoderma gangrenosum	Bowel-associated dermatosis-arthritis syndrome
Erythema nodosum	Sweet's syndrome
Psoriasis	Epidermolysis bullosa acquisita
Cutaneous Crohn's disease	Pyostomatitis vegetans
Aphthous stomatitis	Mucosal cobblestoning of buccal mucosa and palate

Erythema Nodosum

Erythema nodosum (EN) is a skin disorder characterized by subcutaneous fat tissue inflammation. It is associated with many other conditions including infections (*Yersinia,* tuberculosis, coccidioidomycosis, histoplasmosis, and blastomycosis), autoimmune disorders (sarcoidosis and Behcet's disease), medications, and IBD. The incidence of EN in IBD patients is higher in CD compared to patients with UC, and in females, ages 24–40 years of age. The prevalence of EN in CD patients is 2–6 %.

EN presents as painful, tender, subcutaneous, erythematous nodules on the lower extremities, most commonly in the pretibial areas (Fig. 19.2a). Diagnosis is based on clinical history. EN parallels the underlying CD activity (present during flares of disease) and therefore responds to the treatment of the underlying CD. EN is typically treated with systemic steroid therapy, and in refractory cases dapsone, cyclosporine, and anti-TNFα agents have been effective. Supportive care for EN includes stockings, elevation of legs, and bed rest. Once treated, these lesions do not result in permanent sequelae.

Pyoderma Gangrenosum

Pyoderma gangrenosum (PG) is a rare, ulcerating, neutrophilic dermatosis with a prevalence of 1–6 % in CD patients. The pathophysiology of PG is poorly understood. Dysfunction of the immune system's neutrophil activity is thought to be the underlying mechanism. It is characterized by necrosis and ulceration of the skin, predominately

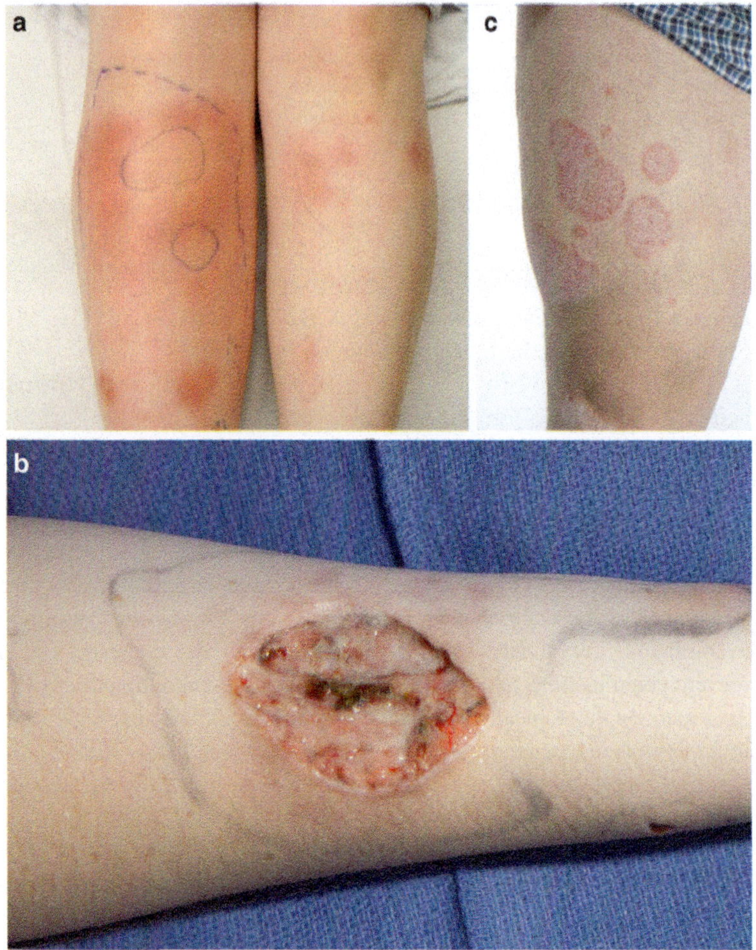

Fig. 19.2 (**a**) Tender, erythematous, subcutaneous nodules on lower extremities. (**b**) Ulcerated lesion with a purulent and necrotic base extending into the subcutaneous fat. (**c**) Well-demarcated, erythematous, scaly plaques on the lower extremity

affecting the lower extremities. Twenty to fifty percent of lesions occur in areas of trauma (e.g., around stomas). The lesions are typically multiple and recur (Fig. 19.2b). Lesions start as a tender nodule, plaque, or pustule, and often enlarge and erode to become a sharply marginated ulcer with surrounding erythema. The skin and subcutis becomes necrotic, friable, hemorrhagic or purulent, with changes extending into the musculature.

PG can be classified into five subtypes: classic (ulcerative), bullous, peristomal, vegetative, and pustular PG. The most common subtype in CD is classic and peristomal PG. Diagnosis of PG is based on clinical history and exam. Diagnosis is reached if a patient meets the following criteria: two major criteria (rapid progression of lesion and exclusion of other causes) and two minor criteria (pathergy, systemic disease associated with PG, histology suggestive of neutrophilic dermatosis, and rapid response to steroid treatment).

PG may or may not parallel CD disease activity. In a cohort of 60 IBD patients with PG, only 58 % had active luminal disease, highlighting that over 40 % of patients did not have active IBD at the time they were experiencing PG lesions [5]. In another cohort study of 270 CD and 125 UC patients including 37 patients with PG or EN, predictors of PG or EN included female sex, younger age, CD, presence of other extraintestinal manifestations, and previous biologic therapy [6].

The goal of treatment is to control inflammation of the wound, reduce pain, optimize wound healing, and minimize exacerbating factors.

Any underlying luminal disease should be treated. Limited small, and slowly progressive PG lesions can be treated with combination therapy including topical agents (steroids or tacrolimus), intralesional agents (steroids), and/or systemic agents (steroids, dapsone, or cyclosporine). Large, rapidly progressive lesions should be treated with systemic therapy (steroids, cyclosporine, anti-TNFα agents, or ustekinumab) with concomitant therapy (azathioprine, methotrexate, mycophenolate mofetil, topical or intralesional steroids).

Psoriasis

Psoriasis occurs in up to 10 % of CD patients. The rash, which may involve any area of the body, is characterized by red, scaly papules, and plaques (Fig. 19.2c). Psoriasis does not parallel CD activity and is often diagnosed prior to the development of CD.

Treatment includes topical agents (steroids, coal tar, retinoids, and vitamin D analogues), phototherapy, and systemic agents (methotrexate, retinoids, cyclosporine, anti-TNFα agents, and ustekinumab).

With increased use of anti-TNFα agents, paradoxical development of de novo psoriasis has been increasingly reported. Most patients respond to discontinuation of anti-TNFα agents and treatment with topical or systemic agents. Not all patients develop recurrent de novo psoriasis when switching to a different anti-TNFα agent [7].

Cutaneous Crohn's Disease

Cutaneous Crohn's disease is a rare condition associated with CD. It presents as subcutaneous nodules, plaques, or ulcers involving the lower extremities and intertriginous areas. Diagnosis is based on clinical suspicion in the setting of underlying CD, however it requires histological confirmation. Biopsies show noncaseating granulomas with multinucleated giant cells in the dermis surrounded by lymphocytes, plasma cells, and eosinophils. Cutaneous Crohn's disease does not parallel CD activity. It is usually diagnosed in those with colonic CD and is rarely the first manifestation of CD. Treatment includes topical and systemic steroids, immunomodulators, and anti-TNFα agents.

Hepatobiliary Manifestations

Hepatic Manifestations

There are few conditions affecting the liver in patients with CD. Although rare, autoimmune hepatitis has been reported in CD patients. The majority of these cases are associated with AIH/PSC overlap syndromes. Granulomatous hepatitis is also rare, but does occur. These cases are thought to be idiopathic and may be associated with mesalamine and sulfasalazine use. Other medications, including corticosteroids and immunomodulators, can cause liver toxicity or steatosis. A careful review of medications should be performed in any CD patient found to have an elevation in liver enzymes (Table 19.4).

Biliary Manifestations

Primary sclerosing cholangitis (PSC) is a chronic cholestatic disease affecting intra- and extrahepatic bile ducts resulting in inflammation and fibrosis of the biliary tree. PSC is most common in UC patients, but can be seen in patients with CD as well. The prevalence of PSC ranges from 1.2 % to 3.4 % in CD. PSC can present before or after the diagnosis of CD. CD patients with elevated liver enzymes, particularly an elevated alkaline phosphatase, should undergo evaluation for PSC with MRCP (Fig. 19.3).

Table 19.4 Hepatobiliary manifestations of CD

Hepatic	Biliary
Autoimmune hepatitis	Primary sclerosing cholangitis
Granulomatous hepatitis	Primary biliary cirrhosis
Steatosis	Cholelithiasis
Drug-induced liver injury	Cholangiocarcinoma

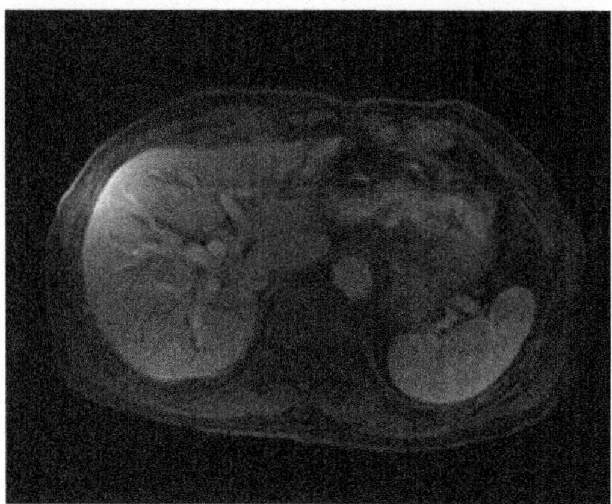

Fig. 19.3 MRCP showing irregular, dilated, and thickened intrahepatic ducts

PSC activity is independent of the underlying CD. Even in the setting of quiescent CD, PSC can progress. PSC patients with progressive liver disease can develop cirrhosis and often require liver transplantation. Interestingly, one study showed that colectomy in UC patients prior to liver transplantation prevented recurrent PSC post-transplant [8].

Patients with CD are twice as likely to develop cholelithiasis compared to the general population with a prevalence of 11–34 %. CD patients are likely at risk for cholelithiasis due to higher bile salt concentration (due to ileal inflammation or resection leading to impaired enterohepatic cycling of bile salts), decrease in gallbladder motility, and more frequent use of total parenteral nutrition.

Neurologic Manifestations

Peripheral Neuropathy

Peripheral neuropathy is the most common neurological manifestation in CD (prevalence of 8.3–39 %). Etiologies include immune-mediated neuropathy, vitamin B12 deficiency, and metronidazole-induced neuropathy. Immune-mediated neuropathy includes chronic inflammatory demyelinating polyneuropathy, large fiber axonal polyneuropathy, and small fiber neuropathy [9]. Peripheral neuropathies are infrequently related to CD disease activity and usually do not respond to treatment of underlying CD. Demyelinating polyneuropathies are typically treated with intravenous immunoglobulins, plasmapheresis, or prednisone. CD patients with signs and symptoms of a possible neuropathy should undergo electromyography and nerve conduction studies with the guidance of neurology (Table 19.5).

Table 19.5 Neurological manifestations of CD

Neurologic manifestations
Peripheral neuropathy
Demyelinating disorders
Cerebrovascular disorders
Medication-induced neurological manifestations

Demyelinating Disorders

Epidemiological studies have suggested an association between CD and multiple sclerosis (MS). Population-based studies have showed an increased risk of MS in CD patients [10]. Incidental focal white matter lesions are also reported more frequently in patients with CD than the general population (Fig. 19.4). Possible explanations of this association include a brain–gut interaction, shared genetic susceptibility, and similar environmental risk factors of disease (smoking, higher socioeconomic status, vitamin D deficiency, and colder climates). MS has also been reported in CD patients treated with anti-TNFα agents. However, there are no conclusive studies showing that anti-TNFα agents cause MS.

Cerebrovascular Disorders

Young CD patients (<50 years of age) have an increased incidence of cerebrovascular accidents compared to the general population. Most of these events are noted in patients with active CD, usually in the postoperative state, and may arise from arterio-arterial embolism, cardioembolism, and in situ cerebral thrombosis [11]. Patients with CD are also at risk for cerebral sinus vein thrombosis.

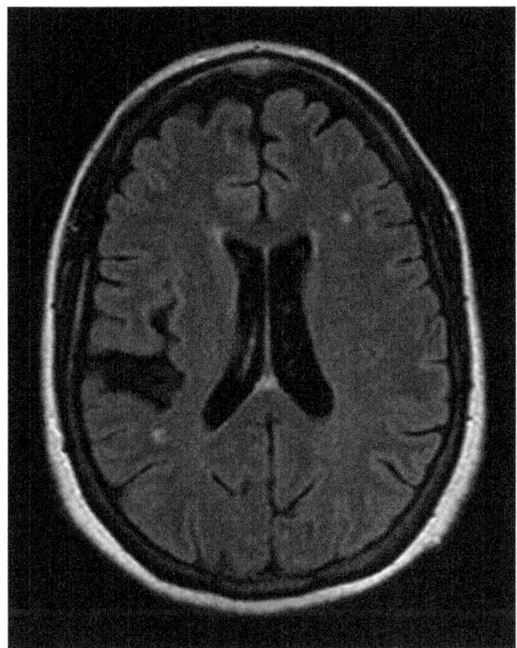

Fig. 19.4 MRI of the head showing focal white matter lesions

Medication-Induced Neurological Manifestations

Metronidazole is frequently used for perianal CD. Metronidazole has been associated with peripheral neuropathy and pure sensory or autonomic neuropathy. The neuropathy is usually transient and resolves upon discontinuing the drug.

Natalizumab is an anti-a4-integrin monoclonal antibody used in the treatment of refractory CD. Natalizumab has been associated with progressive multifocal leukoencephalopathy (PML). PML is a rare and usually fatal viral (JC virus) disease that results in inflammatory demyelination of the CNS white matter resulting in permanent weakness or paralysis, vision loss, impaired speech, and cognitive deterioration. Diagnosis is made by performing a JC virus PCR of the cerebrospinal fluid. Patients should be risk-stratified prior to using natalizumab for their CD. Prior immunosuppressive medications, JC virus positive serum antibody, and duration of natalizumab use are all factors that increase the risk of natalizumab-induced PML [12].

Table 19.6 Hematologic manifestations of CD

Hematologic manifestations
Anemia
Iron deficiency
Vitamin B12 deficiency
Folic acid deficiency
Anemia of chronic disease
Autoimmune hemolytic anemia
Myelodysplastic syndrome
Promyelocytic leukemia

Central demyelinating diseases (optic neuritis and MS) and peripheral neuropathy have been associated with the use of anti-TNFα agents [13]. While an increased incidence of central and peripheral demyelinating diseases has been described in patients with CD, it is not entirely clear if anti-TNFα agents cause demyelinating disease, increase the risk of developing demyelination, or unmask subclinical central/peripheral demyelination in genetically susceptible individuals. Current guidelines recommend discontinuing anti-TNFα agents in patients with neurological symptoms found to have demyelination.

Hematologic Manifestations

Anemia is common in patients with CD. The underlying etiology may be multifactorial and includes iron deficiency, vitamin B12 deficiency, folate deficiency, and anemia of chronic disease. Autoimmune hemolytic anemia, myelodysplastic syndrome, and promyelocytic leukemia are rare associations with CD (Table 19.6).

Thromboembolic Manifestations

Patients with CD have a markedly increased risk of acute mesenteric ischemia. They are also at risk for myocardial infarction and stroke [14].

CD patients are at an increased risk of sustaining venous thromboembolisms compared to the general population. CD disease activity is an independent risk factor for venous thromboembolisms [15]. Current guidelines strongly

Table 19.7 Thromboembolic manifestations of CD

Thromboembolic manifestations
Arterial
Venous

Table 19.8 Cardiopulmonary manifestations of CD

Cardiopulmonary manifestations
Pericarditis
Myocarditis
Pneumonitis
Eosinophilic pneumonia

Table 19.9 Renal manifestations of CD

Renal manifestations
Nephrolithiasis
Glomerulonephritis
Urinary system fistulas
5-Aminosalicylate induced tubulointerstitial nephritis

recommend venous thromboembolism prophylaxis in acutely ill CD patients admitted to the hospital (Table 19.7).

Cardiopulmonary Manifestations

Various cardiopulmonary manifestations have been associated with CD (Table 19.8). Pneumonitis and pericarditis are also a rare side effect of treatment with 5-aminosalicylates.

Renal Manifestations

Calcium oxalate stones are commonly seen in CD patients with small intestinal inflammation or resection resulting in an increase of oxalate absorption in the colon [16]. Tubulointerstitial nephritis is a rare but serious side effect of 5-aminosalicylates. Renal function should be monitored periodically in patients on 5-aminosalicylates (Table 19.9).

Table 19.10 Pancreatic manifestations of CD

Pancreatic manifestations
Acute pancreatitis
Drug-induced
Granulomatous involvement of pancreas
Duodenal Crohn's disease
Chronic pancreatitis
Autoimmune pancreatitis

Pancreatic Manifestations

The most common cause of acute pancreatitis in CD patients is a result of treatment with azathioprine, 6-mercaptopurine, and 5-aminosalicylates. Rarely, acute pancreatitis is a result of CD involving the pancreas itself or the duodenum, leading to swelling, scarring, and obstruction of the ampulla of Vater. Autoimmune pancreatitis has been increasingly recognized in patients with CD [17] (Table 19.10).

References

1. Steer S, et al. Low back pain, sacroiliitis, and the relationship with HLA-B27 in Crohn's disease. J Rheumatol. 2003;30:518–22.
2. Orchard T, Wordsworth B, Jewell D. Peripheral arthropathies in inflammatory bowel disease: their articular distribution and natural history. Gut. 1998;42:387–91. doi:10.1136/gut.42.3.387.
3. Bernstein C, Leslie W, Leboff M. AGA technical review on osteoporosis in gastrointestinal diseases. Gastroenterology. 2003;124:795–841. doi:10.1053/gast.2003.50106.
4. Orchard T, et al. Uveitis and erythema nodosum in inflammatory bowel disease: clinical features and the role of HLA genes. Gastroenterology. 2002;123:714–8. doi:10.1053/gast.2002.35396.
5. Agarwal A, Andrews J. Systematic review: IBD-associated pyoderma gangrenosum in the biologic era, the response to therapy. Aliment Pharmacol Ther. 2013;38:563–72. doi:10.1111/apt.12431.
6. Ampuero J, Rojas-Feria M, Castro-Fernández M, Cano C, Romero-Gómez M. Predictive factors for erythema nodosum and pyoderma gangrenosum in inflammatory bowel disease. J Gastroenterol Hepatol. 2014;29:291–5. doi:10.1111/jgh.12352.
7. Cullen G, Kroshinsky D, Cheifetz A, Korzenik J. Psoriasis associated with anti-tumour necrosis factor therapy in inflammatory bowel disease: a new series and a review of 120 cases from the literature.

Aliment Pharmacol Ther. 2011;34:1318–27. doi:10.1111/j.1365-2036.2011.04866.x.

8. Singh S, Talwalkar J. Primary sclerosing cholangitis: diagnosis, prognosis, and management. Clin Gastroenterol Hepatol. 2013;11:898–907. doi:10.1016/j.cgh.2013.02.016.
9. Gondim FAA, Brannagan TH, Sander HW, Chin RL, Latov N. Peripheral neuropathy in patients with inflammatory bowel disease. Brain. 2005;128:867–79. doi:10.1093/brain/awh429.
10. Kimura K, et al. Concurrence of inflammatory bowel disease and multiple sclerosis. Mayo Clin Proc. 2000;75:802–6. doi:10.4065/75.8.802.
11. Andersohn F, Waring M, Garbe E. Risk of ischemic stroke in patients with Crohn's disease: a population-based nested case-control study. Inflamm Bowel Dis. 2010;16:1387–92. doi:10.1002/ibd.21187.
12. Gorelik L, et al. Anti-JC virus antibodies: implications for PML risk stratification. Ann Neurol. 2010;68:295–303. doi:10.1002/ana.22128.
13. Deepak P, Stobaugh D, Sherid M, Sifuentes H, Ehrenpreis E. Neurological events with tumour necrosis factor alpha inhibitors reported to the food and drug administration adverse event reporting system. Aliment Pharmacol Ther. 2013;38:388–96. doi:10.1111/apt.12385.
14. Ha C, Magowan S, Accortt NA, Chen J, Stone CD. Risk of arterial thrombotic events in inflammatory bowel disease. Am J Gastroenterol. 2009;104:1445–51. doi:10.1038/ajg.2009.81.
15. Murthy SK, Nguyen GC. Venous thromboembolism in inflammatory bowel disease: an epidemiological review. Am J Gastroenterol. 2011;106:713–8. doi:10.1038/ajg.2011.53.
16. Caudarella R, et al. Renal stone formation in patients with inflammatory bowel disease. Scanning Microsc. 1993;7:371.
17. Pitchumoni CS, Rubin A, Das K. Pancreatitis in inflammatory bowel diseases. J Clin Gastroenterol. 2010;44:246–53. doi:10.1097/MCG.0b013e3181cadbe1.

Enterostomal Therapy in the Management of the Patient with Crohn's Disease

20

Janice C. Colwell

Despite advances in medical therapy for Crohn's disease (CD) surgical intervention is still required for many patients. Patients with colonic or perianal disease may require a proctocolectomy. An end ileostomy is recommended since refractory colonic disease frequently involves the rectum, limiting the possibilities of restorative surgery [1]. For some patients with Crohn's disease a temporary loop stoma may be created. Permanent or temporary, the creation of a stoma can be frightening to a patient living with Crohn's disease. A recent study by Krouse et al. [2] found that coping and acceptance were the most common issues that a person with an ostomy described as their greatest challenge. The health care team can offer care coordination to help provide the CD patient with the tools needed to make the adjustment. The team members should include: surgeons, wound ostomy and continence nurses, inflammatory bowel disease (IBD) physicians, and the patient and their support members. This chapter will cover the pre-operative preparation of the patient anticipating ostomy surgery, stoma site marking, stoma creation considerations, post-operative care, pouching systems, post discharge care, and stoma and peristomal complications.

Pre-operative Preparation

When helping to prepare a patient to live with a stoma, there are several considerations. The patient and their support (family, significant other, etc.) should receive a thorough explanation of the surgical procedure, information on how a stoma is managed and the adjustments they will need to make and the stoma site should be chosen before the surgical procedure. If at all possible the pre-operative session should be held several days or weeks before the surgery to allow the patient to hear this information in a setting where they can have a discussion with the health care team. Key points related to the stoma will include what the stoma looks like, how it functions, how it will be managed, what skills they will need to acquire and answering all of their questions related to living with a stoma. Commonly asked questions include: Will I have odor and will everyone know that I have a stoma? A brief explanation about odor and concealment will help to alleviate the fears that many people have who undergo ostomy surgery. There are kits that can be used during the pre-operative session that contain a GI anatomy illustration, pouches, reading material on general ostomy concepts as well as materials that can be used to site the stoma (see Table 20.1).

J.C. Colwell, RN, MS, CWOCN, FAAN (✉)
Advanced Practice Nurse: Wound Ostomy and Skin Care, Department of General Surgery, The University of Chicago Medicine, 5841 S. Maryland Avenue, MC1083, 60637 Chicago, IL, USA
e-mail: janice.colwell@uchospitals.edu

A. Fichera and M.K. Krane (eds.), *Crohn's Disease: Basic Principles*,
DOI 10.1007/978-3-319-14181-7_20, © Springer International Publishing Switzerland 2015

Table 20.1 Pre-operative ostomy teaching kits

Source	Product description	Use
American College of Surgeons https://www.facs.org/education/patient-education/skills-programs/ostomy-program • Available to college members free of charge • Available from Coloplast (manufacturer of ostomy products contained in kit). www.coloplast.com	*Home ostomy skill kit* Topics covered: • Your operation • Pouching systems • Emptying • Changing • Problem solving • Life with an ostomy Includes: • A booklet with information on the operation, home skills such as emptying and changing a pouch, problem solving, and home management • A DVD with demonstration of each skill • Stoma practice model • Stoma supplies (measurement guide, marking pen, scissors, sample pouch) • Ostomy self-care checklist	Can be used as part of pre-operative teaching session, kit can be sent home for the patient to work on skills before surgery
Hollister, Inc. www.hollister.com Available from Hollister representative	*Pre-operative kit* Topics covered: • What is an ostomy • How is it managed • Image of pouches/stoma Includes: • Two pouches • Marking pen • Educational booklet	Can be used as part of pre-operative teaching session, pouch can be used to determine stoma site, pen to mark stoma site. Booklet and pouches can be sent home with patient to practice

Pre-operative Stoma Site Marking

All patients who will have a stoma created should have the stoma site marked before surgery. The American Society of Colon and Rectal Surgeons and the Wound Ostomy and Continence Nurses Society have developed a consensus statement of the value of pre-operative stoma site marking [3]. The consensus statement supports the need for pre-operative stoma site marking and provides a template for the selection of the proposed stoma site to be used by the clinician marking the stoma site. Person et al. [4] evaluated the impact of pre-operative stoma site marking on patients and reported an improved quality of life, an increase in independence and a reduction in the post-operative complications in the population that had their stoma site marked before the surgical intervention. Pre-operative stoma site marking has also been associated with less difficulty adjusting to an ostomy and with less post-operative ostomy complications [5, 6].

Stoma Site Selection

Once the procedure has been explained to the patient, examine the patients' abdomen in a sitting position fully clothed (feet on the ground). Note the presences of belts, or other devices near or on the abdomen such as a brace. Ask the patient if they need to wear special equipment such as tool belt or a uniform that may use a belt on or around the mid abdomen. Observe for creases, scars, folds and overall abdominal contours. Be sure the patient's abdomen is relaxed; encourage a deep breath and that will slowly release tension to provide muscle relaxation. The ideal spot will be 2–3 in. that remain flat in all positions and on which a pouching system adhesive can be placed. If the stoma is placed in or near a crease, the pouching system adhesive will crease and cause a break in the seal with leakage. Determine the location of the rectus muscle as placement within the rectus muscle may prevent the development of a peristomal hernia.

Once a proposed stoma site is determined, place a light pen mark in the area and ask the patient to stand, bend forward, and lay flat. Watch the contours of the abdomen in the area of the stoma mark in all of these positions. If there are dominant creases, consider another location. While standing, ask the patient if they can see the proposed site and do the same in sitting position. It is important that the patient easily see and access the stoma site to achieve independence in stoma care. While it is ideal that the stoma site not be at the belt line, in many cases this may be the best location and the patient can be instructed in ways to wear a belt over the pouching system. Once the site has been chosen, use a surgical marking pen to create a round circle and cover with a transparent dressing. For many patients an ideal site can be at the apex of the infra-abdominal bulge. However for the patient with an obese abdomen they may not see the lower abdomen and an upper abdominal site may be visible and has less adipose tissue in which to bring up the intestine. In some cases it may be necessary to choose more than one site. Numbering the sites to identify the preferred site is helpful. In situations where there are limited sites (previous surgeries with scarring, significant weight loss creating folds and creases) it may be helpful to identify creases with a dotted pen marked line (in order to avoid if at all possible). Patients who are wheelchair dependent should have their stoma site marked sitting in their chair and the site maybe easier for self-care if in the upper abdominal quadrant. In a situation in which the patient will have two stomas, it is preferable not to have both stomas on the same abdominal plane, because a belt may need to be worn for at least one pouch and if the stomas are on the same plane it may prevent the use of a pouching system belt used for pouch adherence. Marking the pregnant patient can be a challenge since the pregnant abdomen is a temporary size and shape and if the stoma is to be permanent it maybe best to consider a site between the umbilicus and the lower abdominal fold knowing (and being sure to let the patient know) that they may need help placing the pouching system until after the end of the pregnancy. Choosing a site while the patient is on the operating table is a challenge, once the rectus muscle is identified, the abdominal area can be pinched to determine the infra-umbilical bulge, or the abdominal tissue pushed upward and down to look for natural creases or folds.

Stoma Creation

A stoma should protrude above the skin 2–3 cm after eversion to allow the stoma effluent to drain into the pouching system [7, 8]. A stoma that is leveled with the pouch adhesive will cause seal issues as the stoma output can undermine the seal causing leakage and skin irritation [9]. There has been some discussion that a colostomy could have less protrusion but that is not advisable in the patient with Crohn's disease as the stoma output can be liquid and cause pouch seal issues.

An ileostomy is the preferred fecal diversion because the stoma output varies from pasty to watery and can easily be emptied from the pouch with little difficulty. A transverse colostomy is a large stoma usually located above the umbilicus making concealment and management difficult, the stool is odoriferous. A left sided stoma can have pasty to formed stool making it difficult for easy drainage from the pouch with odor. The preferable stoma would be a small bowel stoma.

Postoperative Care

In the postoperative period a clear drainable cut to fit pouch should be used. A cut to fit pouch allows the user to cut the skin barrier on the pouch the same size and shape as the stoma to provide skin protection. As the stoma heals and the postoperative edema subsides the opening in the skin barrier can be changed to match the size of the stoma. If and when the stoma becomes round a precut skin barrier can be used. A clear pouch allows the staff to assess the stoma for color and presence of stoma function (gas and effluent). The first indication of return of bowel function will be the presence of gas in the pouch and this will be evident by gently pressing on the pouch to see if gas has been trapped in the pouch. If the pouching system does not have a secure seal, the gas will exit the pouch, causing odor and preventing an important post-operative observation. The pouch should be placed in the operating room, an opening made in the skin barrier to match the stoma size and the seal should be secured upon application.

Education on self-ostomy care should begin as soon as the person is able to participate and in most cases this should be the first day after surgery. With average length of stay 6 days, teaching should start immediately after surgery. The patient's identified support person should be present for the education as it may be difficult for the patient to retain all of the information on self-care. The patient will need to acquire two skills, to empty the pouch and to change the pouch. All patients or a designated person should know how to empty the pouch before discharge. The pouch is emptied when 1/3rd full and for a person with an ileostomy this would be 5–6 times a day. The routine wear time for a pouching system is 4 days and while it is ideal that the patient knows how to and feels confident that they can change the pouch before discharge this is unlikely. They should have participated in at least one pouch change prior to discharge and in most cases should have a home care nursing service arranged that can continue lessons until they return to the stoma clinic.

In the postoperative period the patient will encounter a large volume of gas as bowel function returns. Because of stoma edema the gas will make noise causing the patient to distress as they may think that the gas amount, volume, and noise will be present moving forward. They need to understand that the volume of gas after abdominal surgery is large and will decrease significantly and that once the post-operative stoma edema decreases there should be no noise from their stoma when gas is released.

Pouching Systems

A pouching system consists of the pouch and any accessory products used to secure the pouch to the skin. A pouch has the following components: a skin barrier, outer water resistant adhesive, the pouch, and a closure. All pouching systems are odor proof when correctly applied. The skin barrier is the most important part of the pouching system as it provides the seal of the system to the skin and protects the skin. The skin barrier is composed of several materials including adhesives and a hydrocolloid. The hydrocolloid will slowly absorb moisture from both the skin and the stoma and over time will erode the adhesive seal, and when this occurs the pouching system will need to be changed. The erosion of the hydrocolloid occurs faster in the presence of moisture such as in a moist humid environment or in the presence of a high liquid stoma output. Once the hydrocolloid significantly erodes, the seal becomes inadequate, allowing stoma effluent to make contact with the skin and causing pouching system adhesive failure. For most fecal stomas wear time (the time between pouch application and erosion of the pouch seal) is 4 days [10]. Frequent removal can cause skin stripping from the aggressive adhesive, allowing the seal to stay in place for a prolonged period of time can cause skin exposure to the stoma output and cause skin damage. Wear time is determined by examining the skin barrier on a removed pouch to determine if the erosion was excessive (the skin barrier next to the stoma will appear discolored and soft). Based upon the degree of erosion, a wear time is determined.

Skin barriers are available in cut to fit, precut or moldable; the opening in the skin barrier should match the size and shape of the stoma (round opening to round stoma, oval opening for oval stoma) [11]. A second characteristic of a skin barrier is the shape, flat or convex (referring to the back of the skin barrier, the adhesive surface toward the skin.) There are several considerations when deciding when to use a flat or convex skin barrier. The peristomal skin should be examined when the person is laying, standing, and sitting. The area is examined for the presence of creases and/or folds. If the area around the stoma is flat in all positions, a flat barrier should be successful in maintaining the skin barrier seal [9]. If creases and folds are found, these can compromise the seal and a convex barrier can help to flatten the creases. The convex shape can help to keep the peristomal skin flat to enhance the seal. A second consideration for the use of convexity would be a stoma that does not protrude above the skin barrier causing a seal problem (the stoma effluent discharges under the skin barrier) [12]. A convex adhesive can apply pressure directly around the stoma to help with stoma protrusion. A third consideration for the use of convexity maybe when the lumen of the stoma is near or flush to the skin. In some cases the stoma has adequate protrusion but the lumen is off to the side close to the skin and the stoma output drains under the skin barrier. The convex skin barrier can help the stoma lumen protrude up over the skin barrier edge.

Accessory items can be used to protect peristomal skin and enhance the seal and include skin barrier paste, rings, liquid skin barriers, and pouch belts. The skin barrier rings and paste are used around the stoma to protect skin and improve the seal, liquid skin barriers provide a protective surface to protect skin from stoma effluent, and a pouch belt can be used to enhance the security of a seal, especially with a convex skin barrier.

The pouch is in many ways the least important part of the pouching system because the skin barrier is the critical component as it provides the seal and security. Pouches collect the stoma effluent and are available in many options including clear, opaque, drainable, non-drainable, various lengths and closures (on a drainable pouch), with and without a gas filter and as a one- or two-piece system. As noted above a clear pouch allows visualization of the stoma and the pouch contents and should be used in the immediate post-operative period and while some patients continue after discharge to use a clear pouch many prefer an opaque pouch. A drainable pouch is used for a person who needs to drain the stool more than twice a day and is most frequently used for a person with an ileostomy; a closed pouch can be removed and discarded when ½ full, and is generally indicated when a person has a left sided colostomy with formed less frequent stoma output. The length of the pouch is usually a patient preference a short pouch (9 in.) may need to be emptied more often than a regular length pouch (12 in.) and the length is a patient decision unless they have high stoma output. A gas filter (a deodorized gas vent) and pouch closures are again a patient preference.

Another pouching system choice is a one- or two-piece pouching system. A one-piece pouching system is constructed with the solid skin barrier and the pouch as one unit, the pouch is heat sealed onto the skin barrier. Considerations of using a one-piece pouching system: a flat peristomal profile with the pouch on as compared to many of the two-piece pouching systems, only a single seal (no risk of detachment of skin barrier to pouch) and the possible difficulty of placing the pouch over the stoma when using an opaque pouch (can't see through the pouch to center the skin barrier opening over the stoma) [13].

A two-piece pouching system consists of a solid skin barrier with a flange that accepts the pouch. Considerations in using a two-piece pouching system: ability to center the skin barrier around the stoma with no pouch in place providing easy visualization, being able to change the pouch without removing the skin barrier, capability to use a pouch liner, profile of the plastic flange under clothing (the coupling mechanism has a slight protrusion), and security of the pouch and flange connection.

Post-Operative Follow-Up

All patients with a new stoma should have follow-up in the stoma clinic 3–4 weeks after surgery. This will give the ostomy nurse the opportunity to assess the patient's ability to self-manage, to resize the stoma and make the necessary adjustments to the pouching system and determine if the patient is working toward integrating the stoma into their daily lives. Most patients don't really know what to ask about living with a stoma while in the hospital but as they live with a stoma they begin to look for answers to questions about diet, clothing, concealment, and return to activities such as sports, work, intimacy, and travel. Ongoing follow-up with the ostomy nurse is key to provide problem solving and continued surveillance. Hurlufsen et al. [14] examined 202 individuals with stomas and found that 57 % of the participants with an ileostomy and 35 % with a colostomy had peristomal skin issues, only 38 % knew they had a problem and more than 80 % did not seek professional help, illustrating the need for continued follow-up and education.

Complications

Reports in the literature note that between 21 and 70 % of all people with an ostomy will develop a peristomal or stoma complication [15]. The reports differ because of varying reporting time frames, lack of a standard definitions, and lack of measurement techniques. However it is clear that many people with a stoma will encounter stoma related complications. Duchesne et al. [16] examined independent predictors of stoma related complications and found obesity and the presence of IBD (no identification of Crohn's disease vs. ulcerative colitis) as risk factors for development of stoma related complications. Carlstedt et al. [17] reported on stoma specific complications in patients with IBD and found a greater proportion of stoma related complications in patients with Crohn's disease. The following complications will be presented: peristomal skin irritation, peristomal fistula, peristomal pyoderma gangrenosum (PPG), stoma stricture, and high output stoma.

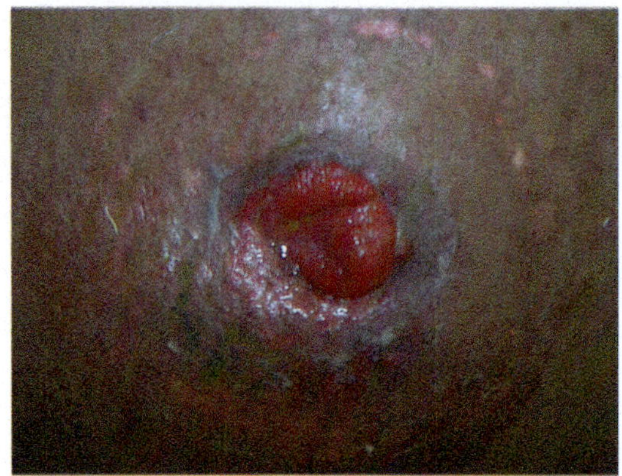

Fig. 20.1 Irritant contact dermatitis: stoma output damaging peristomal skin [28, with permission]

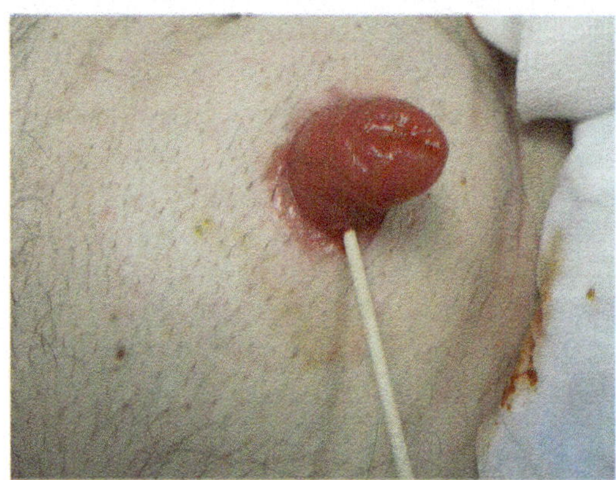

Fig. 20.2 Stoma fistula

Peristomal skin irritation (Fig. 20.1) is described as irritant contact dermatitis (ICD) or allergic contact dermatitis. ICD is defined as damage to the peristomal skin resulting from exposure to fecal effluent or chemical preparations [18]. The etiology of ICD is a poor pouching system fit (not matching the shape or size of the skin barrier opening to the stoma shape or size or not matching the shape of the skin barrier to the peristomal skin [flat versus convex]) or prolonged wear time (allowing the skin barrier to erode and allow the stoma effluent to contact the skin). Patients with difficult to fit and/or poorly located stomas are at highest risk for developing skin complications [19]. Once the etiology is determined and corrected the skin can be treated with a skin barrier powder to absorb the moisture of the denuded skin and the area should progress toward healing.

A *peristomal fistula* is the abnormal opening in or next to the stoma that drains stool. This finding may indicate recurrence of CD [20], either with active disease or a proximal stricture. Another cause of a peristomal fistula can be a suture placed full thickness through the side of the stoma at the time of creation. The fistula opening is either on the peristomal skin (Fig. 20.2) or on the stoma (Fig. 20.3). In some cases the patient reports peristomal tenderness accompanied by erythema and warmth. This type of finding may indicate a peristomal abscess or the impending development of a peristomal fistula. While the patient is worked up for disease activity,

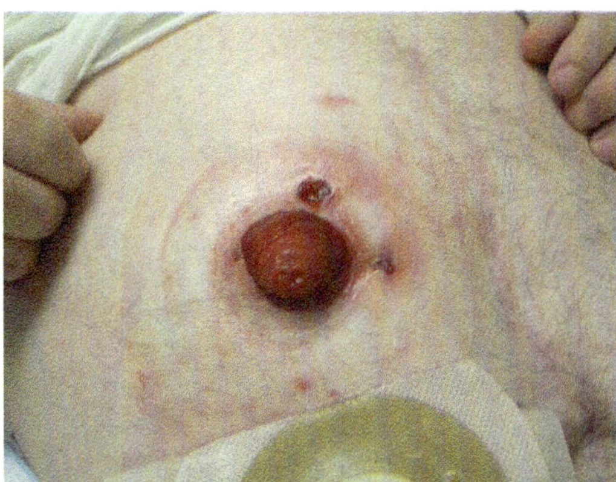

Fig. 20.3 Peristomal fistula

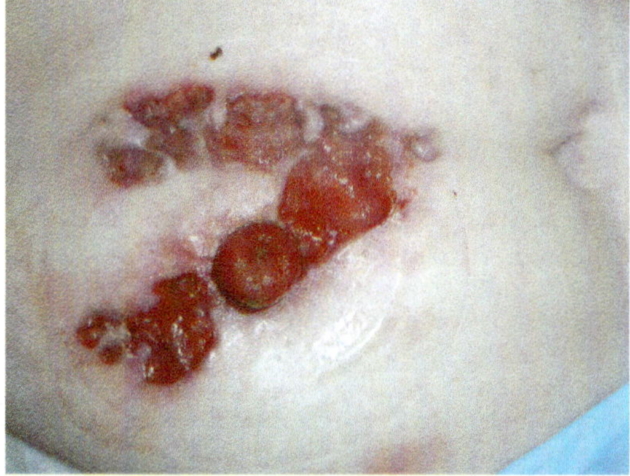

Fig. 20.4 Peristomal pyoderma

the area that is draining the stool will need to be accommodated by the pouch with an opening created in the skin barrier to allow the stool to drain in the pouch. In some instances if the fistula is more than 4 in. out from the stoma a separate pouching system will need to be used, generally a challenge since the two pouches can be difficult to utilize in a small area with little room for both adhesives.

PPG is a rare complication thought to be seen more frequently in the patient with ulcerative colitis than Crohn's disease [21] (Fig. 20.4). The true incidence is unknown with only a limited amount of cases reported in the literature [22]. This inflammatory ulcerative condition frequently begins as a pustule, and quickly becomes a painful full thickness ulcer. The patient may note a sore red area on the peristomal skin and at the next pouch change notes a much larger area that has a purple area surrounding the ulcer, with a deep painful ulcer or ulcers, undermining and skin bridges. While there is no diagnostic tool to identify PPG, some clinicians will perform a biopsy to rule out other etiologies. The cause of PPG is unclear, thought to be related to pathergy (pouch adhesive skin injury) [21] and also thought to relate to disease activity. Topical treatment is aimed toward decreasing the inflammatory response by using topical immunomodulators such as tacrolimus [23] or steroids (injection or paste). The challenge is to maintain a seal on the pouch despite a moist wet wound that loosens the skin barrier. To absorb the moisture and assist with the seal, there are several options that can be considered. An alginate dressing can be placed into the wound base to absorb the excessive moisture and this can be covered by a thin hydrocolloid (when the moisture is controlled with the alginate dressing) or a small piece of non-adhesive foam (for further moisture control when there is an overwhelming amount of moisture). The pouching system may need to be changed more often as the seal can be undermined by the drainage. A topical gel anesthetic can be used at pouch change in order to cleanse the wound without excessive pain. Systemic therapy should be considered along with topical therapy and can include high dose steroids and/or infliximab [24]. As the area(s) heal, scar tissue can develop which will leave the area with uneven contours necessitating a change in the type or shape of the skin barrier.

Stoma stenosis is a narrowing or contracting of the stoma at skin or fascial level. Stomal stenosis is reported in 2–15 % of the stoma and is more common in Crohn's patients [25]. While it is rare for the stenosis to present an acute obstruction, the patient may initially report a "noisy stoma" when stool or gas passes, or pain when a high fiber food is eaten. The stoma may appear to have retracted and when a digital exam is attempted the stoma lumen may not easily be digitalized.

The stoma should be examined closely for signs of recurrence of disease; a referral for workup of recurrence of disease is warranted as the stenosis may reflect inflammatory activity [26].

High stoma output has been identified as a management issue for patients and clinicians but is poorly reported in the literature. Tilney et al. [27] reported in a meta-analysis four studies that included high stoma output as a complication. Dehydration from high ostomy output can result in early readmission, electrolyte imbalances, and renal impairment. Normal ileostomy output (total small intestine intact) varies between 1,000 and 1,200 ml/24 h. It is imperative that ostomy output be measured and recorded in the post-operative period to determine if the patient is at risk for high output. If high ostomy output is found, it will be important to rule out a partial or intermittent bowel obstruction (due to bowel edema), abdominal sepsis, enteritis (such as c diff.), or sudden drug withdrawal (opiates or corticosteroids). Patient education is key to prevent or for early identification of dehydration as this frequently occurs post discharge. The plan of care may include the following: the use of isotonic fluids, restriction of hypo and hyper tonic fluids, dietary restrictions of high sugar foods and fluids, dietary inclusions of starch based foods, the use of antidiarrheal medications [28, 29].

Conclusion

Helping a patient with a new ostomy takes a coordinated team approach and ongoing access to an ostomy nurse specialist. It is the health care team's responsibility on not just "curing" the disease by removing the diseased bowel, but to help the patient move through the adjustment of living with a stoma and help them return to an optimal psychological and social well-being [2]. This will include a thorough pre-operative preparation, the best location and creation of the stoma, post op education, adequate follow-up and a program that provides for long-term follow-up of the person with a stoma.

References

1. Hoentjen F, Colwell JC, Hanauer SB. Complications of peristomal recurrence of Crohn's disease: a case report and a review of literature. J Wound Ostomy Continence Nurs. 2012;39:297–301.
2. Krouse RS, Grant M, Rawl SM, et al. Coping and acceptance: the greatest challenge for veterans with intestinal stoma. J Psychosom Res. 2009;66:227–33.
3. American Society of Colon and Rectal Surgeons Committee Members, Wound Ostomy Continence Nurses Society Committee Members. ASCRS and WOCN joint position statement on the value of preoperative stoma marking for patients undergoing fecal ostomy surgery. J Wound Ostomy Continence Nurs. 2007;34:627–8. http://www.fascrs.org/physicians/position_statements/stoma_siting/. Accessed Oct 2014.
4. Person B, Benjamin MD, Ifargan R, Lachter J, Duek S, et al. The impact of preoperative stoma site marking on the incidence of complications, quality of life, and patient's independence. Dis Colon Rectum. 2012; 55:783–7.
5. Bass EM, Del Pino A, Tan A, Pearl RK, Orsay CP, Abcarian H. Does preoperative stoma marking and education by the enterostomal therapist affect outcome? Dis Colon Rectum. 1997;40:440–2.
6. Pittman J, Rawl S, Schmidt C, Grant M, Ko CY, Wendel C, Krouse R. Demographic and clinical factors related to ostomy complications and quality of life in veterans with an ostomy. J Wound Ostomy Continence Nurs. 2008;35:493–503.
7. Cottam J, Richards K, Hasted A, Blackman A. Results of a nationwide prospective audit of stoma complications within 3 weeks of surgery. Colorectal Dis. 2007;9:834–8.
8. Geisler D, Glennon E. Intestinal stomas and their complications. In: Bailey HR, Billingham RP, Stamos MJ, Snyder MJ, editors. Colorectal surgery: expert consult. Philadelphia, PA: Elsevier Health Sciences; 2013.
9. Gray M, Colwell J, Doughty D, Goldberg M, Hoeflok J, Manson A, McNichol L, Rao S. Peristomal moisture-associated skin damage in adults with fecal ostomies: a comprehensive review and consensus. J Wound Ostomy Continence Nurs. 2013;40:389–99.
10. Richbourg L, Fellows J, Arroyave W. Ostomy pouch wear time in the United States. J Wound Ostomy Continence Nurs. 2008;35:504–8.
11. Wound Ostomy and Continence Nurses Society. Colostomy and ileostomy products and tips: best practice for clinicians. Mount Laurel, NJ: Wound Ostomy and Continence Nurses Society; 2013.
12. Colwell JC. Pouching systems. In: Colwell JC, Carmel J, Goldberg MC, editors. Principles of ostomy care. Philadelphia, PA: Wolters Kluwer; 2015 (in press).
13. Wound Ostomy and Continence Nurses Society. Management of the patient with a fecal ostomy: best practice guidelines for clinicians. Mount Laurel, NJ: Wound Ostomy and Continence Nurses Society; 2010.

14. Herlufsen P, Olsen AG, Carlsen B, et al. Study of peristomal skin disorders in patients with permanent stomas. Br J Nurs. 2006;15:854–62.
15. Salvadalena G. Incidence of complications of the stoma and peristomal skin in individuals with colostomy, ileostomy and urostomy: a systematic review. J Wound Ostomy Continence Nurs. 2008;35:596–607.
16. Dushesne JC, Wang Y, Weintraub SL, et al. Stoma complications: a multivariate analysis. Am Surg. 2002;68:961–6.
17. Carlstedt A, Fasth S, Hutlon L, et al. Long term ileostomy complications in patients with ulcerative colitis and Crohn's disease. Int J Colorectal Dis. 1987;2:22–5.
18. Colwell JC, Beitz J. Survey of wound, ostomy and continence (WOC) nurse clinicians on stomal and peristomal complications: a content validation study. J Wound Ostomy Continence Nurs. 2007;34:57–69.
19. Argumugam PJ, Bevan L, Macdonald L, et al. A prospective audit of stomas-analysis of risk factors and complications and their management. Colorectal Dis. 2003;5:49–52.
20. Kann BR. Early stoma complications. Clin Colon Rectal Surg. 2008;21:23–30.
21. Marzano AV, Borghi A, Stadnicki A, et al. Cutaneous manifestations in patients with inflammatory bowel diseases: pathophysiology, clinical features and therapy. Inflamm Bowel Dis. 2014;20(1):213–27.
22. Kwiatt M, Kawata M. Avoidance and management of stomal complications. Clin Colon Rectal Surg. 2013; 26:112–21.
23. Lyon CC, Stapleton M, Smith AJ, Mendelsohn S, et al. Topical tacrolimus in the management of peristomal pyoderma gangrenosum. J Dermatolog Treat. 2001;12:13–7.
24. Brooklyn TN, Dunmill MG, Shetty A, et al. Infliximab for the treatment of pyoderma gangrenosum: a randomized, double blind placebo controlled trial. Gut. 2006;55:505–9.
25. Beraldo S, Titley G, Allan A. Use of W-plasty in stenotic stoma: a new solution for an old problem. Colorectal Dis. 2006;8:715–6.
26. Ecker KW, Gierend M, Kreissler-Haag D, Feifel G. Reoperations at the ileostomy in Crohn's disease reflect inflammatory activity rather than surgical stoma complications alone. Int J Colorectal Dis. 2001;16:76–80.
27. Tilney HA, Sains PS, Lovegrove RE, et al. Comparison of outcomes following ileostomy versus colostomy for defunctioning colorectal anastomosie. World J Surg. 2007;31:1142–51.
28. Baker ML, Williams RN, Nightingale JM. Causes and management of a high output stoma. Colorectal Dis. 2011;13:191–7.
29. Colwell J, Goldberg M, Carmel J. Fecal & urinary diversions. New York, NY: Elsevier; 2004.

Diet and Nutrition in the Treatment of Crohn's Disease

21

Diane R. Javelli

Abbreviations

CD	Crohn's disease
EN	Enteral nutrition
FODMAPS	Fermentable oligo- di-mono saccharides and polyols
IBD	Inflammatory bowel disease
MSVS	Multivitamin mineral supplement
SCFA	Short chain fatty acids
TPN	Total parenteral nutrition
UC	Ulcerative colitis

Diet and Nutrition in the Treatment of Crohn's Disease

Chronic inflammatory disorders such as CD affect the intestinal tract and digestive system in a myriad of ways that can lead to suboptimal nutrition [1]. Intestinal inflammation and diarrhea may cause malabsorption of macro and micro nutrients leading to weight loss, nutrient deficiencies, and development of malnutrition in up to 85 % of patients [2]. Food ingestion itself is often associated with undesirable symptoms such as abdominal pain, nausea, vomiting, and diarrhea which in turn may decrease nutrient intake. Other clinical manifestations of CD such as anorexia, oral ulcers, and fatigue can further decrease patient ability or desire to eat [3].

Following a proper diet may improve symptoms of CD, enable healing of intestinal mucosa by providing adequate nutrients, and gives patients a sense of control in the management of their disease. Patients in good nutritional status are more likely to utilize their medications, have higher energy levels, exhibit fewer gastrointestinal symptoms, and have better immunity to fight infections and heal intestinal mucosa [4].

However, patients often follow self-imposed restrictive diets in an effort to feel better and on the advice of friends, family, healthcare professionals, or the Internet. Websites and social media have increased patient access to medical and nutritional resources but unfortunately they also serve as a source of confusing and unreliable information. Many of these diet approaches only serve to put patients at further risk of nutrient deficiencies by encouraging them to unnecessarily avoid foods or whole groups of foods thereby eliminating valuable nutrients, calories, and protein. The healthcare professional can guide patients toward reliable sources of information. Patients newly diagnosed with CD, nutritional complications, or those seeking nutritional advice should be guided to establish care with a Registered Dietitian Nutritionist [1].

A recent review of diet and IBD found diets high in fat and meat consumption like those consumed

D.R. Javelli, RDCD (✉)
Department of Outpatient Nutrition, University of Washington Medical Center,
1959 NE Pacific Street, 98195 Seattle, WA, USA
e-mail: djavelli@uw.edu

A. Fichera and M.K. Krane (eds.), *Crohn's Disease: Basic Principles*,
DOI 10.1007/978-3-319-14181-7_21, © Springer International Publishing Switzerland 2015

in westernized countries were associated with an increased disease risk while diets high in fiber, fruits, and vegetables were linked to lower disease risk [5]. However the effect of this type of diet on current disease activity was not studied.

The goals of diet therapy should be aimed at meeting nutritional needs to optimize body weight and muscle mass, prevent and correct nutrient deficiencies, prevent dehydration, and minimize gastrointestinal symptoms. The diet prescription should be individually tailored to provide adequate calories, carbohydrate, protein, fats, vitamins, minerals, fluid and address symptom management [6]. While no specific food or type of diet has been proven to cure CD, excluding certain foods has been shown to be beneficial during a disease flare. Limiting insoluble fiber from whole grains, fruits, and vegetables is advised during a flare, as is decreasing caffeine and alcohol intake. Lactose may also need to be reduced or avoided. Foods to consume during a flare include diluted juices, canned fruit, lean poultry and fish, eggs, potatoes, white bread, rice, and noodles [7]. In this chapter we will examine the dietary needs of patients with CD, common nutritional complications, how to identify and treat nutrient deficiencies, and specific recommendations for patients with particular types or complications of CD.

Calories

Obtaining adequate caloric intake can be difficult when poor appetite is present or eating leads to increased symptoms. Achieving optimal caloric intake is important to provide energy to fuel body functions, daily activities, and promote healing. Caloric needs can be estimated at 25–35 kcals/kg for those patients that are underweight or normal weight. Diet should be advanced slowly in order to not overfeed patients that are severely underweight. A calorie range of 15–25 kcals/kg may be more appropriate for obese individuals (BMI > 30) but caution should be used to not restrict calories at the expense of providing adequate nutrients for healing [8]. Small, frequent meals throughout the day should be encouraged as the intestinal tract may better tolerate smaller volumes. Calorically dense foods should be offered when tolerated to enhance the ability to meet nutritional needs with smaller volumes of food.

Carbohydrates

The body's preferred fuel source is carbohydrate which includes foods such as rice, bread, grains, potatoes, cereals, crackers, fruits, and vegetables. During a flare low fiber refined grains and peeled cooked vegetables are frequently recommended. While there is no evidence that such foods prevent or cure CD, patients frequently report symptom reduction with this type of diet [9].

Sugar is often claimed to be responsible for a host of health problems including a role in development of inflammation. Many high sugar foods have a high glycemic load that can cause dramatic changes in insulin levels that may lead to increased inflammation. There also seems to be a correlation between high refined sugar consumption and development of CD [10]. In contrast, interventional studies have not proven that avoidance of sugar is beneficial in the treatment of CD [11]. Foods containing sugars provide a source of calories which may be beneficial for patients struggling to meet caloric needs. However, diets high in sugar are often lower in vitamins, minerals, and protein; therefore, moderate sugar consumption is likely a prudent long-term goal.

There is evidence that monosaccharides such as fructose may be poorly absorbed in the small intestine therefore leading to symptoms of gas, bloating, diarrhea, or even constipation. In these instances an elimination diet to remove or reduce these types of sugars may be useful [12].

Protein

Patients with CD often have increased protein needs particularly during a flare because intestinal inflammation impairs nutrient absorption leading to possible protein malabsorption. Protein requirements are also elevated due to losses from severe diarrhea and high output fistulas. It is important to help patients achieve maximal protein needs to support healing. Protein requirements should be evaluated individually based on current intake as well as disease state and may be up to 50 % higher (or 1.0–1.5 g/kg body weight) in a patient experiencing a severe flare [8].

Unfortunately, many IBD patients find they don't have an appetite for, don't tolerate, or choose not to eat meat. The practitioner must look for creative ways to help the patient meet protein needs. Lean sources of protein are typically tolerated best such as chicken, turkey, fish, and eggs. Low-fat milk, yogurt, and cheeses are good protein sources if individual tolerates lactose. Nut butters while higher in fat may also be well tolerated.

If patient can tolerate eggs, dairy, or soy foods, they may be added to diet. Use of a protein powder or nutritional supplement drink can also be encouraged to help maximize protein intake. Vegetarian patients, especially Vegans may have a more difficult time meeting protein needs since the diet restricts many of the common protein containing foods. However, it is important to honor individual food preferences and guide patients toward food sources that both meet their personal preferences and nutritional needs.

Fat

High fat or greasy foods can be problematic because they may exacerbate symptoms of diarrhea, gas, and bloating. A low fat diet is also advised when fat malabsorption is present. Patients often identify deep fried foods, foods rich in butter or cream, or cheese dishes as symptom provoking foods [9, 11]. Intolerance to lactose could be a factor in some of these foods as well. It is important to note that not all patients get symptoms from high fat foods and for these patients fat can be a good source of calories, especially if they are struggling to maintain weight. In addition olive oil, avocado, nut butters, and sources of omega 3 fats such as tuna and salmon may have anti-inflammatory properties [2].

Fiber

A low fiber diet is the most common diet recommended for treatment of CD symptoms. However, low fiber diets have not shown a definite benefit to control disease or inflammation. In fact some researchers have concluded that including fiber in the diet may have beneficial effects because digestion of dietary fiber produces short chain fatty acids (SCFA) in the colon which may help restore immune tolerance and decrease intestinal inflammation [13]. SCFAs include lactic, formic, acetic, propionic, isobutyric, butyric, and pyruvic acids. SCFA are found both in foods and produced in the colon when bacteria digest non-absorbable carbohydrates. However, despite these conclusions many patients correlate increased pain and diarrhea with an increased fiber intake and note a decrease in these symptoms when dietary fiber is limited, especially raw fruits, vegetables, nuts, seeds, and whole grains. Therefore a low fiber diet is reasonable in a patient with active disease [9]. Insoluble fibers such as seeds, strings, i.e. from beans or celery, and thick fruit skins are especially difficult to tolerate while soluble fiber may be better tolerated because of its ability to absorb water softening the fiber into a gel. This in turn may change the consistency of the stool and slow intestinal transit and diarrhea [1]. Soluble fiber examples include: pectin and gums which are found mainly in the flesh of fruits and vegetables as well as some grains such as oats. Beans are a good source of soluble fiber but may not be tolerated due to the insoluble fiber present in the bean skin. Hummus, pureed refried beans, and pea soup may be tolerated due to the processing of that skin. However, beans and legumes can lead to increased intestinal gas and bloating. In an effort to increase the fiber content of packaged foods many manufacturers are adding soluble fiber to their products. Inulin and chicory root are two types of soluble fiber that are now being added to foods such as yogurt, yogurt drinks, meal replacement bars, and fiber bars. While these types of soluble fibers may be tolerated in small amounts, the large amounts being added to packaged foods often cause more gas and bloating in patients.

In general a low fiber diet should be recommended when patients are symptomatic and diet should be liberalized as their condition improves per patient tolerance. Exceptions include patients with new ostomies, recent intestinal surgery, or intestinal narrowing due to inflammation or strictures, which often requires a low fiber or liquid diet [11].

Lactose

Studies have shown lactose and dairy products to be frequently reported intolerances among patients with CD. Common complaints include gas, bloating, and diarrhea likely due to poor absorbability in the small intestine [14]. It can be difficult to distinguish between lactose intolerance and symptoms of active disease. However, dairy products are rich in calcium, vitamin D, and protein and should not be restricted unless patient has known symptoms with ingestion. Patients may exhibit lactose intolerance during a flare but not in remission [4]. Lactose intolerance is dose dependent and people are often able to tolerate small servings of dairy products. For those with frank lactose intolerance lactose free dairy products and lactase enzyme supplements are available.

Caffeine and Alcohol

Caffeine can act as a stimulant to the intestinal tract, increasing frequency of diarrhea. In addition, caffeinated drinks are less hydrating due to their diuretic effect. In cases with severe diarrhea a decrease in caffeine may be beneficial. Alcohol can also irritate the GI tract and can interfere with the action of some medications [1]. One study concluded that patients were more likely to report intolerance to energy drinks, diet colas, colas, champagne, red wine, and beer [6]. Since individual tolerance varies greatly complete avoidance of caffeine and alcohol may not be necessary.

Nutritional Assessment

CD patients are at risk for poor nutritional status and should therefore be screened for nutritional complications at the time of diagnosis, during flare ups, when strictures are present, if surgery is required and at least annually. Validated nutrition screening tools have been developed that ask a series of questions to guide the practitioner in determining if patients are currently at nutritional risk. Subjective global assessment (SGA), nutrition risk screening 2002 (NRS-2002), malnutrition universal screening tool (MUST), and nutritional risk index (NRI) are examples of these tools and can be incorporated into practice to determine nutritional status of the patient. These screening tools include questions to help the practitioner identify changes indicating an increased risk for malnutrition such as weight loss, decrease in appetite, or inability to take food orally due to nausea, swallowing difficulty, fatigue, or diarrhea. Calculation of the Body Mass Index alone is often misleading because it may not accurately distinguish between well-nourished patients and those that are undernourished. If a patient is identified at nutritional risk, a complete nutritional assessment, review of diet history, and development of an individual care plan by a Registered Dietitian is recommended [15].

Collecting lab data is essential to identify nutrient deficiencies such as iron, B12, and zinc but is not particularly helpful in diagnosing protein calorie malnutrition. A serum albumin level was once thought to be the gold standard for identifying protein malnutrition. However, using albumin level as an indicator of protein status is ineffective in the presence of chronic inflammation. Inflammation in the body triggers the liver to reduce production of negative acute phase proteins such as albumin, prealbumin, and transferrin in favor of manufacturing positive acute phase proteins such as C-reactive protein to help fight inflammation. Albumin, like the other negative acute phase proteins is expected to return to normal as the inflammatory response resolves [16]. Therefore a low albumin does not always indicate a malnourished state or an inadequate intake of protein, nor does a normal albumin level indicate that the patient is well nourished. However, protein needs are elevated in patients with chronic inflammation. A thorough diet history should be completed and if intake found to be inadequate an effort should be made to add high protein foods, protein powders, or nutritional supplement drinks. In some cases enteral or total parenteral nutrition (TPN) may be needed but only if the patient is unable to meet nutritional needs with oral intake. A low albumin level in isolation is not an indicator for initiation of TPN.

Nutritional Complications and Deficiencies

Nutritional deficiencies in CD are common for a number of reasons: decreased appetite leading to inadequate intake of nutrients, decreased nutrient absorption due to small bowel inflammation, reduced intestinal transit time due to diarrhea which can limit absorption of nutrients, and surgical resection. Additionally, a decreased desire to eat to prevent extra trips to the bathroom, restricted diets, and pain/discomfort with meals or after eating can also lead to deficiencies. The most common nutrient deficiencies found in patients with CD are iron, vitamin B12, vitamin D, calcium, magnesium, folic acid, and zinc. Anemia is frequently associated with CD and while most often related to iron deficiency, anemia related to folic acid and vitamin B12 deficiencies are also common occurrences. A thorough workup should be completed to determine the type of anemia to ensure proper treatment. The prevalence of anemia is higher in CD patients than in UC but can be present in both, leading to fatigue, hospitalization, and delay of discharge [17]. Anemia of chronic disease is another common occurrence and should be considered as well. Inadequate intake of vitamin D and calcium as well as malabsorption can lead to osteoporosis.

Since nutrient deficiencies are common in patients with active inflammation and poor oral intake a daily multivitamin (with or without iron) as well as calcium and vitamin D is typically prescribed. In some cases a patient may require additional iron. Lab data should be collected to establish baseline nutritional status at initial appointment and at least annually. If nutrient deficiency is detected, then follow-up blood work should be obtained to ascertain correction of the deficiency.

Iron

Iron deficiency anemia is common in patients with CD and is most often linked to blood loss from the intestinal tract, poor absorption due to rapid transit time, and a poor quality diet. The primary site of iron absorption is the duodenum. The active bleeding that may occur with CD makes it difficult for duodenal absorption to keep up with actual losses. Iron deficiency anemia can result and supplementation with 60–120 mg elemental iron daily is recommended [17]. It is advised to co-administer a source of vitamin C with ferrous forms of iron such as a standard 250 mg vitamin C tablet or 3 ounces of a beverage containing vitamin C. However oral iron is often poorly tolerated causing symptoms of nausea, abdominal pain, diarrhea, or constipation which makes it difficult to distinguish between the disease and tolerability of iron supplementation. IV iron infusions may be indicated in those with intolerance to oral iron, moderate to severe anemia <10.5 Hgb, or inefficacy of oral iron [18, 19]. A standard infusion of iron sucrose twice a week for 2 weeks followed by once weekly for additional 6 weeks is typically adequate to see improvement in iron stores [17].

Vitamin B12 (Cobalamin)

Vitamin B12 deficiency has been noted in up to 48 % of patients. The primary absorption site for vitamin B12 is the terminal ileum, therefore vitamin B12 deficiency is more common in patients with Crohn's disease than ulcerative colitis. Vitamin B12 levels should be monitored and if below normal range should be treated with intra-muscular injection of 1,000 μg vitamin B12 monthly.

Oral vitamin B12 may be administered at dosages of 1,000 μg daily but may not be effective in those with inflammation of the ileum due to impaired absorption. Sublingual or intra-nasal vitamin B12 may be good options as well. Patients with areas of resected ileum >30 cm, jejunostomies, and some ileostomies are also more susceptible to vitamin B12 deficiency and should be supplemented [20].

Vitamin D

Vitamin D absorption takes place in the small intestine so inflammation at this site can lead to deficiency. In addition many people are prone to vitamin D deficiency, especially in northern latitudes. Furthermore patients with fatigue may spend less time outdoors leading to less vitamin D exposure from the sun. Poor appetite and restricted diets, especially in those avoiding dairy products due to lactose intolerance may be an additional cause for deficiency [21]. As a precaution all patients with active CD can be given a daily vitamin D supplement of 1,000–2,000 IU daily of vitamin D3 (cholecalciferol). Vitamin D can be given separately or in combination with calcium or multivitamin supplement. A vitamin 25 OH level should be tested and if found to be deficient(<20 ng/ml) patient should be treated with a recommended dosage of 50,000 IU vitamin D2 (ergocalciferol) once weekly for 6–8 weeks. Check vitamin D level after 8 weeks and if within normal limits reduce dosage to 1,000–2,000 IU daily of vitamin D3. Vitamin D levels of <30 mg/dl are considered suboptimal and may respond to treatment with 2,000 IU daily [22].

Calcium

CD can lead to a loss of bone, osteopenia, and osteoporosis by a variety of mechanisms. Calcium absorption occurs both through active transport in the duodenum and upper jejunum as well as passive absorption throughout the small bowel. Intestinal inflammation, rapid transit of nutrients through the small bowel, and inadequate intake of calcium containing foods due to lactose avoidance further place patient at risk for decreased bone density. Patients requiring steroid therapy such as prednisone are at additional risk for bone loss. A daily dosage of 1,500–2,000 mg is recommended. Calcium is most efficiently absorbed in doses of 500 mg TID. Adequate vitamin D intake is crucial for absorption of calcium.

Zinc

Absorption of zinc occurs predominantly in the jejunum but also throughout the small intestine, therefore inflammation and diarrhea can cause excess zinc losses. Serum levels of zinc should be tested but because zinc is transported in part by albumin, low levels may be indicative of active inflammation or hypoalbuminemia. If the serum zinc level is <60 mcg/dl, supplementation of 50 mg of elemental zinc in the form of 220 mg zinc sulfate or 350 mg zinc gluconate should be prescribed. Zinc has an inverse relationship to copper and therefore high dosages of zinc can lead to copper deficiency. Retest zinc level after 6–8 weeks. Once inflammation is resolved normal zinc levels should be achieved by taking a daily multivitamin/mineral supplement that contains zinc [23, 24].

Copper

Copper deficiency is not typically noted in CD but can be caused by severe diarrhea, fistulas, ostomies, or zinc supplementation. If a patient is on high dosages of zinc, testing of serum copper is advised. Supplemental dosage to correct copper deficiency is 2–4 mg daily [25, 26].

Magnesium

Assessment of magnesium status is challenging because much of our body stores of magnesium are inside the cell or bone. Serum magnesium level is the most common measurement of magnesium concentration; however, a correlation with total body stores may be inaccurate.

Frequent diarrhea, inadequate oral intake, and/or treatment with immune suppressors such as tacrolimus or cyclosporine can cause reduced serum levels of magnesium [27]. If serum magnesium level is determined to be low supplemental magnesium chloride or magnesium oxide may be used. A dosage of 64 mg elemental magnesium has been suggested [28]. Severe hypomagnesiumemia often requires IV administration of magnesium.

Fat Soluble Vitamins ADEK

Deficiency of vitamins ADE and K may occur due to fat malabsorption. Water soluble vitamins ADEK may be more absorbable in these patients. However no standardized recommendations are available to guide practitioners as to optimal dosages specifically to prevent or treat deficiencies associated with CD [8].

Folate

Folate deficiency has been reported in up to 67 % of patients with CD. Decreased intake of folate containing foods such as green leafy vegetables or beans is common in CD patients. Furthermore a number of medications used to treat CD such as sulfasalazine and methotrexate can impair absorption of folate. Therefore folic acid supplementation of 1–2 mg/day is advised to prevent deficiency [29].

Complications of IBD Requiring Special Diet

Food Allergies/Food Intolerances

Food Allergies have not been positively linked to the development of CD. While CD is not caused by food allergies some people with CD do have allergies to certain foods and this should be taken into consideration when making dietary recommendations. Food intolerances are much more common in the patient with CD than are food allergies. Food allergies affect about 4–8 % of the population and are immune mediated, while food intolerances are much more prevalent and do not involve the immune system. The most common food allergens are proteins found in dairy products, wheat, soy, eggs, tree nuts, peanuts, fish, and shellfish. Food intolerances or non-allergic food hypersensitivity are usually diagnosed after food allergies and other gastrointestinal conditions have been ruled out [30]. Many patients with CD have food intolerances. Common food intolerances include lactose, fructose, and gluten.

Gluten

While many patients report good tolerance to refined grain products and starches some patients report a decrease in symptoms with exclusion of grains. One study in a subgroup of IBD patients found that those with significant intestinal symptoms reported a decrease in those symptoms and a decrease in numbers of reported flares while following a gluten free diet. Researchers did note a possible link to fermentable Oligo, Di, Mono saccharides, and polyols (FODMAPs), i.e. fructans, a fermentable carbohydrate found in wheat and other grains rather than gluten itself [31]. While patients often correlate symptom improvement to the exclusion of gluten it may actually be related to a decrease in fructans [14]. To date a gluten free diet has not been indicated for use in treatment of CD except in those patients with known celiac or non celiac gluten sensitivity.

Fermentable Oligo, Di, Mono Saccharides and Polyols

The most typical approach to managing food intolerances is to initiate a food elimination diet to determine if symptoms improve when foods are removed from the diet. Foods are then added back to the diet systematically to determine which foods produce symptoms. One elimination diet in particular has been researched thoroughly and is becoming standard of practice for management of food intolerance. FODMAPs are categories of sugars and starches found commonly in the diet. In CD patients that struggle with gas, bloating, diarrhea, or even constipation especially in a state of disease remission, reduction of these fermentable carbohydrates may be beneficial. In the past decade considerable research has shown that eliminating sources of fermentable saccharides can help reduce these symptoms. FODMAPs include sugars found in milk, fruit, honey, high fructose corn syrup, and fibers found in foods like wheat, onions, vegetables, and beans. These FODMAPs may be poorly absorbed in the small intestine leaving them to travel down to the large intestine where colonic bacteria feed on them and produce carbon dioxide, hydrogen, and methane gas. This malabsorption can lead to development of excessive gas, painful bloating, diarrhea, or constipation. Diet treatment involves following a FODMAPs Elimination diet to remove all sources of FODMAPs from the diet for at least 2 weeks and observing the patient to see if symptoms improve. After an elimination period, a FODMAPs Challenge diet is implemented by adding specific groups back into diet and observing for return of symptoms [14]. A telephone survey of 72 Australian participants found that a majority of those queried had significant improvement of symptoms when adherent to a low FODMAP diet. Symptomatic improvement included a decrease in abdominal pain, bloating, gas, and diarrhea [32]. A Registered Dietitian should be consulted to help patients understand and adhere to the diet without imposing too many additional restrictions and further risking nutrient deficiencies.

Calcium Oxalate Stones

Kidney stones occur in up to 18 % of adult patients with IBD especially in those with inflammation or resection of the small bowel [33]. Typically calcium binds to oxalate to be excreted from the body but in the presence of fat malabsorption calcium binds to fat instead. Circulating oxalate is then available to be absorbed and deposited in the kidney causing stone formation. Dehydration is also a factor in development of stones because highly concentrated urine is more likely to lead to stone formation. Dietary therapy includes a low oxalate, low fat diet with adequate fluid intake to help lower urine concentration [34]. Reducing sodium intake to $<3,000$ mg/day may put more calcium into circulation to bind oxalate. Avoidance of vitamin C supplements is recommended to help reduce levels of oxalates in the urine and calcium supplementation is advised to help bind oxalate in the intestine. Other factors such as hypocitraturia, hypomagnesuria, and uric acid stones should be considered as well in those with kidney stone formation [35].

Strictures

Narrowing of the intestinal lumen due to scar tissue or strictures often causes pain with eating and impacts ability to maintain nutritional status requiring special dietary considerations. A low fiber diet is typically recommended for patients with strictures. Ingestion of vegetable and fruit skins or strings, nuts, seeds, popcorn, and possibly large chunks of fibrous meats can be problematic in a narrowed intestinal tract if they are too large to pass through the strictured area. In cases of severe strictures a soft or liquid diet may be recommended until resolution of inflammation or surgical repair of strictured site. Pain at the site of the stricture is sometimes severe and can diminish patient desire to eat. Use of nutritional supplement drinks or supplemental nutrition such as TPN or EN may be necessary if severe [8].

Ostomies

Complications of CD can lead to the need for surgical resection of the small intestine or colon requiring the creation of an ostomy. Most nutrient absorption occurs in the upper small intestine so those patients with end ileostomies and colostomies are likely to remain well nourished. Shorter ileostomies and jejunostomies often require additional nutritional support and vitamin supplementation due to loss of absorptive capacity. Therefore strategies similar to those used by patients with short bowel syndrome (SBS) may be beneficial. While there are no specific standards set for diet after ostomy a low fiber diet is often recommended for the first 4–6 weeks with most patients able to return to a normal diet after this time [36]. However due to variations between patients a trial and error period of eating is often needed to identify foods that may cause increased discomfort and stool output.

Nutritional supplements can be useful to provide an additional source of calories, protein, and nutrients especially in the first few weeks after surgery. Many commercial products are high in sugar which due to the osmotic load may increase stool output, especially in those with ileostomies. However, nutritional supplements come in a variety of formulations which may be better tolerated. For example, a high protein lower carbohydrate formula like those available for diabetic patients may increase tolerance. Patients should be encouraged to sip supplements slowly and experiment with different formula preparations until they find one that meets their needs.

Colostomies that are created toward the distal end of the colon are more likely to retain their absorptive capability of fluid, sodium, and potassium, so stool output is closer to normal consistency in these patients. Since stool output is thicker it is important to consume adequate amounts of fluid and fiber to prevent constipation [37].

People with ileostomies lack the benefit of the colon's absorptive capacity of fluid and electrolytes. Sodium and potassium losses can occur due to absence of a functioning colon, therefore salt intake should be liberalized. Foods that are high in potassium such as bananas, cantaloupe, milk, yogurt, and cooked vegetables should be encouraged if tolerated. Ileostomies are also more prone to dehydration and extra fluid may need to be consumed to compensate for losses. However, drinking plain water may lead to an increase in stool output [37]. In those with high stool output it may be beneficial to consume a hypotonic oral rehydration solution (ORS) which contains electrolytes to improve fluid absorption in the ileum. Limiting quantities of fluids consumed at one time and restricting fluid intake to 30 min before and after meals may be beneficial especially in the initial postoperative period [38].

Since decreased fluid absorption in the small intestine creates more liquid stool, thickening the stool effluent may slow down the transit time and allow for better nutrient absorption. Some foods have been found to thicken stool output in the ileostomy patient. Potatoes, white rice, oatmeal, applesauce, peanut butter, bananas, white bread, low fiber crackers, and marshmallows are examples [37].

It is possible that foods that do not get digested well can cause obstruction of the stoma. Blockages occur more frequently in ileostomies than colostomies but can occur in either. Foods such as popcorn, mushrooms, corn, beans, stringy vegetables like celery or sprouts, and dried fruit can be problematic. Peeling fruits and vegetables, cooking foods thoroughly, and chewing well can all help minimize incidence of blockage. Odor can also be a problem for the ostomy patient and therefore elimination of certain foods such as garlic, onions, eggs, beans, and asparagus may be helpful [39].

Short Bowel Syndrome

A detailed discussion of SBS is beyond the scope of this chapter but deserves mention due to prevalence in CD. Patients that have had one or more surgical resections can be at risk for complications due to SBS. SBS can be defined in a number of ways but typically exists when only 100–120 cm of small bowel remains without an intact colon, or 50 cm small bowel with colon. SBS has also been defined as the inability of the bowel to function in a capacity to support fluid and nutrient requirements despite adequate oral intake and regardless of length of intact bowel [40]. In other words, patients with CD can exhibit symptoms of SBS due to marked inflammation encompassing a large area of the GI tract. Symptoms of SBS include increased stool output, steatorrhea, electrolyte imbalance, decreased appetite, weight loss, malabsorption of nutrients [41]. Pt with SBS should be monitored for fat malabsorption and are at special risk for deficiencies of fat soluble vitamins A, D, E, and K. Some patients with SBS may benefit from a small dose of cholestyramine to help bind bile salts if unable to absorb due to missing or non-functioning ileum but caution should be taken because it can also bind vitamins A, D, E, and K furthering risk of deficiency.

Many patients with SBS will require TPN at least initially. However, even patients with as little as 50–60 cm small bowel left may be able to consume an oral diet to partially meet nutritional needs [42]. The ability of patients to return to a normal diet after surgical resection leading to SBS depends on a number of variables: the length of small bowel that remains, the section of the small bowel that remains, whether colon is present with an intact ileocecal valve, and the length of time it takes the remaining intestine to adapt and become more absorptive. Patients with ileal resections greater than 60 cm are more likely to have problems with malabsorption of nutrients, especially vitamin B12. Presence of an intact colon is advantageous to help prevent dehydration and depletion of electrolytes. Food choices, beverages, and composition of diet can all impact stool output and nutrient absorption. Carbohydrates and fermentable fibers can produce SCFA in the colon which can provide a significant source of calories for the patient.

Diet therapy for the patient with SBS is often divided by category: those with an intact colon and those without a colon in continuity. Patients with intact colon are advised to follow a diet that is low in fat and high in carbohydrate with protein to meet individual goals. Patients without a colon should include a higher amount of fat and lower amount of carbohydrate again with adequate protein to meet nutritional needs [40].

Other diet related suggestions for SBS include limiting fluid intake with meals to slow transit time, reduce intake of hypertonic fluids and include isotonic fluids such as ORSs which are better absorbed. A Registered Dietitian should be consulted to assist patients with diet and fluid management and may be able to suggest changes to maximize nutrient intake and reduce amount of required parenteral nutrition. It is important not to underestimate the benefits of small decreases in TPN. Reducing infusion of TPN even a few hours can give patient more freedom to take short trips, do errands, reduces time spent in the bathroom, and carries less risk to the liver.

Nutritional Support: TPN/TF/ Nutritional Supplement Drinks

Weight loss affects up to 80 % of patients with CD. Poor appetite, abdominal pain, and diarrhea are a few of the contributing factors [2]. When patients are unable to meet nutrient needs with regular diet enteral supplementation may be necessary. Enteral nutrition can be delivered orally or via a feeding tube placed in the stomach or small intestine. Enteral nutrition can supplement all or part of one's nutritional needs. There are a variety of commercial nutritional supplement drinks available which offer quick convenient sources of calories, protein, fatty acids, vitamins, and minerals in a form that is typically well tolerated. Homemade protein drinks or smoothies can also be nutritious alternatives. If the patient is unable to tolerate drinking supplements, tube feeding formulas can be introduced.

Exclusive enteral nutrition (EEN) has been particularly effective in pediatric patients to achieve remission and found to be more useful than corticosteroids [43]. However, use of EEN in the adult population has not provided such clear results with some studies suggesting that EEN is not as effective in adults while others have found clear benefits of enteral nutrition to induce clinical remission and promote healing of the mucosa [11, 44]. Additionally elemental products have not been shown to be superior to standard polymeric formulas. Unfortunately intolerance to formulas and inconvenience of tube feeding regimen leads to poor compliance in the adult population [45].

TPN may be indicated when a patient is unable to tolerate enteral feedings. TPN may also be useful in the case of high output diarrhea, stricturing disease, fistulas or in patients with SBS. TPN is very effective in improving nutritional status in patients but has not been shown to be more efficacious than enteral feeding or corticosteroids in inducing remission. TPN is expensive, presents a higher infection risk, and can lead to cholestatic liver disease. In addition complete bowel rest may result in atrophy of intestinal mucosa further decreasing absorptive capacity and may have negative effects on gut microbiota [45]. Therefore, every effort should be made to meet nutritional needs of patient with enteral nutrition prior to initiating TPN [46].

Nutritional Intervention When Surgery Is Required

Up to 66 % of CD patients will need surgical intervention to help control disease or development of strictures [47]. The stress of surgery increases protein, calorie and vitamin/mineral requirements by creating a catabolic and hypermetabolic state. Dependent on nutritional status of the patient prior to surgery malnutrition can result after surgery. Additionally, major surgery can temporarily weaken the immune system making the body more prone to infection. Studies have shown that patients who consume special supplement drinks called immune-modulating supplements prior to surgery have lower complication and infection rates, and may have a shorter hospital stay [48, 49].

In 2009 the Society of Critical Care Medicine (SCCM), in conjunction with the American Society of Parenteral and Enteral Nutrition (A.S.P.E.N.), published guidelines discussing appropriate use of immune-modulating formulas. There are several ingredients that have been shown to support the immune system including arginine, glutamine, dietary nucleotides, omega-3 fatty acids, and antioxidants. The indications for use of these various immune ingredients are discussed at length in their report and are beyond the scope of this chapter. However, in their report SCCM and A.S.P.E.N. make a Grade A recommendation for use of these ingredients with the following patient populations "major elective surgery, trauma, burns, head and neck cancer, and critically ill patients on mechanical ventilation, with caution in patients with severe sepsis" [50].

There are a number of commercial formulas available that contain ingredients shown to have immune-modulating effects. However, only immunonutrition containing supplemental arginine, omega-3 fatty acids, and nucleotides has level 1 evidence showing a significant reduction in risk of infectious complication rates after major surgery [51]. Immune-modulating formulas are available for purchase through a variety of sources, for use under medical supervision. Products can be delivered orally or via tube feedings and should be given several days prior to surgery and again 3–4 days post operatively. It is important to note that the research did not specifically study the CD population but included bowel resection surgeries similar to those done in patients with CD.

Surgeons should be encouraged to actively assess patients for risk of malnutrition by using one of the many nutrition screening tools available: NRS 2002, MUST, SGA, or Strong for Surgery Nutrition checklist [52]. Patients that are determined to be at nutritional risk should be referred to an RD for interventions to improve food, nutrient, fluid intake and discuss available options for immune-modulating formulas immediately pre-op and consideration of use post operatively [53]. Energy needs after surgery have been estimated to be up to 50 % higher than normal energy needs. If oral intake will be delayed due to surgery, a nasogastric tube can be placed and feeding started within 36 h to preserve gut integrity and promote healing [54].

Pre- and Probiotics

Given the association between development of CD and the gut microbiota dietary research has centered on the use of pre and probiotics [11]. Prebiotics are non-digestible food components which help stimulate growth of beneficial bacteria. Examples of prebiotics include fructooligosaccharides (FOS), galactoligosaccharides (GOS), and inulin. Probiotics are microbial ingredients found in foods such as yogurt with live cultures, kefir, and fermented vegetables [8, 9].

FOS and GOS prebiotics may enhance growth of beneficial probiotic bacteria, in particular bifidobacteria and lactobacilli which may have immune regulatory effects. However study results have been mixed with exacerbation of symptoms seen in some subjects [11]. It is also important to note that most prebiotics are FODMAPs and therefore symptoms of gas, bloating, diarrhea, or constipation may occur if incomplete absorption occurs [14]. Pre and probiotics could possibly be used to alter the gut microbiome and used in the treatment of CD but studies to date have only shown clear evidence in patients with UC and pouchitis, not in CD. Additionally, improvement of symptoms with probiotics was more likely to occur in mild disease with better efficacy in maintaining remission rather than inducing remission [55].

Omega 3 and Omega 6 Poly Unsaturated Fatty Acids

Omega 3 fatty acids EPA and DHA are known to have anti-inflammatory effects while omega 6 fatty acids have pro-inflammatory effects. Diets containing higher amounts of omega 6 fatty acids are associated with higher incidence of IBD [56]. Fish oil supplements are high in EPA and DHA and have been shown to decrease the production of some inflammatory mediators. However, studies using fish oil supplements to induce and maintain remission of IBD have shown disappointing results [57]. In an effort to reduce omega 6 fatty acids and increase omega 3 fatty acids patients can be encouraged to include more fatty fish such as salmon and tuna in their diets along with other omega 3 sources including flax oil, flax meal, and omega 3 fortified foods such as cereal and eggs.

Special Diets

Diets that seek to exclude carbohydrates have remained popular over the years. These diets claim that reducing carbohydrate intake will cure IBD by changing the population of gut bacteria. The specific carbohydrate diet (SCD) is one diet that reduces intake of carbohydrates, and grains in particular. The SCD was developed more than 50 years ago and was originally used to treat those with celiac disease. It has gained popularity over the past 20 years in the CD populations due to its claims to reduce intestinal inflammation [58]. These claims have yet to be validated in the adult population but are being studied in pediatric patients and have shown promising results of inducing remission [59]. However, this diet has not adequately been studied outside the pediatric population and more research will need to be done to determine if these diets will provide similar response in adults.

Diet and the Gut Microbiome

Increasing evidence suggests that the microbiome of the gastrointestinal tract plays an important role in triggering, maintaining, and exacerbating illnesses including inflammatory diseases such as CD. A decrease in microbiome diversity may be partially to blame. Some gut bacteria have been found to be beneficial while others may be harmful when overabundant in the gut [55]. However, the type and amount of organisms required to make up a healthy microbiome is not known and may differ between individuals. Healthy persons may have a different microbiome than people with pre-existing illnesses.

There may also be differences in the gut microbiota of different races, i.e. Asians and Africans have been noted to have a more diverse microbiome and more SCFAs present than Europeans. However, it is not known how environmental factors such as sanitation, food storage, and diet play into this [60]. Fermentation is a common practice of food preservation in many parts of the world. Fermentation increases the content of probiotics and SCFAs in foods which may be beneficial to the gut microbiome. However, more reliance on refrigeration for food storage and decreased vegetable intake has led to a decrease in fermented food consumption.

There is increasing evidence that diet itself can change the composition of microbiota in the gut [13] but at present the roles of nutrients, gut microbiome, and environmental factors, i.e. diet have not been clearly defined [10]. There is interest in how absorption of carbohydrates may change the bacterial population of the intestine. Further studies are needed to fully understand the link between diet, the gut microbiome, and CD, and may provide new information about disease pathogenesis and treatment. Additionally more research is needed in all areas of diet to understand other possible links between food consumption, food additives, nutrient intake, nutrient deficiencies and their role in the development and treatment of CD.

The Role of the Registered Dietitian as Part of Multidisciplinary Team

Registered dietitians/nutritionists (RDN) are specially trained in Medical Nutrition Therapy and offer the most comprehensive and safe approach to treating nutritional deficiencies, managing symptoms, and assisting with meal planning in the IBD patient. Patients with IBD are often eager to embrace any lifestyle change they believe will lead to a cure. As a result they are susceptible to questionable advice. Encourage patients to thoroughly review the credentials of anyone claiming to be a "Nutritionist." Many states have no regulations preventing individuals with minimal or no training to call themselves Nutritionists. RD/RDNs are clinically trained to work with patients in conjunction with the health care provider to review labs, nutrient needs, drug nutrient interactions, and prescribe an individual diet plan to treat symptoms associated with CD such as weight loss, gas, bloating, diarrhea, and loss of appetite.

Summary

While diet and nutrition are not known to be curative in CD, the role they play in symptom management and overall wellness is vital to the treatment of any patient with CD. Nutrition does not replace medication or surgical procedures but should be considered a complementary part of treatment. Malnourished patients or those seeking to educate themselves about diet and nutrition can benefit from working with a Registered Dietitian to obtain a nutritional assessment and individualized treatment plan. While to date there is not one specific diet proven to offer sustainable disease control research is offering valuable information to the link between diet and CD. Further exploration is needed to continue to look for answers in order to help find the best treatment and a cure for this disease.

References

1. Diet, nutrition, and inflammatory bowel disease. Crohn's and Colitis Foundation of America. Available at http://www.ccfa.org/assets/pdfs/diet-nutrition-2013.pdf.
2. Lomer M. Symposium 7: nutrition in inflammatory bowel disease dietary and nutritional considerations for inflammatory bowel disease. Proc Nutr Soc. 2011; 70:329–35.
3. Lichtenstein G, et al. Management of Crohn's disease in adults. American College of Gastroenterology. Available at: www.gicare.org/guidelines/management-of-crohn's-disease-in-adults/. 2009.
4. Long M, Cimperman L. Food for thought: nutrition & IBD. Crohn's and Colitis Foundation of America; 2013 Sept 4. www.ccfa.org. Available at www.ccfa.org/resources/food-for-thought.html.
5. Hou JK. Am J Gastroenterol. 2011;106(4):563–73.
6. Triggs C. Dietary factors in chronic inflammation: food tolerances and intolerances of a New Zealand Caucasian Crohn's disease population. Mutat Res. 2010;690:123–38.
7. Dalessandro T. What to eat with IBD a comprehensive nutrition and recipe guide for Crohn's disease and ulcerative colitis. Briarcliff Manor, New York. CMG Publishing 2006.
8. Eiden KA. Nutritional considerations in inflammatory bowel disease. Nutrition Issues in Pract Gastroenterol. Series 5 2003:34–54.
9. Cohen AB, et al. Dietary patterns and self reported associations of diet with symptoms of IBD. Dig Dis Sci May, 58(5):1322–1328.
10. Gentschew L, et al. Role of nutrition and microbiota insusceptibility to inflammatory bowel diseases. Mol Nutr Food Res. 2012;56:524–35.
11. Richman E. Review article: evidence-based dietary advice for patients with inflammatory bowel disease. Aliment Pharmacol Ther. 2013;38:1156–71.
12. Barrett JS, Gibson PR. Clinical ramifications of malabsorption of fructose and other short-chain carbohydrates. Nutrition Issues in Pract Gastroenterol. Series 53 2007;51–65.
13. Albenberg LG, et al. Food and the gut microbiota in IBD: a critical connection. Curr Opin Gastroenterol. 2012;28(4):314–20.
14. Barrett JS, Gibson PR. Fermentable oligosaccharides, disaccharides, monosaccharides and polyols (FODMAPs) and non-allergic food intolerance.

FODMAPs or food chemicals? Ther Adv Gastroenterol. 2012;5(4):261–8.
15. Almeida AI, Correia M, et al. Nutritional risk screening in surgery: valid, feasible, easy! Clin Nutr. 2012;31:206–11.
16. Banh L. Serum proteins as markers of nutrition: what are we treating? Nutrition Issues in Pract Gastroenterol. 2006:46–64.
17. Guagnozzi D, et al. Anemia in inflammatory bowel disease: a neglected issue with relevant effects. World J Gastroenterol. 2014;20(13):3542–51.
18. Gomollon F, et al. Current management of iron deficiency anemia in inflammatory bowel disease: a practical guide. Drugs. doi:10.1007/s40265-013-013102.
19. Gasche C, et al. Iron, anemia, and inflammatory bowel diseases. Gut. 2004;53(8):1190–7.
20. Battat R, et al. Vitamin B12 deficiency in inflammatory bowel disease: prevalence, risk factors, evaluation, and management. Inflamm Bowel Dis. 2014;20(6):1120–8.
21. Pappa H. Vitamin D deficiency and supplementation in patients with IBD. Gastroenterol Hepatol (N Y). 2014;10(2):127–9.
22. Naik AS, et al. Nutritional care in adult inflammatory bowel disease. Pract Gastroenterol. 2012;36(6):18–27.
23. Lee HH, et al. Zinc absorption in human small intestine. Am J Physiol. 1989;256:G87–91.
24. Zinc, serum, random urine. Test catalog, Test ID: ZNS, ZNSU. Rochester, MN: Mayo Medical Laboratories. Available at: http://www.mayomedicallaboritories.com/test-catalog/Overview/8620. 2014.
25. Wapnir RA. Copper absorption and bioavailability. Am J Clin Nutr. 1998;67:1054S–60.
26. O'Donnell K. Severe micronutrient deficiencies in RYGB patients: rare but potentially devastating. Pract Gastroenterol. 2011;35(11):13–27.
27. Treatment of magnesium deficiency. Available at: www.nih.gov. 2014.
28. Treatment of magnesium deficiency. Available at: www.Mayoclinic.com. 2014.
29. Buchman AL. Nutritional therapy for Crohn's disease. Nutrition Issues in Pract Gastroenterol. 2005:17–28.
30. Food allergy research and education. Available at: www.foodallergy.org. 2014.
31. Herfarth H. Prevalence of a gluten–free diet and improvement of clinical symptoms in patients with inflammatory bowel diseases. Inflamm Bowel Dis. 2014;20(7):1194–7.
32. Eswaran S, et al. Food: the forgotten factor in the irritable bowel syndrome. Gastrolenterol Clin North Am 2011 Mar:40(1):141–62.
33. Torio M. Nephrolithiasis as an extra-intestinal presentation of pediatric inflammatory bowel disease unclassified. J Crohns Colitis 2010 Dec; 4(6):674–8.
34. Crohn's and Colitis Foundation. Extra intestinal complications: kidney disorders; Available at http://www.ccfa.org/resources/kidney-disorders.html. 2009.
35. McConell N. Risk factors for developing renal stones in inflammatory bowel disease. BJU Int. 2002;89(9):835–41.
36. Nutrition for people with stomas 2: an overview of dietary advice. Nursing Times. 2008 Dec 104:49, 26–27.
37. Fulham J. Providing dietary advice for the individual with a stoma. Br J Nurs. 2008;17(2):S22–7.
38. Ostomy nutrition guide. University of Pittsburgh Medical Center; Available at http://www.upmc.com/patients-visitors/education/nutrition/pages/ostomy-nutrition-guide.aspx. 2014.
39. Burch J. Nutrition and the ostomate: input, output and absorption. Br J Community Nurs. 2006;11(8):349–51.
40. Parrish C. The clinicians guide to short bowel syndrome. Nutrition issues in gastroenterology series. Pract Gastroenterol. 2005:67–106.
41. Matarese L. Nutrition and fluid optimization for patients with short bowel syndrome. JPEN J Parenter Enteral Nutr. 2013;37(2):161–70.
42. DiBaise JK, Young RJ, Vanderhoof JA. Intestinal Rehab & the Short Bowel Syndrome: Part 1. Am J Gastro 2004;99:1386.
43. Day AS, et al. Exclusive enteral feeding as primary therapy for Crohn's disease in Australian children and adolescents: a feasible and effective approach. J Gastroenterol Hepatol. 2006;21:1609–14.
44. Wild G, et al. World J Gastroenterol. 2007;13(1):1–7.
45. Bayless T, Hanauer S. Advanced therapy in inflammatory bowel disease. Volume II: IBD and Crohn's disease. Perioperative Nutrition Supoort 2011;131:815–18.
46. Guagnozzi D, Gonzalez-Castillo S, et al. Nutritional treatment in inflammatory bowel disease, an update. Rev Esp Enferm Dig. 2012;104(9):479–88.
47. Engstrom P, Goosenberg E. Diagnosis and management of bowel diseases. 3rd ed. United Kingdom. Professional Communications. 2007.
48. Braga M, et al. Surgery. 2002;132:805–14.
49. Waitzberg DL, et al. World J Surg. 2006;30:1592–604.
50. McClave, Stephen A, Martindale, Robert G, et al. Guidelines for the provision and assessment of nutrition support therapy in the adult critically ill patient: society of critical care medicine (SCCM) and American society of parenteral and enteral nutrition A.S.P.E.N. JPEN J Parenter Enter Nutr 2009. May-Jun;33(3): 277–316.
51. Drover JW, et al. J Am Coll Surg. 2011;212:385–99.
52. Strong for surgery nutrition checklist. Available at www.strongforsurgery.org. 2014.
53. Almeida, A et al. Nutritional Screening in Surgery: Valid, Feasible, Easy. Clin Nutr. 31(2012):206–11.
54. Abrahao V. Nourishing the dysfunctional gut with whey protein. Curr Opin Clin Nutr Metab Care. 2012;15:480–4.
55. Scaldaferri F. Gut microbial flora, prebiotics, and probiotics in IBD: their current usage and utility. BioMed Res Int. Article ID 435268. 2013.
56. Shoda R, et al. Epidemiologic analysis of Crohn's disease in Japan: increased dietary intake of n-6 polyunsaturated fatty acids and animal protein relates to the increased incidence of Crohn's disease in Japan. Am J Clin Nutr. 1996;63:741–5.

57. Goh J. Review article: nutrition and adult inflammatory bowel disease. Aliment Pharmacol Ther. 2003;17: 307–20.
58. Gottschall E. Breaking the vicious cycle intestinal health through diet. Ontario, Canada. The Kirkton Press. 1994.
59. Suskind D, et al. Nutritional therapy in pediatric Crohn disease: the specific carbohydrate diet. J Pediatr Gastroenterol Nutr. 2014;58(1):87–92.
60. Kanai T, et al. Diet, microbiota, and inflammatory bowel disease: lessons from Japanese foods. Korean J Intern Med. 2014;29(4):409–15.

Fertility/Sexual Function

22

Julia Berian and Mukta K. Krane

Introduction

Advances in the surgical and medical management of Crohn's disease (CD) continue to improve clinical control highlighting the need for an increased focus on patient quality of life and functional outcomes. Patients with CD are often diagnosed in their late adolescence or early adulthood when body image, sexuality, sexual function, and fertility are of particular concern.

Sexuality and sexual function are dependent on a complex interplay of biological, anatomical, psychological, and social aspects. Symptoms and treatment related factors of CD have a significant effect on both physiologic and psychosocial aspects. The impact of CD on sexual function and fertility was first reported in the 1970s, but the majority of available literature is limited by small sample sizes, use of non-validated survey instruments, heterogeneous patient population, absence of baseline data, and low response rates. The focus of this chapter is to review the influence of CD on sexual function and fertility and illustrate areas of future research.

J. Berian, MD
Department of Surgery, University of Chicago,
5841 S. Maryland Avenue, Chicago, IL 60637, USA
e-mail: Julia.Berian@uchospitals.edu

M.K. Krane, MD (✉)
Department of Surgery, University of Washington
School of Medicine, 1959 NE Pacific Street,
Box 356410, Seattle, WA 98195-6410, USA
e-mail: mkrane@uw.edu

Affect of Clinical Manifestations of Crohn's Disease on Sexual Function

CD is a chronic illness consisting of a constellation of symptoms including abdominal and joint pain, increased bowel frequency, perianal fistulas, abscesses, skin tags, and incontinence which may lead to embarrassment, decreased libido, and sexual impairment. Similar to other chronic diseases, CD is often accompanied by fatigue and chronic pain profoundly affecting all domains of quality of life including sexual desire and performance. The stress of dealing with CD and its physical impairments can lead to depression and anxiety further decreasing sexual activity and compounding the strain on intimate relationships.

Seventy-seven to eighty percent of patients with IBD are in an intimate relationship, which is similar to the general population [1–3]. The type of disease (Crohn's disease vs. ulcerative colitis), gender, and operative history do not appear to make a difference in terms of partnership status [1]. About 50 % of patients feel that the disease has an adverse impact on relationship status due to stigma and difficulties with sexual intimacy. While gender does not seem to make a difference,

A. Fichera and M.K. Krane (eds.), *Crohn's Disease: Basic Principles*,
DOI 10.1007/978-3-319-14181-7_22, © Springer International Publishing Switzerland 2015

patients who have undergone surgical treatment of their disease report a greater negative affect on intimate relationships.

Patient perceptions on sexuality and sexual function were first evaluated by Gazzard et al. who found that of 52 patients surveyed who had been married before developing CD, 54 % stated that sexual intercourse had become less frequent after the diagnosis and 23 % stated that sexual intercourse had ceased completely. In fact, only 12 of the 52 patients (23 %) reported that their sexual drive and frequency of intercourse had not changed after developing CD [4]. Several years later Moody et al. published similar findings in a study where 45 women with CD in a stable relationship were compared to age-match controls. Twenty-four percent of women with CD reported infrequent or no sexual intercourse compared to 4 % of controls. However, the frequency of sexual intercourse was similar among those sexually active regardless of the presence or absence of CD. The most common reasons for sexual inactivity were abdominal pain (24 %), diarrhea (20 %), and fear of fecal incontinence (14 %). In addition, dyspareunia was commonly reported, particularly in patients with perianal disease and the presence of fistulas [5]. These results are consistent with those of Muller et al. who found that 54 % of women and 43 % of men in a population of 217 IBD patients felt that IBD negatively affected their intimate relationships. Fifty-eight percent of those that were sexually active reported a reduction in sexual frequency and libido due to their disease [1].

Recently, a large study by Marin et al. compared sexual function in male and female patients with IBD to matched controls using the International Index of Erectile Function (IIEF) in males and the Female Sexual Function Index (FSFI) in females [6]. Of the 355 patients (202 female and 153 male) and the 200 controls (127 female and 73 male) who made up the study population, most were sexually active at the time of the survey. However, 39 % of women and 35 % of men acknowledged that IBD had worsened their sexual function in terms of decreased sexual desire (47 % of women and 29 % of men) and sexual satisfaction (46 % of women and 30 % of men). Of those patients who had completely ceased sexual intercourse, half of them stated that IBD was responsible for their sexual inactivity. While a significantly lower mean IIEF score was recorded in men with IBD compared to controls (59.1 vs. 63.1 respectively, $p=0.03$), there was not a significant difference in the proportion of abnormal IIEF scores. However, when individual domains were evaluated, a greater portion of abnormal scores was observed in erectile function ($p=0.044$) and desire ($p=0.031$) in patients with IBD. In women, mean scores in global FSFI and in each individual domain were significantly lower in patients with IBD compared to controls. In addition, 49 % of patients with IBD reported an abnormal FISI score compared to 19 % of controls ($p<0.0001$). In univariate analysis, CD was one of the factors associated with lower FSFI scores. This data is consistent with the few other studies conducted using validated survey instruments that have demonstrated that CD may have a significant direct impact on sexual function, particularly in women. Surprisingly, the negative affect of certain manifestations of the disease including incontinence and perineal complications did not reach statistical significance. Instead as with most other chronic diseases, depression is the strongest risk factor for sexual dysfunction in the CD population [2, 3, 7].

Disease activity seems to have a significant influence of sexual function by impacting frequency of sexual activity, libido, body image, and sexual satisfaction. Timmer et al. found that of 280 male patients, severe sexual compromise was reported in 67 % of patients with active disease compared to 21 % of patients in remission [2, 3]. In fact, men in remission or with mildly active disease scored similarly to controls on the IIEF. Sexual impairment was attributed to erectile/ejaculatory dysfunction and fear of intimacy due to unpredictable bowel movements, flatus, and concern of fecal incontinence during sexual intercourse. In addition, disease severity is linked to more severe depression and fatigue, which are known to have a significant impact of sexual function.

Influence of Crohn's Disease Treatment on Sexual Function

Medical Management

The literature available on the influence of medical management of CD on sexual function is limited. Although medications are responsible for up to 25 % of cases of erectile dysfunction (ED) in the general population, CD medications do not appear to cause an increased frequency of ED. A few studies have demonstrated an association between methotrexate and ED and one case of sulfasalazine causing impotence has been reported [8–11]. Sexual dysfunction has not been associated with other commonly used CD medications including: 6-MP, azathioprine, prednisone, infliximab, or adalimumab [12]. Interesting up to 10 % of patients are reportedly non-compliant with medications due to a perceived detrimental effect on sexual function [1]. However, medications that are often prescribed in the CD population, particularly antidepressants and antianxiety medications commonly diminish sexual function.

Surgical Management

An estimated 70 % of patients with CD will require surgery within 20 years of their diagnosis. Several studies have found that patients experience sexual dysfunction and body image derangements post-operatively, particularly if they have undergone pelvic surgery. However, there is also evidence in the literature that some aspects of sexual function may improve after surgical intervention especially if the patient experiences improvement of their general health.

Patients with Crohn's colitis refractory to medical management, colorectal dysplasia or cancer, or severe perianal or rectal disease often require a proctocolectomy with an end ileostomy. In these cases, disturbances in sexual function and sexuality may be due to the rectal dissection itself and/or the presence of a stoma.

Pelvic dissection during proctectomy may lead to injury of the presacral nerves and the pelvic plexus. In men this has been shown to lead to sexual dysfunction manifested by erectile and/or ejaculatory dysfunction. The effect of nerve injury in women is not well understood and more difficult to ascertain because objective criteria to assess sexual function in women are not well defined.

While most patients with CD will not undergo a restorative proctocolectomy with ileal pouch anal anastomosis (IPAA), the majority of the literature on the effects of pelvic surgery on sexual function in IBD patients is conducted on patients undergoing IPAA. As sexual dysfunction in these studies is most often attributed to the proctectomy, this data can be extrapolated to CD patients undergoing a total proctocolectomy and end ileostomy.

Erectile dysfunction and retrograde or loss of ejaculation has been reported in men undergoing proctectomy for benign conditions with an incidence of 0–25 % and up to 15 %, respectively [13]. A large study conducted by the Mayo Clinic surveyed sexual function in 762 men before and after total proctocolectomy with IPAA using a non-validated sexual function questionnaire. Nineteen percent of patients reported deterioration, 25 % improvement, and 56 % no change post-operatively when compared to pre-operative sexual function. Three percent of patients reported retrograde or no ejaculation after IPAA [14]. Lindsey et al. compared the incidence of sexual dysfunction in male patients undergoing rectal dissection for IBD using the standard total mesorectal excision technique versus a close rectal dissection approach where the rectum is mobilized close to the rectal wall in order to minimize damage to the pelvic nerves [15]. They found that of 156 patients 3.8 % experienced complete impotence and 13.5 % of men reported partial diminution of erectile function but were still able to participate in sexual intercourse. No ejaculatory dysfunction was observed. Interestingly, there were no statistically significant differences in the rate of complete or partial impotence between the total mesorectal and close rectal dissection techniques (2.2 % vs. 4.5 %, $P=0.67$ and 13.5 % and 13.3 %, $P=0.99$, respectively). In a meta-analysis, which included 43 studies, the pooled incidence of sexual dysfunction after IPAA was 3.6 % [16].

Among women undergoing proctocolectomy for IBD, several studies have demonstrated disturbances in sexual function including dyspareunia, inability to achieve orgasm, and decreased libido [17, 18]. In a study of 71 women, Scaglia et al. found that 33 % of women reported impaired sexual function and 22 % reduced sexual satisfaction post-operatively. In addition, 12 % of women reported dyspareunia pre-operatively compared to 27 % after surgery [19]. Using the FSFI, Ogilvie et al. found that of 83 sexual active women with IBD who had undergone proctectomy, 47 % reported scores consistent with sexual dysfunction [20]. On the other hand, a number of studies have shown an improvement in sexual function post-operatively including increased frequency of sexual intercourse, decreased incidence of dyspareunia, and increased overall sexual satisfaction [21, 22]. Among male patients, despite the known risk of injury to pelvic nerves, one recent study indicated improvement in sexual function after IPAA. In a survey of 122 men, IIEF domains for erectile function, sexual desire, intercourse satisfaction, and overall satisfaction showed significant increases from pre to post-operative assessments [23].

Inconsistencies in the rate of post-operative dysfunction reported in the literature are often attributed to improved general health from baseline, which in some cases may outweigh anatomic disturbances in sexual function caused by proctectomy. To examine the influence of the pre-operative health status and sexual dysfunction on post-operative sexual function, Wang et al. conducted a prospective study using validated surveys to examine post-proctectomy sexual function in the IBD population [24]. The study included 66 patients who had completed surveys pre- and post-operatively. For men, median IIEF overall scores and scores in the domains for sexual desire, satisfaction with intercourse, and erectile function significantly improved from baseline 6 months post-operatively. Overall and individual domain scores on the Sexual Function Questionnaire (SFQ) also significantly improved in men after proctectomy. While FSFI sexual desire scores significantly improved from baseline in women, there was no statistically significant difference in the SFQ scores or for the FSFI domains of lubrication, satisfaction, pain, orgasm, or arousal in women post-proctectomy.

Impact of Stoma

Fear of having a stoma is a common concern in patients with CD. In fact, in a prospective study evaluating disease-related concerns, having a stoma was the biggest fear in IBD patients ranking higher than concern over medication side effects and the need for surgery itself [25]. Most studies comparing quality of life in patients undergoing proctocolectomy with IPAA versus proctocolectomy with end ileostomy demonstrate diminished sexual function and body image scores in those with a stoma. In the study above by Wang et al, in contrast to men undergoing IPAA, men with permanent end ileostomies only showed improvements in the IIEF orgasmic function domain and total IIEF score. It should be noted, however, that patients in the end ileostomy group were older and had lower baseline IIEF scores. Women with permanent end ileostomies demonstrated no significant change in any of the FSFI domains measured [24].

Overview Crohn's Disease and Fertility

The literature on fertility in Crohn's disease (CD) has evolved over the past several decades. Many early studies relied on pregnancy rates alone to evaluate fertility, a method which fails to account for desire for pregnancy and advice against pregnancy. Therefore the true numbers of patients attempting conception are not taken into account. Infertility is commonly defined as the inability to conceive a pregnancy within 1 year without contraceptive measures.

A review of the literature from the 1970s and 1980s initially suggested that Crohn's disease contributed to infertility or sub-fertility [26]. Early studies were, however, commonly characterized by biased samples (e.g., referral-center based selection), small sample sizes, and unclear definitions of fertility.

One of the larger studies by Mayberry et al. in 1986 compared 224 married female CD patients with 208 age-matched, married controls, where 182 of the pairs status was married at the time of the survey [27]. Findings indicated that prior to diagnosis pregnancy rates were similar between female Crohn's patients and controls, while following diagnosis Crohn's patients had lower pregnancy rates. In this study, however, infertility was defined as failure to become pregnant among married women not using contraceptive methods for 6 months or longer duration. Desire for pregnancy was not taken into account and it was recognized that study patients did receive advice against pregnancy. The infertility rate among controls was 28–29 %, with rates of infertility among Crohn's cases measured at 25 % and 42 % pre- and post-diagnosis, respectively.

A similar case–control study was conducted among male CD patients. Fertility was estimated by comparing the number of children born to the wives of CD patients both before and after diagnosis to the number born to the wives of age-matched controls before and after an equivalent "critical date." Among 42 married, age-matched pairs, the mean number of children in CD patients prior to diagnosis was 1.2 compared to 1.5 for controls, and after diagnosis that number dropped to 0.4 compared to 0.8 in controls [28].

By 1989, Narendranthan et al. recognized the potential inaccuracies of assessing fertility by pregnancy rate alone. Their publication of a case–control study of men with CD and ulcerative colitis attempted to better assess fertility by inquiring about attempts at conception for 1 year or longer, any fertility consultation with a physician, any reproductive advice they had received and finally fears regarding childbearing. The analysis was limited to IBD males with female spouses who had no known fertility problems. Of the 106 men with Crohn's disease, the number of children was less than controls, though not statistically significant (mean of 2.11 pregnancies vs 1.75 in controls and CD patients, respectively). Further analysis of time-to-conception revealed that there was no significant difference between CD patients and controls: 92 % and 95 % had spouses conceive, controls and CD patients, respectively. Disease duration, treatment, and the presence of an ostomy were also included in the analysis without any effect on the time-to-conception, thereby leading the authors to conclude that fecundity, or the probability of conception in each menstrual cycle was not different between men with IBD and controls [29].

The studies which emerged in the 1990s were generally drawn from larger populations and more detailed, refined definitions of fertility. Survey data from Hudson's 1997 study of Scottish women with IBD indicated that conception rates between CD and controls were similar. The rate of involuntary infertility found amongst the CD population (14 %) did not differ from involuntary infertility amongst the control population. In this study, desire for pregnancy was taken into account, with "voluntary infertility" found to be higher among CD and UC patients than the control population. In a smaller subset analysis, disease activity seemed to play a role in the course of a pregnancy; those with remission or mild disease were more likely to have a normal delivery, whereas severe exacerbation carried an increased risk of preterm labor [30].

Recent studies continue to confirm similar findings. A survey by Mañosa et al. of 503 IBD patients in Spain reports that the pregnancy rate among IBD patients (47 % CD and 53 % UC) is comparable to controls. The survey further evaluated the 148 childless patients and found that 78 % cited personal choice as their reason, followed by self-reported infertility in 14 % and "other IBD-related causes" in 8 %. Of note, 6 % of these patients had consulted with a physician and undergone further studies for infertility [31].

The phenomenon of "voluntary childlessness" may explain early studies' initial interpretation of reduced fertility in Crohn's patients, given the heavy reliance on pregnancy rates. Current literature has turned focused attention to the reasons behind voluntary childlessness in IBD patients. In a survey of Illinois CCFA members, voluntary childlessness was found among 18 and 14 % of CD and UC patients, respectively. This was significantly higher than the rate of the general population, which was estimated at 6.2 % based on national data. The rate of non-voluntary childlessness was similar to the general population (5 % in CD, 1.7 % in UC, and 2.5 % in the general population). The most commonly cited reasons for voluntary childlessness included concern regarding worsening or recurrence of disease due to the pregnancy, fear over passing the disease to progeny, worry over the stress of raising a child or being unable to care for the child. On average women with CD and UC had fewer children (average of 0.8 and 0.6, respectively) compared with 1.18 average births per woman from national and Illinois-level census data. Given a higher level of education among the sample, the authors posit that voluntary childlessness is likely multifactorial and that educational attainment may contribute [32].

An Australian survey aimed to characterize patients' concerns related to IBD and pregnancy, their perceptions of infertility risk, and the influence of those perceptions on reproductive behavior. Respondents reported a fear of infertility in 47.2 % of CD patients and 25.8 % of UC patients. Concerns regarding infertility were significantly higher among female than male CD patients and those with history of surgery compared to those managed medically. Despite these differences, however, the rate of consultation with a physician for fertility related concerns did not differ between CD or UC respondents and population-based estimates. Patient-reported reasons for voluntary childlessness included fear of IBD-related congenital abnormalities, concern for IBD in child, concern for medication teratogenicity, receipt of advice that conception may be difficult or inadvisable [33].

Generally, Crohn's patients fertility is comparable to that of the general population. The birth rate among these patients, however, reflects an increase in "voluntary childlessness" which is often attributed to disease-related concerns.

Influence of Medical Management of Crohn's Disease on Fertility

There are myriad studies addressing different CD therapies and their impact on fertility. Sulfasalazine and 5-aminosalicylates are well studied and recognized to have negative effects on male fertility, attributed to oligospermia with inhibited sperm morphology and motility [34]. These effects are known to abate with discontinuation of therapy.

While Sulfasalazine and 5-ASA have been well studied with consistent results, a review of additional CD therapies, such as corticosteroids and biologic agents reveals conflicting studies or limited data [35]. While rat studies suggest negative effects of corticosteroids on fertility, there are limited data in human studies. Increased steroid levels in men may result in decreased sperm concentration, which argues to limit steroid treatment to short durations in order to control active disease. Immunosuppressive agents such as mercaptopurine (6-MP) and azathioprine (AZA) are characterized by conflicting data and, as such, are believed unlikely to have significant effects on fertility. Biologic agents such as infliximab and adalimumab are poorly studied and, therefore, effects on fertility are generally unknown. Regarding medication effects on female fertility, most IBD medications have not been shown to have a detrimental effect, excepting the known teratogenic and mutagenic effects of methotrexate [35].

The importance of pre-conception medications in the female CD patient cannot be underestimated. One review indicates that regardless of fertility effects, the treating provider must review the FDA classification of drugs which may safely be used in pregnancy [36]. Sulfasalazine and 5-ASA are characterized by initial reports of teratogenicity and congenital defects, however, later, larger studies have not supported these findings. Use of antibiotics should be carefully guided; there is a low teratogenic risk of metronidazole, quinolones, and rifaxamin. In the face of alternative agents, medications with an unknown safety profile should be avoided. Biologic agents are generally considered low risk, with infliximab supported by more data than adalimumab. As in male fertility studies, AZA and 6MP are controversial, with some data suggesting teratogenicity, but additional data from transplant literature supporting the safety of their use. The teratogenicity of medications such as thalidomide and methotrexate precludes their use in a pre-conception patient [36].

The Role of Surgical Treatment of Crohn's Disease on Infertility

As discussed previously, much of the literature on surgical management of IBD focuses on proctocolectomy with IPAA. Though this operation is usually limited to UC patients, instances of indeterminate colitis and the shared pathophysiology of post-operative adhesions make a discussion of proctocolectomy with or without IPAA an important part of understanding the role of surgery as it relates to infertility in Crohn's disease.

A 1990 study by Wikland included 41 female UC patients and 31 female CD patients after proctocolectomy with end ileostomy in evaluating gynecologic problems and fertility post-operatively. Data were gathered both through self-report questionnaire and correlation with gynecologic examination. The most common gynecologic problem reported was a significant increase in vaginal discharge in 49 % of these women post-operatively, compared to 9 % pre-operatively. Anatomic changes were observed on gynecologic exam in 81 % of the patients, with the most common change being caudal fixation and dilation of the posterior vaginal fornix. Fertility was assessed via self-report of pregnancies conceived over those attempting conception. Survey findings indicate that pregnancy rate before and after surgery differed significantly, with 72 % of patients (39/54) becoming pregnant before surgery compared to 37 % (10/27) after surgery [37]. Given the anatomic changes observed, the source of the decreased fertility is presumed due to adhesions within the pelvis. A similar study evaluated patients following restorative proctocolectomy with IPAA. Anatomic changes were evaluated with hysterosalpingography, which revealed that of 21 IPAA patients, two patients had bilateral occlusion of the fallopian tubes and 9 had unilateral occlusion [38].

In a questionnaire survey of men and women in Finland, 95 UC patients who had undergone proctocolectomy with IPAA reported an infertility rate of 20 % among females and a rate of erectile dysfunction of 14.6 % among males. The infertility rate in this study was slightly higher than established population rates at the time, with infertility reported from 6 to 10.6 % in Nordic populations [39].

Recent data from North America supports these findings, with increased infertility rates observed among surgically treated UC patients. Several studies compare the rate of infertility within the same patients both pre- and post-operatively. A Cleveland Clinic study of 300 patients confirmed reduced fertility among women following restorative proctocolectomy with IPAA. This survey found that among UC and FAP patients who attempted to conceive prior to surgery, 48 out of 127 were unsuccessful after 1 year without contraception (38 %). This was compared with 76 out of 135 women unable to conceive for a similar duration after surgery (56 %). It is worth noting that both pre- and post-operative infertility rates are higher than the US average, estimated at 13.8 % [40]. A recent meta-analysis focused on a comparison between pre- and post-IPAA patients, confirming that the relative risk of infertility was significantly increased at 3.91 (95 % CI 2.06, 7.44) [41].

Other studies focus on comparison between surgical patients and medically managed counterparts. A Canadian study found that the infertility rate among UC females following IPAA (38.1 %) was significantly higher than in UC females managed nonoperatively (13.3 %) [42]. Focusing on comparison between surgical and medical treatment of UC, a meta-analysis concerning fertility changes showed relative risk of infertility after surgery was 3.17, with a 95 % confidence interval of 2.41–4.18. Raw data was used from the included studies to calculate the weighted average infertility rate among non-surgical UC (15 %) and among post-operative patients (48 %) [43].

As laparoscopy becomes more widely utilized, however, new data suggest that the negative impact of IPAA on fertility may be curtailed with a minimally invasive approach. A cross-sectional study across three centers in the Netherlands and Belgium found that among laparoscopic IPAA patients, 19 of 27 (70 %) females attempting conception after surgery became pregnant compared to open IPAA patients, in which 9 of 23 (39 %)

achieved pregnancy [44]. A study of 2 centers in France reported preserved fertility among women following laparoscopic IPAA in comparison with controls following laparoscopic appendectomy. The pregnancy rate among female laparoscopic IPAA patients was 73 %, with 11 of the 15 patients achieving conception naturally; this did not significantly differ from the pregnancy rate among laparoscopic appendectomy controls [45].

Fertility in Crohn's disease is, therefore, similar to the general population, with the exception of the subset of patients who are surgically managed with pelvic dissections. Even among this subset, there are opportunities for improvement with the advance of laparoscopic techniques and mechanisms to decrease the extent of dissection and adhesion formation.

Addressing Sexual Dysfunction and Infertility with Patients

While the true incidence of sexual dysfunction and infertility in patients with CD is unknown it is clear that they are concerned with the impact of the disease on their relationships, self-image, fecundity, and sexual function. Unfortunately, health care professionals do not adequately address sexual health in the context of disease activity or the effects of treatment on sexual function. In a study by Borum et al, women with IBD were surveyed regarding whether their physicians discussed sexual function and sexuality and with what frequency. Twelve of sixty-four women reported that the issue had been addressed by their gastroenterologist but in all cases the discussion had been initiated by the patient [46]. Patients are generally uncomfortable discussing sexual function and sexuality and therefore are unlikely to volunteer information regarding sexual dysfunction. It is therefore the burden of the healthcare professional to create a supportive environment in which to discuss relationships, sexual function, and fertility and to provide disease specific information on sexual dysfunction and infertility to patients with CD in order to facilitate the psychosocial adjustment required with this disease.

Conclusion

Patient related and treatment factors associated with CD have a significant impact on sexual function and fertility. Patients need to be counseled on the affect of their disease process and various treatment regimens on functional outcomes and feel comfortable discussing these issues with their healthcare providers.

References

1. Muller KR, Prosser R, Brampton P, Mountifield R, Andrews JM. Female gender and surgery impair relationships, body image, and sexuality in inflammatory bowel disease: patient perceptions. Inflamm Bowel Dis. 2010;16(4):657–63.
2. Timmer A, Bauer A, Dignass A, Rogler G. Sexual function in persons with inflammatory bowel disease: a survey with matched controls. Clin Gastroenterol Hepatol. 2007;5(1):87–94.
3. Timmer A, Bauer A, Kemptner D, Furst A, Rogler G. Determinants of male sexualfunction in inflammatory bowel disease: a survey based cross-sectional analysis in 280 men. Inflamm Bowel Dis. 2007;13(10): 1236–43.
4. Gazzard BG, Price HL, Libby GW, Dawson AM. The social toll of Crohn's disease. Br Med J. 1978;2: 1117–9.
5. Moody G, Probert CSJ, Strivastava EM, RHodes J, Mayberry JF. Sexual dysfunction amongst women with Crohn's disease: a hidden problem. Digestion. 1992;52:179–83.
6. Marin L, Manosa M, Garcia-Planella E, Gordillo J, Zabana Y, Cabre E, Domenech E. Sexual function and patients' perceptions in inflammatory bowel disease: a case control survey. J Gastroenterol. 2013;48: 713–20.
7. Timmer A, Kemptner D, Bauer A, Takses A, Ott C, Furst A. Determinants of female sexual function in inflammatory bowel disease: a survey based cross-sectional analysis. BMC Gastroenterol. 2008;8:45.
8. Blackburn Jr WD, Alarcon GS. Impotence in three rheumatoid arthritis patients treated with methotrexate. Arthritis Rheum. 1989;32:1341–2.
9. Ireland A, Jewell DP. Sulfasalazine-induced impotence: a beneficial resolution with olsalazine? J Clin Gastroenterol. 1989;11:711.
10. Riba N, Moreno F, Costa J, Olive A. Appearance of impotence in relation to the use of methotrexate. Med Clin (Barc). 1996;106(14):558.
11. Thomas E, Koumouvi K, Blotman E. Impotence in a patient with rheumatoid arthritis treated with methotrexate. J Rheumatol. 2000;27:1821–2.

12. Feagins LA, Kane SV. Sexual and reproductive issues for men with inflammatory bowel disease. Am J Gastroenterol. 2009;104:768–73.
13. Bauer JJ, Gelernt IM, Salky B, Kreel I. Sexual dysfunction following proctocolectomy for benign disease of the colon and rectum. Ann Surg. 1983;197:363–7.
14. Farouk R, Pemberton JH, Wolff BG, Dozois RR, Browning S, Larson D. Functional outcomes after ileal pouch-anal anastomosis for chronic ulcerative colitis. Ann Surg. 2000;231:919–26.
15. Lindsey I, George BD, Kettlewell MG, Mortensen NJ. Impotence after mesorectal and close rectal dissection for inflammatory bowel disease. Dis Colon Rectum. 2001;44(6):831–5.
16. Hueting WE, Buskens E, van der Tweel I. Results and complications after ileal pouch anal anastomosis: a meta-analysis of 43 observational studies compromising 9,317 patients. Dig Surg. 2005;22:69–79.
17. Bambrick M, Fazio VW, Hull TL, Pucel G. Sexual function following restorative proctocolectomy in women. Dis Colon Rectum. 1996;39:610–4.
18. Hueting WE, Gooszen HG, van Laarhoven CJ. Sexual function and continence after ileo pouch anal anastomosis: a comparison between a meta-analysis and a questionnaire survey. Int J Colorectal Dis. 2004;19:215–8.
19. Scaglia M, Delaini GG, Hulten L. Sexual dysfunctions after conventional proctectomy. Chir Ital. 1992;44:230–42.
20. Ogilvie JW, Goetz L, Baxter NN, Park J, Minami S, Madoff RD. Female sexual function after ileal pouch-anal anastomosis. Br J Surg. 2008;95:887–92.
21. Metcalf AM, Dozois RR, Kelly KA. Sexual function in women after proctocolectomy. Ann Surg. 1986;204(6):624–7.
22. Damgaard B, Wettergren A, Kirkegaard P. Social and sexual function following ileal pouch-anal anastomosis. Dis Colon Rectum. 1995;38:286–9.
23. Gorgun E, Remzi FH, Montague DK, Connor JT, O'Brien K, Loparo B, Fazio VW. Male sexual function improves after ileal pouch anal anastomosis. Colorectal Dis. 2005;7(6):545–50.
24. Wang JY, Hart SL, Wilkowski KSY, Lee JW, Delmotte EC, del Rosario KM, del Rosario AS, Varma MG. Gender-specific difference in pelvic organ function after proctectomy for inflammatory bowel disease. Dis Colon Rectum. 2011;54:66–76.
25. Moser G, Tillinger W, Sachs G, Genser D, Maier-Dobersberger T, Spiess K, Wyatt J, Vogelsang H, Lochs H, Gangl A. Disease-related worries and concerns: a study on out-patients with inflammatory bowel disease. Eur J Gastroenterol Hepatol. 1995;7:853–8.
26. Fielding JF. Pregnancy and inflammatory bowel disease. Ir J Med Sci. 1982;151:194–202.
27. Mayberry JF, Weterman IT. European survey of fertility and pregnancy in women with Crohn's disease: a case control study by European collaborative group. Gut. 1986;27:821–5.
28. Burnell D, Mayberry J, Calcraft BJ, Morris JS, Rhodes J. Male fertility in Crohn's disease. Postgrad Med J. 1986;62:269–72.
29. Narendranathan M, Sandler RS, Suchindran CM, Savitz DA. Male infertility in inflammatory bowel disease. J Clin Gastroenterol. 1989;11:403–6.
30. Hudson M, Flett G, Sinclair TS, Brunt PW, Templeton A, Mowat NA. Fertility and pregnancy in inflammatory bowel disease. Int J Gynaecol Obstet. 1997;58(2):229–37.
31. Mañosa M, Navarro-Llavat M, Marín L, Zabana Y, Cabré E, Domènech E. Fecundity, pregnancy outcomes, and breastfeeding in patients with inflammatory bowel disease: a large cohort survey. Scand J Gastroenterol. 2013;48(4):427–32.
32. Marri SR, Ahn C, Buchman AL. Voluntary childlessness is increased in women with inflammatory bowel disease. Inflamm Bowel Dis. 2007;13(5):591–9.
33. Mountifield R, Bampton P, Prosser R, Muller K, Andrews JM. Fear and fertility in inflammatory bowel disease: a mismatch of perception and reality affects family planning decisions. Inflamm Bowel Dis. 2009;15(5):720–5.
34. Alonso V, Linares V, Belles M, Albina ML, Sirvent JJ, Domingo JL, Sanchez DJ. Sulfasalazine induced oxidative stress: a possible mechanism of male infertility. Reprod Toxicol. 2009;27(1):35–40.
35. Heetun ZS, Byrnes C, Neary P, O'Marain C. Review article: reproduction in the patient with inflammatory bowel disease. Aliment Pharmacol Ther. 2007;26(4):513–33.
36. Mahadevan U. Fertility and pregnancy in the patient with inflammatory bowel disease. Gut. 2006;55(8):1198–206.
37. Wikland M, Jansson I, Asztély M, Palselius I, Svaninger G, Magnusson O, Hultén L. Gynaecological problems related to anatomical changes after conventional proctocolectomy and ileostomy. Int J Colorectal Dis. 1990;5(1):49–52.
38. Oresland T, Palmblad S, Ellström M, Berndtsson I, Crona N, Hultén L. Gynaecological and sexual function related to anatomical changes in the female pelvis after restorative proctocolectomy. Int J Colorectal Dis. 1994;9(2):77–81.
39. Tiainen J, Matikainen M, Hiltunen KM. Ileal J-pouch-anal anastomosis, sexual dysfunction, and fertility. Scand J Gastroenterol. 1999;34(2):185–8.
40. Gorgun E, Remzi FH, Goldberg JM, Thornton J, Bast J, Hull TL, Loparo B, Fazio VW. Fertility is reduced after restorative proctocolectomy with ileal pouch anal anastomosis: a study of 300 patients. Surgery. 2004;136(4):795–803.
41. Rajaratnam SG, Eglinton TW, Hider P, Fearnhead NS. Impact of ileal pouch-anal anastomosis on female fertility: meta-analysis and systematic review. Int J Colorectal Dis. 2011;26(11):1365–74.

42. Johnson P, Richard C, Ravid A, Spencer L, Pinto E, Hanna M, Cohen Z, McLeod R. Female infertility after ileal pouch-anal anastomosis for ulcerative colitis. Dis Colon Rectum. 2004;47(7):1119–26.
43. Waljee A, Walljee J, Morris AM, Higgins PD. Threefold increased risk of fertility: a meta-analysis of infertility after ileal pouch anal anastomosis in ulcerative colitis. Gut. 2006;55(11):1575–80.
44. Bartels SA, D'Hoore A, Cuesta MA, Bensdorp AJ, Lucas C, Bemelman WA. Significantly increased pregnancy rates after laparoscopic restorative proctocolectomy: a cross-sectional study. Ann Surg. 2012; 256(6):1045–8.
45. Beyer-Berjot L, Maggiori L, Birnbaum D, Lefevre JH, Berdah S, Panis Y. A total laparoscopic approach reduces the infertility rate after ileal pouch-anal anastomosis: a 2-center study. Ann Surg. 2013;258(2): 275–8.
46. Borum ML, Igiehon E, Shafa S. Physicians may inadequately address sexuality in women with inflammatory bowel disease. Inflamm Bowel Dis. 2007;13(10): 1236–43.

Quality of Life in Patients with Crohn's Disease

23

Felipe Bellolio-Roth and Robin S. McLeod

Quality of life is an important outcome in clinical medicine. Despite this, there is little consensus on its definition or on the optimal method for measuring it. In 1947, the World Health Organization (WHO) introduced a broadened definition of health as "a state of complete physical, mental and social well-being and not merely the absence of disease" which has been adopted by many [1]. It incorporates the domains of physical, emotional, and social well-being into the concept of quality of life. Somatic sensation (i.e., presence or absence of pain) is sometimes included [2]. Others have added economic well-being (i.e., the ability to earn a living or perform work) but some have rejected this domain since it then implies that quality of life varies with the level of remuneration one receives for that work. It is also accepted that quality of life should be assessed by or considered from the patient's perspective, that quality of life may fluctuate over time and there may be cross cultural differences. Calman has also proposed the definition of quality of life as "the gap between a person's expectations and achievements" which seems appropriate and also incorporates the concept that quality of life is personal and may vary among individuals [3].

F. Bellolio-Roth, MD
Department of Digestive Surgery, Pontificia Universidad Catolica de Chile, Santiago, Chile

R.S. McLeod, MD, FRCSC, FACS (✉)
Department of Surgery, University of Toronto, Room 16-1612 620 University Avenue, Toronto, ON, Canada M5G 1L7
e-mail: robin.mcleod@cancercare.on.ca

Methods for Assessing Quality of Life

In general, there are two different types of instruments used to measure quality of life: psychometrically and utility based measures [4]. There are advantages and disadvantages to both. Psychometrically based measures of quality of life attempt to quantify this phenomenon using a range of questions from the various domains being assessed. The ratings or scores of the individual items are usually summated to give an overall measure of quality of life. Items can be equally weighted to derive a summary score or they can be differentially weighted in accordance with the importance of each item. There are two types of psychometric measures. Generic measures have been designed to be applicable to individuals with a broad range of diseases and impairments, undergoing varied treatments. Their usefulness is that they are applicable to a wide range of groups and therefore quality of life between these groups can be compared. The disadvantage is that they may lack the sensitivity to detect small but clinically important differences in a particular group of patients. Other advantages of the generic instruments are that they often have

A. Fichera and M.K. Krane (eds.), *Crohn's Disease: Basic Principles*,
DOI 10.1007/978-3-319-14181-7_23, © Springer International Publishing Switzerland 2015

been used extensively and therefore their validity and reliability have been well established in varied populations, they can be used to compare outcomes among different groups and they can be useful in cost-effectiveness studies and health policy analysis. They can also detect and measure unexpected treatment effects. Some examples of generic instruments are the Medical Outcomes Trust SF-36 [5], the Sickness Impact Profile [6], and the Nottingham Health Profile [7].

Disease-specific instruments have been designed to measure those areas of quality of life of importance to specific patient populations. Usually these instruments contain items of importance to this population, so disease-specific measures may be more responsive to small, clinically important changes and may better discriminate between individuals within the population. They may also appear more relevant to clinicians and patients. However, they tend to have less established reliability and validity than generic measures and cannot be used to compare different populations to whom disease-specific instruments are not applicable.

There are several disease-specific instruments that have been developed for assessing patients with inflammatory bowel disease. The Cleveland Clinic Questionnaire for IBD was developed for use in daily clinical practice and as a quality assurance tool [8]. It has 18 items sampling functional performance, social function, life in general, and medical symptoms. It is limited in its usefulness in that the scores from each item cannot be summated. In a small sample of 164 patients, patients with ulcerative colitis experienced superior quality of life to that of patients with Crohn's disease, as did patients who had never required surgery compared to those who had undergone surgery previously. Otherwise, its use has been limited and it has not been formally tested for validity and reliability.

Drossman and colleagues developed the Rating Form of Inflammatory Bowel Disease Patient Concerns (RFIPC) [9]. It is a 25-item measure assessing 4 domains including the impact of disease, sexual intimacy, complications of disease, and body stigma. Responses are recorded on a 10 cm visual analogue scale. These investigators have used this instrument to assess both ulcerative colitis and Crohn's disease patients. Patients' greatest concerns were observed to be related to surgery, energy level, and body image. As well, the severity of their concerns correlated with psychological well-being and daily function. They also correlated better with health-care utilization than with disease activity scores.

The Inflammatory Bowel Disease Questionnaire (IBDQ) was developed by Irvine and colleagues from McMaster University [10, 11]. The original instrument included 32 questions grouped into 4 categories, including bowel symptoms (10 questions), systemic symptoms (5 questions), emotional function (12 questions), and social function (5 questions). Response options are rated in terms of frequency on a 7-point Likert scale so the summary score may range from 32 to 224. More recently a shortened version has been developed. The IBDQ has been tested in multiple cohorts of patients and randomized controlled trials [11–16]. It has been shown to be both reliable and valid and responsive to change in outpatients being treated medically for Crohn's disease. In 42 patients in the Canadian Crohn's Relapse Prevention Trial, who were clinically stable over 8 weeks, an intra-class correlation coefficient of 0.67 was obtained. In the same study, changes in the IBDQ correlated with changes in disease activity scores and patient global assessments so patients who had exacerbation of their disease also had substantial worsening of the IBDQ scores. While the validity of this instrument has been established in patients who have Crohn's disease, it has not been formally assessed for evaluating post-operative patients. However, the IBDQ now would be regarded as the gold standard for assessing quality of life in patients with Crohn's disease and over the years it has been used extensively in clinical trials as well as for comparing outcome in cohorts of patients with various patterns of disease and disease activity [17]. More recently two shorter instruments have been developed. The obvious benefits are that they are easier to administer. These include the Short Health Scale which includes only four items each of which are scored on a visual analogue scale [18]. It was validated against the IBDQ and was found to correlate well with a correlation coefficient of −0.836. Surti and colleagues also developed a "Novel Single-Item Rating Scale" which includes only one item and has been validated in only a small sample of patients with moderately good correlation [19].

The alternative to measuring quality of life psychometrically is using utility based measures [20, 21]. Utilities represent individual's preferences for a given state relative to death or perfect health. Complete wellness is given a utility value of 1.0 and death 0. A health state less than completely well is given a value between 0 and 1.0. Utilities may be assigned using either a decomposed or holistic approach. In the decomposed method, an individual is asked to rate his/her functioning in a number of health domains or attributes. For each specific category, a utility value is generated from a defined population and they can then be combined. In the holistic approach, an individual assigns a utility to his/her health status taking into consideration all aspects of quality of life. Two methods for generating utilities are the standard gamble method or time trade-off technique. In the standard gamble, a utility is calculated based on how much risk the patient would be willing to take to have normal health rather than his/her present health state while in the time trade-off, the utility is calculated based on how many years of life the patient would be willing to give up. Utility assessments tend to be less sensitive in detecting differences or changes than psychometrically based measures. As well, if the holistic approach is used to generate utilities, it is not possible to discern which domain or aspect of health is affected. Their main use has been in the field of health economics and policy making in performing cost utility studies.

Quality of Life in Patients with Crohn's Disease

Understanding and assessing quality of life in individuals with Crohn's disease is difficult because the disease is chronic; the patterns, site, and manifestations of disease are quite variable and finally the activity of the disease may vary over time. Thus, quality of life may vary amongst individuals as well as within individuals, depending on the activity when it is measured. It appears that disease activity has the greatest impact on quality of life although some studies have reported decreased quality of life in patients even when the disease is not active. Reduced quality of life in individuals who are in remission is attributed to concerns regarding the uncertainty of the disease and the future, particularly the need for surgery and an ostomy [16]. In addition, many patients complain of chronic fatigue and this may impact on their general well-being and quality of life.

The IBSEN study is a population based prospective cohort study which included 144 newly diagnosed patients between 1990 and 1993. The investigators reported outcome after 10 years of follow-up including quality of life in 99 patients who completed the SF-36 and a Norwegian version of the IBDQ [15]. After adjusting for age, gender and education, the Crohn's patients were found to have lower SF-36 scores on the general health and vitality dimensions compared to population controls. The mean IBDQ score was 183 (95 % CI 178–189) which is similar to reported scores of patients in remission. However, patients who reported current symptoms related to their Crohn's disease had lower scores on seven of the eight dimensions of the IBDQ. On multiple linear regression analysis, only current symptoms were associated with reduced IBDQ scores.

Blondel-Kucharski and colleagues followed a cohort of 231 patients with Crohn's disease who were identified by 23 gastroenterologists who practice in 19 hospitals in France [22]. They also found significantly lower SF-36 scores compared to the standard population and noted that patients worried about having an ostomy, the uncertainty of the disease, their energy level, and the need for surgery. Of note, compared with patients' assessments, physicians underestimated the impact of Crohn's disease on quality of life.

Guassora and colleagues also compared quality of life with a modified IBDQ in 94 Crohn's patients followed in Copenhagen to that of matched controls [23]. Contrary to the findings of the other studies described above, although these investigators observed differences between the scores in the two groups, the differences were small and not considered clinically significant. This may be due to the fact that 74 % of the Crohn's patients were in remission when the assessment was completed. Disease activity again was the main determinant affecting quality of life.

Disease activity seems to be the biggest determinant of quality of life. Cohen performed a systematic review of 10 studies which assessed the effect of disease activity on quality of life [17]. In eight of the studies, validated instruments were used including one study which measured disease activity with utility scores [24]. In nine of the ten studies disease activity correlated with quality of life. This included correlation with global as well as all dimensional scores of the disease-specific questionnaires.

In the ACCENT I trial, which assessed the efficacy and safety of maintenance therapy with infliximab, patients had elevated Crohn's Disease Activity Index (CDAI) scores of 220–400 at entry [14]. The primary outcome was a change in CDAI scores but in addition, the physical and mental components of the SF-36 were administered at baseline, week 10, 30, and 54 so quality of life could be assessed prospectively. At baseline, patients had severely impaired quality of life with mean scores of 34 ± 8 and 39 ± 11 (out of 50) for physical and mental components, respectively. At week 54, the mean physical and mental component scores for those in remission were 46.6 and 49.8, respectively, which are similar to that of the general US population whereas for those who were not in remission the mean scores were 37.4 and 41.3, respectively. As well, this trend was observed in employment rates. At baseline, 38.4 % of patients were unemployed whereas the unemployment rate decreased to 26.4 % in the group in remission and only to 33.5 % in the group who were not in remission.

Castillo-Cejas and colleagues looked at the effect of fatigue on quality of life in 99 patients who had Crohn's disease [25]. Not only did they find that fatigue correlated significantly with disease activity, it also correlated with quality of life. Zhang and colleagues, in a study of 105 patients, found that depression was the most significant predictor of poor quality of life and in this study disease activity was only weakly correlated with quality of life [26].

Quality of Life in Patients having Surgery for Crohn's Disease

Quality of life is an important consideration in patients having surgery for Crohn's disease. Whereas morbidity and mortality were appropriate measures to assess outcome 50 years ago when, for instance, the accepted mortality for toxic megacolon was 30–50 %, today deaths following elective and emergency surgery are rare. Furthermore, surgery is rarely performed for a life saving indication. Rather, one of the most common indications for surgery in patients with Crohn's disease is failure of medical therapy, or in effect, poor quality of life. Thus, if one wishes to assess whether surgery has been successful, then it is imperative that quality of life be measured. Finally, because Crohn's is a chronic disease and occurs in young individuals, it is very important that surgery does more good than harm since surgery is not curative.

Several studies have shown that quality of life is improved following surgery [27–29]. Thus, whether patients have a medically or surgically induced remission, quality of life is improved compared with the status of patients with active disease. Furthermore, a high quality of life following surgery can be sustained as long as the patient is in remission. Conversely, if the disease does recur, quality of life worsens. This has been shown in multiple studies using a range of instruments including the IBDQ, The Cleveland Clinic Global Quality of Life (CGQL), the RIFPC, The Psychological General Well Being Index (PGWBI), and the EuroQol. As well, utility studies using the time trade-off technique and direct questioning of objectives have been used.

Yazdanpanah and colleagues assessed a small cohort of 26 patients with the RFIBDPC as well as the SF-36 [30]. They were able to show that quality of life improved post-operatively but interestingly patients' concerns were unchanged.

The five most common concerns were having an ostomy, requiring further surgery, energy level, uncertainty of the disease, and pain and suffering. Scarpa and colleagues also reported improvement in quality of life after surgery in a cohort of 97 patients but in addition to disease activity, the number of daily stools was found to impact on quality of life [31]. Finally, Delaney and colleagues assessed quality of life 30 days postoperatively and not surprisingly found that development of complications also affected quality of life [32]. However, this does not seem to affect long-term quality of life. Kasparek and colleagues assessed quality of life using a variety of validated instruments in a cohort of 48 patients who had suffered complications and a control group of 43 patients whose surgery was uncomplicated [33]. Quality of life was comparable in the two groups except for the physical functioning subscale of the SF-36.

Bellolio-Roth and colleagues reported on the long-term outcome and quality of life in a cohort of 207 patients who had an ileocolic resection with a mean follow-up of 96.1 months [34]. Of these, 88 (42.7 %) patients self-reported clinically recurrent disease and 17 (19.8 %) had undergone a second operation. The median total score was 5.5 on the short IBDQ out of a possible 7. This is similar to scores reported by Irvine and colleagues and Shirbel and colleagues in patients with a medically induced remission: (4.67–5.83 and 5.3, respectively) [35, 36]. On multivariable linear regression, Bellolio-Roth and colleagues found that self-reported recurrence of Crohn's disease and non-perforating disease as an indication at the original surgery were associated with decreased SIBDQ scores. Thus, this study suggests that long-term patients can expect to have a good quality of life as long as the disease does not recur.

Multiple studies have shown that short-term outcomes are improved in those who have had surgery performed laparoscopically [37]. However, there does not seem to be any long-term benefits with regard to quality of life. Patel and colleagues combined 34 studies which included 2,519 patients [37]. Complications were significantly lower in patients having surgery laparoscopically (RR 0.71, 95 % CI 0.58–0.86) but there was no significant difference in recurrence. Quality of life was not measured in any of these studies. In a separate study reported by Thaler and colleagues, 37 individuals who had elective laparoscopic (21) or open (16) resections were followed for a mean follow-up of 42.6 months [38]. Patients completed the SF-36 Health Surgery and the Gastrointestinal Quality of Life Index (GIQLI). The mean physical (PCS) and mental component summary (MCS) scales of the SF-36 were 47.2 and 49.2, respectively (range 0–50). The overall mean score on the GIQLI was 103 (possible range 0–144). There was no significant difference in mean scores in those who had open compared with laparoscopic surgery. As in other studies, recurrence was also the only factor associated with a decreased quality of life.

Although quality of life appears to be similar irrespective of the surgical approach, Dunker and colleagues have reported that body image and cosmesis is superior in patients having a laparoscopic surgical approach [39]. The results of this study are limited, though, because only 11 patients in each group were surveyed using a non-validated instrument.

Despite patients' concerns and fears about an ostomy, many studies have suggested that quality of life is good in individuals that have a stoma [40, 41]. This likely is due to an improvement in physical well-being due to eradication of disease activity. On the other hand, Knowles and colleagues reported on a small sample of 31 patients who had Crohn's disease and a stoma. Using three validated instruments, they found that approximately half reported having anxiety and depression related to the stoma [42].

Quality of Life of Patients with Perianal Disease

Perianal disease is a common manifestation of Crohn's disease. Manifestations may range from skin tags to complex and multiple fistulas. Patients with fistulas, especially, may suffer significantly with pain and discharge despite medical and surgical treatment. Although most clinicians would likely feel that the presence of perianal disease has a significant negative impact on quality of life, little has been written on this topic. Riss and colleagues surveyed 69 patients who had perianal disease and had undergone surgery for simple (11) or complex (58) fistulous disease and compared their results to healthy controls [43]. Not surprisingly, the physical health component was significantly lower in the patients compared with the controls. However, there was no significant difference in the mental health component. The mean IBDQ score of the patients with perianal disease was also lower (mean 157) than the controls (mean 189). With regard to sexual activity, only 59.4 % of patients stated they were sexually active in the last 4 weeks compared with 73.9 % of the controls. However, the overall score of the Female Sexual Function Index (FSFI) which was used to assess sexual function in female patients and the International Index of Erectile Function (IIEF) which was used to assess sexual function in males were not significantly different between the patients and the controls. Another study reported by Kasparek and colleagues found that the quality of life of patients who had a diverting stoma because of severe perianal disease was similar to those who were not diverted [44]. This likely reflects the improvement in symptoms due to the defunctioning stoma.

Conclusion

Quality of life is an important metric for the assessment of Crohn's disease. Furthermore, it should be a major consideration in ensuring patients receive patient centered care. Multiple studies show that quality of life is good in patients where the disease is in remission—whether it is induced medically or surgically and worsens significantly if the disease is active. Thus, a major therapeutic goal should be to ensure patients are and stay in remission.

Despite this, however, quality of life is lower in Crohn's patients than the normal population. In part this seems to be due to fatigue as well as concerns and uncertainty about the disease. Thus, psychosocial support should be available to assist patients in achieving optimal well-being and quality of life.

References

1. World Health Organization. The first 10 years of the World Health Organization. Geneva: WHO; 1958.
2. Schipper H, Clinch JJ, Olweny CLM. Quality of life studies: definitions and conceptual issues. In: Spilker B, editor. Quality of life and pharmacoeconomics in clinical trials. Second Edition. New York-Philadelphia: Lippincott-Raven; 1996.
3. Calman KC. Quality of life in cancer patients – an hypothesis. J Med Ethics. 1984;10:124–7.
4. Patrick DL, Deyo RA. Generic and disease-specific measures in assessing health status and quality of life. Med Care. 1989;27:S217–32.
5. Ware JE, Sherbourne CD. The MOS 36-Item Short-Form Health Status Survey (SF- 36): 1. Conceptual framework and item selection. Med Care. 1992;30(6): 473–83.
6. Bergner M, Bobbitt RA, Carter WB, Gilson BS. The sickness impact profile: development and final revision of a health status measure. Med Care. 1981;19: 787–805.
7. Jenkinson C, Fitzpatrick R, Argyle M. The Nottingham Health Profile. An analysis of its sensitivity in differentiating illness groups. Soc Sci Med. 1988;27: 1411–4.
8. Farmer RG, Wesley KA, Farmer JM. Quality of life assessment by patients with IBD. Cleve Clin J Med. 1992;59:35–52.
9. Drossman DA, Patrick DL, Mitchell CM, Zagami EA, Appelbaum MI. Health related quality of life in IBD. Functional status and patient worries and concerns. Dig Dis Sci. 1989;34:1379–86.
10. Guyatt G, Mitchell A, Irvine EJ, Singer J, Williams N, Goodache R, Tompkins C. A new measure of health status for clinical trials in IBD. Gastroenterology. 1989;96:904–10.
11. Irvine EJ, Feagan B, Rochon J, Archambuitt A, Fedork RN, Groll A, Kinnear D, Saibil F, McDonald JWD. Quality of life: a valid and reliable measure of therapeutic efficacy in the treatment of IBD. Gastroenterology. 1994;106:287–96.
12. Love JR, Irvine EJ, Fedorak RN. Quality of life in IBD. J Clin Gastroenterol. 1992;14:15–9.
13. Martin F, Sutherland L, Beck IT, et al. Oral 5-ASA versus prednisone in short-term treatment of Crohn's disease: a multicentre controlled trial. Can J Gastroenterol. 1990;4:452–7.
14. Lichtenstein GR, Yan S, Bala M, Hanauer S. Remission in patients with Crohn's disease is associated with improvement in employment and quality of life and a decrease in hospitalizations and surgeries. Am J Gastroenterol. 2004;99:91–6.

15. Hoivik ML, Bernklev T, Solberg IC, Cvancarova M, Lygren I, Jahnsen J, Moum B. The IBSEN Study Group: patients with Crohn's disease experience reduced general health and vitality in the chronic stage: ten-year results from the IBSEN study. J Crohns Colitis. 2012;6:441–53.
16. Lesage A-C, Hagege H, Tucat G, Gendre J-P. Results of a national survey on quality of life in inflammatory bowel diseases. Clin Res Hepatol Gastroenterol. 2011;35:117–24.
17. Cohen RD. The quality of life in patients with Crohn's disease. Aliment Pharmacol Ther. 2002;16:1603–9.
18. McDermott E, Keegan D, Byrne K, Doherty GS, Mulcahy HE. The short health scale: a valid and reliable measure of health related quality of life in English speaking inflammatory bowel disease patients. J Crohns Colitis. 2013;7:616–21.
19. Surti B, Spiegel B, Ippoliti A, Valiliauskas EA, Simpson P, Shih DQ, Targan SR, McGovern DPB, Melmed GY. Assessing health status in inflammatory bowel disease using a novel single-item numeric rating scale. Dig Dis Sci. 2013;58:1313–21.
20. Torrance GW. Measurement of health state utilities for economic appraisal. A review. J Health Econ. 1986;5:1–30.
21. Torrance GW, Thomas WH, Sackett DLS. A utility maximization model for evaluation of health care progress. Health Serv Res. 1972;7:118–33.
22. Blondel-Kucharski R, Chircop C, Marquis P, Cortot A, Baron F, Gendre JP, Colombel JF. Health related quality of life in Crohn's disease: a prospective longitudinal study in 231 patients. Am J Gastroenterol. 2001;96:2915–20.
23. Gaussora AD, Kruuse C, Thomsen OO, Binder V. Quality of life study in a regional group of patients with Crohn disease. Scand J Gastroenterol. 2000; 35(10):1068–74.
24. Gregor JC, MacDonald JWD, Klar N, et al. An evaluation of utility measurement in Crohn's disease. Inflamm Bowel Dis. 1997;3:265–76.
25. Castillo-Cejas MD, Robles V, Borruel N, Torrejon A, Navarro E, Pelaez A, Casellas F. Questionnaires for measuring fatigue and its impact on health perception in inflammatory bowel disease. Rev Esp Enferm Dig. 2013;105:144–53.
26. Zhang CK, Hewett J, Hemming J, Grant T, Zhaeo H, Abraham C, Oikonomou K, Kanakia M, Cho JH, Proctor DD. The influence of depression on quality of life in patients with inflammatory bowel disease. Inflamm Bowel Dis. 2013;19:1732–9.
27. Broering DC, Eisenberger CF, Kock A, Bloechle C, Knoefel WT. Quality of life after surgical therapy of small bowel stenosis in Crohn's disease. Dig Surg. 2001;18:124–30.
28. Tillinger W, Mittermaier C, Lochs H, Moser G. Health-related quality of life in patients with Crohn's disease. Influence of surgical operation-a prospective trial. Dig Dis Sci. 1999;44:932–8.
29. Thirlby RC, Sobrino MA, Randall JB. The long term benefit of surgery on health related quality of life in patients with inflammatory bowel disease. Arch Surg. 2001;136:521–7.
30. Yazdanpanah Y, Klein O, Gambiez L, Baron P, Desreumaux P, Marquis P, Cortot A, Quandalle P, Colombel JF. Impact of surgery on quality of life in Crohn's disease. Am J Gastroenterol. 1997;92: 1897–900.
31. Scarpa M, Ruffolo C, D'Inca R, Filosa T, Bertin E, Ferraro S, Polese L, Martin A, Sturniolo GS, Frego M, D'Amico DF, Angriman I. Health-related quality of life after ileocolonic resection for Crohn's disease: long term results. Inflamm Bowel Dis. 2007;13: 462–9.
32. Delaney CP, Kiran R, Senagore AJ, O'Brien-Ermlich B, Church J, Hull TL, Remzi FH, Fazio VW. Quality of life improves within 30 days of surgery for Crohn's disease. J Am Coll Surg. 2003;196:714–21.
33. Kasparek MS, Glatzlo J, Mueller MH, Schneider A, Koenigsrainer A, Kreis ME. Post-operative complications have little influence on long term quality of life in Crohn's patients. J Gastrointest Surg. 2008;12: 569–76.
34. Bellolio-Roth F, Cohen Z, MacRae HM, O'Connor BI, Huang H, Victor JC, McLeod RS. Patients requiring ileocolic resection for Crohn's disease have excellent long-term outcome (accepted for publication Ann Surg)
35. Irvine EJ, Zhou Q, Thompson AK. The short inflammatory bowel disease questionnaire: a quality of life instrument for community physicians managing inflammatory bowel disease. CCRPT Investigators Canadian Crohn's Relapse Prevention Trial. Am J Gastroenterol. 1996;91:1571–8.
36. Shirbel A, Rechert A, Roll S, et al. Impact of pain on health-related quality of life in patients with inflammatory bowel disease. World J Gastroenterol. 2010; 16:3168–77.
37. Patel SV, Patel SVB, Ramagopalan SV, Ott MC. Laparoscopic surgery for Crohn's disease: a meta-analysis of perioperative complications and long term outcomes compared with open surgery. BMC Surg. 2013;13:14–27.
38. Thaler K, Dinnewitzer A, Oberwalder M, Weiss EG, Nogueras JJ, Wexner SD. Assessment of long-term quality of life after laparoscopic and open surgery for Crohn's disease. Colorectal Dis. 2005;7:375–81.
39. Dunker MS, Stiggelbout AM, van Hogezand RA, Ringers J, Griffioen G, Bemelman WA. Cosmesis and body image after laparoscopic-assisted and open ileocolic resection for Crohn's disease. Surg Endosc. 1998;12:1334–40.
40. Jimmo B, Hyman NH. Is ileal pouch anal anastomosis really the procedure of choice for patients with ulcerative colitis? Dis Colon Rectum. 1998;41:41–5.
41. McLeod RS, Churchill DN, Lock AM, Vanderburgh S, Cohen Z. Quality of life of patients with ulcerative colitis preoperatively and postoperatively. Gastroenterology. 1991;80:1307–13.
42. Knowles SR, Wilson J, Wilkinson A, Connell W, Salzberg M, Castle D, Desmond P, Kamm MA.

Psychological well-being and quality of life in Crohn's disease patients with an ostomy: a preliminary investigation. J Wound Ostomy Continence Nurs. 2013;40:623–9.
43. Riss S, Schwameis K, Mittlbock M, Pones M, Vogelsang H, Reinisch W, Riedl M, Stift A. Sexual function and quality of life after surgical treatment for anal fistulas in Crohn's disease. Tech Coloproctol. 2013;17:89–94.
44. Kasparek MS, Glatzle J, Temeltcheva T, Mueller MH, Koenigsrainer A, Kreis ME. Long-term quality of life in patients with Crohn's disease and perianal fistulas. Influence of fecal diversion. Dis Colon Rectum. 2007;50:2067–74.

Index

A. Fichera and M.K. Krane (eds.), *Crohn's Disease: Basic Principles*,
DOI 10.1007/978-3-319-14181-7, © Springer International Publishing Switzerland 2015

The manufacturer's authorised representative in the EU is Springer Nature Customer Service Centre GmbH, Europaplatz 3, 69115 Heidelberg, Germany. If you have any concerns regarding our products, please contact ProductSafety@springernature.com

Printed and bound by CPI Group (UK) Ltd, Croydon, CR0 4YY

15/07/2026

02167625-0001